ʖhiffman

-319-43885-6 ISBN 978-3-319-43887-0 (eBook)
7/978-3-319-43887-0

ngress Control Number: 2017937947

d-free paper

imprint is published by Springer Nature
company is Springer International Publishing AG
company address is: Gewerbestrasse 11, 6330 Cham, Switzerland

Adult Umbilical Reconstruction

Melvin A. Shiffman
Editor

Adult Umbilical Reconstruction

Principles and Techniques

Springer

Editor
Melvin A
Tustin
Californi
USA

ISBN 97
DOI 10.

Library o

Foreword

The umbilicus is the first cutaneous scar on the human body. It is the final result of the natural necrotic phenomenon of the umbilical cord, which occurs few days after birth. Nature defies the surgeon whenever performing an operation on it due to its peculiar skin around the cavity with scar tissue in the depth. The umbilicus is strategically located at the center of the abdomen and harmoniously balanced with the body which is always noticed but not easily imitated. Several kinds of alterations may damage its appearance, causing physical and psychological repercussion to the patient. Quite often, redundancy of skin, hernia, diastasis of the rectus abdominis, unaesthetic surgical scars, deviation from the midline of the abdomen, flat surface, and some other situations may disturb the anatomy of the umbilicus.

There are basically two groups of surgeries to perform on the umbilicus. The first group includes the surgical approaches to several problems located on the umbilicus and umbilical region. Dr. Melvin Shiffman presents in this book a wide variety of the abnormalities and provides peculiar and adequate surgical treatment under very high technical standards. The second group regards the creation of a new umbilicus during abdominoplasty. It is well known that the transposition of the umbilicus was not performed during surgery in the first publication by Kelly in 1899 and several authors many decades afterwards. Nevertheless, Vernon in 1957 opened a new era describing the first transposition of the navel during surgery by removing a round piece of skin and subcutaneous tissue to suture to the skin of the abdominal wall. Afterwards, some authors introduced other approaches pulling the umbilicus in order to suture on the abdominal wall and doing other types of incisions such as vertical, horizontal, circular, and semicircular ones. The final scar is a circular one with a very high incidence of scar retraction and contraction, as mentioned by Grazer and Goldwing in 1977. In the meantime, looking for ways on how to avoid these complications, I developed personal techniques to create a natural umbilicus during full abdominoplasty when it is mandatory to perform transposition of the umbilicus. Based on my approach, some surgical principles represent significant differences in comparison to the others: (a) the cutaneous incisions on the umbilicus are done following the direction lines of the skin inward; (b) the final scars make an atypical Z-plasty which avoids unaesthetic appearance as well as scar retraction and contraction; (c) the skin of the abdominal wall is pushed to depth in order to be sutured to the umbilicus; (d) the final appearance is a natural deep cavity on the new umbilical region; (e) the final scars rest smoothly on the interior side of the umbilical cavity.

Due to my intensive work in this small area of the human body, I recognized the importance of this book edited by Dr. Melvin Shiffman. In fact, he presents a fascinating Table of Contents encompassing multiple pathologies and deformities that frequently affect the umbilicus. Dr. Shiffman and the outstanding authors involved in this book describe meticulous and sophisticated techniques presenting excellent results. The high-level presentations and photographic illustrations show appropriate solutions which are to be commended. Finally, I congratulate Dr. Melvin Shiffman for such great effort dedicated to an arduous field. This work will be very useful to all plastic surgeons, encouraging them to improve surgical techniques, leading to better surgical results. Also, I recommend this book to all general surgeons who are concerned or interested about the subject, which is carefully described and very well illustrated. I am sure Dr. Shiffman has achieved his goal: perfecting the art of creating an aesthetic well-balanced and harmonious umbilical region.

São Paulo, Juarez M. Avelar

Preface

This book is the first book to be completely about adult umbilical reconstruction. There are chapters in many books but not extensive information contained in one volume. The contributing international experts have chapters on anatomy, umbilical shape and position, history of umbilicoplasty, history of techniques, a large variety of techniques, history of tumors of the umbilicus, malignant tumors of the umbilicus, complications, and outcomes.

Plastic surgeons, general surgeons, gynecologists, and family practitioners will be interested in the information contained in the book that may relate to their practices. Any surgeon performing abdominoplasty will get practical knowledge from the book.

Tustin, CA Melvin A. Shiffman

Contents

Contributors

Fikri M. Abu-Zidan Department of Surgery, College of Medicine and Health Sciences, UAE University, Al-Ain, UAE

Nezih Akkapulu Department of General Surgery, Ordu Teaching and Research Hospital, Ordu, Turkey

Ammar Al-Dhamin Tawam Hospital, Al Ain, UAE

Koshiro Arai Department of Plastic and Reconstructive Surgery, Otaru General Hospital, Otaru, Hokkaido, Japan

Juarez M. Avelar Alameda Gabriel Monteiro da Silva, Sao Paulo, Brazil

Guillermo Blugerman B & S Center of Excellence in Plastic Surgery, Buenos Aires, Argentina

Claudio Cannistrá Department of Plastic Surgery, Centre Hôspitalier Universitaire Bichat Claude Bernard, Paris, France

Ernando Luiz Ferraz Cavalcanti Instituto de Medicina Integrada Professor Fernando Figueira, Recife, Pernambuco, Brazil

Amy S. Colwell Division of Plastic Surgery, Massachusetts General Hospital, Harvard Medical School, Boston, MA, USA

Marco Conte Department of Surgery "Pietro Valdoni", "Sapienza" Università di Roma, Roma, Italy

Joey Corkum Private Practice, Halifax, NS, Canada

Andrew L. Da Lio Department of Plastic Surgery, Ronald Reagan UCLA Medical Center, UCLA Medical Center, Santa Monica, Beverly Hills, CA, USA

Fabio Neves da Silva Department of Plastic Surgery, Hospital Federal de Ipanema, Rio de Janeiro, Brazil

Adrien Daigeler Department of Plastic Surgery, Burn Center, Hand Center, BG-University Hospital Bergmannsheil, Bochum, Germany

Emmanuel A. de la Cruz Department of Plastic Surgery, Burn Center, Hand Center, BG-University Hospital Bergmannsheil, The Woodlands, TX, USA

Everardo Abramo de Oliveira Private Practice, Rio de Janeiro, Brazil

Ibrahim Orgun Deren Plastic Surgery Department, Near East University, PK, Lefkosa, Turkey

Luca A. Dessy Department of Plastic and Reconstructive Surgery, "La Sapienza" University of Rome, Assemini, CA, Italy

Edgar Dippel Skin Cancer Center, Ludwigshafen Hospital, Ludwigshafen, Germany

Alfredo Donnabella Brazilian Society of Plastic Surgery, Private Practice, Belo Horizonte, MG, Brazil

Saleh Abdel-Kader Department of Surgery, Faculty of Medicine, Ain Shams University, Cairo, Egypt

General Surgery, Al-Ain Hospital, Al-Ain, UAE

Surak Eo Plastic and Reconstructive Surgery, DongGuk University Medical Center, DongGuk University Graduate School of Medicine, Goyang, South Korea

Mohammad S. Fazeli Department of Surgery, Imam Hospital Complex, Tehran University of Medical Sciences, Keshavarz Boulevard, Tehran, Iran

Randall S. Feingold Aesthetic Plastic Surgery, P.C., Great Neck, NY, USA

Diogo Franco Hospital da Fundão, HUCFF – UFRJ, Serviço de Cirurgia Plástica, Rio de Janeiro, Brazil

Department of Plastic Surgery, Federal University of Rio de Janeiro, Rio de Janeiro, Brazil

Talita Franco Department of Plastic Surgery, Federal University of Rio de Janeiro (UFRJ), Rio de Janeiro, Brazil

Michael J. Frederick Department of Plastic Surgery, Massachusetts General Hospital, Harvard Medical School, Boston, MA, USA

Raimondo Gabriele Department of Surgery, "P.Valdoni", University of Rome "La Sapienz", Roma, Italy

Thomas J. Gampper Department of Plastic and Maxillofacial Surgery, University of Virginia Health System, Charlottesville, VA, USA

Joshua A. Gillis Department of Surgery, Section of Plastic Surgery, Dalhousie University, Halifax, NS, Canada

Vimal J. Gokani St Andrews Centre for Plastic Surgery and Burns, Chelmsford, UK

Vidal Guerreiro Department Plastic Surgery, Federal University of Mato Grosso, Cuiaba, MT, Brazil

Alexander R. Gupta MS4 at University of Texas Medical Branch at Galveston, Dallas, TX, USA

Sanaz Hatami Department of Surgery, University of Alberta, Edmonton, AB, Canada

2-132 Li Ka Shing Centre for Health Research Innovation, University of Alberta, Edmonton, AB, Canada

Ron Hazani Hazani Plastic Surgery, Beverly Hills, CA, USA

Darryl J. Hodgkinson Cosmetic and Restorative Surgery Clinic, Sydney, NSW, Australia

Ronald E. Hoxworth Department of Plastic Surgery, University Hospitals, UT Southwestern Medical Center, Dallas, TX, USA

Frank F.A. IJpma Department of Surgery, Isala Klinieken, Zwolle, Netherlands

Department of Surgery, Scheper Hospital, Emmen, Netherlands

Department of Surgery, Academic Medical Center/University, Amsterdam, Netherlands

Ron Israeli Aesthetic Plastic Surgery, P.C., Private Practice, Great Neck, NY, USA

Durdane Keskin Ataturk Training and Research Hospital, Plastic Surgery Department PK, Cankaya, Ankara, Turkey

Kensuke Kiyokawa Department of Plastic and Reconstructive Surgery, and Maxillofacial Surgery, Kurume University School of Medicine, Fukuoka-ken, Japan

Erwin A. Kruger Division of Plastic Surgery, David Geffen School of Medicine at UCLA, Los Angeles, CA, USA

Amir Lebaschi Department of Tissue Engineering, Repair, and Regeneration, Hospital for Special Surgery, New York, NY, USA

Malcolm A. Lesavoy UCLA School of Medicine, Los Angeles, CA, USA

Christoph Löser Skin Cancer Center, Ludwigshafen Hospital, Ludwigshafen, Germany

Marcelo Lotocky B & S Center of Excellence in Plastic Surgery, Private Practice, Buenos Aires, Argentina

J. Bastos Martins Plastic and Reconstructive Surgery Department, Hospital São José (Central Lisbon Hospital Center), Lisbon, Portugal

Marco Mazzocchi Department of Surgery and Biomedical Science, Section of Plastic Surgery, University of Perugia, Perugia, Italy

João Medeiros Plastic Surgery Department, Federal University of Rio de Janeiro (UFRJ), Rio de Janeiro, Brazil

André Luis Rosenhaim Monte Private Practice, Porto Alegre, Brazil

Steven F. Morris Department of Surgery, Division of Plastic Surgery, Dalhousie University, Halifax, NS, Canada

Paul G. Morrison Department of Urology, University of Iowa, Iowa City, IA, USA

Ghada Morshed Department of Surgery, Fayoum University, Cairo, Egypt

Soraya Navysany Skin Cancer Center, Ludwigshafen Hospital, Ludwigshafen, Germany

Niri S. Niranjan St. Andrew's Centre for Plastic Surgery and Burns, Broomfield Hospital, Chelmsford, Essex, UK

Wendy M. Novicoff Department of Public Health Sciences and Orthopaedic Surgery, University of Virginia, Charlottesville, VA, USA

Norbert Pallua Department for Plastic Surgery, Hand Surgery, Burn Center, University Hospital of the RWTH Aachen University, Aachen, Germany

Michel E. Pfulg Laclinic Montreux, Montreux-Territet, Switzerland

Oscar Ramirez Private Practice, "Ramirez Plastic Surgery" at Elite Center for Cosmetic Surgery, Weston, FL, USA

Private Practice, Clinica Corporacion de Cirujanos Plasticos, Miraflores, Peru

Fernanda Parentoni Santos Barbacena Medical School, Barbacena, Brazil

Diego Schavelzon Private Practice, Buenos Aires, Argentina

Laurenz Schmitt Clinical Centre Dermatology and Allergology, Department Dermatosurgery Pauwelsstr, University Hospital Aachen, Aachen, Germany

Nariman Sepehrvand Department of Medicine, University of Alberta, Edmonton, AB, Canada

2–132 Li Ka Shing Centre for Health Research Innovation, University of Alberta, Edmonton, AB, Canada

Asuman Sevin Plastic Surgery Department, Cayyolu Guven Medical Center, Cayyolu, Ankara, Turkey

Kutlu Sevin Ankara University, Cankaya, Ankara, Turkey

Melvin A. Shiffman Tustin, CA, USA

Carla I.J.M. Theunissen Plastic Surgery, Isala Klinieken, Zwolle, Netherlands

Mehmet Bulent Tirnaksiz Department of General Surgery, Hacettepe University School of Medicine, Ankara, Turkey

Chad R. Tracy Departments of Urology, University of Iowa, Iowa City, IA, USA

Koichi Watanabe Department of Plastic and Reconstructive Surgery and Maxillofacial Surgery, Kurume University School of Medicine, Kurume, Fukuoka, Japan

Gabriel Wexler B & S Center of Excellence in Plastic Surgery, Private Practice, Buenos Aires, Argentina

Andrew Michael Williams Department of Plastic, Reconstructive and Aesthetic Surgery, Bradford Royal Infirmary, Bradford, UK

Ken Yamashita Department of Plastic and Reconstructive Surgery, Sapporo Medical University School of Medicine, Sapporo, Hokkaido, Japan

Charlotte W. Ying The Cosmetic and Restorative Surgery Clinic, Private Practice, Sydney, NSW, Australia

Takatoshi Yotsuyanagi Department of Plastic and Reconstructive Surgery, Sapporo Medical University School of Medicine, Sapporo, Hokkaido, Japan

Deborah Yu Department of Plastic and Maxillofacial Surgery, University of Virginia Health System, Charlottesville, VA, USA

Departments of Public Health Sciences and Orthopaedic Surgery, University of Virginia Health System, Charlottesville, VA, USA

Verena-Constanze Buchinger-Kähler Department for Plastic Surgery, Hand Surgery, Burn Center, University Hospital of the RWTH Aachen University, Aachen, Germany

Part I
Anatomy

Chapter 1
The Anatomy of the Umbilicus

Ronald E. Hoxworth and Alexander R. Gupta

1.1 Introduction

The umbilicus is a median depression in the abdomen, located above the pubis about one third of the distance from the pubic symphysis to the xiphoid process which is a relatively consistent position in adults. It is the remnant site for attachment of the umbilical cord in utero, which functions as the nutritional conduit between the developing fetus and the placenta during development. Though largely extraneous in function during adulthood, the umbilicus serves as an important landmark in the anatomy of the abdomen, specifically with regard to the abdominal wall pathology and surgical approach.

This chapter will describe the normal anatomy of the umbilicus, including the layers of the abdominal wall, vascular components, and neurologic aspects of the umbilicus and stalk. In addition, a brief review of the umbilicus during development will be discussed, with an emphasis on congenital abnormalities and the subsequent consequence in postpartum life.

R.E. Hoxworth, M.D., M.B.A. (✉)
Department of Plastic Surgery, University of Texas Southwestern Medical Center,
1801 Inwood Rd., Dallas, TX 75390-9132, USA
e-mail: ron.hoxworth@utsouthwestern.edu

A.R. Gupta, M.D.
Department of Surgery, University of California San Francisco,
513 Parnassus Ave., San Francisco, CA 94143, USA
e-mail: alexgupta1@gmail.com

M.A. Shiffman (ed.), *Adult Umbilical Reconstruction*,
DOI 10.1007/978-3-319-43887-0_1

1.2 Location

The position of the umbilicus within the abdomen is relatively undeviating among human adults, typically observed on a transverse line drawn between the level of the superior point of the iliac crest. This site corresponds with the level of the intervertebral disk of the third and fourth lumbar vertebrae, though normal variation in position of the umbilicus may lie anywhere between the circumferential lines of the third and the fifth lumbar vertebrae. The dermatome of the tenth thoracic spinal nerve (T10 dermatome) is responsible for sensory of the skin at the level of the umbilicus.

It should be noted that the vertical position of the umbilicus is not absolute; some circumstances that may lead to variation in position of the umbilicus include hereditary conditions (e.g., achondroplasia), pathologic states (e.g., ascites), and normal physiologic changes (e.g., pregnancy).

While there may be variation in the vertical position of the umbilicus, on a horizontal plane, it will be consistently found within the linea alba, a fibrous structure running vertically down the midline of the abdomen, spanning the gap between the xiphoid process and the pubic symphysis. The structure of the linea alba, along with the other components of the abdominal wall, will be described more fully in the following sections.

1.3 Basic Anatomic Overview of the Abdominal Wall

The abdominal wall is composed structurally of nine basic units. Arranged from superficial to deep, the layers are as follows: skin; subcutaneous tissue, including Camper's fascia and Scarpa's fascia; external oblique muscle; internal oblique muscle; transversus abdominis muscle; transversalis fascia; extraperitoneal adipose tissue; and peritoneum.

The external oblique muscle, internal oblique muscle, and transversus abdominis muscle bodies are responsible for the enclosure of the lateral circumference of the abdominal contents and, as they approach the midline of the abdomen anteriorly, give rise to large aponeuroses. These aponeuroses are the components responsible for the formation of the rectus sheath, which encloses the rectus abdominis muscles. At the level of the umbilicus, the fibers of the aponeuroses of the external oblique muscle and those of the anterior lamellae of the internal oblique muscle course anteriorly to the rectus abdominis muscle, forming the anterior portion of the rectus sheath. Along the midsternal line, these aponeuroses from one half of the abdomen join those from the other half of the abdomen to form a fibrous structure called the linea alba, which demarcates the midline of the abdomen. Meanwhile, the posterior lamellae of the aponeurosis of the internal oblique muscle, in conjunction with the aponeurosis of the transversus abdominis muscle, pass posteriorly to the rectus abdominis muscle to form the posterior aspect of the rectus sheath. The concomitance of these three aponeurotic layers fully envelops the rectus abdominis muscle at the level of the umbilicus. Located deep to the transversus abdominis muscle and its aponeurosis is the transversalis fascia, which reinforces the other layers of the abdominal cavity. It is ultimately responsible for the structural integrity of the abdominal wall, and defects within it allow herniation of abdominal contents.

The rectus abdominis muscle is composed of paired bodies of parallel muscle fascicles running along the craniocaudal axis. Each of this pair is interrupted by a number of tendinous intersections, which are fibrous bands that course laterally to medially, where they intersect with the linea alba at the midline of the abdomen. These tendinous intersections serve the function of forming fibrous attachments between the rectus abdominis muscle and the anterior portion of the rectus sheath, which aids in anchoring the muscle into its place in the midline. The left and right halves of the rectus abdominis muscle are split vertically into two adjacent muscle bodies by the linea alba. At the level of the umbilicus, the rectus sheath lines the rectus abdominis muscle at both the anterior and the posterior aspects, though there are no fibrous attachments between it and the muscle on the posterior side as is the case with the anterior portion. More inferior on the abdominal compartment (caudal to the arcuate line of the abdomen), there is no posterior aspect to the rectus sheath, and the rectus abdominis muscle lies directly superficial to the transversalis fascia.

Deep to the transversalis fascia lies the extraperitoneal space, which contains the remnants of three structures that were part of the fetal-placental umbilical cord conduit. The first of these structures is the falciform ligament, which lies in the anteroposterior plane, where it anchors together the liver and the ventral body wall. Its reach extends superiorly from its origin at the umbilicus, where it attaches to the left lobe of the liver and eventually to the diaphragm. Contained within the free edge of the falciform ligament of the liver is the round ligament of the liver (*ligamentum teres hepatis*), which is the remnant of the obliterated fetal umbilical vein. This vessel coursed in utero from the umbilicus to the left portal vein as it carried oxygenated blood returning from the placenta. The second of these vestigial bodies within the extraperitoneal space is the medial umbilical ligament, which is a paired structure contained within the medial umbilical folds (*plica umbilicalis medialis*) on the deep ventral surface of the abdominal wall. These structures represent the remnant of the fetal umbilical arteries, which coursed in utero from the internal iliac vessels to the umbilicus as they carried deoxygenated blood toward the placenta. The final structure of interest is the median umbilical ligament (not to be confused with the medial umbilical ligaments), which is a midline fibrous structure contained within the median umbilical fold. The median umbilical ligament extends from the apex of the bladder to the umbilicus as it tracks on the deep ventral surface of the abdominal wall. This structure represents the remnant of the fetal urachus, which drained the urinary bladder through the umbilicus in utero.

1.4 Vascular and Lymphatic Components of the Periumbilical Region

The vascularity of the abdominal wall is complex, as the tissues receive blood supply from a variety of sources, including the epigastric arteries, intercostal and lumbar arteries, deep circumflex iliac artery, and the musculophrenic artery. Though each of these vessels is important in supplying the various anatomic regions of the abdominal wall, this section will focus on those that are enclosed within the rectus sheath or are directly involved with umbilical components. The lymphatic system of the abdominal wall will also be mentioned in brief.

The inferior epigastric artery supplies, under normal conditions, the dominant vascular supply of the anterior abdominal wall. It is a branch of the external iliac artery, and it arises on the proximal aspect of the inguinal ligament. The artery courses anteriorly and superiorly along the inferomedial margin of the deep inguinal ring and continues through the extraperitoneal space to the transversalis fascia. As it continues superiorly, it pierces the said fascial layer so that it runs in between it and the posterior aspect of the rectus abdominis muscle. Ultimately, the artery passes anteriorly at the arcuate line of the abdomen, such that it ascends between the posterior rectus sheath and the rectus abdominis muscle. Once within the rectus sheath, the vessel divides extensively to supply the lower portions of the rectus abdominis muscle and other inferomedial aspects of the abdominal wall through its musculocutaneous perforating branches. Ultimately, the distal branches of the inferior epigastric artery anastomose with branches of the superior epigastric artery near the level of the umbilicus.

These aforementioned musculocutaneous perforating branches of the inferior epigastric artery are of particular interest in this setting, as they have a significant impact on surgical method within the region of the umbilicus. The branches are widely variable in both number and location, creating a necessity for particular care when dissecting the region; this is due to their role in providing a large portion of the blood supply to superficial tissues within periumbilical space. A surgeon creating a tissue flap within the anterior abdominal region in reconstructive surgery must keep this principle in mind, as the survival of any flap could be largely dependent on these musculocutaneous perforators.

The superior epigastric artery is a terminal branch of the internal thoracic artery, usually arising at the level of the sixth or seventh costal cartilage. From its origin, the artery descends and courses anteriorly until it crosses the diaphragm through the sternocostal triangle. From here, it enters through the posterior rectus sheath to run along the posterior aspect of the rectus abdominis muscle. The vessel branches soon after entering the rectus sheath to supply the upper portions of the rectus abdominis muscle and other superomedial tissues within the abdominal wall. The distal branches continue inferiorly, until they ultimately anastomose with branches of the inferior epigastric artery as previously described.

Though the inferior and superior epigastric arteries are the primary vessels responsible for the arterial supply of the rectus abdominis muscle, it should be noted that the intercostal and lumbar arteries also have some significance in this region. As they course medially in the plane between the transversus abdominis muscle and the internal oblique muscle, these arteries give rise to distal branches that penetrate the lateral aspects of the rectus sheath at the level corresponding to each vessel's origin. Here, they form anastomoses with the distal branches of the superior and inferior epigastric arteries to supply a nominal amount of blood to the circuit.

Though the musculocutaneous perforators of the inferior and superior epigastric vessels are responsible for a large portion of the arterial supply to the skin and subcutaneous layers of the abdominal wall, it should be appreciated that a noteworthy portion comes from superficial arteries that supply the region. Of primary interest in the umbilical region is the superficial inferior epigastric artery, which branches from the femoral artery just inferior to the inguinal ligament. This vessel runs superomedially within the subcutaneous tissue toward the umbilicus, where it branches extensively to supply the integument surrounding the umbilicus.

Normal venous drainage of the anterior abdominal wall is relatively simple, with veins tending to course alongside their named arterial counterparts. In general, drainage of venous blood at levels superior to the umbilicus empties into the superior vena cava via the subclavian vessels, while drainage of venous blood at levels inferior to the umbilicus empties into the inferior vena cava via the external iliac veins.

Numerous venous anastomoses exist between the infraumbilical and supraumbilical systems, which allow collateral venous return, even in the case of obstruction of the superior or inferior vena cava. Of particular relevance in this discussion is the paraumbilical vein, which courses within the falciform ligament of the liver to connect the umbilical circulation with the left portal vein. This collateral connection between the portal venous system and the superficial anterior abdominal wall becomes essential for patients with portal venous hypertension. In this setting, the paraumbilical veins will engorge to allow a reduction in portal venous pressure via the shunt of blood to the inferior epigastric vein, ultimately bypassing the liver. This well-documented phenomenon, termed *caput medusae*, is a classic syndrome of portal hypertension and one of the best documented cases involving this shunt.

The lymphatic drainage of the abdominal wall typically follows the direction of venous drainage, such that supraumbilical channels will lead superiorly toward the axillary lymph nodes, while infraumbilical channels tend to drain inferiorly toward the inguinal lymph nodes. The lymphatic channels immediately adjacent to the umbilicus drain toward the liver through the falciform ligament.

1.5 Innervation of the Periumbilical Region

The innervation of the abdominal wall is comparatively simple, as the majority of sensory and motor function stems from branches of the intercostal nerves and the subcostal nerves, which originate at the anterior rami of the spinal nerve. Other named nerves, including the iliohypogastric nerves and the ilioinguinal nerves merit comment, as they have a role in the innervation of the inferior aspects of the abdominal wall and pelvis; however this discussion will focus on the seventh through eleventh intercostal nerves (thoracoabdominal nerves), as well as the subcostal nerves, as these are the ones responsible for the abdominal wall in the periumbilical region.

Within the abdominal wall, the primary route of innervation arises from the seventh through twelfth thoracic branches of the spinal nerve (thoracoabdominal and subcostal nerves). Each of these originates from the anterior ramus of the spinal nerve in the posterior midline, at a vertical level immediately inferior to its corresponding thoracic vertebrae (e.g., the seventh thoracic spinal nerve originates just below the seventh thoracic vertebrae). As each thoracic spinal nerve leaves the spinal column, it courses circumferentially within its intercostal space toward the anterior midline. Each nerve passes deep to the costal cartilage and continues inferiorly to enter the abdominal wall in the plane between the transversus abdominis muscle and the internal oblique muscle. Each thoracoabdominal nerve, including the subcostal nerves, gives numerous branches within this plane, including the lateral cutaneous branch, which innervates the skin on the lateral aspect of the abdomen through its anterior and posterior branches; the anterior cutaneous branch, which is the terminal portion of the thoracoabdominal nerves and innervate the skin at the midline of the abdomen through its medial and lateral branches; and the muscular branches, which supply the musculature of the anterior abdominal wall, including the external oblique muscle, the internal oblique muscle, the transversus abdominis muscle, and the rectus abdominis muscle. Each of these nerves is primarily responsible for motor and sensory on one vertical level corresponding with a specific dermatome, with some overlap occurring between each one. Of particular interest in this discussion, the tenth thoracoabdominal nerve supplies the dermatome involving the integument at the level of the umbilicus.

Due to the course of these nerve fibers, a special deliberation must be made when considering longitudinal incisions within the abdomen. If such an incision is made at the midline, it may be assumed that no significant sensory impairment will result, as each half of the abdomen is supplied individually by the left- and the right-sided intercostal nerves – no nerve bundles would be transected. Contrarily, longitudinal incisions made lateral to the midline would result in sensory impairment within regions inferior and medial to the level of the incision (within the respective dermatome), as this would lead to disruption of the anterior or lateral cutaneous branches as they course through this superficial abdominal plane.

The iliohypogastric and the ilioinguinal nerves do not play a role in sensory or motor function of the periumbilical region; however, they deserve brief mention in this discussion based on their role toward this end within the hypogastrium. As was the case with the thoracoabdominal and subcostal nerves, transection of these nerves through poorly designed incisions may lead to permanent sensory loss within their supplied regions. This is of particular interest when performing inguinal herniorrhaphy and may also play a role in creating abdominal tissue flaps and potential innervation.

1.6 Discussion

1.6.1 Normal Development of the Umbilicus and Abdominal Wall

In order to obtain an appreciation for the various congenital abnormalities that may arise during the development of the abdominal wall and umbilicus, a basic understanding of the normal process must be pursued. This section will describe the basic structures involved in the umbilical cord as it relates to the abdominal wall development under normal conditions but is not meant to be a comprehensive embryologic review of the trunk and abdomen.

The development of the abdominal wall begins early in the gestational period, occurring between the fourth and eighth weeks after conception. Differentiation of the abdominal wall structures begins from the paraxial and lateral plate mesoderm, which initially aligns down the posterior midline, just lateral to the neural tube, into the segmental blocks known as somites. These somites are split functionally into two different groups; the dorsolateral subgroup is the dermomyotome group, and the ventromedial subgroup is the sclerotome group. The latter develops into the ribs and vertebrae of the embryo, while the former differentiates into the skeletal musculature and the skin of the trunk, which will be the focus of this discussion.

Following the maturation of the sclerotome into definitive vertebrae, each dermomyotome migrates to cover each intervertebral disk, where it gives rise to a new cellular line of myoblasts. As part of this differentiation, the remaining part of the dermomyotome becomes known as the dermatome. These myoblasts eventually split into three distinct layers, which give rise to the external oblique muscles, internal oblique muscles, and transversus abdominis muscle; this begins by the seventh week of development. The dermatomes are responsible for the development of the overlying dermis associated with each myotome. At this time in the development of these cell lines, a nerve branch becomes associated with each dermatome and myotome, in so forming the framework for the segmental association of each intercostal nerve with overlying skin and musculature. Fusion of the abdominal wall muscles at the anterior midline occurs by the eighth week in development under normal conditions.

Concurrent with the emergence of the newly materializing abdominal wall is the formation of the umbilical cord. The earliest form of the umbilical cord arises when the expanding amnion grows to envelop the tissues of the body stalk, the vitelline duct (omphalomesenteric duct), and the umbilical coelom, beginning around the fourth week in development. Blood flow through the umbilical cord, between the embryo and the placenta, is expected to commence one week later. As the growing fetus matures, so does the umbilical cord as the structures contained within it change, as detailed below.

In the beginning of umbilical development, the stalk contains the allantois, two umbilical arteries, and two umbilical veins. The allantois develops as a diverticulum from the yolk sac, which extends from the body stalk to the fetal bladder to help with gas exchange and liquid waste elimination during the early parts of development. By the end of the eighth week of development, the allantois will normally regress in full, leaving behind an intra-abdominal remnant, known as the urachus. Failure of this process to occur as expected would lead to one of many umbilical abnormalities, which will be discussed as a group in the subsequent section. The second change occurring within the stalk as the cord matures is the urachus of the right umbilical vein, which occurs by the sixth week of development. The obliteration of these early cord features leaves behind a host of remnants that may be seen on anatomic examination of an adult abdomen, as was discussed in the vascular section.

The vitelline duct component of the umbilical cord is responsible for the early connection between the primitive intestines and the yolk sac. Under normal conditions, it will regress by the tenth week of development, leaving a solid, fibrous remnant between the ileum and the umbilicus. Failure of the vitelline duct to fully obliterate can lead to a host of umbilical abnormalities, which can vary in presentation depending on which aspects of the fetal structure remains. These abnormal variations will be discussed more completely in an upcoming section.

The umbilical coelom is the final structure housed within the umbilical cord at the initial stage, and it serves to connect the intraembryonic coelom with the extra-embryonic coelom. Early in the growth of the alimentary tract, the size of the abdominal cavity is relatively slow to enlarge, such that the budding abdominal contents cannot be retained entirely within it. The existence of the umbilical coelom allows the protrusion of the developing gut through the umbilical ring into the extra-embryonic coelom until the intraembryonic cavity can become sufficient in size to accommodate all of the contents on its own. Once the abdominal contents have reentered the abdominal cavity in full, the umbilical coelom regresses, which allows the complete fusion of the ventral abdominal wall. This normally occurs around the 12th week of development.

At the time of birth, all of these umbilical structures should have regressed under normal conditions, except for the two umbilical arteries and one umbilical vein. When the umbilical cord is split at the time of delivery, the flow of blood across the cord is discontinued, and these vessels quickly degenerate into their mature remnants. The umbilical ring closes in short order through scarring, leaving no opening between the intra-abdominal and extra-abdominal compartments. If the closure of the umbilical ring does not occur completely, a congenital umbilical hernia will be present.

1.6.2 Congenital Anatomic Abnormalities of the Umbilicus and Abdominal Wall

Congenital disorders of the umbilicus come from a variety of different developmental sources and may present as a protruding mass, umbilical drainage, or both. Some of these disorders, including persistence of the vitelline duct and persistence of the allantois, have already been mentioned, but another common umbilical abnormality, the umbilical hernia, may also be present. This section will examine these problems in greater depth, in conjunction with two congenital defects related to the abdominal wall – omphalocele and gastroschisis.

One relatively common form of umbilical deformity is the infantile umbilical hernia. This type of defect will appear as a mass protruding in the umbilical region, most often in its superior portions. It usually occurs within weeks of the sloughing of the umbilical cord, though may be evident within a few days of life. This type of hernia occurs when the closure of the umbilical ring through physiologic scarring produces a weak and ineffective seal, and intra-abdominal contents are able to pass into the subcutaneous layer. Critical in the distinction here is the fact that a normal layer of the skin overlies the herniated contents. This type of hernia will often resolve spontaneously within the first few years of life, since the mechanism of the defect is the incomplete scarring of the umbilical remnant, which will heal naturally with age. This is in contrast to omphalocele, which is a more involved version of umbilical herniation.

Omphalocele is the result of a defect during the formation of the abdominal wall, which allows the passage of abdominal contents into the umbilical cord. It differs from a simple umbilical hernia in its structure, in that it is the result of the incomplete fusion of the muscles of the abdominal wall in the midline, not simply the scarring within the umbilical ring. As previously discussed, a part of normal alimentary development entails the passage of growing viscera into the extraembryonic coelom; under normal conditions, these contents will return to the abdominal compartment by week 12 of development, to allow the normal fusion of the abdominal wall to occur. In this case, the abdominal contents do not return as expected, and the abdominal wall remains patent as a result. The problem presents as viscera visibly protruding through a defect into the umbilical cord and will vary in severity based on the amount of abdominal contents within the umbilical cord. This is different from the simple umbilical hernia, as there is no skin overlying the protruding viscera; however, it is covered by normal peritoneum and amnion. This covering is key in the classification of an omphalocele, as it helps to differentiate this disorder from a related abdominal wall defect, termed gastroschisis. Gastroschisis, like omphalocele, is a defect in the formation of the abdominal wall; however, gastroschisis presents with completely exposed bowel, which is uncovered by the skin, peritoneum, or amnion. This defect is appreciated at the junction of the umbilicus and the normal skin of the abdominal wall and is almost always located to the right of the umbilicus. This site represents the location of the obliterated right umbilical vein. The size of the defect is usually relatively small in comparison to omphalocele (less than 4 cm). Though the mechanism for the development of this defect has not been defined conclusively, it is likely related to disruption of normal blood supply from the omphalomesenteric duct artery to the developing abdominal wall. The result is improper nutrition to the developing area, with the small right-sided patency occurring.

The vitelline duct, which under normal conditions will regress by the tenth week of development, can result in a variety of congenital umbilical abnormalities if it fails to obliterate as expected. The specific presentation related to this condition will vary based on the portion of the duct that is retained. One of the most familiar forms of this abnormal regression, a Meckel's diverticulum, results from the persistence of the intestinal end of the vitelline duct. This true diverticulum usually arises near the distal end of the ileum, which is the most common site of embryonic attachment of the vitelline duct to the small bowel. A second variant results from complete patency through the entirety of the track of the duct, resulting in a fistula between the distal ileum and the umbilicus (enterocutaneous fistula). This type of deformity is uncommon and presents with the passage of stool and intestinal contents through the umbilicus shortly after birth. Other uncommon presentations of vitelline remnants include an umbilical polyp or vitelline duct cyst, which result from persistence of the distal aspect of the vitelline duct or accumulation of mucus in a medially retained portion of the duct, respectively. Finally, persistence of the allantois, which under normal conditions will regress into a fibrous cord by the end of development, may result in a vesicocutaneous fistula (connection between the urinary bladder and the umbilicus). If the allantois remains fully patent, this condition will present with the passage of urine through the defect in the umbilicus. Alternatively, a urachal cyst, which presents as a palpable lower abdominal mass, or a urachal sinus, presenting as a chronic drainage of small amounts of mucus through the umbilicus, may be present if only a portion of the allantois is retained.

These umbilical and abdominal wall malformations are in many cases complicated, requiring further work-up and intricate management in order to resolve the issue at hand. These considerations are beyond the scope of this discussion, however should be reviewed for a full appreciation of the problems created by these aberrations.

1.7 Conclusions

The umbilicus has a well-studied and well-described embryonic origin. The complexity of the anatomy as it relates to the abdomen collectively is essential for the appropriate diagnosis and treatment of congenital and acquired deformities.

Chapter 2
The Arterial Vascularization of the Abdominal Wall with Special Regard to the Umbilicus

Norbert Pallua and Verena-Constanze Buchinger-Kähler

2.1 Introduction

The blood supply of the abdominal wall is focus of many anatomical studies [1–3]. By understanding the blood supply, a surgeon can minimize the risk of postoperative necrosis, wound healing disorders, and conspicuous scars.

Serious postoperative complications can be avoided, if surgical incisions and maneuvers are adopted to the important vascular architecture of the abdominal wall. Due to this concept, surgeons started to study the arterial blood supply thoroughly [4–6]. This chapter will focus on the normal anatomy as well as on the blood supply after surgical intervention.

2.2 Preoperative Conditions

The vessels of the abdominal wall arise from the thoracic and pelvic arteries and perform multiple anastomoses with tremendous importance for surgical dissection or flap creation. The major blood supply is provided by the deep epigastric arcade, formed by the deep superior and inferior epigastric arteries [1, 7]. Additional blood supply emerges from the following arteries: intercostal, subcostal, musculophrenic, lumbar, superficial epigastric, superficial external pudendal, and superficial and deep circumflex iliac arteries (Fig. 2.1).

N. Pallua, M.D., Ph.D. (✉) • Dr. V.-C. Buchinger-Kähler
Department for Plastic Surgery, Hand Surgery, Burn Center,
University Hospital of the RWTH Aachen University, Pauwelsstr. 30, D-52074,
Aachen, Germany
e-mail: npallua@ukaachen.de

M.A. Shiffman (ed.), *Adult Umbilical Reconstruction*,
DOI 10.1007/978-3-319-43887-0_2

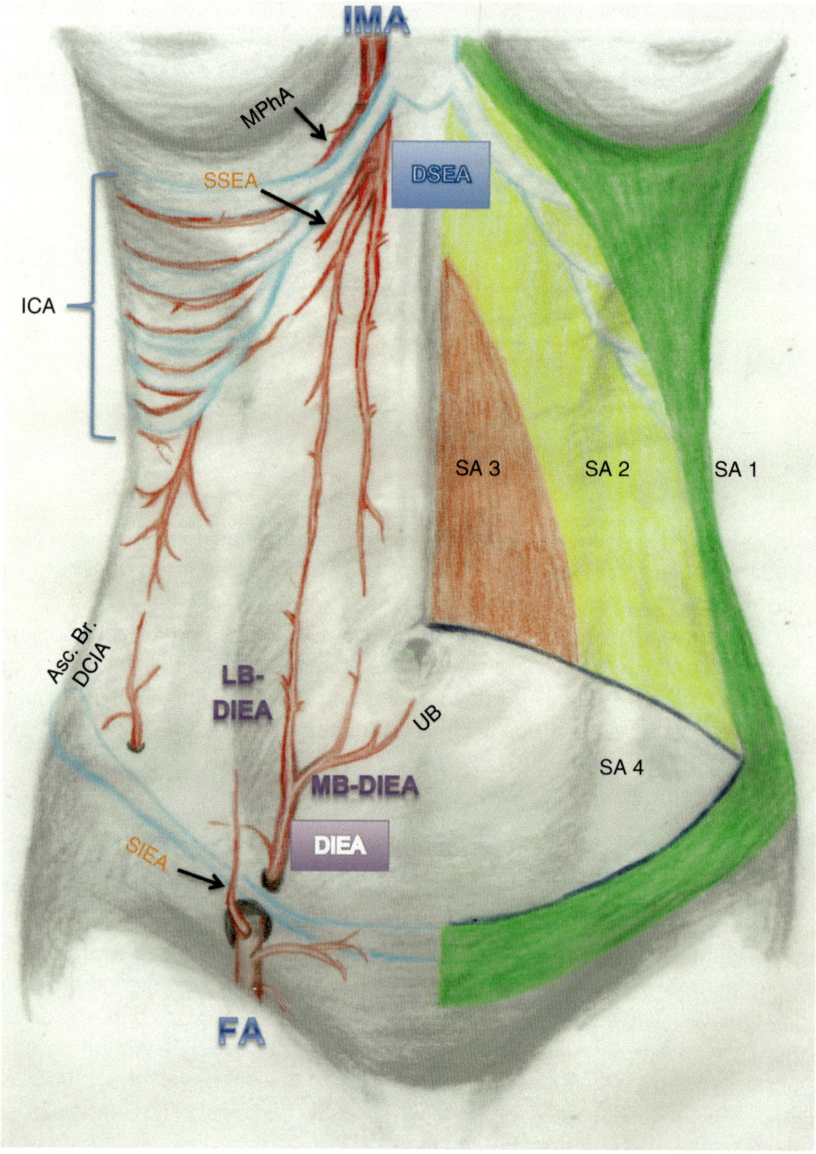

Fig. 2.1 Arterial blood supply of the anterior abdominal wall. *Right*: arterial branches and important anastomoses. *DSEA* deep inferior epigastric artery, *SSEA* superficial superior epigastric artery, *MPhA* musculophrenic artery, *Asc. Br. DCIA* ascending branch of deep circumflex iliac artery, *DSEA* deep superior epigastric artery, *SIEA* superficial inferior epigastric artery, *ICA* intercostal arteries, *UB* umbilical branch. *Left*: Matarasso's suction areas 1–4 (*SA 1–4*). Note that SA 4 can be excised in full abdominoplasty. If excision is not recommended, liposuction can be performed unrestricted in this area

2.3 The Deep Epigastric Arcade

The *deep superior epigastric artery* (*DSEA*) derives from the internal mammary artery at the level of the sixth rib, profound to the xiphoid process and the costal margin (Fig. 2.2). It passes the sternocostal triangle (Larry/Morgagni space) covered by the transverse thoracic muscle [8]. Here the *superficial superior epigastric artery* (*SSEA*) departs, perforates the anterior rectus sheath, and follows subcutaneously in the course of the eighth rib. The DSEA descends laterally oblique before dividing into a medial and a lateral branch with similar calibers [9] and gaining the posterior aspect of the rectus abdominis muscle in its own muscular fascia groove. Mu found an anastomosis with the ninth posterior intercostal artery [10]. This connection between the DSEA and the lateral intercostal circulation is of clinical interest during extended undermining of the abdominal wall. Four large (≥0.5 mm) perforators of the DSEA pierce the rectus sheet 4–6 cm of the costal margin in each hemiabdomen [11]. Note that perforators of the DSEA have a predictable occurrence and course. These perforators run caudally orientated and are forming conspicuous anastomoses across the midline in the subdermal plexus [11]. They provide the blood supply for the supraumbilical abdominal wall.

The *deep inferior epigastric artery* (*DIEA*) arises from the external iliac artery and enters the abdominal wall posterior to the inguinal ligament. Before entering the rectus sheath, a branch separates to anastomose with the deep circumflex iliac artery. A clinically important anastomosis may be present as a connection between the external iliac artery and DIEA with the obturator artery of the internal iliac system, due to a variation of origin of the obturator artery. This connection, generally known as corona mortis, can be identified in 10–70 % of cases [12–14]. Injury with severe to potentially lethal bleeding could occur during femoral or obturator hernia repair or pelvic trauma [14]. The DIEA continues in the posterior rectus sheet, lying there in a muscular rim and supplying the rectus muscle with several muscular branches. In the middle third of the muscle below the umbilicus, the artery divides into two main branches: a smaller medial (MB-DIEA) and dominant lateral branch (LB-DIEA) (Fig. 2.3) [2, 9].

The *lateral branch* of the DIEA emits the majority of perforators. O'Dey et al. [9] observed – similar to studies of Mu et al. [10] and Taylor et al. [15] – an anastomosis of the lateral branch of the DIEA and the DSEA around 4 cm above the umbilicus, whereas the MB-DIEA faded on the level of the umbilicus. O'Dey et al. [9] showed nine rows of perforators, located caudal to cranial in 2–3 cm distance. Mu et al. [10] found two parallel lines of perforators at 2.4–4.9 cm from the midline. The lateral branch of the DIEA is seen as the leading vessel for the blood supply of the skin of the central anterior abdominal wall.

The importance of perforators of the *MB-DIEA* has been recognized for breast reconstruction [16]. Perforators of the MB-DIEA have indirect connections with the contralateral (across the midline) medial row perforators via the subdermal plexus, whereas medial and lateral row perforators have direct and indirect connections within the same hemiabdomen [16, 17].

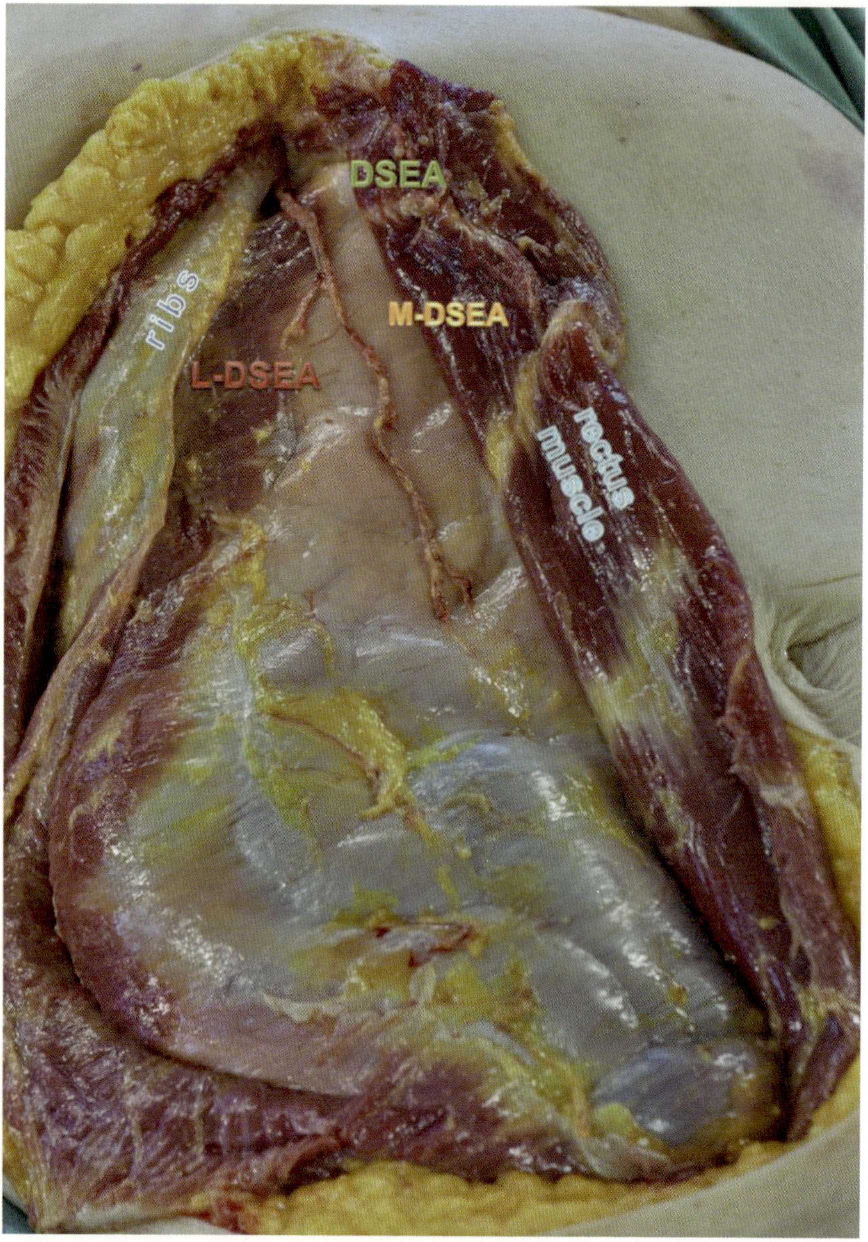

Fig. 2.2 The DSEA emerges below the sixth rib and runs oblique before dividing into equal-sized medial and lateral branches. The rectus muscle is turned over to expose the deep vascular arcade

Perforators of the DIEA follow no predictable paradigm or regularity in their angle or branching pattern [11]. In conclusion, these perforators form extensive anastomoses with one another in the subcutaneous layer, mostly at the level of the subdermal plexus [11, 18]. Note that the medial perforators superior to the

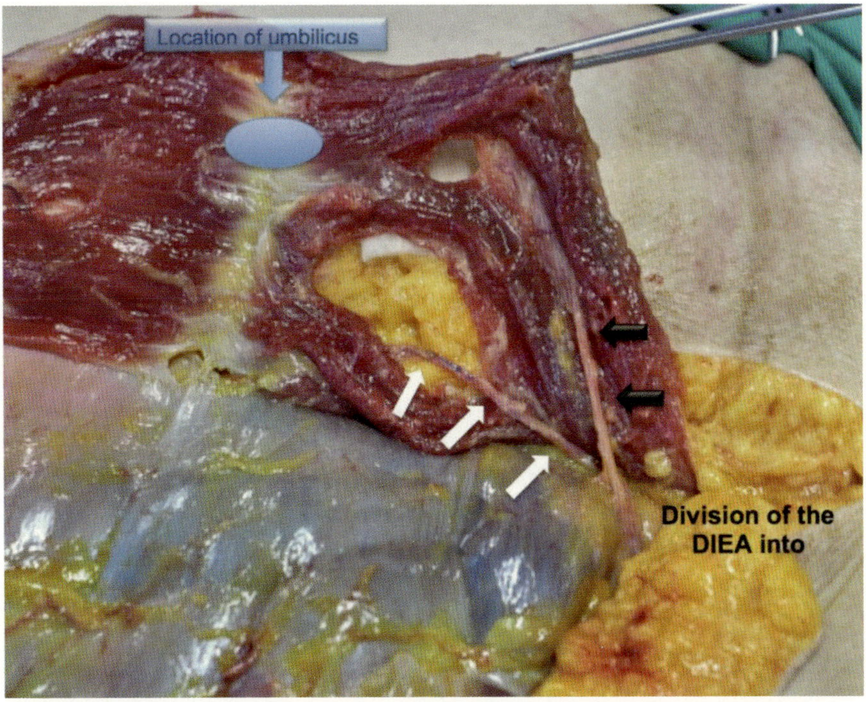

Fig. 2.3 Dissection of a fresh corps: *Left* margin of photo represents cranial, *right* margin is caudally orientated. The DIEA ascends from caudal and divides below the umbilicus into a smaller medial (*white arrows*) and a thicker lateral branch (*black arrows*). The lateral branch emits the majority of perforators, running below the rectus muscle as shown in the photo

umbilical level are considerably smaller in number and caliber than those of the lower abdomen [1].

The umbilicus is supplied by *Rr. umbilicales*, arising from the *MB-DIEA* (Fig. 2.4). The umbilical perforators pierce the linea alba and enter the anulus umbilicalis, resembling the bottom of the papilla umbilicalis. Mostly one perforator advances the papilla umbilicalis (67 %), whereas in 33 %, two perforators pierced the papilla [9]. These perforators run either as septo-cutaneous perforators under the rectus muscle or pierce the muscle as musculo-cutaneous perforators. Both types enter the papilla from the inferolateral and ascend diverging to the skin.

2.4 The Superficial Inferior Epigastric Artery (SIEA)

This vessel originates 2–3 cm below the inguinal ligament from the femoral artery or the common trunk with the superficial circumflex iliac artery [19]. Then the SIEA crosses the inguinal ligament at its midpoint, lying deep to Scarpa's fascia (Fig. 2.1). It continues superomedially, penetrating Scarpa's fascia above

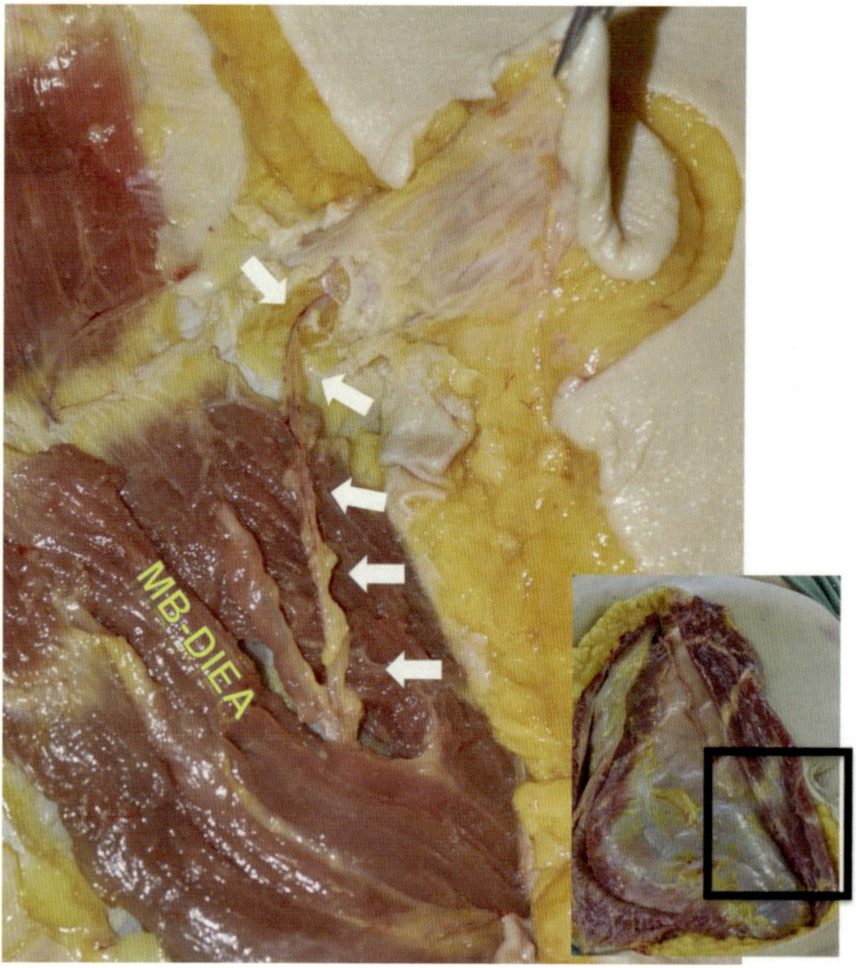

Fig. 2.4 Dissection of a fresh corps. Large image: The umbilical branch (*white arrows*) derives from the MB-DIEA (medial branch of the deep inferior epigastric artery) below the level of the navel. It enters the bottom of the umbilical papilla from inferior to laterally. Note the diverging vessels to the skin. The MB-DIEA fades at the level of the umbilicus. Small image: Overview of the trunk. The *black box* outlines the area of interest, magnified above

the inguinal ligament to run in a superficial subcutaneous plane. The supplied territory overlaps the other major vascular systems of blood supply to the anterior abdominal wall [19].

This vessel is of great interest for breast reconstruction because flap harvesting does not violate the rectus fascia, minimizing donor-site morbidity [20, 21]. Unfortunately several studies point out an inconsistency of the pedicle in 13–42 % as the major disadvantage of the SIEA flap. Taylor and Daniel (1975) [22] described 35 %, while Chevray [23] found it absent in 30 %.

2.5 Vascular Territories and Alterations Due to Periumbilical Surgery

Maintenance of umbilical blood supply is often challenging in periumbilical surgery. Especially when the patient presents with the following conditions: smoker, adipositas, extended abdominal apron, hernia, advanced age, diabetes, and cardiovascular disease. Interestingly, most surveys cannot detect a correlation between the incidence of complication and the professional experiences of the surgeon [24, 25]. In conclusion, circulatory problems of the abdominal flap may be inherent by the procedure itself and not associated with surgical skills.

In an abdominoplastic procedure, the skin inferior to the umbilicus is normally resected. Intraoperatively, the medial perforator row is dissected and severed. A large amount of periumbilical perforators can be observed (and cauterized) whose number decrease as the dissection proceeds superiorly. Boyd et al. [1] detected a watershed area above the umbilicus with extensive arborization and rather small caliber vessels. Only a few numbers of large vessels can be found above the umbilical level.

The blood supply of the adipose layers is also of clinical importance. Scarpa's fascia separates the deep layer supported by the muscle perforators – from superficial fat – supplied by the subdermal plexus. Assuming this bimodal blood supply, the level of dissection bears tremendous risks for circulatory problems [26]. Undermining the deep fat during abdominoplasty disrupts this primary blood supply and makes it prone to ischemia or eventually supports a steeling effect on the upper layers. Therefore, the superficial fat should not be excised, whereas the deep layer can be removed if needed [27].

2.6 Huger Zones

Huger [5] studied the modification of blood supply during abdominal dermolipectomy and revealed three vascular territories (Fig. 2.5). Zone I extends from the xiphoid process to the os pubis between the lateral borders of the rectus muscle. The deep arcade supplies this area. Zone II represents the inferior aspect of the abdomen, between the anterior superior iliac spine, the groin, and the pubic crests. This area is supplied by the superficial epigastric artery, the superficial circumflex iliac artery, and the external pudendal artery (superficial system), as well as by the deep inferior epigastric vessels. Zone III covers the lateral abdomen and flanks and is provided by segmental intercostal, subcostal, and lumbar arteries.

Traditional abdominoplasty combines extended abdominal dissection to the lateral costal margin and resection of Scarpa's fascia with attached fat, preserving only the lateral perforators (Zone III) [28]. In contrast, limited dissection abdominoplasty preserves Scarpa's fascia below the umbilicus and extends as a tunnel superior to the umbilicus on the linea alba between the rectus sheets.

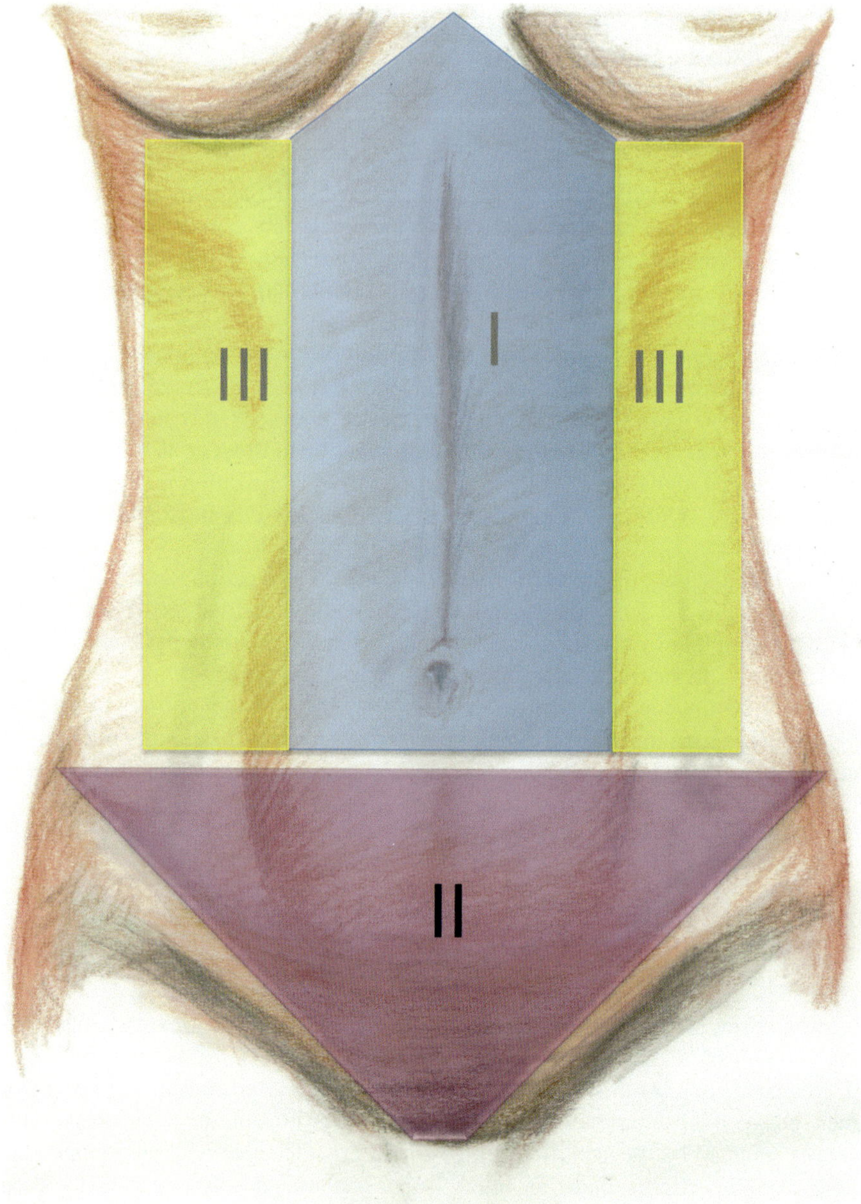

Fig. 2.5 Vascular zones by Huger [5]. Zone I represents the area between the lateral borders of rectus muscle and comprises the deep epigastric arcade. The blood supply in this area is sacrificed in traditional abdominoplasty

The goal of limited dissection [29] is preservation of the medial perforators and – by respecting Scarpa's fascia – preserving the anastomosis of DSEA and DIEA. A study of Munhoz et al. [30] proved that 80 % of perforators, lymphatic vessels, and nerves could be preserved by limited dissection. As previously mentioned, the perforators of the DSEA are more predictable. Therefore Zone I and III remain for blood supply.

2.7 Alterations Due to Dissection Technique and the Role of Scarpa's Fascia

In 2014, Roostaeian et al. [31] evaluated the flap perfusion by using laser fluorescence imaging and found no significant difference between traditional abdominoplasty and limited-undermining lipoabdominoplasty. The study protocols of those two studied groups differed substantially (infiltration of tumescence and liposuction versus none), reducing the comparableness.

Recently Swanson [32] published his results using the same imaging technique but reducing the variables, comparing limited dissection with preservation of Scarpa's fascia to full dissection. He was not able to show a significant improvement of perfusion or a lower seroma rate. In contrast, Saldanha [29] reported a seroma rate of 60 % performing the classical technique in contrast to only 1 % after switching to limited dissection. Swanson [32] further propagated limited dissection would lead to tension on the inferior skin flap with reduced blood supply. Le Louarn and Pascal [33] therefore perform the "high-superior-tension" technique to reduce the tension of the distal abdominal flap by using paraumbilical high-tension sutures in combination with liposuction and limited epigastric dissection. By this procedure, they tighten the epigastric skin and decrease tension on the hypogastrium, resulting in decreased risk of hypoperfusion.

Mayr et al. [28] assessed the infraumbilical perfusion rate (Zone I) after conventional, extended abdominoplasty [34] by laser fluorescence angiography. They measured an alarming decrease of over 80 % compared to untouched skin and a compensatory blood inflow from subcostal and intercostal branches. They suggest dissection and preservation of a perforator of the DSEA.

The flap-raising technique can also reduce risks of decreased perfusion after abdominoplasty. Dissection by electrosurgery is associated with a pronounced collateral damage compared to sharp (scalpel) preparation, due to thermal injury [35]. Therefore we prefer sharp dissection, especially in the delicate umbilical area.

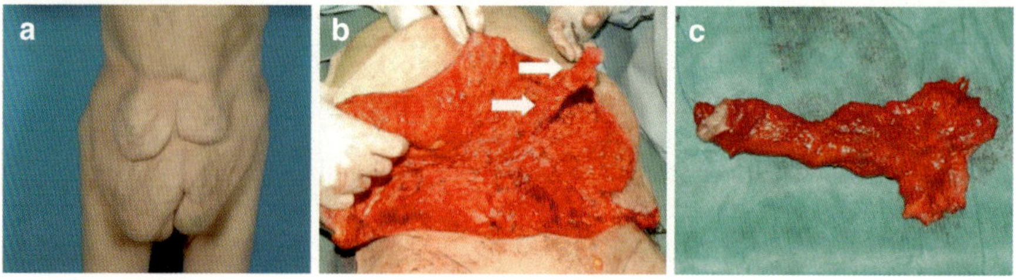

Fig. 2.6 (**a**) A 69-year-old patient after 70 kg weight loss. The patient suffered from incarcerated umbilical hernia 6 months before. (**b**) The umbilical stalk is tremendously elongated (*white arrows*). (**c**) Excision of nearly 20 cm of the insufficiently perfused and scarified stalk

2.8 Massive Weight Loss Patients and Blood Supply

Postbariatric patients are challenging patients with higher complication rates from 30 to 80 % [36–38]. Information about the percentage of umbilical necrosis due to postbariatric abdominoplasty is rare. Grieco et al. [39] showed 4 % of umbilical necrosis in a small-sized study on massive weight loss patients. Dellon [40] reported 12.5 % navel necrosis, who had also associated an umbilical hernia. The majority of studies summarize loss of umbilical in wound healing complication [38]. Nevertheless, an elongated navel stalk evidently bears an increased risk of impaired circulation after circumcision analogue to large ptotic breast and their multi-agent chemotherapy (MAC) (Fig. 2.6).

2.9 The Influence of Liposuction

Many authors elaborated the effects of liposuction to the abdominal circulation. Matarasso [6] based his reflection on the work of Huger and defined four "suction areas" (Fig. 2.1). As discussed previously, in traditional abdominoplasty, Huger Zone I is sacrificed, and blood enters postoperatively from the lateral aspect (Huger Zone III). Suction area 3 represents the triangular shaped middle of the undermined flap that will cover the umbilical to pubic area and requires precautious liposuction, without thinning the subcutaneous fat layer (above Scarpa's fascia). He also dissuades from any interruption of the midline crossover of blood flow (as a Fleur-de-lis/T-shaped scar) in this triangle [6]. Suction area hosts the segmental lumbar, subcostal, and intercostal arteries and is a safe and favored area for liposuction. It is recommendable to remove fat parallel to the vessels.

Saldanha [29] prefers liposuction above and below Scarpa's fascia to facilitate its visualization and preservation. Smith and Smith [40] developed a combination technique of extensive liposuction and abdominoplasty by preserving a perforator of the DSEA. They located this vessel consistently in a 2 cm radius area 6 cm below the subcostal margin and 4 cm lateral to the midline (Fig. 2.7). The risks increase with the amount of flap undermining, the quantity of liposuction, and the tension on wound closure [41, 42].

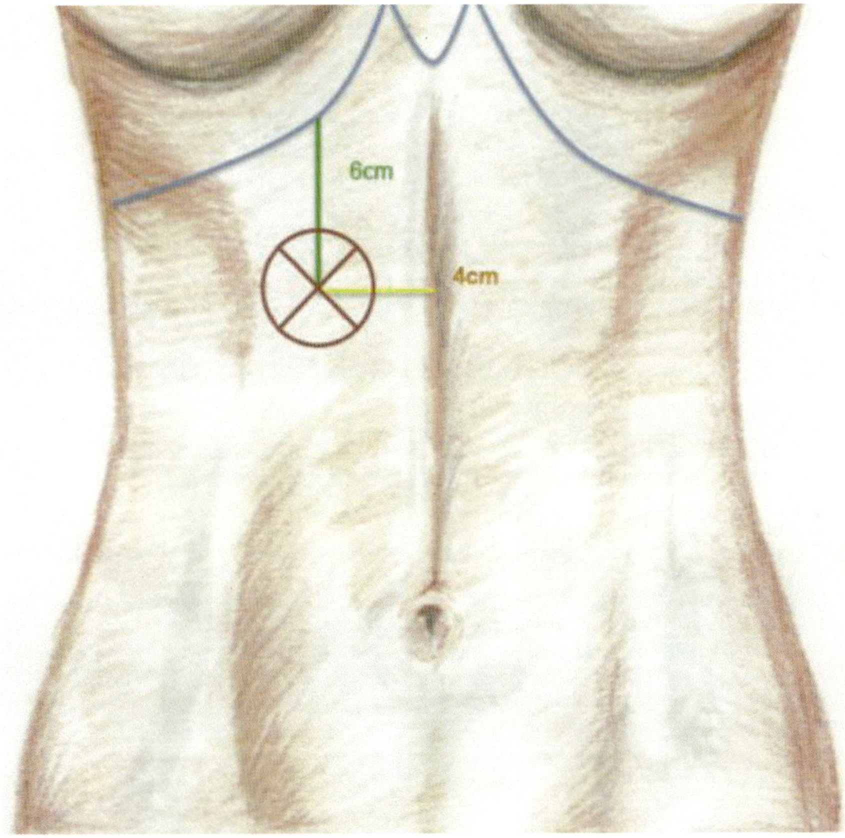

Fig. 2.7 The perforator of the deep superior epigastric artery is found 6 cm below the costal margin and 4 cm laterally to the midline, in a radius of 2 cm

2.10 Conclusions

1. Major blood supply of the abdomen is performed by the deep epigastric arcade.
2. Both DSEA and DIEA divide into a medial and a lateral branch.
3. The upper third of the abdominal integument is supported by DSEA perforators exclusively, while the central region perforators of the DIEA dominate.
4. In the *native* abdomen, the major blood supply arises from the DIEA.
5. Perforators of the DSEA are more predictable in their course, which is important for dissection during abdominoplasty.
6. The MB-DIEA perforators support the medial periumbilical abdomen and the umbilicus and connect with the contralateral MB-DIEA perforators that lead attention for utilization for large breast reconstruction.
7. The lateral branch of the DIEA anastomoses 4 cm above the umbilicus with the DSEA, whereas the MB-DIEA fades on the level of the umbilicus, arises from the MB-DIEA, pierces the linea alba, and enters the papilla umbilicalis from inferolateral to ascend to the umbilical skin.

8. During circumferential umbilical incision, the blood supply from subdermal plexus is interrupted, leading to a sole nutrition by the perforators of the MB-DIEA.
9. Huger's Zone III represents the lateral arc (segmental lumbar, subcostal, and intercostal arteries) that remains after extensive undermining in classical abdominoplasty and provides blood supply to the medial flap like a random pattern flap.
10. Limited dissection preserves Huger's Zones I and III with the reliable perforators of the DSEA.
11. Sharp dissection in the periumbilical area is advisable to protect the blood supply.
12. Liposuction in the middle triangle can compromise circulation and should solely be applied in the deep adipose layer.

References

1. Boyd JB, Taylor GI, Corlett R. The vascular territories of the superior epigastric and the deep inferior epigastric systems. Plast Reconstr Surg. 1984;73(1):1–16.
2. El-Mrakby HH, Milner RH. The vascular anatomy of the lower anterior abdominal wall: a microdissection study on the deep inferior epigastric vessels and the perforator branches. Plast Reconstr Surg. 2001;109:539–43.
3. O'Dey DM, Heimburg DV, Prescher A, Pallua N. The arterial vascularisation of the abdominal wall with special regard to the umbilicus. Br J Plast Surg. 2004;57(5):392–7.
4. Masterton JP. Necrosis of the abdominal wall following operations. Aust N Z J Surg. 1967;37(2):183–7.
5. Huger WE. The anatomic rationale for abdominal lipectomy. Ann Surg. 1979;45:612–7.
6. Matarasso A. Liposuction as an adjunct to a full abdominoplasty. Plast Reconstr Surg. 1995;95(5):829–36.
7. Taylor GI, Corlett R, Boyd JB. The extended deep inferior epigastric flap: a clinical technique. Plast Reconstr Surg. 1983;72(6):751–65.
8. Gilkeson RC, Basile V, Sands MJ, Hsu JT. Chest case of the day. Morgagni's hernia. Am J Roentgenol. 1997;169(1):268–70.
9. O'Dey DM, Okafor CA, Bozkurt A, Prescher A, Pallua N. Perforator vessel anatomy of the papilla umbilicalis: topography and importance for reconstructive abdominal wall surgery. Langenbecks Arch Surg. 2010;395(8):1121–7.
10. Mu L, Yan Y, Li S, Li Y, Huang L, Ling Y. Transparent morphology of the thoracoabdominal wall. J Reconstr Microsurg. 2001;17(8):611–4.
11. Tregaskiss AP, Goodwin AN, Acland RD. The cutaneous arteries of the anterior abdominal wall: a three-dimensional study. Plast Reconstr Surg. 2007;120(2):442–50.
12. Braithewaite JL. Variations in origin of the parietal branches of the internal iliac artery. Am J Anat. 1952;86:423–30.
13. Hong HX, Pan ZJ, Chen X, Huang ZJ. An anatomical study of corona mortis and its clinical significance. Chin J Traumatol. 2004;7:165–9.
14. Ates M, Kinaci E, Kose E, Soyer V, Sarici B, Cuglan S, Korkmaz F, Dirican A. Corona mortis: in vivo anatomical knowledge and the risk of injury in totally extraperitoneal inguinal hernia repair. Hernia. 2016;20(5):659–65.
15. Taylor GI, Corlett RJ, Dhar SC, Ashton MW. The anatomical (angiosome) and clinical territories of cutaneous perforating arteries: development of the concept and designing safe flaps. Plast Reconstr Surg. 2011;127(4):1447–59.

16. Wong C, Saint-Cyr M, Mojallal A, Schaub T, Bailey SH, Myers S, Brown S, Rohrich RJ. Perforasomes of the DIEP flap: vascular anatomy of the lateral versus medial row perforators and clinical implications. Plast Reconstr Surg. 2010;125(3):772–82.
17. Moon KH, Taylor GI. The vascular anatomy of rectus abdominis musculocutaneous flaps based on the deep superior epigastric system. Plast Reconstr Surg. 1988;82:815–30.
18. Taylor GI, Corlett RJ, Boyd JB. The versatile deep epigastric (inferior rectus abdominis) flap. Br J Plast Surg. 1984;37:330–50.
19. Hester Jr TR, Nahai F, Beegle PE, Bostwick 3rd J. Blood supply of the abdomen revisited, with emphasis on the superficial inferior epigastric artery. Plast Reconstr Surg. 1984;74(5):657–70.
20. Wu LC, Bajaj A, Chang DW, Chevray PM. Comparison of donor-site morbidity of SIEA, DIEP, and muscle-sparing TRAM flaps for breast reconstruction. Plast Reconstr Surg. 2008;122:702–9.
21. Coroneos CJ, Heller AM, Voineskos SH, Avram R. SIEA versus DIEP Arterial Complications: a cohort study. Plast Reconstr Surg. 2015;135(5):802–7.
22. Taylor G, Daniel R. The anatomy of several free flap donor sites. Plast Reconstr Surg. 1975;56:243–53.
23. Chevray PM. Breast reconstruction with superficial inferior epigastric artery (SIEA) flaps: a prospective comparison with TRAM and DIEP flaps. Plast Reconstr Surg. 2004;114:1077–83.
24. Floros C, Davis PK. Complications and long-term results following abdominoplasty: a retrospective study. Br J Plast Surg. 1991;44:190–4.
25. Uchelen JH, Werker PN, Kon M. Complications of abdominoplasty in 86 patients. Plast Reconstr Surg. 2001;107:1869–73.
26. El-Mrakby HH, Milner RH. Bimodal distribution of the blood supply to lower abdominal fat: histological study of the microcirculation of the lower abdominal wall. Ann Plast Surg. 2003;50(2):165–70.
27. Nahai FR. Anatomic considerations in abdominoplasty. Clin Plast Surg. 2010;37:407–14.
28. Mayr M, Holm C, Höfter E, Becker A, Pfeiffer U, Mühlbauer W. Effects of aesthetic abdominoplasty on abdominal wall perfusion: a quantitative evaluation. Plast Reconstr Surg. 2004;114:1586–94.
29. Saldanha OR, Federico R, Daher PF. Lipoabdominoplasty. Plast Reconstr Surg. 2009;124:934–45.
30. Munhoz AM, Kamamoto F, Saito FL, Menezes M, Gemperli R. Anatomical mapping of the perforant abdominal vessels and clinical application in the treatment of aesthetic deformities of the abdominal wall through lipoabdominoplasty. In: Saldanha O, editor. Lipoabdominoplasty. Rio de Janeiro: Di Livros; 2006. p. 103–13.
31. Roostaeian J, Harris R, Farkas J. Comparison of limited undermining Lipoabdominoplasty and traditional abdominoplasty using laser fluorescence imaging. Aesthet Surg J. 2014;34:741–7.
32. Swanson E. Comparison of limited and full dissection abdominoplasty using laser fluorescence imaging to evaluate perfusion of the abdominal skin. Plast Reconstr Surg. 2015;136(1):31–43.
33. Le Louarn C, Pascal JF. The high-superior-tension technique: evolution of lipoabdominoplasty. Aesthetic Plast Surg. 2010;34(6):773–81.
34. Regnault P. Abdominal lipectomy, a low "W" incision. New York: New York International Society of Aesthetic Plastic Surgery; 1972.
35. Valença-Filipe R, Martins A, Silva Á, Vásconez LO, Amarante J, Costa-Ferreira A. Dissection technique for abdominoplasty: a prospective study on scalpel versus diathermocoagulation (coagulation mode). Plast Reconstr Surg Glob Open. 2015;3(1):e299.
36. Gmur RU, Banic A, Erni D. Is it safe to combine abdominoplasty with other dermolipectomy procedures to correct skin excess after weight loss? Ann Plast Surg. 2003;51:353–7.
37. Taylor J, Shermak M. Body contouring following massive weight loss. Obes Surg. 2004;14:1080–5.
38. Greco 3rd JA, Castaldo ET, Nanney LB, Wendel JJ, Summitt JB, Kelly KJ, Braun SA, Hagan KF, Shack RB. The effect of weight loss surgery and body mass index on wound complications after abdominal contouring operations. Ann Plast Surg. 2008;61(3):235–42.

39. Grieco M, Grignaffini E, Simonacci F, Raposio E. Analysis of complications in postbariatric abdominoplasty: our experience. Plast Surg Int. 2015;(2015):209173. http://www.hindawi.com/journals/psi/2015/209173 Accessed 15 Feb 2016.
40. Dellon A. Fleur-de-Lis Abdominoplasty. Aesthetic Plast Surg. 1985;9:27–32.
41. Smith LF, Smith Jr LF. Safely combining abdominoplasty with aggressive abdominal liposuction based on perforator vessels: technique and a review of 300 consecutive cases. Plast Reconstr Surg. 2015;135(5):1357–66.
42. Matarasso A. Liposuction as an adjunct to full abdominoplasty revisited. Plast Reconstr Surg. 2000;106:1197–202.

Part II
Shape and Position of the Umbilicus

Chapter 3
Ideal Position and Shape of the Umbilicus

Melvin A. Shiffman

3.1 Introduction

The position and shape of the umbilicus is extremely important in the aspect of the beauty of the abdomen. The umbilicus is exposed by bathing suits (especially bikini), shorts, short blouses, and exposed midriff. Many young women are happy to expose their umbilical region if there is no scar or distortion of the umbilicus.

3.2 Umbilical Position

3.2.1 Author's Technique

The author uses the base of the pedicle to determine the ideal position of the umbilicus [1] in the linea alba. The midline of the umbilical stalk opening is in the midline of the abdomen skin from birth. In the standing position, marking of the midline is done from the xiphoid process to the center of the pubis detected by the parting of the hair in slightly different directions. This avoids the different positions of the umbilicus in the lower abdominal flap when there is a long pedicle especially in the obese patients. The level of the new umbilicus is marked at the level of the base of the pedicle. The incision of the skin should be performed about 1–2 cm lower than the marking. This will allow an upward tilt to the pedicle and allow a superior hooded appearance. The umbilical pedicle should be short. This necessitates shortening the pedicle by suturing to the fascia around the pedicle base.

M.A. Shiffman, M.D., J.D.
Private Practice, 17501 Chatham Drive, Tustin, CA 92780-2302, USA
e-mail: shiffmanmdjd@gmail.com

M.A. Shiffman (ed.), *Adult Umbilical Reconstruction*,
DOI 10.1007/978-3-319-43887-0_3

3.2.2 History

Rohrich et al. [2] found that the umbilicus was not at the midline in nearly 100 % of subjects. Editorial comment: "This is because the umbilical stalk normally moves in the subcutaneous tissues despite its deep attachment to the deep fascia. The fact is that the adipose subcutaneous layer is loose and because of the length of the umbilical stalk the umbilicus does not necessarily fall straight down when standing or supine but arbitrarily falls to one side or the other, more so with obesity. However, the aesthetic appearance is better when the umbilicus is in the midline."

There are a number of ways to determine the best position of the umbilicus [3–14], but the simplest method is using the level of the iliac crests at the midline (the xipho-pubic line) [15–19]. Sabatier et al. [19] described the midline for the umbilicus as the xipho-pubic line and a transverse line that joins the iliac crest about 2 cm above each anterior superior iliac spine.

In fact Dubou and Ousterhout [16] found that a line drawn from the highest level of the crest of one ilium to the same point on the other side will transect the umbilicus in 96 % of the subjects.

Daher et al. [20] utilized the measurement of 18–20 cm from the anterior vulvar commissure along the xipho-pubic line to position the umbilicus. Baroudi [1], however, stated that the umbilical pedicle base is the level for the placement of the umbilicus. Cammarota [21] used the position on the xipho-pubic line 18–20 cm from the anterior vulvar commissure.

There is a difference in the position of the umbilicus in a newborn compared to an adult. The position of the umbilicus in an infant is the most aesthetically pleasing if the umbilicus is placed 60 % of the way from the xipho-sternum to the pubis [6].

3.3 Umbilical Shape

The ideal umbilicus is a small T or vertically oriented umbilicus with the addition of a superior hood or shelf according to Craig et al. [22], while the oval shape was superior according to Pallua [3]. Baack et al. [15] stated that the normal umbilicus is hooded superiorly, has a central opening, and proceeds slightly superiorly as it approaches the abdominal wall fascia.

References

1. Baroudi R. Umbilicaplasty. Clin Plast Surg. 1975;2(3):431–48.
2. Rohrich RJ, Sorokin ES, Brown SA, Gibby DL. Is the umbilicus truly midline? Clinical and medicolegal implications. Plast Reconstr Surg. 2003;112(1):259–63.
3. Pallua N, Markowicz MP, Grosse F, Walter S. Aesthetically pleasant umbilicoplasty. Ann Plast Surg. 2010;64(6):722–5.

4. Avelar JM. Abdominoplasty: technical refinement and analysis of 130 cases in 8 years' follow-up. Aesthetic Plast Surg. 1983;7(4):205–12.
5. Park S, Hata Y, Ito O, Tokioka K, Kagawa K. Umbilical reconstruction after repair of omphalocele and gastroschisis. Plast Reconstr Surg. 1999;104(1):204–7.
6. Williams AM, Brain JL. The normal position of the umbilicus in the newborn: an aid to improving the cosmetic result in exomphalos major. J Pediatr Surg. 2001;36(7):1045–6.
7. Rosenfeld LK. Comprehensive abdominoplasty approaches using complementary techniques. In: Nahai F, editor. The Art of aesthetic surgery: principles & techniques. St. Louis: Quality Medical Publishing, Inc; 2005. p. 2384–422.
8. Kakudo N, Kusumoto K, Fujimori S, Shimotsuma A, Ogawa Y. Reconstruction of a natural-appearing umbilicus using an island flap: case report. J Plast Reconstr Aesthet Surg. 2006;59(9):999–1002.
9. Abhyankar SV, Rajguru AG, Patil PA. Anatomical localization of the umbilicus: an Indian study. Plast Reconstr Surg. 2006;117(4):1153–7.
10. Williams AM, Platt AJ. Relocating the umbilicus in abdominal surgery. Plast Reconstr Surg. 2006;117(7):2528.
11. Thomas M, DSilva JA, Menon H, Padubidri R. Deciding the position of neoumbilicus in abdominoplasty: a novel idea. Am J Cosm Surg. 2007;24(4):181–2.
12. Colwell A, Kpodzo D, Gallico 3rd GG. Low scar abdominoplasty with inferior positioning of the umbilicus. Ann Plast Surg. 2010;64(5):639–44.
13. Kinoshita M, Park S, Shiraishi T, Ueno S. Thoracoabdominoplasty with umbilicoplasty for Cantrell's syndrome. J Plast Surg Hand Surg. 2012;46(5):367–70.
14. Parnia R, Ghorbani L, Sepehrvand N, Hatami S, Bazargan-Hejazi S. Determining anatomical position of the umbilicus in Iranian girls, and providing quantitative indices and formula to determine neo-umbilicus during abdominoplasty. Indian J Plast Surg. 2012;45(1):94–6.
15. Baack BR, Anson G, Nachbar JM, White DJ. Umbilicoplasty: the construction of a new umbilicus and correction of umbilical stenosis without external scars. Plast Reconstr Surg. 1996;97(1):227–32.
16. Dubou R, Ousterhout DK. Placement of the umbilicus in an abdominoplasty. Plast Reconstr Surg. 1978;61(2):291–3.
17. Regnault P, Daniel RK. Abdominoplasty. In: Regnault P, Daniel RK, editors. Aesthetic plastic surgery: principles and techniques. Boston: Little, Brown and Company; 1984. p. 617–54.
18. Lopez-Tallaj L, Gervain J. Restaurção umbilical na abdominoplastia: uma simples técnica rectangular. Rev Soc Bras Cir Plast. 2001;16(3):39–46.
19. Sabatier PH, Barray L, Picaud AJ. Une technique originale de refection de l'ombilic. Ann Chir Plast. 1978;23(4):245–8.
20. Daher JC, Benedik A, Ceva Faria CAD, Di Lamartine J, Neto JNR, Cosa OM, Cammarota MC. Umbilicoplasty: experience with the skin mini-circle technique. Rev Bras Cir Plast 2011;26(2).
21. Cammarota MC. Umbilicoplastia: experiência com a técnica do minicirculo de pele. Rev Bras Cir Plast. 2011;26(2):302–5.
22. Craig SB, Faller MS, Puckett CL. In search of the ideal female umbilicus. Plast Reconstr Surg. 2000;105(1):389–92.

Chapter 4
The Aesthetically Pleasant Umbilicus

Norbert Pallua and Verena-Constanze Buchinger-Kähler

4.1 Introduction

The umbilicus represents the only natural scar of the body. Its configuration and position are essential to the aesthetic appearance of the abdomen. Absence or deformity of this cavitation draws unwanted attention and may lead to emotional distress [1]. The navel has been an object of interest though the history of art or cultural believes. Leonardo Da Vinci set the umbilicus as the center of his Vitruvian Man.

Statistically abdominoplasty was ranked as the sixth most performed cosmetic surgery in 2014 with nearly 700,000 procedures in a worldwide survey of plastic surgeons by ISAPS International Survey on Aesthetic/Cosmetic Procedures [2]. As the umbilicus is the major aesthetic component of the abdomen, its influence on the satisfaction of patients undergoing abdominoplasty is obvious. Therefore acquiring deep knowledge of location, shape, size, depth, and tilting angle of the "normal" umbilicus helps to understand the difference and alteration due to aging, pregnancy, weight fluctuation, or hernias.

4.2 Aesthetic Importance of the Umbilicus Throughout the Course of History to Modern

In the early techniques of abdominoplasty, the navel was neglected. Kelly (1899) [3] excised the umbilicus in an elliptical transversal incision. In 1924 Thorek [4] described umbilical preservation in abdominoplasty by placing the incision

N. Pallua, M.D., Ph.D. (✉) • Dr. V.-C. Buchinger-Kähler
Department for Plastic Surgery, Hand Surgery, Burn Center,
University Hospital of the RWTH Aachen University, Pauwelsstr. 30, D-52074,
Aachen, Germany
e-mail: npallua@ukaachen.de

M.A. Shiffman (ed.), *Adult Umbilical Reconstruction*,
DOI 10.1007/978-3-319-43887-0_4

below the navel. If larger excisions were required, he advised to include the umbilicus and transplant it later as a composite graft. First attention to the preservation of the umbilicus was paid by Prudente in 1943 [5], emphasizing that he had been using this technique since 1936. An important landmark for umbilicoplasty was published by Vernon in 1957 [1], who combined the transverse incision of Thorek [4] with undermining the abdominal flap and umbilical transposition.

4.3 Techniques of Umbilicoplasty

The W-technique of Regnault (1975) [6] recommends a 2 cm horizontal incision across the midline, 2 cm below the waistline. Pulling on the flap would open up the incision and create a "marquise" shape. In contrast Grazer (1973) [7] performed a 1–1.5 cm transverse incision close to Pitanguy's [8] but with an elliptical removal of skin. A circular skin excision was recommended by Gonzalez-Ulloa in 1960 [9]. In 1967 Pitanguy [8] introduced a *U-shaped* incision in the abdominal wall to reinsert the umbilicus.

Baroudi et al. [10] drew particular attention to the aesthetical importance of the umbilicus. He shortened the umbilical pedicle by suturing it to the abdominal fascia and resected a ring of fat around the skin incision to create a fold and the natural depression of the umbilicus. The *Ω-shaped* incision was published by Freeman in 1978 [11]. Juri et al. [12] set the next landmark by performing a *V-incision*. He also thinned the periumbilical fat layer 6 cm above the umbilicus and 3 cm below to create a natural periumbilical depression. The circular scar after navel reinsertion was indicated as one of the most obvious signs for a tummy tuck. Delerm [13] published his technique in 1982. He put emphasis on cutting the umbilical stalk vertically to its aponeurotic attachments and suture a superior-based *round skin flap* of the abdominal wall to the aponeurosis to provide more stability to the upper part. In 1998 Choudhary and Taams [14] presented their technique of "umbilicosculpture" with a horizontal abdominal incision, shortening of the umbilical stalk, and teardrop-shaped periumbilical fat excision.

Nowadays a variety of techniques are utilized, and most surgeons have their own notion of a pleasant umbilicus. The shape of abdominal incision varies and occasionally the ways of shortening the umbilical stalk or fixation techniques to the fascia differ.

Niranjan and Staiano [15] recognized the importance of the superficial fascia (Scarpa) to the blood supply of the navel flap. They performed a *U-shaped* incision and sutured the superficial fascia to the dermis of the U-flap instead of fixating the umbilicus itself to the rectus fascia. By this maneuver, they wanted to avoid the feeling of tethering of the umbilicus. *A triangular skin* incision was introduced by Avelar (1978) [16] and later by Massiha (1997) [17]. The latter sutured the shortened umbilicus to the rectus sheet and the three abdominal flaps to the umbilicus to hide the incision lines in the depth of the umbilical crater. Ramirez [18] left the decision to the patient whether to have a frowning inversed V-incision or his preferred *V-shaped/heart-shaped* incision to create a "smiling" umbilicus.

The *inverted U-flap* was introduced by Malic [1]. She secured the cranial tip of the inverted U and the stalk at 6-o'clock to the rectus fascia. Saldanha et al. [19] advised *star-shaped* incisions to evade postoperative scar retraction.

Pitanguy preferred a transverse reimplanted umbilicus, whereas Lee and Mustoe [20] propagated the vertical orientated umbilicus without superior hooding to create a youthful navel. Schoeller et al. [21] defatted a 6–7 cm diameter round area of the abdominal flap and created a new navel by tying this round patch with purse-string sutures to a deepithelialized original navel stalk.

In 2010 Pallua et al. [22] published their technique to create a natural, aesthetically pleasant umbilicus. To achieve this result *an inverted V-incision* with a corresponding triangle excised in the inferior portion of the umbilicus is performed. Respecting gender differences following suture techniques can lead to a more feminine or masculine abdominal surface: to create a natural supraumbilical depression for a female abdomen, the subdermal layer of the umbilical disk is only fixed by a permanent suture to the fascia in the upper pole (at 12.00 o'clock). This maneuver also leads to a natural tilting angle of the umbilicus (Fig. 4.1). In women the infraumbilical area is rather slightly curved than tight and straight. The scar is hidden from the patients view because the abdominal flap is sutured to the depth of the umbilical dimple. For a straighter and more masculine surface, the subdermal layer needs fixation at 3.00, 9.00, and 12.00 o'clock.

Visconti and Salgarello in 2015 [23] incised the abdominal wall in an "ace of spades" figure to create an oval shape with a natural superior hooding.

In most papers special attention is advised for patients with thin abdominal fat layers. Irregularities in the periumbilical fat, shallow umbilical depression, and umbilical scarring are more obvious. Therefore, the technique has to be adjusted to the anatomical circumstances.

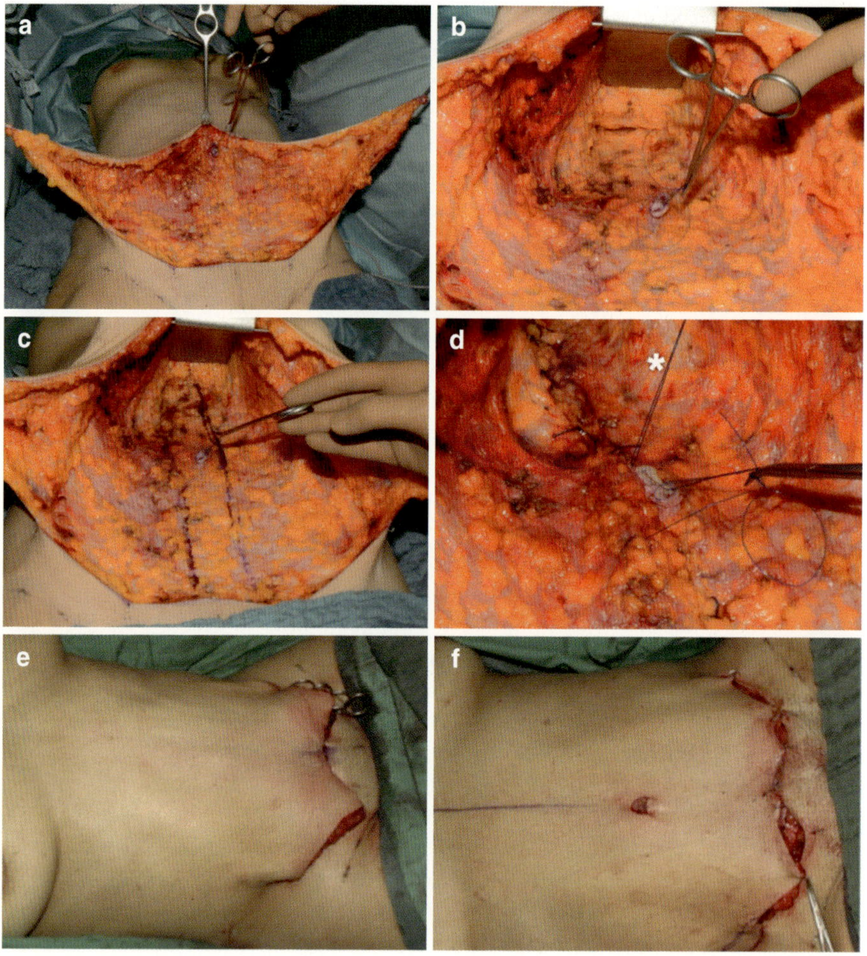

Fig. 4.1 Limited dissection abdominoplasty. (**a**) Preservation of the Scarpa's fascia. (**b**) The dissection proceeds in a small tunnel supraumbilical. (**c**) The diastasis of the rectus muscle is marked. (**d**) The upper pole of the umbilicus is fixed subdermal to the fascia with nonabsorbable sutures (= *). This suture is guided through the skin flap incision, as you can see in (**f**) and sutured to the dermis edge of the inverted V. (**e**, **f**) In a beach chair position, the resection area is measured, and the placement of the umbilicus is marked, mostly slightly above the palpated stalk

References

1. Vernon S. Umbilical transplantation upward and abdominal contouring in lipectomy. Am J Surg. 1957;94(3):490–2.
2. ISAPS International Survey on Aesthetic/Cosmetic. Procedures performed in 2014. http://www.isaps.org/Media/Default/global-statistics/2015%20ISAPS%20Results.pdf. Accessed 15 Feb 2016.

3. Kelly HA. Report of gynecological cases excessive growth of fat. Johns Hopkins Med J. 1899;10:197.
4. Thorek M. Plastic surgery of the breast and abdominal wall. Springfield, IL: Charles C Thomas; 1924.
5. Prudente A. Dermolipectomia abdominal comconservação da cicatriz umbilical. Buenos Aires: Anais II Cong Latino-Americano Cir Plast; 1943.
6. Regnault P. Abdominoplasty by the W technique. Plast Reconstr Surg. 1975;55:265–74.
7. Grazer FM. Abdominoplasty. Plast Reconstr Surg. 1973;51:617–23.
8. Pitanguy I. Abdominal lipectomy: an approach to it through an analysis of 300 consecutive cases. Plast Reconstr Surg. 1967;40:384.
9. Gonzalez-Ulloa M. Belt lipectomy. Br J Plast Surg. 1960;13:179–86.
10. Baroudi R, Keppke EM, Netto FT. Abdominoplasty. Plast Reconstr Surg. 1974;54:161–8.
11. Freeman BS, Wiemer DR. Abdominoplasty with special attention to construction of the umbilicus: technique and complications. Aesthetic Plast Surg. 1978;2(1):65–74.
12. Juri J, Juri C, Raiden G. Reconstruction of the umbilicus in abdominoplasty. Plast Reconstr Surg. 1979;63:580–2.
13. Delerm A. Refinements in abdominoplasty with emphasis in reimplantation of the umbilicus. Plast Reconstr Surg. 1982;70:632–7.
14. Choudhary S, Taams K. Umbilicosculpture: a concept revisited. Br J Plast Surg. 1998;51: 538–41.
15. Niranjan N, Staiano J. An anatomical method for re-siting the umbilicus. Plast Reconstr Surg. 2004;113:2194–8.
16. Avelar JM. Abdominoplasty: systematization of a technique without external umbilical scar. Aesthetic Plast Surg. 1978;2:141.
17. Massiha H, Montegut W, Phillips R. A method of reconstructing a natural-looking umbilicus in abdominoplasty. Ann Plast Surg. 1997;38(3):228–31.
18. Ramirez OM. Abdominoplasty and abdominal wall rehabilitation: a comprehensive approach. Plast Reconstr Surg. 2000;105(1):425–35.
19. Saldanha OR, Azevedo SF, Delboni PS, SaldanhaFilho OR, Saldanha CB, Uribe LH. Lipoabdominoplasty: the Saldanha technique. Clin Plast Surg. 2010;37(3):469–81.
20. Lee MJ, Mustoe TA. Simplified technique for creating a youthful umbilicus in abdominoplasty. Plast Reconstr Surg. 2002;109:2136.
21. Schoeller T, Wechselberger G, Otto A, Rainer C, Schwabegger A, Lille S, Ninković M. New technique for scarless umbilical reinsertion in abdominoplasty procedures. Plast Reconstr Surg. 1998;102:1720–3.
22. Pallua N, Markowicz M, Grosse F, Walter S. Aesthetically pleasant umbilicoplasty. Ann Plast Surg. 2010;64(6):722–5.
23. Visconti G, Salgarello M. The Divine Proportion "Ace of Spades" Umbilicoplasty: A New Method of Navel Positioning and Plasty in Abdominoplasty. Ann Plast Surg. 2016;76(3): 265–9.

Chapter 5
Relocating the Umbilicus in Abdominal Surgery

Andrew Michael Williams

5.1 Introduction

Individuals may require relocation of the umbilicus following surgery which has excised or repositioned the lower abdominal skin. The formation of a new umbilicus may be required due to excision of the native umbilicus or developmental absence of the umbilicus in conditions such as exomphalos major. In each of these scenarios, deciding on the correct location for the umbilicus is essential in achieving the optimum cosmetic result. Not only must the umbilicus be of an appropriate morphology and size, but it must also be accurately located according to fixed anatomical landmarks which help the surgeon define the correct position.

5.2 Technique

The position of the umbilicus depends upon both a craniocaudal and lateral coordinates, both of which must be accurately defined in order to maximise the aesthetic outcome. In the adult male and female patient, the midline can be found by a variety of techniques. The apex of the xiphisternum will usually run in a straight line to the centre of the symphysis pubis. In the erect patient, this will be a plumb line from the xiphisternum. This technique is best used when skin is excised or repositioned on the anterior abdomen as it uses independent, fixed reference points. Alternatively if the anterior abdominal skin has not been relocated, the symphysis pubis on the adult abdomen can be used to indicate the midline. This method relies upon the fine hair on the lower abdomen, pointing towards the midline and that in the midline,

A.M. Williams, M.A., M.B. BChir.
Department of Plastic, Reconstructive and Aesthetic Surgery Bradford Royal Infirmary, Duckworth Lane, Bradford BD9 6RJ, UK
e-mail: andrew.williams1@bthft.nhs.uk

M.A. Shiffman (ed.), *Adult Umbilical Reconstruction*,
DOI 10.1007/978-3-319-43887-0_5

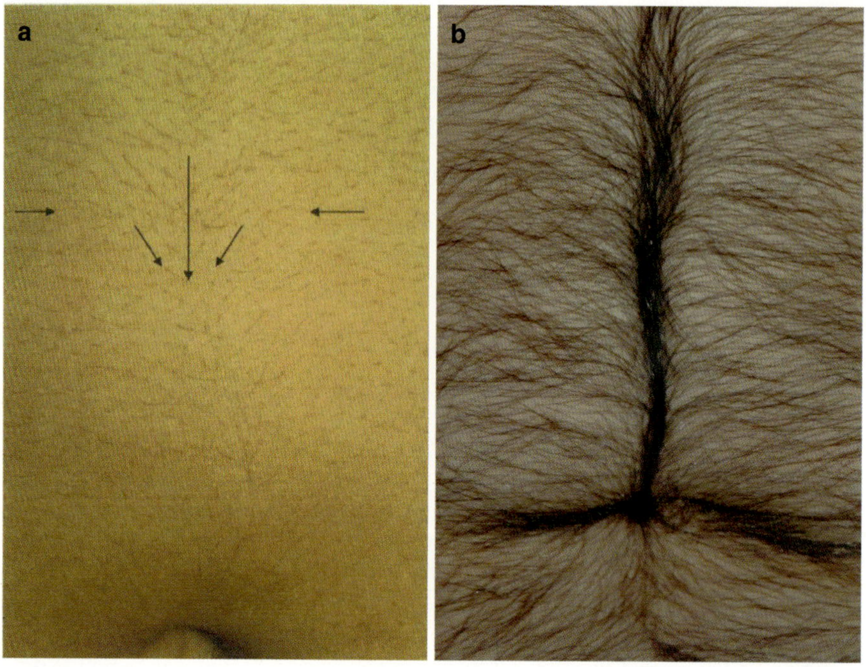

Fig. 5.1 (**a**) The position of the new umbilicus. (**b**) Can be estimated by following the direction of the fine lanugo hair which will point towards the site in the male and to a lesser extent the female patient

pointing in an inferior direction [1]. Both these methods can have their accuracy checked by measuring from bilateral fixed anatomical sites, such as the anterior superior iliac spines, with the new umbilical position lying half way between these sites (Fig. 5.1). The craniocaudal position is slightly harder to define. In the neonate with exomphalos major, who requires complete reconstruction of a neo-umbilicus and anterior abdominal wall, the position of the umbilical reconstruction is suggested as being 60 % of the way from the xiphisternum to the symphysis pubis [2]. This was determined by measuring the position of the umbilicus in fifty newborn babies with "normal"-appearing umbilical positions. Records have shown that it is easy to position the neo-umbilicus too cranially, at approximately 50 % of the distance between the xiphisternum and symphysis, as opposed to the two thirds rule which is suggested elsewhere [3]. This may result in an abnormal appearance. In the adult population, the position is harder still to define, often because of the differing abdominal dimensions and morphologies of the adult abdomen. In a slim individual, the position may be easier to define, at a location similar to the paediatric position, previously described. This may be at the level of the anterior superior iliac spines. In a more protuberant abdomen, the position may be less easy to define and may be further complicated in patients with massive weight loss who have a significant abdominal panniculus. The likelihood is, however, in this latter group that the need for repositioning of the umbilicus is due to the excision of the excess skin and the restoration of a flatter anterior abdominal wall. While the umbilical stalk in these circumstances often requires shortening, it too may act as a useful guide to the ideal position of the new umbilicus if it is brought forward perpendicular to the rectus sheath. Finally, it goes without saying that the ultimate goal of umbilical repositioning is patient satisfaction, and therefore, allowing the competent patient to be involved in deciding the final, new position of the umbilicus is essential in achieving the best aesthetic outcome and psychological outcome for the patient.

5.3 Conclusions

Locating the umbilicus in the midline using fixed, anatomical, midline structures or bisecting bilateral symmetrical structures and checking this using lanugo hair in the adult population is relatively straightforward. Measurable dimensions in the neonate (60–66 % of the way from the xiphisternum to symphysis pubis) and fixed anatomical structures in the adult (anterior superior iliac spine) may guide the craniocaudal position, but this may require more of a surgeon's skill in deciding the best position of the umbilicus, while being cognisant of the patient's opinion.

References

1. Williams AM, Platt AJ. Relocating the umbilicus in abdominal surgery. Plast Reconstr Surg. 2006;117(7):2528.
2. Williams AM, Brain JL. The normal position of the umbilicus in the newborn: an aid to improving the cosmetic result in exomphalos major. J Pediatr Surg. 2001;36(7):1045–6.
3. Lee SL, DuBois JJ, Greenholz SK, Huffman SG. Advancement flap umbilicoplasty after abdominal wall closure: postoperative results compared with normal umbilical anatomy. J Pediatr Surg. 2001;36(8):1168–70.

Chapter 6
The Average Size and Position of the Umbilicus in Young Men and Women

Deborah Yu, Wendy M. Novicoff, and Thomas J. Gampper

6.1 Introduction

In 2014, abdominoplasty ranked as the fourth most common cosmetic surgical procedure with 164,021 procedures performed that year [1]. The procedure has steadily risen in the ranks of most common aesthetic procedure performed [1]. The umbilicus is transposed within the abdominal skin flap as part of the abdominoplasty procedure. Despite the prevalence of this procedure, few publications address the size, shape, and location of the umbilicus.

In 1975, Baroudi [2] described a normal navel as having "a round, depressed scar, surrounded by a natural skin fold, measuring 1.5–2 cm in diameter." These characteristics were not based on any objective data taken from subjects. Baroudi remarked that the absence of an umbilicus is "distressing" and even "a deformed one" would affect the "self-image and psychologic balance of its carrier." He does not distinguish between men and women when making these statements.

Three years later, in 1978, Dubou and Ousterhout [3] published their study of the umbilicus placement of 100 randomly chosen, nonobese patients (no BMI reported), of whom 36% were male and 64% female, ranging from 18 to 69 years of age. The results were provided as means of the whole group and not separated according to subject gender. Dubou and Ousterhout reported that the horizontal level of 96% of their subjects' umbilicuses were at the height of the iliac crest, with the mean distance from the umbilicus to the xiphoid was 15.5 cm (range 11–20 cm) and from the umbi-

D. Yu, M.D. (✉) • T.J. Gampper
Department of Plastic and Maxillofacial Surgery, University of Virginia Health System, P.O. Box 800376, Charlottesville, VA 22908, USA
e-mail: drdeborahyu@gmail.com; tjg6f@hscmail.mcc.virginia.edu

W.M. Novicoff
Departments of Public Health Sciences and Orthopaedic Surgery, University of Virginia Health System, P.O. Box 800717 Health Sciences Center, Charlottesville, VA 22908, USA
e-mail: wmn2v@virginia.edu

M.A. Shiffman (ed.), *Adult Umbilical Reconstruction*,
DOI 10.1007/978-3-319-43887-0_6

licus to the pubis was 15.03 cm (range 10–18 cm). The mean position of the umbilicus in relation to the iliac crest was 0.1 cm below the iliac crest (range of 2.5 cm below to 2 cm above). No surgical or pregnancy histories were noted for the subjects.

More recently, in 2000, Craig et al. [4] described the "ideal" female umbilicus based on a panel's review of photographs. This group's results suggested that a small, T- or vertical-shaped umbilicus that had a superior hood or shelf was the most aesthetically appealing. No quantitative measurements were reported in their study.

The authors' group [5] recently published a study reporting the average size and position of the umbilicus in young men and women. The resulting data was to aid in umbilical transposition during abdominoplasty as well as any other abdominal wall reconstruction procedures.

6.2 Technique

A study to measure the average size and position of the umbilicus in young males and females was approved by the University of Virginia Institutional Review Board for Health Sciences Research (IRB HSR) [5]. Participants were screened prior to the study for exclusion criteria that could affect the size, shape, or location of the umbilicus: no history of scars on the abdomen (striae, operative scars, etc.), no history of pregnancy, and no weight loss of more than 10 pounds. Demographics (age, sex, race, height, and weight) were recorded. In addition to measurements for umbilical height, width, and overall shape, the following measurements were also taken to denote the position of the umbilicus in relation to existing landmarks: transverse distance of the umbilicus to the right and left iliac crests, umbilicus position relative to the iliac crest level (iliac crest was 0), umbilicus to xiphoid, and umbilicus to pubis. All measurements were taken by one of two investigators. All photographs were taken by one investigator.

A total of 80 subjects met the inclusion criteria, 43 females and 37 males [5]. The majority of subjects (72.5 %) were Caucasian. The remaining 22 subjects encompassed 3.8 % African Americans, 21.3 % Asians, and 2.5 % Hispanics. The mean age for all subjects was 22.4 years, and the mean BMI was 22.4 kg/m^2. The mean height of the umbilicus was 2.1 cm and the mean width was 2.3 cm. There were a variety of umbilical shapes recorded by the investigators, including crescent, round, triangular, and oval (vertical, transverse, or oblique).

The umbilicus was located at a mean of −0.7 cm in relation to the iliac crest (crest = 0) [5]. The mean distance from the right iliac crest to the umbilicus center for all subjects was 14.5 cm and from the left iliac crest to the umbilicus center was 14.4 cm. The mean distance from the superior edge of the umbilicus to the xiphoid was 17.5 cm. The mean distance from the inferior edge of umbilicus to the superior edge of the pubis was 13.9. The only measurements that had a significant correlation with body mass index (BMI) were the distances from the umbilicus center to the right and left iliac crests. No measurement was significantly correlated with age.

6.3 Young Men

In the study, the mean age of the male subjects was 22.5 years with a mean BMI of 23.0 kg/m^2 [5]. The mean height of the umbilicus in males was 2.1 cm and the mean width was 2.1 cm (Fig. 6.1). The umbilicus was located at a mean of 1.0 cm inferior to the iliac crest in males.

The mean distance from the right iliac crest to the umbilicus center was 15.1 cm, and the mean distance from the left iliac crest to the umbilicus center was 14.9 cm in males. The mean distance from the superior edge of the umbilicus to the xiphoid was 18.0 cm, and the mean distance from the inferior edge of umbilicus to the superior edge of the pubis was 14.1 cm (Fig. 6.2).

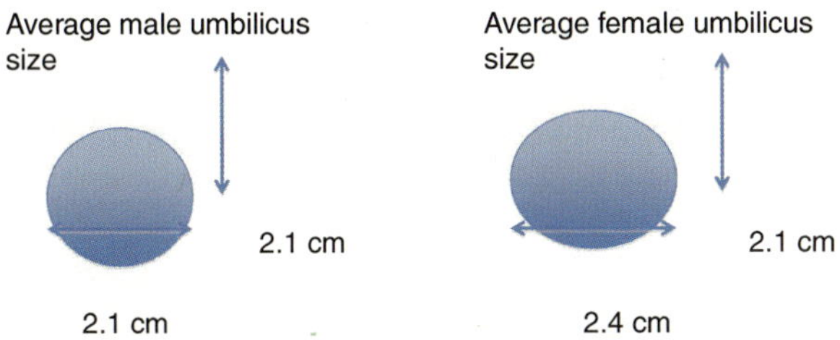

Fig. 6.1 The mean measurements of the umbilicus in young males and females

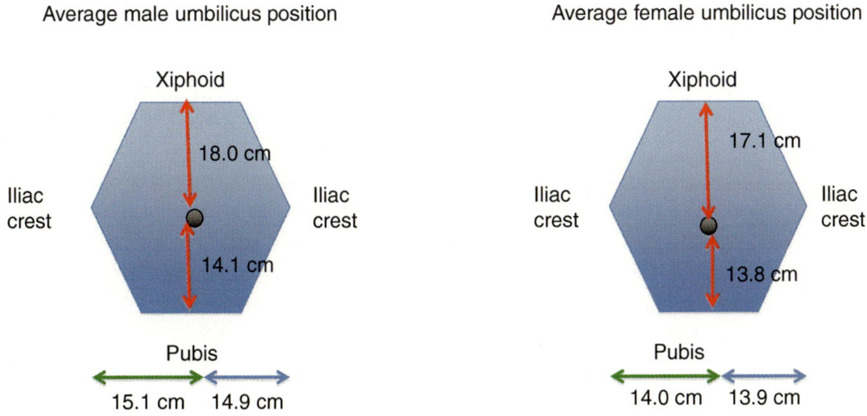

Fig. 6.2 The mean position of the umbilicus in young males and females with respect to right and left iliac crests, the xiphoid, and the pubis

6.4 Young Women

The mean age of the female subjects was 22.4 years with a mean BMI of 21.9 kg/m^2 [5]. The mean height of the umbilicus was 2.1 cm and the mean width of the umbilicus was 2.4 cm in females (Fig. 6.1). The umbilicus was located at a mean of 0.4 cm inferior to the iliac crest in females.

The mean distance from the right iliac crest to the umbilicus center was 14.0 cm, and the mean distance from the left iliac crest to the umbilicus center was 13.9 cm in females. The mean distance from the superior edge of the umbilicus to the xiphoid was 17.1 cm, and the mean distance from the inferior edge of umbilicus to the superior edge of the pubis was 13.8 cm in females (Fig. 6.2).

6.5 Comparison of the Two Genders

There was a significant difference in BMI between the genders with males having a slightly higher BMI for the authors' study group [5]. The measurements of statistically significant difference between the two genders were related to the umbilicus position: the distance above/below in relation to the iliac crest, the distance from the iliac crests to the umbilicus center, and the distance from the xiphoid to the superior aspect of the umbilicus.

6.6 Discussion

Prior reports of umbilical position were either subjective or nondiscriminatory with respect to age, weight, or previous pregnancy, surgery, and significant weight loss. The authors' previous study quantified the size and position of the umbilicus in young healthy subjects to serve as a reference because the goal of abdominoplasty is to restore youthful contours [5]. There were a variety of umbilical shapes encountered, including crescent, round, triangular, and oval (vertical, transverse, or oblique). The most common umbilical shape noted in the authors' study was a round shape in both males and females, with the oval shape being the second most common. This result was consistent with Baroudi's [2] previously described "normal" umbilicus shape as a "round, depressed scar." However, the mean height of the umbilicus in the authors' study was 2.1 cm and the mean width was 2.3 cm, which was consistent with a transverse oval shape [5]. Interestingly, in Craig et al.'s [4] study, neither the round or transverse oval shapes scored the highest in aesthetic appeal. The mean size of the umbilicus in the authors' study was consistent with previously described normal umbilicus by Baroudi [2].

The authors reported that the umbilicus was located at a mean of –0.7 cm in relation to the iliac crest (crest=0), which was similar to previous publications but slightly different from the prevailing school of thought of placement of the umbilicus at the iliac crest [3, 5]. The umbilicus was midline as the measurements from umbilicus center to right and left iliac crests were similar [5]. The umbilicus was closer to the pubis compared with the xiphoid in the authors' study [5]. The proximity to the pubis was also found by Dobou and Ousterhout, but the difference between the two mean measurements was smaller in their study (difference of only 0.25 cm in their study versus nearly 4 cm in the authors' study) [3, 5].

The authors' study was unique in that we separated the measurements according to gender and race, which had not been published previously [5]. There were several statistically significant measurements that differed between the two genders: the distance above/below in relation to the iliac crest, the distance from the iliac crests to the umbilicus center, and the distance from the xiphoid to the superior aspect of the umbilicus.

The authors concluded that the umbilicus is located more inferiorly in males compared with females and that on average the distance to the iliac crests is shorter in females, the latter of which is likely related to differing body types by gender, specifically the wider hips in females compared with males [5].

6.7 Conclusions

The authors found in the previous study that the mean height of the umbilicus in young men and women is very similar and the mean width slightly greater in women [5]. Young women have an umbilicus that is positioned more superiorly than young men. The umbilicus in both genders is typically found in the midline in relation to bilateral iliac crests and in the inferior half of the abdomen, closer to the pubis. The measurements on the average size and position of the umbilicus in young males and females can serve as a guide for umbilical reconstruction.

References

1. The American Society for Aesthetic Plastic Surgery Cosmetic Surgery National Data Bank Statistics 2014, Accessed 17 July 2015.
2. Baroudi R. Umbilicaplasty. Clin Plast Surg. 1975;2(3):431–48.
3. Dubou R, Ousterhout DK. Placement of the umbilicus in an abdominoplasty. Plast Reconstr Surg. 1978;61(2):291–3.
4. Craig SB, Faller MS, Pucket CL. In search of the ideal female umbilicus. Plast Reconstr Surg. 2000;105(1):389–92.
5. Yu D, Novicoff WM, Gampper TJ. The average size and position of the umbilicus in young men and women. Ann Plast Surg. 2016;76(3):346–8.

Chapter 7
Formula for Positioning the Umbilicus

Norbert Pallua

7.1 Introduction

Today a wide range of configurations exists. The goal is not only to preserve the umbilicus but also to create an aesthetically pleasant – maybe ideal – umbilicus.

During the course of decades the concept of umbilicoplasty was elaborated. The appearance of the three-dimensional umbilicus is influenced by:

1. Abdominal incision (height, width, shape)
2. Length of umbilical stalk
3. Diameter of the umbilical disk and shape
4. Periumbilical fat distribution

7.2 The Positioning of the New Umbilicus

During reinsertion of the umbilicus in abdominoplasties, special attention needs to be given to the aspects of localization. The umbilicus is an essential feature of the abdominal wall and is decisive for the contour and harmony of it.

To elaborate the perfect location, it is important to note that the height is subject to the force of gravity. The shape and height differ in standing versus lying position. In an upright position, the umbilicus has a small natural-looking superior hood and is slightly inferior tilted. This tilt and the contribution of the navel to the abdominal surface is a contribution to embryology. Based on Dick's [1] study, there are four fibrous cords attached to the umbilical base which represent remnants of the

N. Pallua, M.D., Ph.D.
Department for Plastic Surgery, Hand Surgery, Burn Center, University Hospital of the RWTH Aachen University, Pauwelsstr. 30, D-52074, Aachen, Germany
e-mail: npallua@ukaachen.de

M.A. Shiffman (ed.), *Adult Umbilical Reconstruction*,
DOI 10.1007/978-3-319-43887-0_7

obliterated umbilical vein, the urachus, and the two umbilical arteries' surface [2]. These cords apply traction from behind and create the inward and upward drag of the umbilical scar, with this the characteristic superior hood.

Based on this knowledge, it becomes obvious that the superior hood disappears in supine position, and the base of the umbilicus becomes visible. In an upside-down position, the navel develops an inferior hooding [3].

In young adults the umbilicus is flat and orientated vertical [4]. Aging and fat accumulation lead to enhanced hooding, a wide orifice of the navel, horizontal orientation, and deepening of the stalk [5]. The location also differs between genders [3].

7.2.1 Regarding the Height

In supine position anatomical texts describe the navel as the level of the disk between the third and fourth lumbar vertebrae, which is inapt in clinical practice [6]. Important for measuring the height and location of the umbilicus is defining the anthropometric points and their distance to the navel: xiphoid process, anterior superior iliac spine, iliac crest, pubic symphysis, and limit of the vulvar cleft.

Baroudi et al. [7] proclaimed the umbilicus as a 1.5–2 cm diameter measuring depressed scar, located in the midline at the level of the superior iliac crest. These data were not survey based. In 1978 Dubou and Ousterhout [8] published their results of 100 nonobese subjects. They found the umbilicus in 96 % (lying position) at the topmost level of the iliac crest, the approximate midpoint between xiphoid and pubis (15.5 cm versus 15.03 cm) in the midline.

The common assumption that the umbilicus is placed in the midline is also controversial. Rohrich's [9] findings suggest that an umbilical deviation of the midline is seen in nearly 100 % of all subjects and asymmetry is normal and therefore should be pointed out before performing abdominoplasty. In the 2010 published article, Pallua et al. [10] measured in supine position the distance between the anatomic landmarks of the trunk in photographs of 137 subjects and set in relation to the body mass index (BMI). By using a regression analysis, it was possible to predict the position of the umbilicus from the BMI (Table 7.1).

Table 7.1 Formula of the position of the umbilicus, referring to BMI. ASISR indicates anterior superior lilac spine right; ASISL: anterior superior lilac spine left [10]

Distance	Formula
Girth of the abdomen	$3.2 \times BMI + 10.04$
Distance ASISL – umbilicus	$0.54 \times BMI + 3.62$
Distance ASISR – umbilicus	$0.49 \times BMI + 4.72$
Distance ASISR – SAISL	$0.88 \times BMI + 8.4$

7.2.2 *Reinserting the Umbilicus*

Existing evidence demonstrates that marking the appropriate position preoperatively is not an ideal method because it can be erased by the time the umbilicus is brought out. Lanugo hair on the abdomen converges over the linea alba in the midline and may help to determine the right place of the umbilicus [11].

Some surgeons developed special devices for reinsertion of the umbilicus, like the umbilicus marker of Avelar [12], a kind of forceps whose lower part is placed on the umbilicus and the upper part on the abdominal flap. Avelar suggests reinserting the umbilicus in the abdominal wall 1 cm lower than its projection, taking account of an upward trend he observed in the follow-up.

In contrast Le Louarna and Pascal [13] advised elevating the site of the new umbilicus by inserting it 2–5 cm higher than the projection of the umbilicus stalk on the skin, as a key element of the high superior tension technique. Paraumbilical sutures were placed lateral to the umbilical stalk to the aponeurosis at 3 and 9 o'clock to improve tightening of epigastric skin and decrease tension in the hypogastrium.

7.2.3 *Umbilicus and the Golden Section*

Abhyankar's [2] study focused on the young (<30 years) female umbilicus of the Indian population. His findings suggested a 1.6:1 ratio between the distance of the xiphisternum and umbilicus and the distance between the umbilicus and the pubic symphysis (Fig. 7.1). Also, the ratio between umbilicus and the anterior superior iliac spine and distance between the right and left anterior superior iliac spine is 0.6:1. Therefore the ideal female umbilicus could be placed in the intersection of two arcs drawn with a radius 0.6 times that of the inter-anterior superior iliac spine distance. One year later Danilla [14] extended Abhyankar's [2] work by an equation to help the surgeon to "be more confident in where to perform umbilical reimplantation": $Xu = -2.32 + 0.91Xp - 0.07H$ (Xu = distance between xiphisternum and umbilicus, Xp = distance between xiphisternum and pubic symphysis, and H = height).

Interestingly multiple plastic surgeons find symmetry and ratios like the golden section (1.6:1) as a symbol for simplified beauty. Parnia in 2012 [15] applied the same principles as those of Danilla [14] to develop a similar equation and applied it to the Iranian female population. Visconti et al. [16] analyzed 81 top bikini models by the ratio of xiphoid-umbilicus distance to umbilicus-abdominal crease distance and concluded that the most attractive position is 1,618 in golden ratio. He suggested using a Fibonacci Caliper intraoperatively to locate the navel in abdominoplasty.

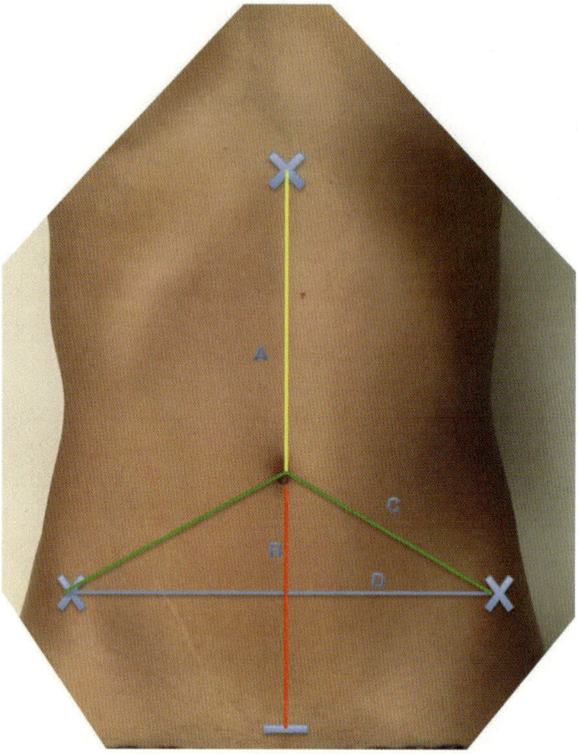

Fig. 7.1 Measurements for locating the umbilicus due to Abhyankar [2]. Golden section (1.6:1) should be present in the relation from distance A to B. (**a**) Distance between the xiphisternum and the umbilicus. (**b**) Distance between the umbilicus and the pubic symphysis. (**c**) Distance between the anterior superior iliac spine and the umbilicus. (**d**) Inter-anterior superior iliac spine distance

7.2.4 Gender Specifics of Localization

In 2015 Dudukovic et al. [17] investigated 98 Croatian women and men between 18 and 49 years in supine position and found differences for male to female and young to middle-aged women. They developed two different regressive equations for exact umbilical localization. In women the best prediction of position was based on the distance from the inter-anterior hypochondrium line to the umbilicus. In men the interspinous line distance to the umbilicus was most reliable. With their complex formula for navel positioning, still a margin of error up to 2.51 cm for women and 1.7 cm for men is measurable. Throughout our research of literature, the male umbilicus is commonly located slightly lower on the abdominal wall than the female [18].

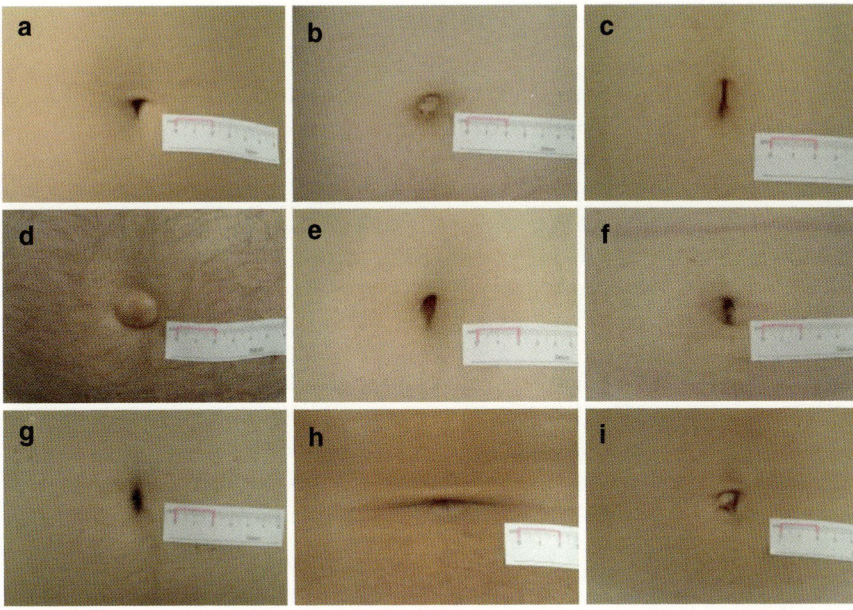

Fig. 7.2 Possible navel shapes: (**a**) T shaped, (**b**)round shaped, (**c**) vertical shaped, (**d**) outie, (**e**) oval with superior hooding, (**f**) oval with inferior hooding, (**g**) oval shaped, (**h**) horizontally shaped, (**i**) distorted shaped navel

7.3 The Ideal Shape

As mentioned above the young and female umbilicus is generally flat, vertically orientated, with a small hood, and slightly inferior tilted. After childbirth a transverse orientation occurs. Sakamoto analyzed Japanese navels from childhood to adolescence and confirmed changing in shape and lengthening of the stalk during growing [19]. Weight gain contributes to a deeper umbilical stalk a widened appearance. Shapes can vary: T-shape, vertical, horizontal, oval, round, protrusion ("outie") (Fig. 7.2). Extremes like a pronounced deep and wide or an exceedingly tiny umbilicus are commonly seen as unappealing. A so-called outie presents like a protuberant mass of subcutaneous scar that fills the normal tube [20]. This protuberance is regarded as a normal variation of umbilical shape and has to be distinguished from an umbilical hernia with a defect of fascia. Outies are mostly considered unattractive in literature [7, 20]. There are ethological differences seen in the distribution of outies and innies.

A prospective observation study on Nigerian children found prevalence of 92 % outies and 49 % for the adult population [21]. Here in contrast the "innie" is the unusual variation.

7.3.1 *Gender Differences in Shape*

Craig et al. [4] studied the shape in 2000 by photographic analyses of 147 Caucasian women, scored by a predominantly male panel. He proclaimed the T-shaped umbilicus as the most attractive form and also as the most frequent one (37 %). A protrusion was seen in 10 % of the studied objects and was rated unappealing. In 2008 Cavale and Butler [22] assessed an online voting for the ideal umbilicus. Both men and women overwhelmingly preferred the oval-shaped and superior hooded navel.

Pallua et al. [10] revealed in their study that the most aesthetically pleasing shape was oval in 60 % for male and 45 % for female patients. The naturally occurring shape differed significantly between the genders. Women showed most frequently a vertical shape (43 %), followed by the T-shape, whereas the oval and vertical shape (both 39 %) dominated the male navel shape. In contrast Freeman and Wiener [23] found no differences between the male and female navel.

Noteworthy is that most literature is focused on the female navel. An explanation is delivered by Iranmanesh et al.'s [24] online survey to the importance of the umbilicus. The majority of women considered their umbilicus "important" or "extremely important" in their overall physical appearance, but only 29 % of the men were concerned. The results were reversed regarding the partner's umbilicus: only 25 % of the women considered their partners umbilicus as "important" or "extremely important" versus 45 % of the men. 35 % of the men voted the umbilicus as sexually important in contrast to only 19 % of the women. Our own study confirmed that females are more critical to their navel than males [10].

Coherent to this tradition, Visconti et al. [16] surveyed bikini models via facebook.com. This analysis revealed that 82 % rated the oval/vertical shape with a superior hooding as aesthetically pleasant. Lee et al. [25] examined images of 37 Playboy models ("Playmates"), presumed to be beautiful, and concluded that the ideal umbilicus is oval shaped, centered horizontally, with either no hooding or a superior hooding and its length is 5 % of the length of the xiphoid.

The *width and length* of the median natural umbilicus differs in literature. In the Pallua et al.'s [10] study, the male height was 1.12 cm versus female 1.05 cm. Width for male participants was 0.92 cm and for female 0.66 cm. Yu et al.'s [18] findings suggest a height of 2.1 cm and width of 2.3 cm without gender differences in width or shape.

A deep and elongated stalk bares functional problems, like difficulties in daily personal hygiene beneath aesthetical deficits. The length of the umbilical stalk should therefore be adjusted to the diameter of the abdominal wall to reduce the risk of troublesome cavity.

7.3.2 *The Tilting Angle*

The aesthetic pleasant umbilicus should have a slightly inferior inclination [12]. There are different possibilities to recreate this tilt during umbilicoplasty:

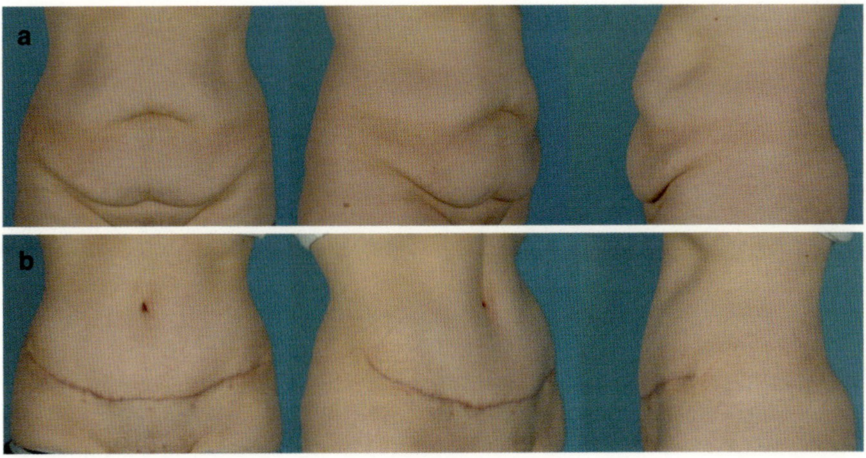

Fig. 7.3 (**a** *Top*) 34-year-old female, primipara, suffering from diastasis recti in the upper abdomen. (**b**) Two months postoperative following lipoabdominoplasty with modified tension technique. The scars are still immature. Note the nice slope in the upper abdomen in the middle (oblique). The umbilicus has the inverted V-shape

1. Forming of the umbilical disk.
2. Liposculpturing the surrounding subcutaneous fat by resection just fat superior to the navel [10].
3. Suturing of the umbilical stalk to the fascia: fixation exclusively the upper pole to the fascia will create a feminine curve infraumbilical [10].

The tilting angle gives a curvature to the supra- and infraumbilical area. Attractive feminine abdomens are more curved, whereas a straight well-trained abdomen is a masculine feature. These requirements can easily be met by fixation points of the umbilicus to the rectus fascia. By liposculpturing, the abdominal wall can be contoured as a slope to the navel. These little hints create easily a tremendous effect and customize your abdominoplasty (Fig. 7.3).

Including the findings in literature and my experience, the beautiful feminine navel is oval to vertical, 1 cm in height, and has a slight inferior tilt (depending on the individual preference and condition). Striving for reconstruction of an aesthetically pleasant navel has a high level of gratitude and patient satisfaction.

7.4 Neoumbilicoplasty

The above-discussed themes involve umbilicoplasty, where the umbilicus remains anchored to the abdominal fascia. In difference, neoumbilicoplasty intends to create an umbilicus de novo in the absence of it due to various reasons. These reasons can be iatrogenic (necrosis after abdominoplasty or after abdominal surgery), tumor, infections, or extended hernias.

A missing navel corresponds to the variety of techniques for re-creation. Umbilico-neoplasty can be performed as purse-string sutures, flaps, and grafts. Determining factors for the choice of technique are:

1. Condition and availability of surrounding tissue
2. Vascularization
3. Scarring of the abdominal wall

7.4.1 Sutures

McMillan [26] reported the first restoration of the navel after hernia repair in 1955. A very simple and effective technique was published by Kirianoff in 1978 [27]. He performed a Y-shaped incision of the abdominal wall in a radius of 2.5 cm, undermined the two lateral flaps, resected the subcutaneous fat to the rectus fascia, and sutured the flaps to the fascia.

A combination of *purse-string suture* and wound *healing by secondary intention* was performed by Bartsich and Schwarz [28] for urachal cyst repair. They placed tracking sutures from the dermis of the abdominal wall defect to the marked umbilical area and tightened the defect with a purse-string suture until the desired umbilical size. The floor of the umbilicus needed secondary wound healing. The disadvantage of purse-string sutures might be a circular scar contraction.

7.4.2 Flaps

Numerous techniques for reconstruction with flaps have been reported. These techniques can be divided into methods for delayed repair, with an intact abdominal surface and methods for immediate reconstruction with an acute defect and missing umbilicus.

7.4.3 Delayed Reconstruction

In case of *delayed repair*, pedicled flaps can partially include the cicatrized area with the advantage of low donor-side morbidity. In 1998 Yotsuyanagi [29] published his technique for vertical scars. The *pedicle flap* was based in the center of the scar as the new bottom, and a cranial and a longer caudal flap were harvested and twisted around each other to create a depression. In their article Itoh and Arai [30] published two methods with island flaps (Fig. 7.4). They formed a triangular flap or alternatively a rhomboid flap into a *cone-shaped* neoumbilicus, leaving a vertical-shaped upper incision for the triangular or a vertical and horizontal incision on the abdominal wall for the rhomboid flap. Sugawara et al. [31]

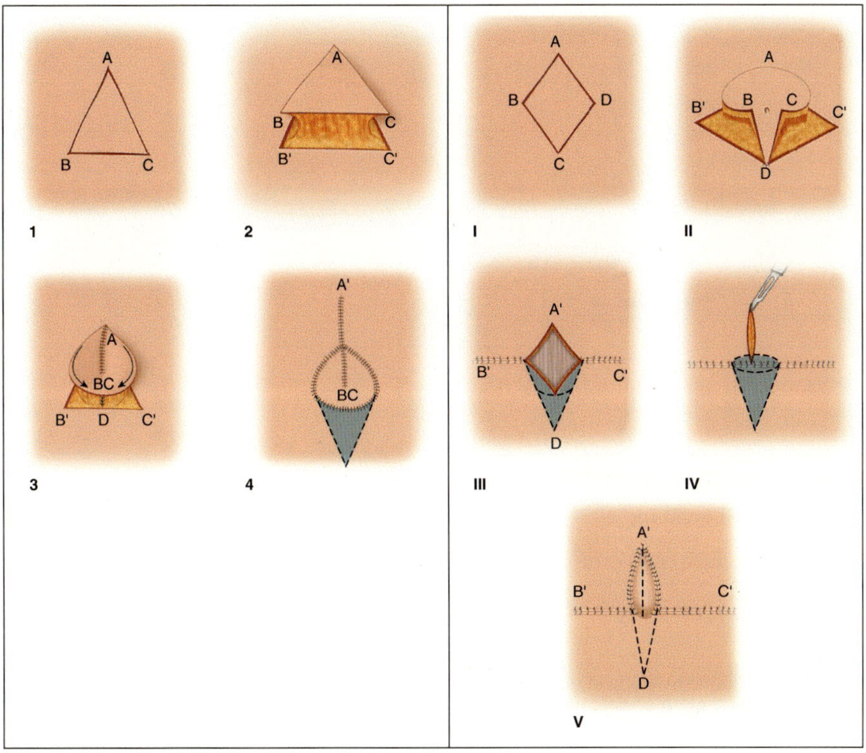

Fig. 7.4 Two neoumbilicoplasty methods by Itoh and Arai [32]. (*Left*) 1. A triangle flap is designed, the apex is pointing in cranially. 2. The subcutaneous fat is preserved below the flap. 3. The conical form is created by connecting points B and C. 4. D is now the apex of the cone and sutured with the BC line. 4. Point D is sutured to the fascia. The skin is closed. (*Right*) I. A rhombic flap is designed. II. Preparation separates the surrounding tissue from the flap. B and C are sutured together. Point D is defatted and sutured to the fascia. III. The donor side is closed above the newly created umbilicus. IV. Cranially a new skin incision is performed and the umbilicus is inserted, placing point a in the upper edge of the skin incision. V. Closure

reconstructed an umbilicus in vertical scars (laparotomy scars) using a superior-based *single triangular flap*, suturing the edges to form a cone. He advised to insert the new molded umbilical bottom down or between the rectus muscles.

Other surgeons refused to rely on the unpredictable vascularization from the deeper abdominal wall (as pedicled flap) and used *skin from the abdominal wall* to create a neoumbilicus. Such a single flap reconstruction from the abdominal wall was described by Pfulg et al. [32]. For vertical laparotomy scars, he designed a triangular skin flap (4×7×6 cm!) within a relatively extended vertical elliptical skin excision. The triangular flap was inverted conically and attached to the fascia. This technique demands extended vertical skin incisions (Fig. 7.5).

Also Barbosa et al. [33] used a single C-flap to correct a vertical scar. He and many others pointed out the importance of postoperative care by placing a spacer (like sterile antibacterial gauze or silicone tubes) to restore a long-term result and prevent scar contracture.

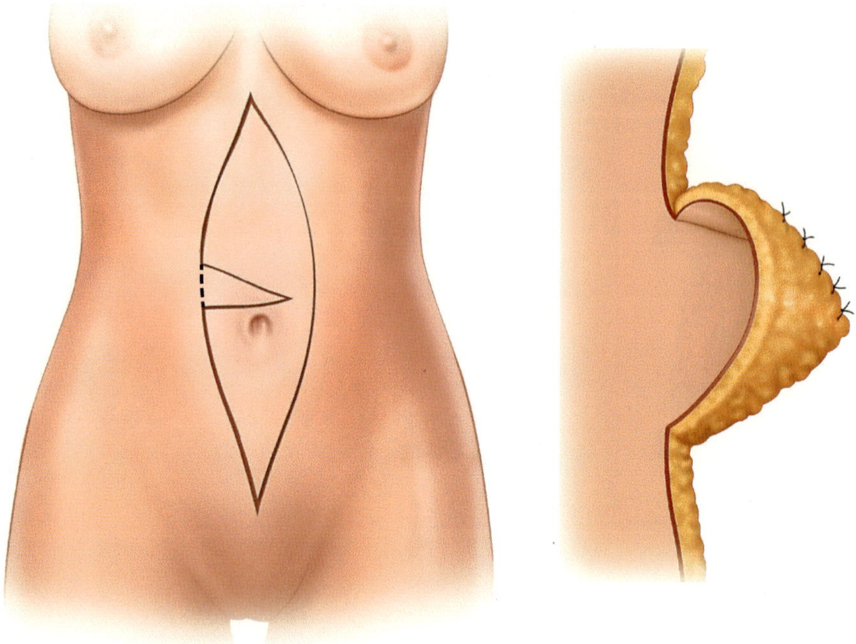

Fig. 7.5 Technique by Pfulg et al. [32] for vertical laparotomy scars. (*Left*) Blue is resection area; black is incision for the large triangular skin flap. (*Right*) The flap was inverted conically and attached to the fascia

7.4.4 Immediate Reconstruction

For immediate reconstruction Hazani et al. [34] used an inferior-based *semicircular/croissant-shaped flap*, transposed the tip to the fascia, and combined it with a *full-thickness skin graft* to create a superior hood (Fig. 7.6). Shrinking might be a potential shortcoming of skin grafts. Therefore they should not use circular. Techniques with two flaps often follow the V to Y pattern. Jamra [35] published his technique for immediate reconstruction in 1979, by defatting two V-shaped flaps, sutured the edges together and to the fascia below, and closed the edges in V-Y pattern. Baack et al. [36] used one inferior- and one superior-based flap and advanced them into a defatted central cylinder to reconstruct a depression and walls (Fig. 7.7).

Accelerating the complexity, *four-flap* techniques have been published, like the "Celtic cross" by De La Cruz et al. [37] for immediate reconstruction (Fig. 7.8). Flaps are harvested vertically and horizontally to the central defect, and the dermis of each flap is sutured toward the center of the underlying muscular fascia. The "iris technique" used the principle of rotation and advancement to minimize the scar size [38].

The "Maltese cross" by Rogliani et al. [39] created four cross-shaped flaps in a circle with circumscribed areas of deepithelialization and normal skin, which are sutured among one other and to the rectus fascia in a specific manner. This complex technique may have a disadvantage by creating a constricted imprint in the margin.

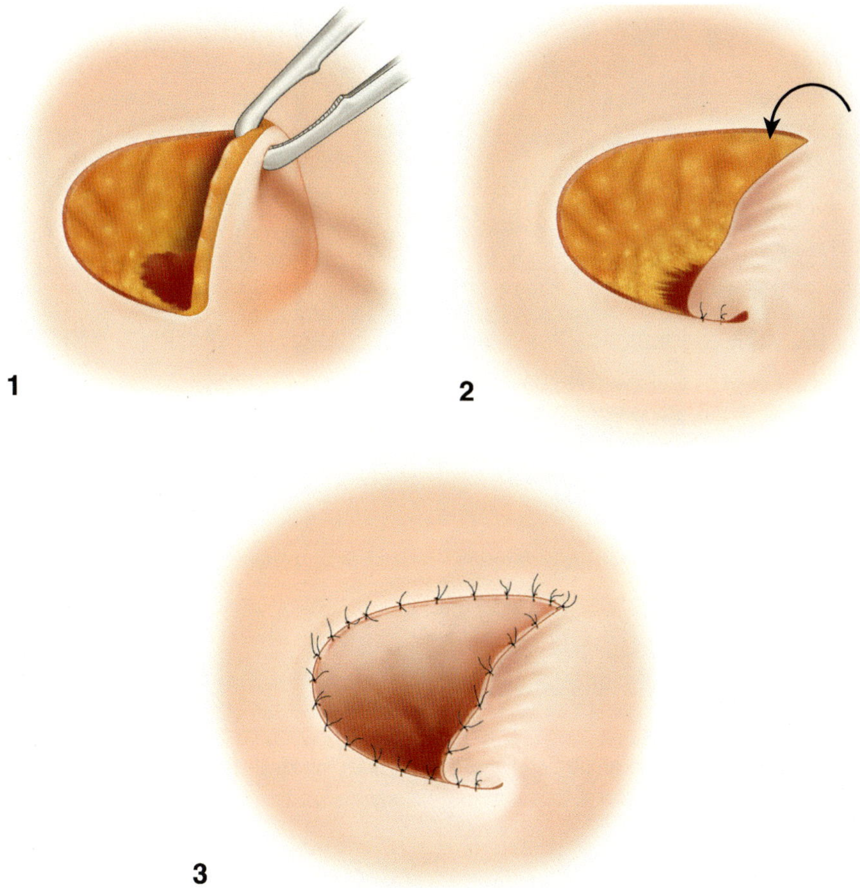

Fig. 7.6 Neoumbilicoplasty by Hazani [34]. (*Top left*) Harvesting of an inferior-based semicircular flap. (*Bottom left*) The flap is sutured to the rectus fascia. (*Right*) Suturing the full-thickness skin graft to the wound margin and bottom

7.5 Conclusions

1. Through the course of history, the aesthetic importance of the umbilicus increased. Nowadays a variety of techniques for reinsertion of the umbilicus are in use. They all intend to hide the scar, prevent umbilical stenosis due to scar contracture, and create an idealized umbilicus.
2. A circular scar after navel reinsertion is indicated as one of the most obvious signs for undergoing a tummy tuck.
3. We prefer the inverted V-technique with periumbilical defatting to create a natural superior hooding and no visible scar for the down looking patient.

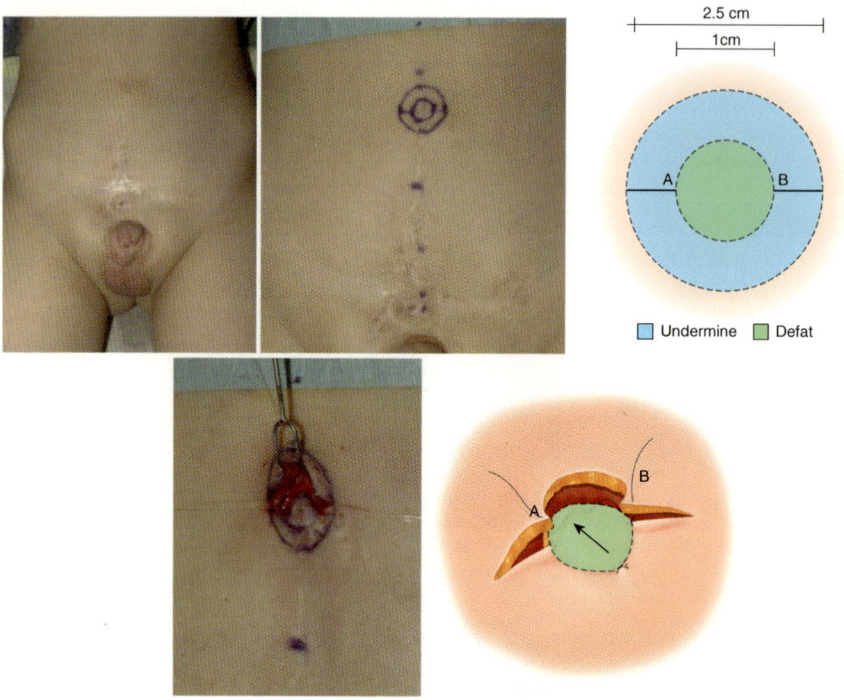

Fig. 7.7 Neoumbilicoplasty technique of Baak et al. [36]. (*Top Left*) Intraoperative 6-year-old boy with status after bladder exstrophy. (*Top middle*, *top right*) Marking. (*Bottom left*) Making flaps. (*Bottom right*) Closure

4. The appearance of the three-dimensional umbilicus is influenced by abdominal incision (height, width, shape), length of umbilical stalk, diameter of the umbilical disk and shape, and the periumbilical fat distribution.
5. The position and shape of the umbilicus differs due to gravity (lying vs standing position).
6. In supine position the navel is mostly located at the topmost level of the iliac crest.
7. The ideal female umbilicus is flat, vertically orientated, and with a small hood and a slightly inferior tilt.
8. The diversity of techniques for neoumbilicoplasty resembles the variety of problems a surgeon is faced within reoperations. Methods range from simple sutures and healing by secondary intent, above local skin flaps to extended excisions and abdominal flaps.
9. Decision-making requires a differentiated analysis of the abdominal conditions including the patient's general habits, conditions, and wishes.
10. Fundamental for successful umbilicoplasty is the above-acquired knowledge of the ideal umbilicus, its location, size, shape, and gender differences.

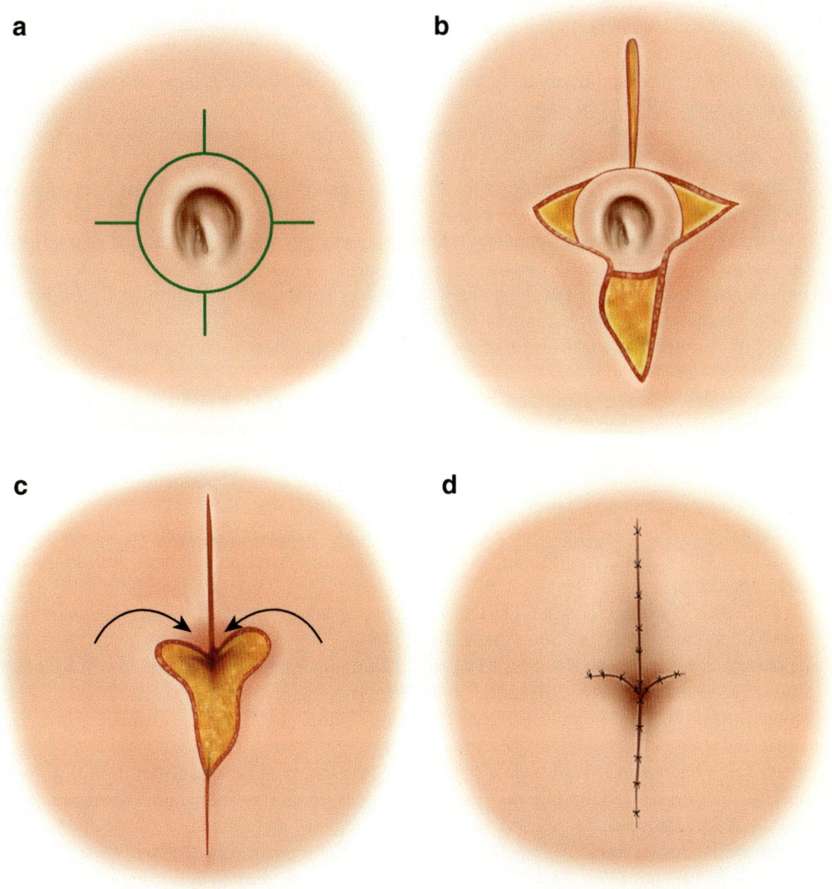

Fig. 7.8 The Celtic cross by De la Cruz [37]. (**a**) Plan for placing the skin incision around a central defect or scar. (**b**) Completed incisions and the central defect is excised and the flaps undermined. (**c**) The upper flaps are fixed to the fascia. (**d**) After suturing

References

1. Dick ET. Umbilicoplasty as a treatment for persistent umbilical infection. Austr N Z J Surg. 1970;39:380–3.
2. Abhyankar SV. Anatomical localization of the umbilicus: an Indian study. Plast Reconstr Surg. 2006;117:1153–7.
3. Choudhary S, Taams K. Umbilicosculpture: a concept revisited. Br J Plast Surg. 1998;51:538–41.
4. Craig SB, Faller MS, Puckett L. In search of the ideal female umbilicus. Plast Reconstr Surg. 2000;105:389–92.
5. Lee MJ, Mustoe TA. Simplified technique for creating a youthful umbilicus in abdominoplasty. Plast Reconstr Surg. 2002;109:2136–40.
6. Gray H. Gray's anatomy of the human body. New York: Grammercy Books; 1977.

7. Baroudi R, Keppke EM, Netto FT. Abdominoplasty. Plast Reconstr Surg. 1974;54:161–8.
8. Dubou R, Ousterhout D. Placement of the umbilicus in an abdominoplasty. Plast Reconstr Surg. 1978;61:291–3.
9. Rohrich RJ. Is the umbilicus truly midline? Clinical and medico legal implications. Plast Reconstr Surg. 2003;112:259–60.
10. Pallua N, Markowicz M, Grosse F, Walter S. Aesthetically pleasant umbilicoplasty. Ann Plast Surg. 2010;64(6):722–5.
11. Williams AM, Platt AJ. Relocating the umbilicus in abdominal surgery. Plast Reconstr Surg. 2006;117:2528.
12. Avelar JM. Abdominoplasty: technical refinement and analysis of 130 cases in 8 years' follow-up. Aesthetic Plast Surg. 1983;7:205–12.
13. Le Louarn C, Pascal JF. The high-superior-tension technique: evolution of lipoabdominoplasty. Aesthetic Plast Surg. 2010;34(6):773–81.
14. Danilla S. Anatomical localization of the umbilicus: a statistical analysis. Plast Reconstr Surg. 2007;119:1123–4.
15. Parnia R. Determining anatomical position of the umbilicus in Iranian girls, and providing quantitative indices and formula to determine neo-umbilicus during abdominoplasty. Indian J Plast Surg. 2012;45:94–6.
16. Visconti G, Visconti E, Bonomo L, Salgarello M. Concepts in navel aesthetic: a comprehensive surface anatomy analysis. Aesthetic Plast Surg. 2015;39(1):43–50.
17. Dudukovic M, Kisic H, Baez ML, Bulic K, Veir Z, Cvjeticanin B, Mijatovic D. Anatomical prediction for surgical positioning of the umbilicus in a white population. Ann Plast Surg. 2015;75:135–9.
18. Yu D, Novicoff WM, Gampper TJ. The average size and position of the umbilicus in young men and women. Ann Plast Surg. 2016;76(3):346–8.
19. Sakamoto Y, Kamagata S, Hirobe S, Hayashi A. Umbilical shape by age and growth: a Japanese study. Plast Reconstr Surg. 2010;126(2):97e–8e.
20. Hodgkinson DJ. Umbilicoplasty: conversion of "outie" to "innie". Aesthetic Plast Surg. 1983;7:221–2.
21. Meier DE, OlaOlorun DA, Omodele RA, Nkor SK, Tarpley JL. Incidence of umbilical hernia in African children: redefinition of "normal" and reevaluation of indications for repair. World J Surg. 2001;25(5):645–8.
22. Cavale N, Butler P. The ideal female umbilicus? Plast Reconstr Surg. 2008;121(5):356e–7e.
23. Freeman BS, Wiemer DR. Abdominoplasty with special attention to construction of the umbilicus: technique and complications. Aesthetic Plast Surg. 1978;2(1):65–74.
24. Iranmanesh P, Morel P, Inan I, Hagen M. Choosing the cosmetically superior laparoscopic access to the abdomen: the importance of the umbilicus. Surg Endosc. 2012;5(8):2578–85.
25. Lee SJ, Garg S, Lee HP. Computer-aided analysis of the "beautiful" umbilicus. Aesthet Surg J. 2014;34(5):748–56.
26. McMillan W. Surgery of umbilical hernia with reconstruction of an artificial umbilicus. Q Bull Northwest Univ Med Sch. 1955;29(4):379–82.
27. Kirianoff TG. Making a new umbilicus when none exists. Plast Reconstr Surg. 1978;61:603–4.
28. Bartsich SA, Schwartz MH. Purse-string method for immediate umbilical reconstruction. Plast Reconstr Surg. 2003;112:1652–5.
29. Yotsuyanagi T, Nihei Y, Sawada Y. A simple technique for reconstruction of the umbilicus, using two twisted flaps. Plast Reconstr Surg. 1998;102:2444–6.
30. Itoh Y, Arai K. Umbilical reconstruction using a cone-shaped flap. Ann Plast Surg. 1992;28:335–8.
31. Sugawara Y, Hirabayashi S, Asato H, Yoshimura K. Reconstruction of the umbilicus using a single triangular flap. Ann Plast Surg. 1995;34:78–80.
32. Pfulg M, Van de Sijpe K, Blondeel P. A simple new technique for neo-umbilicoplasty. Br J Plast Surg. 2005;58:688–91.
33. Barbosa MVJ, Hahas FX, Neto MAS. Strategies in umbilical reconstruction. J Plast Reconstr Aesthet Surg. 2009;62:147–50.

34. Hazani R, Israeli R, Feingold RS. Reconstructing a natural looking umbilicus: a new technique. Ann Plast Surg. 2009;63(4):358–60.
35. Jamra FA. Reconstruction of the umbilicus by a double V – Y procedure. Plast Reconstr Surg. 1979;64(1):106–7.
36. Baack BR, Anson G, Nachbar JM. Umbilicoplasty: the construction of a new umbilicus and the correction of umbilical stenosis without external scars. Plast Reconstr Surg. 1996;97:227–32.
37. De La Cruz EA, Jaber RK, Tabuenca AD, Joe VC. The 'Celtic cross' technique for immediate umbilical reconstruction post-laparotomy and surgical ablation of the umbilicus. J Plast Reconstr Aesthet Surg. 2009;62(2):258–61.
38. Miller MJ, Balch CM. "Iris" technique for immediate umbilical reconstruction. Plast Reconstr Surg. 1993;92(4):754–6.
39. Rogliani M, Silvi E, Arpino A. The Maltese cross technique: umbilical reconstruction after dermolipectomy. J Plast Reconstr Aesthet Surg. 2007;60:1036–8.

Chapter 8
Quantitative Indices and Formula for Localizing the Neo-umbilicus During Abdominoplasty

Nariman Sepehrvand and Sanaz Hatami

8.1 Introduction

Umbilicus is an abdominal structure which is connected to the linea alba by the umbilical stalk [1]. It has been consisted of four fibrous cords which are the remnants of an obliterated umbilical vein, the urachus, and two umbilical arteries [2]. Before the 1950s, it was the norm to sacrifice the umbilicus during an abdominoplasty surgery [3]. In last several decades however, surgeons and researchers made tremendous efforts to find the best way to preserve the umbilicus and its natural look during the surgery, since its presence was perceived to be essential for the aesthetic appearance of the abdomen.

There are several aesthetic considerations for umbilicoplasty including position, depth, shape of the neo-umbilicus, and location of the scar [4]. An aesthetically pleasing umbilicus was described to be small (1.5–2 cm in diameter), oval shaped, depressed, vertically oriented with no hooding, or superiorly hooded [5–7]. The smooth transition from the abdominal wall to the umbilicus through a periumbilical concavity or skinfold is another essential commodity to the aesthetically pleasing appearance of the umbilicus [8]. Its appearance usually changes with factors like gravity, aging, weight gaining, pregnancy, hernia,

N. Sepehrvand, M.D. (✉)
Department of Medicine, University of Alberta, Edmonton, AB, Canada

2-132 Li Ka Shing Centre for Health Research Innovation, University of Alberta, Edmonton, AB, Canada, T6G 2E1
e-mail: sepehrva@ualberta.ca

S. Hatami, M.D.
Department of Surgery, University of Alberta, Edmonton, AB, Canada

4-050 Li Ka Shing Centre for Health Research Innovation, University of Alberta, Edmonton, AB, Canada, T6G 2E1
e-mail: hatami@ualberta.ca

M.A. Shiffman (ed.), *Adult Umbilical Reconstruction*,
DOI 10.1007/978-3-319-43887-0_8

severe abdominal trauma, etc. [9]. It's been reported to be flat and vertically oriented in young and thin individuals, whereas in old and obese patients, it is rounded and transversely oriented [10]. The measures that can be taken to have the most aesthetically pleasing shape for neo-umbilicus have been addressed extensively in other chapters.

Location of the neo-umbilicus is important since a misplaced umbilicus can draw undue attention and consequently may impose undue psychological distress [4]. Patients who are unsatisfied with the postoperative position of their umbilicus, aside from tolerating the emotional toll of an unsatisfactory outcome and/or extra expenses and discomfort of having a corrective procedure, may sue the surgeon [11, 12]. Hence, the surgeons require evidence-based methods to guide them during the surgery for localizing the neo-umbilicus and to let them defend against potential allegations. The traditional approach for determining the proper location for neo-umbilicus was to mark the new umbilical position by palpation under the abdominal flap during abdominoplasty which was tedious and also was subject to errors and were likely to be erased during the process of surgery. For that reason, investigators have conducted several studies to find expeditious and quick but at the same time safe and evidence-based methods for determining the proper location for the neo-umbilicus during surgery.

The aim of this chapter is to describe the natural location of the umbilicus on horizontal and vertical planes of the anterior abdominal wall and to summarize the efforts that have been made so far for developing a mathematical formula for determining the proper and aesthetically pleasing location of the neo-umbilicus during abdominal reconstructive surgeries. The information provided in this chapter could be helpful not only for determining the location of neo-umbilicus during abdominoplasty but also for appraising the position of the umbilicus and the abdominal contour after abdominoplasty to help us to identify the cases that may need a revision abdominoplasty.

8.2 Does Umbilical Position Really Change with Abdominoplasty?

In aesthetic and reconstructive surgeries of the anterior abdominal wall, the position and shape of the umbilicus usually changes. Chin et al. [13] showed a significant net reduction in trunk's circumferential and vertical dimensions. They concluded that the umbilicus displaced cephalically post-abdominoplasty. In cases that the patient is not satisfied with the ultimate postoperative look of the abdomen and in the lack of evidences showing the appropriate place of a normal umbilicus, the abovementioned changes may open up the surgeons to the allegations of medical malpractice [12].

8.3 Position of the Umbilicus on Horizontal Plane

The anatomy textbooks as well as the majority of literature claimed that the umbilicus is located anatomically at the midline [4, 7, 12]. Rohrich et al. [14], however, have conducted two studies and suggested that the umbilicus is not necessarily located in the midline. Based on their report, the umbilicus was more than 2 % away from the midline for more than 50 % of their subjects (136 subjects in total) and was truly at the midline in only 1.7 % of their study population. Although the slight asymmetry, like 2 % deviation from the midline, is not that significant to endanger the pleasing postoperative appearance of the abdomen, these issues should be discussed with patients as a part of patients' preoperative education and informed consent process to prevent unrealistic expectations on the patient side. It should be noted that their study has a limitation which is using the photographic measurements in majority of subjects (116 subjects) and direct measurements only in a very small group (20 subjects).

8.4 Position of the Umbilicus on Vertical Plane

Umbilicus has been suggested to be located at the level of fibrocartilage between the third and fourth lumbar vertebrae when the patient is in supine position [2, 10, 15, 16]. Dobou and Ousterhout [10] studied 100 randomly selected healthy subjects and described the umbilicus to be located at the topmost level of the iliac crest for majority of subjects regardless of their sex, age, or race. Hinderer [17] reported the umbilicus to be located 3 cm above the level of the anterior iliac crest.

Umbilicus is demonstrated to be low riding in almost all of the available studies and reported to be high riding only in a few. In the study of Lee et al. [7], the vertical ratio between above umbilicus and below umbilicus portions was reported to be 46:54. However it should be noted that they used the lower limit of the vulvar cleft instead of the pubic symphysis as the lower landmark for their abdominal length measurements. As a sensitivity analysis, when measured the distance from umbilicus to the top of the vulvar cleft, they found the vertical position of the umbilicus to be at center or slightly above the center, in consistence with other studies.

Rodriguez-Feliz et al. [18] have assessed the umbilicopubic distance (distance between mid-umbilical stalk and the pubic symphysis) intraoperatively in a group of patients who underwent abdominoplasty or panniculectomy and showed the intraoperative umbilicopubic distance to be almost 15 cm in patients with a stature of 145–178 cm. This was similar to the findings of previous studies that measured it in healthy subjects over the abdominal skin [4, 10, 12, 19, 20]. However they also showed an increase in the umbilicopubic distance with increase in patient's height [18].

8.5 Fixed Boney Points Versus Soft Tissue Landmarks

Majority of studies have used the boney points like the xiphoid process or anterior superior iliac spine for their measurements. One of the landmark points that was widely used throughout the studies was pubic symphysis. Some studies questioned the use of pubic symphysis, with alluding to that it reflects an almost wide region rather than a single point. It should be noted that when talking about pubic symphysis in these studies, it actually denotes the midpoint of the upper border of the pubic symphysis.

Few studies have used the soft tissue points as their landmarks for anthropometric measurements [7, 13]. In the study of Lee et al. [7], they used the images of the Playboy centerfold models to delineate the position and shape parameters of an aesthetically pleasing umbilicus. In that study, the abdomen length was defined as the distance between the xiphoid process and the lower limit of the vulvar cleft. The authors admitted the higher advantage of using fixed boney points over soft tissue landmarks, but they used lower limit of vulvar cleft, because despite the pubic symphysis, this soft tissue landmark could be marked easily on images.

8.6 Mathematical Equations for Determining the Proper Location of Neo-umbilicus

Abhyankar et al. [4] performed a study in the Indian population to localize the normal place of umbilicus during the surgery, and they concluded that the ratio between the distance from umbilicus to the xiphisternum and the distance from umbilicus to the pubic symphysis is almost 1.6:1 and the ratio between the distance from umbilicus to anterior superior iliac spine (ASIS) and inter-ASIS distance is 0.6:1 in Indian population. They contend that this can help the plastic surgeons to find the proper position of the umbilicus during abdominoplasty. When each ASIS is taken as the center and the arcs are drawn with a radius of 0.6 times that of the inter-ASIS distance, the intersection point of these two arcs would be the location of the umbilicus.

Subsequently, Danilla et al. [21] had further analyzed the data from the study of Abhyankar et al. [4] and published the following regression equation for localizing the place for neo-umbilicus during surgery:

$$\mathrm{Xu} = -2.32 + 0.91 \times \mathrm{Xp} - 0.07 \times \mathrm{H}$$

where *Xu* is the distance between the xiphisternum and the umbilicus, *Xp* is the distance between the xiphisternum and the pubic symphysis, and *H* is the height, all measured in centimeters.

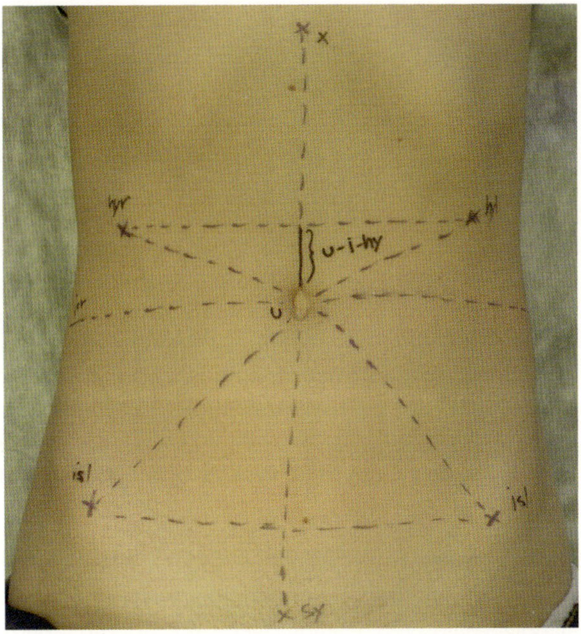

Fig. 8.1 The distance between the umbilicus and the inter-hypochondrium line marked as "u-i-hy." Also the right (hyr) and left (hyl) hypochondriums, xiphoid process (x), pubic symphysis (Sy), and the right and left anterior superior iliac spines (isr and isl) were depicted. Reproduced with permission from Dudukovic et al. [1]

Parnia et al. [12] studied a healthy young population of Iranian girls and applied the same principles that were used by Danilla to come up with a similar formula which could be applicable for the Iranian population.

All abovementioned equations were generated from the data of studies that included only female subjects. Dudukovic et al. [1] have studied a group of random young healthy subjects from both sexes with a comparator group of middle-age female candidates of the abdominoplasty surgery in Croatia, and they showed that, in Croatian women, the distance between the umbilicus and the inter-anterior hypochondrium line (Fig. 8.1) and, in Croatian men, the distance between the umbilicus and the interspinous line (inter-ASIS line) were the most predictive indices for umbilical positioning. Although their aim was to develop a predictive model that is applicable to both sexes, they found that the use of a distinct formula for each sex group would generate the most accurate predictive results. They also showed that age and anthropometric dimensions like body height or body mass could affect the position of the umbilicus on the anterior abdominal wall. Below we provided the mathematical equations that were reported by Dudukovic et al. [1] for predicting proper location of umbilicus in Croatian population:

Regression equation for young women:

$$u - i - hy = BM \times -0.1116 + WC \times 0.0706 - 4.5510$$

Regression equation for young men:

$$u-i-is=age\times 0.2033+BM\times 0.6445+BH\times -0.5692+BMI\times -2.2802+WC\times -0.0911+101.9408$$

where u-i-hy denotes the distance from umbilicus to inter-anterior hypochondrium line (Fig. 8.1) and u-i-is denotes the distance between umbilicus and inter-ASIS line. BM, BH, BMI, and WC are reflecting body mass, body height, body mass index, and waist circumference, respectively [1].

With the aim of including a group of middle-age women to make the study population more representative for the real-world clinical environment, Dudukovic et al. [1] have also included a group of 46 middle-age female patients who were candidates awaiting abdominal surgery. Although the idea of including the middle-age women is a valid and legitimate one, we assume the patients who are awaiting abdominoplasty procedure are not good representatives for the middle-age women population. Hence, the prediction models that were developed using the data of this specific subgroup were not presented here.

Table 8.1 summarizes different studies that have investigated the vertical position of umbilicus in the anterior abdominal wall and shows a variation across the studies and different populations. The BMI difference between different study populations could be a potential factor for this variation. It also reflects a geographic variation for these anthropometric features and proposes a potential role for ethnicity and genetic factors as well.

Table 8.1 Variation of vertical umbilical position in relation to xiphoid process and pubic symphysis across the literature

Author	Country	Study population	No. of patients	Average age	Average BMI	XP-U distance to U-PS distance ratio
El-Sharkawy et al. [20]	Egypt	Healthy volunteers	20 females	23.1	23.1	1.35
			20 males	23.7	23.8	1.14
Abhyankar et al. [4]	India	Healthy subjects	75	19.6	29.9	1.59
Ambardar et al. [19]	USA	Normal patients subgroup	96		22.2	1.12
Parnia et al. [12]	Iran	Healthy subjects	65	22.7	21.2	1.13
Dudukovic et al. [1]	Croatia	Healthy subjects subgroup	49 females	21.9	20.9	0.67
			49 males	22.8	23.9	1.05

BMI body mass index, *PS* pubic symphysis, *U* umbilicus, *XP* xiphoid process

8.7 Statistical Analysis and Formula Development

After collecting the data regarding the anthropometric indices in the study population, the investigators need to undertake linear regression analysis to assess the association between specific variables and the prediction of the position of umbilicus in the derivation cohort. For general information regarding the related statistical analysis methods and prediction models, please refer to the second edition of the textbook of *Categorical Data Analysis* by Agresti [22]. The precision of prediction is better to be tested in a separate but similar validation cohort. This precision could be assessed by comparing the performance of different models in predicting the position of the umbilicus and by comparing the predicted position with the actual observed one.

8.8 Limitations

Although the aforementioned mathematical equations are evidence-based and expeditious ways that can facilitate the localization of neo-umbilicus during surgery, it should be noted that they have been derived generally in studies with small sample sizes.

The data are not generalizable to other regions all around the world, considering the substantial geographic variation between different study populations, mentioned above. Development of new models through international multi-central studies which include ethnically diverse group of subjects from all around the world may be warranted to maximize the generalizability of findings. A good example for such international studies resulted in a widely accepted formula are the efforts that have been made to provide a formula for calculating estimated glomerular filtration rate (eGFR). The CKD-EPI (Chronic Kidney Disease Epidemiology Collaboration) equation was developed in 2009 [23] and is demonstrated to be more accurate than the MDRD formula in estimating the renal function [24]. The equation, expressed as below:

$$\text{eGFR} = 141 \times \min(\text{SCr}/\text{k},1)^{a} \times \max(\text{SCr}/\text{k},1)^{-1.209} \times 0.993^{Age} \times \\ [1.018\, \textit{if Female}] \times [1.159\, \textit{if Black}]$$

Where SCr is serum creatinine (mg/dL), k is 0.7 for females and 0.9 for males, a is −0.329 for females and −0.411 for males, min indicates the minimum of SCr/k or 1, and max indicates the maximum of SCr/k or 1. The CKD-EPI derivation population was consisted of various racial and ethnic subgroups, and various factors including the sex and race were taken into account in this equation [23]. This generalizability guarantees the wide applicability of this prediction model.

The other limitation for the use of these prediction models is the lack of external validation studies. None of the studies that have developed a formula for predicting the location of umbilicus on the anterior abdominal wall has validated the model in a separate validation cohort or externally in other relevant settings.

8.9 Conclusions

The abovementioned mathematical models and equations are useful, evidence based, and expeditious methods for determining the proper location of the neo-umbilicus during the surgery. All surgeries in which the original umbilical location is affected can be benefited from these mathematical formulas for predicting the proper location of neo-umbilicus. This includes a broad spectrum of procedures from abdominoplasties to reconstructive surgeries after penetrating trauma to the abdominal wall or large ventral or umbilical hernia repairs, etc. So far there is no superiority for any of those models over the other because they have been derived in small and local populations. There is a geographic variation in anthropometric features and position of the umbilicus on the anterior abdominal wall across different study populations. Further studies with larger and ethnically diverse study populations as well as validation studies are needed to allow us to endorse the use of these formulas in all umbilicoplasty patients.

References

1. Dudukovic M, Kisic H, Baez ML, Bulic K, Veir Z, Cvjeticanin B, Dujmovic A, Stipic I, Suman O, Mijatovic D. Anatomical prediction for surgical positioning of the umbilicus in a Croatian population. Ann Plast Surg. 2015;75(2):135–9.
2. Baroudi R. Umbilicoplasty. Clin Plast Surg. 1975;2:431.
3. Vernon S. Umbilical transplantation upward and abdominal contouring in lipectomy. Am J Surg. 1957;94(3):490–2.
4. Abhyankar SV, Rajguru AG, Patil PA. Anatomical localization of the umbilicus: an Indian study. Plast Reconstr Surg. 2006;117(4):1153–7.
5. Cavale N, Butler PE. The ideal female umbilicus? Plast Reconstr Surg. 2008;121(5):356e–7e.
6. Craig SB, Faller MS, Puckett CL. In search of the ideal female umbilicus. Plast Reconstr Surg. 2000;105:389.
7. Lee SJ, Garg S, Lee HP. Computer-aided analysis of the "beautiful" umbilicus. Aesthet Surg J. 2014;34(5):748–56.
8. Rozen SM, Redett R. The two-dermal-flap umbilical transposition: a natural and aesthetic umbilicus after abdominoplasty. Plast Reconstr Surg. 2007;119(7):2255–62.
9. Choudhary S, Taams KO. Umbilicosculpture: a concept revisited. Br J Plast Surg. 1998;51(7):538–41.
10. Dubou R, Ousterhout DK. Placement of the umbilicus in an abdominoplasty. Plast Reconstr Surg. 1978;61(2):291–3.
11. Dellon AL. The midline umbilicus. Plast Reconstr Surg. 2004;113(4):1301–2; author reply 1302.

12. Parnia R, Ghorbani L, Sepehrvand N, Hatami S, Bazargan-Hejazi S. Determining anatomical position of the umbilicus in Iranian girls, and providing quantitative indices and formula to determine neo-umbilicus during abdominoplasty. Indian J Plast Surg. 2012;45(1):94–6.
13. Chin SH, Martin WJ, Matarasso A. Do waistline and umbilical position really change after abdominoplasty? Plast Reconstr Surg. 2010;125(1):27e–8e.
14. Rohrich RJ, Sorokin ES, Brown SA, Gibby DL. Is the umbilicus truly midline? Clinical and medicolegal implications. Plast Reconstr Surg. 2003;112(1):259–63.
15. Dick ET. Umbilicoplasty as a treatment for persistent umbilical infection. Aust N Z J Surg. 1970;39:380.
16. Grant B. Grant's method of anatomy. Baltimore: Williams & Wilkins; 1965.
17. Hinderer UT. The dermolipectomy approach for augmentation mammaplasty. Clin Plast Surg. 1975;2(3):359–69.
18. Rodriguez-Feliz JR, Makhijani S, Przybyla A, Hill D, Chao J. Intraoperative assessment of the umbilicopubic distance: a reliable anatomic landmark for transposition of the umbilicus. Aesthetic Plast Surg. 2012;36(1):8–17.
19. Ambardar S, Cabot J, Cekic V, Baxter K, Arnell TD, Forde KA, Nihalani A, Whelan RL. Abdominal wall dimensions and umbilical position vary widely with BMI and should be taken into account when choosing port locations. Surg Endosc. 2009;23(9):1995–2000.
20. El-Sharkawy A, Said T, Shafik I, Khalifa H. A study of the aesthetic patterns of the umbilicus among Egyptians with a new technique for umbilical reconstruction de novo. Kasr El-Aini J Surg. 2004;5(3):87–99.
21. Danilla S, Bonasic S. Anatomical localization of the umbilicus: a statistical analysis. Plast Reconstr Surg. 2007;119(3):1123–4.
22. Agresti A. Categorical data analysis. 2nd ed. Hoboken, NJ: Wiley; 2002.
23. Levey AS, Stevens LA, Schmid CH, Zhang YL, Castro 3rd AF, Feldman HI, Kusek JW, Eggers P, Van Lente F, Greene T, et al. A new equation to estimate glomerular filtration rate. Ann Intern Med. 2009;150(9):604–12.
24. Stevens LA, Schmid CH, Greene T, Zhang YL, Beck GJ, Froissart M, Hamm LL, Lewis table JB, Mauer M, Navis GJ, et al. Comparative performance of the CKD Epidemiology Collaboration (CKD-EPI) and the Modification of Diet in Renal Disease (MDRD) Study equations for estimating GFR levels above 60 mL/min/1.73 m2. Am J Kidney Dis. 2010;56(3):486–95.

Chapter 9
Umbilical Resiting and Reconstruction

Vimal J. Gokani and Niri S. Niranjan

9.1 Introduction

The umbilicus, or navel, is the scar resulting from the transection of the cord attaching a foetus to its placenta. The term 'umbilicus' itself comes from the Latin pertaining to the 'navel' or the 'centre'. In anatomical drawings and art such as Leonardo da Vinci's *Vitruvian Man* that depicts the centre of the abdomen, however, its significance appears to be much deeper rooted. Importance has been placed on the umbilicus for centuries. Early Japanese art, dating to the Jomon period (14,000 BC) depicts three balls, representing the breasts and the umbilicus. Even before this, the 11 cm-high statue *Venus of Willendorf*, a prehistoric female figurine dating back to 28,000–25,000 BC, featured an umbilicus.

9.2 Anatomy and Physiology

The umbilicus is shallow, round or elliptical, and either concave or convex. The inferior pole is retracted compared to its hooded superior pole [1]. In the non-obese person, the umbilicus is located at the level of the iliac crests [2]. It migrates caudally with increasing age and is commonly located between the level of the bodies of the third and fifth lumbar vertebrae. It lies approximately in the midline, however is precisely in the midline in under 2 % of the population [3]. The sensation to the skin overlying this level is provided by the tenth thoracic spinal nerve. The umbilical ring overlies the linea alba, onto which it is attached, with an absence of subcutaneous fat. The umbilicus is attached to the linea alba by a fibrous stalk of cicatrix

V.J. Gokani • N.S. Niranjan, M.S. (✉)
St Andrews Centre for Plastic Surgery and Burns, Broomfield Hospital,
Court Road, Chelmsford CM1 7ET, UK
e-mail: niriniranjan@hotmail.com

M.A. Shiffman (ed.), *Adult Umbilical Reconstruction*,
DOI 10.1007/978-3-319-43887-0_9

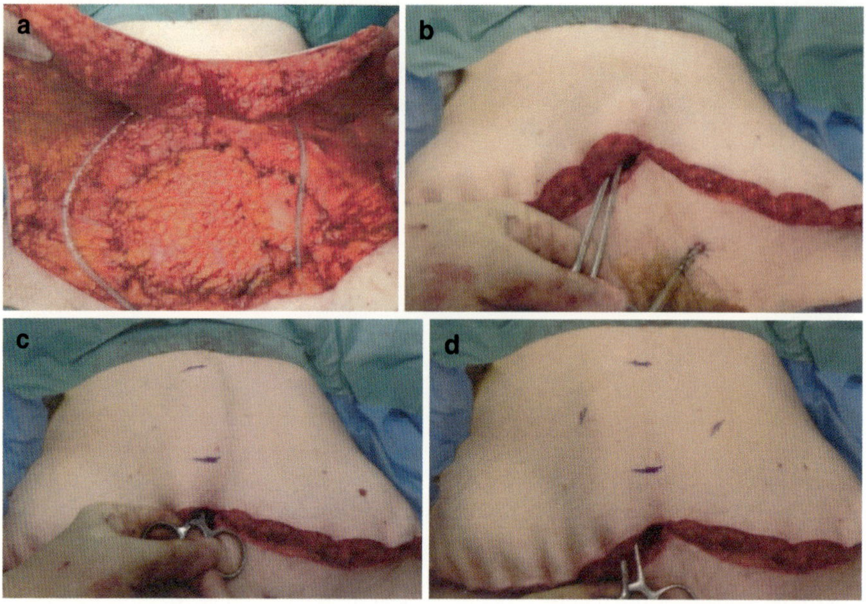

Fig. 9.1 (**a**) The fascial lining surrounding the umbilical cicatrix is demonstrated. (**b**) The Lanes issue forceps applied to the umbilicus. (**c**) The umbilicus pushed cranially in the midline and marked. (**d**) The umbilicus tented to the right of the midline and marked to identify the position of the neo-umbilicus

which itself is surrounded by a distinct fascial plane which extends into the superficial Scarpa's fascia (Fig. 9.1) [4]. This cicatrix gives the umbilicus its natural mobile nature. Deep to the linea alba lie five peritoneal folds, one of which extends cranially. The median umbilical ligament contains the urachal remnant, leading to the bladder; the medial umbilical folds contain the obliterated umbilical arteries which pass to the external iliac arteries; and the lateral umbilical folds, which are formed by the peritoneal folds, cover the inferior epigastric arteries. The ligamentum teres extends cranially to form the ligamentum teres hepatis which transmits the obliterated left umbilical vein. Each of these peritoneal folds contains small arteries which supply blood to the umbilicus, which also derives blood supply through a subdermal plexus and perforators from the deep inferior epigastric artery.

In utero, the umbilicus allows nutrients to pass into the foetus and waste products to be excreted. At approximately day 32 of uterine development, the umbilical loop extends from the umbilical coelom. This tract further extends to form the omphalomesenteric duct, which extends further to produce a physiological herniation of the midgut. The midgut rotates approximately 270° and has re-entered the abdominal cavity by day 59.

This region which is physically significant in utero seals off the abdominal cavity in life. The aesthetic function of the umbilicus is well documented, and it is a surface landmark of the abdominal wall. Despite variability in its normal appearance, reconstruction is remarkably difficult with numerous techniques having been described [5–7]. Its absence or abnormal appearance plays a significant part in the reconstruction of the abdominal wall following reconstructive surgery.

9.3 Resiting of the Umbilicus

9.3.1 Indications

Resiting of the umbilicus is common following abdominoplasty and DIEP, SIEA or TRAM flap procedures.

The umbilicus was routinely discarded in abdominoplasty until the late 1950s. A number of techniques have been described to resite the umbilicus [5–7]. One common technique involves the thinning of the abdominal skin around the umbilicus, which is then attached to the rectus sheath by means of ligature (Fig. 9.2).

This, however, does not restore normal anatomy. The native umbilicus is attached to a mobile stalk. This technique tethers this skin flap to the rectus sheath which can be uncomfortable. Moreover, over-thinning of the skin flap can result in necrosis.

9.3.2 Operative Technique

The technique described here avoids such tethering or stenosis, producing a more natural umbilicus.

Following excision of excess skin following abdominoplasty, a pair of long tissue forceps is applied to the umbilicus, which maintains its normal cicatrized attachment within the fascia (Fig. 9.1). The wound is closed using sutures or staples, as per surgeon preference. To define the position of the neo-umbilicus, a pair of Lanes tissue forceps is applied to the umbilicus and pushed upwards and superiorly in the midline, and the point of maximal tenting is marked on the skin (Fig. 9.1). The same is performed on the right, on the left, and inferiorly. These four points are joined, and the centre of these is marked to yield the centre of the neo-umbilicus (Fig. 9.1).

A U-shaped incision is made, measuring a third of the circumference of a circle, and the U-flap skin is elevated and thinned (Figs. 9.2 and 9.3).

A conical area of fat with a diameter of 1–2 cm, depending on the thickness of the abdominal pannus, is dissected out. Following haemostasis the superficial fascia is sutured to the deep dermis at the base of the U-flap and the edges of the wound (Fig. 9.1d). This results in a hollow around the umbilicus allowing it to remain mobile without tethering the skin to the underlying rectus sheath (Fig. 9.3).

The distal skin of the U-flap is sutured to the umbilicus, creating the superior hood. The inferior circumference of the umbilicus is sutured to the abdominal skin only, with no non-anatomical attachment to the fascia (Figs. 9.2 and 9.3). Neither the umbilicus nor the abdominal skin is sutured to the underlying rectus sheath, and normal anatomical attachments are restored.

After cleaning the skin with normal saline to wash away any surgical skin preparatory solution, the umbilicus is packed with paraffin-soaked gauze, covered with dressing gauze to soak up any ooze, and adhesive tape applied.

Postoperatively, the umbilicus maintains its natural superior hooding, is centred within the abdomen and maintains its natural mobility (Figs. 9.4 and 9.5).

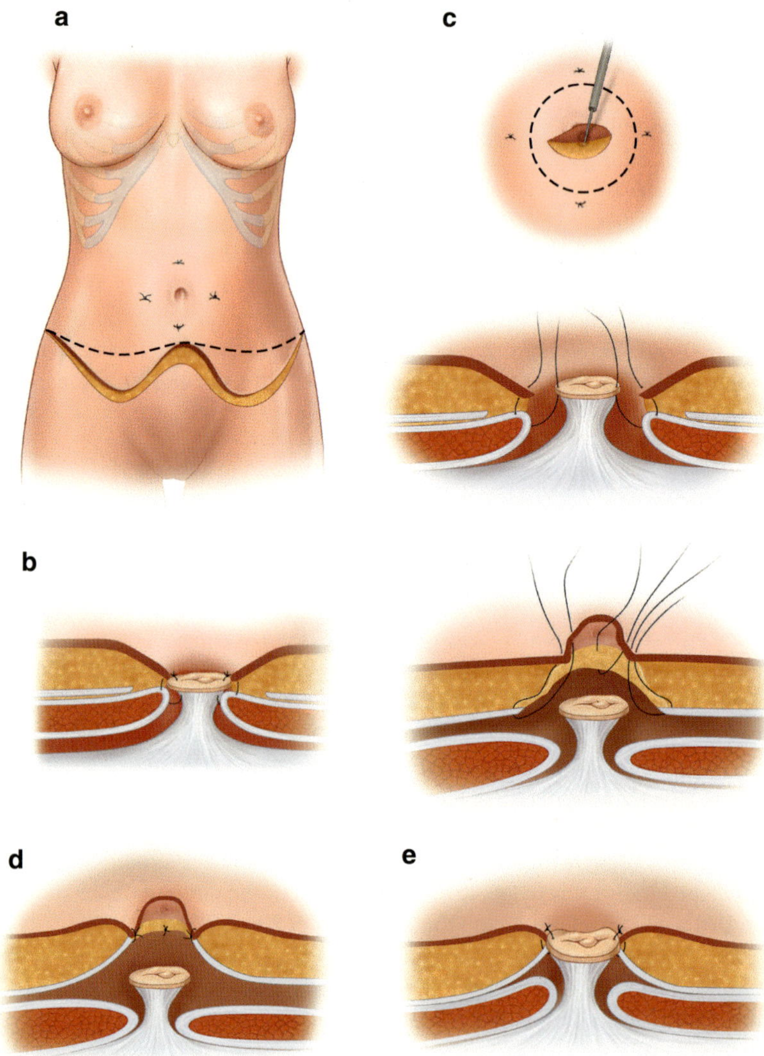

Fig. 9.2 (**a**, **b**) Attachment of the umbilical skin to the rectus sheath (in *green*), resulting in tethering of the umbilicus. (**c**, **d**) Anatomical technique for resiting the umbilicus. (**e**) The skin attached to Scarpa's fascia (in *blue*), resulting in a mobile umbilicus

9.4 Reconstruction of the Umbilicus

9.4.1 Indications

The umbilicus is reconstructed in cases of congenial absence of the umbilicus such as in omphalocoele or when the primary surgical procedure results in destruction of

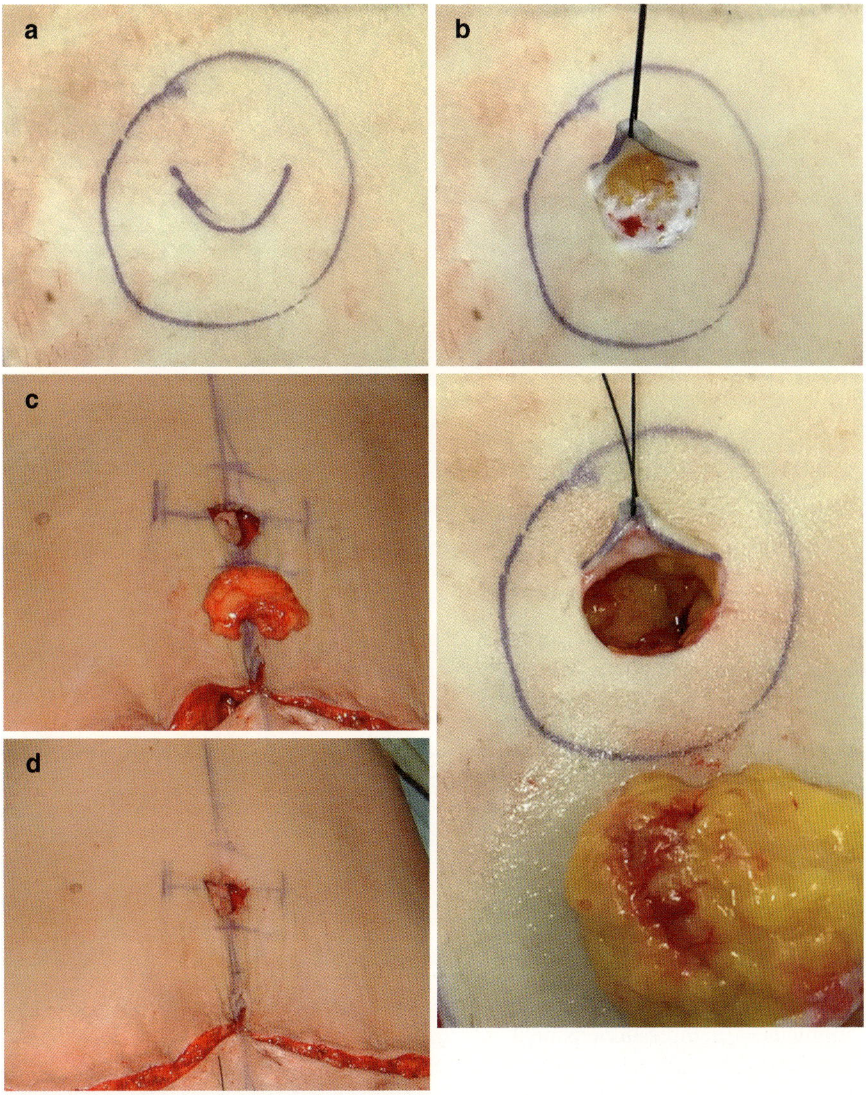

Fig. 9.3 (**a**, **b**) The U-shaped incision in the skin is made and the skin defatted. (**c**) A conical volume of subcutaneous fat is excised, with the base at the rectus sheath. (**d**) The umbilicus is delivered through the anterior abdominal wall. The peri-umbilical skin and the base of the U-flap are sutured to Scarpa's fascia, and the umbilical disc is sutured to the peri-umbilical skin

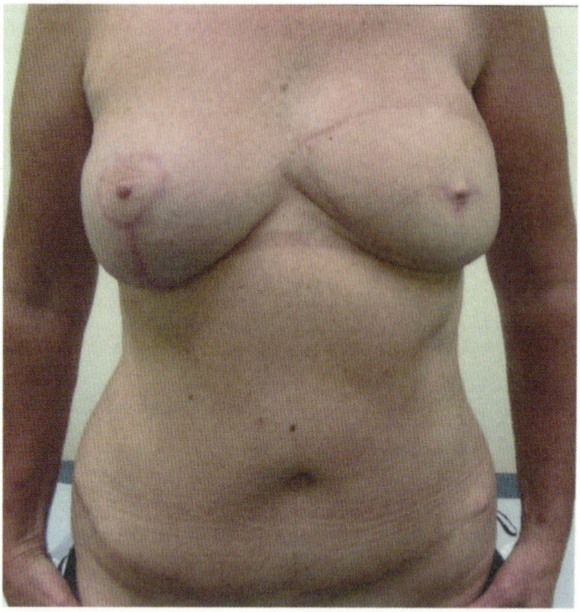

Fig. 9.4 Six months post-DIEP reconstruction of the left breast and umbilical resiting using the anatomical technique

the umbilicus. Such procedures include abdominal wall reconstructions, abdominoplasty, laparotomy or certain laparoscopic procedures.

9.4.2 *Operative Technique*

Umbilical reconstruction was first described in the 1950s [8, 9], and a number of techniques using skin grafts or local flaps have since been described [10–13]. The umbilicus is a three-dimensional structure, and techniques used to describe its reconstruction result in scars which heal to produce such a result.

An early technique described by Baroudi in 1975 [10] involved the excision of a circle of skin and the cylinder of underlying fat at the site of the neo-umbilicus. The surrounding skin is then sutured to the underlying fascia with a purse-string suture, to allow the wound to heal by cicatrization. One criticism of this technique is the potential for umbilical stenosis (Fig. 9.6).

Another technique employs the creation of an x-shaped incision at the site of the neo-umbilicus. Each flap is defatted, and the fat separating the skin flaps and the linea alba is excised. Following haemostasis, the flaps are sutured to the underlying fascia with non-absorbable material. The flaps are inset slightly higher than the centre of the 'X' to facilitate the scar to heal with an aesthetically pleasing superior hooding. The wound is packed with a proflavin-soaked cotton ball which can be readily removed during routine review [14].

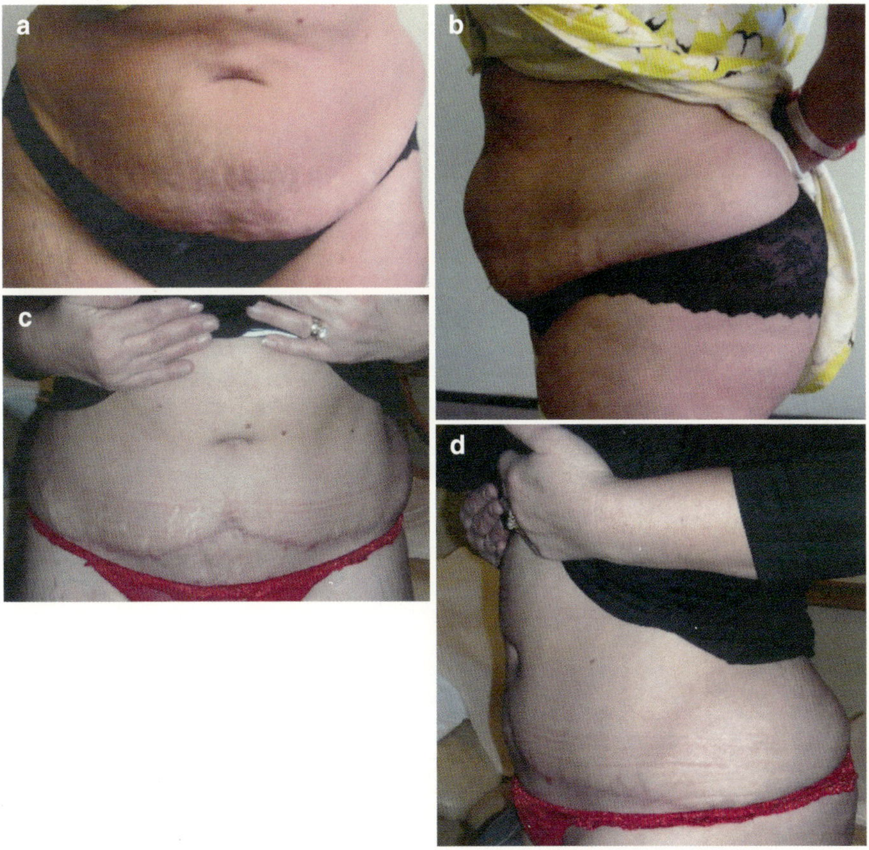

Fig. 9.5 (**a**, **b**) Pre-abdominoplasty. (**c**, **d**) Three months post-abdominoplasty

9.4.3 Postoperative Management

The wound is reviewed at day 3–5 for signs of infection.

9.5 Complications

Umbilicoplasty or reconstruction of the umbilicus is rarely performed alone, and therefore the risks and complications of the procedure are related to the adjunctive surgery. The native umbilicus is a scar which heals by secondary intention during the neonatal period. It is therefore the only scar which a plastic surgeon demands heal by scarring. There is a small risk of infection. Aesthetically, patients' expectations must still be managed.

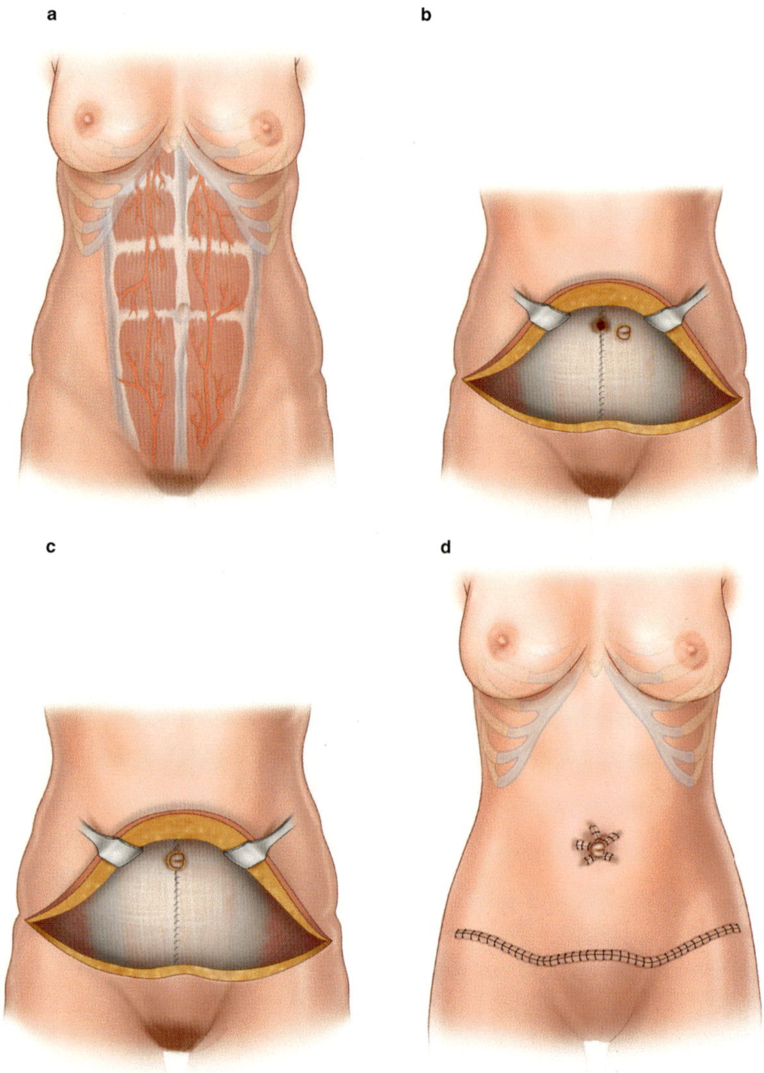

Fig. 9.6 Reconstruction of the umbilicus. (**a**) DIEP perfortators in the anterior abdominal wall. (**b**) The umbilical disc. (**c**) Transfer of the umbilical disc. (**d**) The end result of reconstruction of the umbilicus

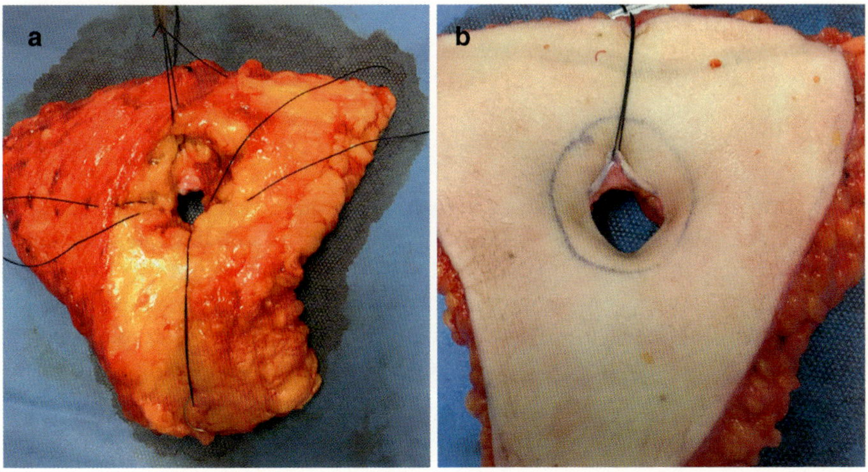

Fig. 9.7 Using the excess skin in an abdominoplasty as a training tool. (**a**) Sutures attaching Scarpa's fascia to the overlying subcuticular skin. (**b**) The resultant umbilicated appearance

9.5.1 Utilizing Excess Tissue as a Training Tool

The authors advocate the tissue excess in abdominoplasty, which would otherwise be discarded, to be used as a training tool on which umbilicoplasty can be practised (Fig. 9.7).

The umbilicus is shallow, round or elliptical, and either concave or convex. The inferior pole is retracted compared to its hooded superior pole [15]. In the non-obese person, the umbilicus is located at the level of the iliac crests [1]. It migrates caudally with increasing age, and is commonly located between the level of the bodies of the third and fifth lumbar vertebrae. It lies approximately in the midline, however is precisely in the midline in under 2 % of the population [2]. The sensation to the skin overlying this level is provided by the tenth thoracic spinal nerve. The umbilical ring overlies the linea alba, onto which it is attached, with an absence of subcutaneous fat. The umbilicus is attached to the linea alba by a fibrous stalk of cicatrix which itself is surrounded by a distinct fascial plane, the fascia of Niranjan. This cicatrix gives the umbilicus its natural mobile nature. Deep to the linea alba lie five peritoneal folds, one of which extends cranially. The median umbilical ligament contains the urachal remnant, leading to the bladder; the medial umbilical folds contain the obliterated umbilical arteries which pass to the external iliac artieries; and the lateral umbilical folds which are formed by the peritoneal folds, cover the inferior epigastric arteries. The ligamentum teres extends cranially to form the ligamentum teres hepatis which transmits the obliterated left umbilical vein. Each of these peritoneal folds contains small arteries which supply blood to the umbilicus, which also derives blood supply through a subdermal plexus and perforators from the deep inferior epigastric artery.

In utero, the umbilicus allows nutrients to pass into the fetus, and waste products to be excreted. At approximately day 32 of uterine development the umbilical loop extends from the umbilical coelom. This tract further extends to form the omphalo-mesenteric duct, which extends further to produce a physiological herniation of the midgut. The midgut rotates approximately 270° and has re-entered the abdominal cavity by day 59.

This region which is physically significant in utero seals off the abdominal cavity in life. The aesthetic function of the umbilicus is well documented, and it is a surface landmark of the abdominal wall. Despite variability in its normal appearance, reconstruction is remarkably difficult with numerous techniques having been described [3–6]. Its absence or abnormal appearance plays a significant part in the reconstruction of the abdominal wall following reconstructive surgery.

9.6 Re-Siting of the Umbilicus

9.6.1 Indications

Re-siting of the umbilicus is common following abdominoplasty and DIEP, SIEA or TRAM flap procedures.

9.6.2 Operative Technique

The umbilicus was routinely discarded in abdominoplasty until the late 1950s. A number of techniques have been described to re-site the umbilicus [3–6]. One common technique involves the thinning of the abdominal skin around the umbilicus, which is then attached to the rectus sheath by means of ligature (Fig. 9.1).

This, however, does not restore normal anatomy. The native umbilicus is attached to a mobile stalk. This technique tethers this skin flap to the rectus sheath which can be uncomfortable. Moreover, over-thinning of the skin flap can result in necrosis. The technique described here avoids such tethering or stenosis, producing a more natural umbilicus.

Following excision of excess skin following abdominoplasty, a pair of long tissue forceps is applied to the umbilicus, which maintains its normal cicatrized attachment within the fascia of Niranjan. The wound is closed using sutures or staples, as per surgeon preference. To define the position of the neo-umbilicus, the forceps tip is pushed upwards and superiorly, and the point of maximal tenting is marked on the skin. The same is performed on the right, on the left, and inferiorly. These four points are joined, and the centre of these is marked to yield the center of the neo-umbilicus (Fig. 9.2). A U-shaped incision is created, measuring a third of the circumference of a circle, and the U-flap is thinned. A conical area of fat with a diameter of 1–2 cm, depending on the thickness of the abdominal pannus, is dissected out (Fig. 9.3). Following hemostasis the superficial fascia is sutured to the deep dermis at the base of the U-flap and the edges of the wound (Fig. 9.4). This results in a hollow around the umbilicus allowing it to remain mobile without tethering the skin to the underlying rectus sheath. The distal skin of the U-flap is sutured to the umbilicus, creating the superior hood. The inferior circumference of the umbilicus is sutured to the abdominal skin only, with no non-anatomical attachment to the fascia. Neither the umbilicus nor the abdominal skin are sutured to the underlying sheath, and only normal anatomical attachments are restored.

After cleaning the skin with normal saline to wash away any surgical skin preparatory solution, the umbilicus is packed with paraffin soaked gauze, covered with dressing gauze to soak up any ooze, and adhesive Microfoam tape (3 M, St. Paul, Minn) applied.

9.7 Reconstruction of the Umbilicus

9.7.1 Indications

The umbilicus is reconstructed in cases of congenial absence of the umbilicus such as in omphalocele or when the primary surgical procedure results in destruction of the umbilicus. Such procedures include abdominal wall reconstructions, abdominoplasty, laparotomy or certain laparoscopic procedures.

9.7.2 Operative Technique

Umbilical reconstruction was first described in the 1950s [7, 16] and a number of techniques using skin grafts or local flaps have since been described [8–11]. The umbilicus is a three dimensional structure, and techniques used to describe its reconstruction result in scars which heal to produce such a result.

An early technique described by Baroudi in 1975 [8] involved the excision of acircle of skin and the cylinder of underlying fat at the site of the neo-umbilicus. The surrounding skin is then sutured to the underlying fascia to allow the wound to heal by cicatrization. One criticism of this technique is the potential for umbilical stenosis.

Another technique employs the creation of an x-shaped incision at the site of the neo-umbilicus. Each flap is defatted, and the fat separating the skin flaps and the linea alba is excised. Following hemostasis, the flaps are sutured to the underlying fascia with non-absorbable material. The flaps are inset slightly higher than the center of the 'X' to facilitate the scar to heal with an aesthetically pleasing superior hooding. The wound is packed with a proflavin soaked cotton ball which can be readily removed during routine review [12].

9.7.3 Postoperative Management

The wound is reviewed at day 3–5 for signs of infection.

References

1. Nahai F. Anatomic considerations in abdominoplasty. Clin Plast Surg. 2010;37(3):407–14.
2. Dubou R, Ousterhout DK. Placement of the umbilicus in an abdominoplasty. Plast Reconstr Surg. 1978;61(2):291–3.
3. Rohrich RJ, Sorokin ES, Brown SA, Gibby DL. Is the umbilicus truly midline. Clinical and medicolegal implications? Plast Reconstr Surg. 2003;112:259–63.
4. Lockwood TE. Superficial fascial system (SFS) of the trunk and extremities: a new concept. Plast Reconstr Surg. 1991;87(6):1009–18.
5. Wilson HK. Reconstruction of umbilicus. Plast Reconstr Surg. 1981;67(4):564–5.
6. De Lacerda DJ, Martins DM, Marques A, Brenda E, De Moura Andrews J. Umbilicoplasty for the abdomen with a thin adipose layer. Br J Plast Surg. 1994;47:386–7.
7. Lim TC, Tan WT. Managing the umbilicus during abdominoplasty. Plast Reconstr Surg. 1996;97:227–32.
8. Andrews JM. Nova técnica de lipectomia abdominal e onfaloplastia. Cuba: Memória do VIII Cong Lat Am Cir Plast; 1956.
9. Vernon S. Umbilical transplantation upward and abdominal contouring in lipectomy. Am J Surg. 1957;94:490–2.
10. Baroudi R. Umbilicoplasty. Clin Plast Surg. 1975;2:431–48.
11. Avelar J. Abdominoplasty: systematization of a technique without external umbilical scar. Aesthetic Plast Surg. 1978;2:141–51.
12. Juri J, Juri C, Raiden G. Reconstruction of the umbilicus in abdominoplasty. Plast Reconstr Surg. 1979;63:580–2.
13. Massiha H, Montegut W, Phillips R. A method of reconstructing a natural-looking umbilicus in abdominoplasty. Ann Plast Surg. 1997;38:228–31.
14. Lee YT, Kwon C, Rhee SC, Cho SH, Eo SR. Four flaps technique for neoumbilicoplasty. Arch Plast Surg. 2015;42(3):351–5.
15. Power ML, Schulkin J. The evolution of obesity. Baltimore, ML: Johns Hopkins University Press; 2009.
16. Suliman M. A simple method for fishing out the umbilicus in abdominoplasty surgery. J Plast Reconstr Aesthet Surg. 2009;62(5):594.

Part III
History

Chapter 10
History of Umbilical Reconstruction Techniques

Melvin A. Shiffman

10.1 Incision to Reinsert the Umbilicus in Abdominoplasty

A variety of abdominal wall incisions are used to reinsert the umbilical stalk onto the abdominal wall during abdominoplasty. These incisions determine to some extent the shape of the new umbilicus when the umbilical stalk is brought out and sutured to the abdominal wall. Other factors include whether or not the umbilical stalk is reshaped, the fixation of the abdominal skin to the underlying fascia or linea alba, and whether or not the umbilical stalk is shortened with sutures from the upper portion of the stalk to the abdominal wall.

Circular excision

Vernon [1]
Lopez-Tallaj and Gervain [2]
Malic [3]

Hexagon excision:

Ng [4]

Horizontal

Daher et al. [5]
Baroudi [6]

Inverted U-shaped incision:

Shiffman [7]
Malic [3]

M.A. Shiffman, M.D., J.D.
Private Practice, 17501 Chatham Drive, Tustin, CA 92780-2302, USA
e-mail: shiffmanmdjd@yahoo.com

M.A. Shiffman (ed.), *Adult Umbilical Reconstruction*,
DOI 10.1007/978-3-319-43887-0_10

Inverted V-shaped incision:

Pallua et al. [8]
Lesavoy [9]

Rectangular excision:

Lopez-Tallaj and Gervain 2]

Round flap:

Delerm [10]
Breukers et al. [11]

Semicircular:

Pitanguy and Radwansky [12]

Shield:

D'Assumpção [13]

Superior V-shaped flap:

Rish and Prado [14]
Ramirez [15]

Transverse (horizontal) incision:

Baroudi [6]
Regnault and Daniel [16]
Pitanguy and Radwansky [12]
Daher et al. [5]
Santanelli et al. [17]

U-shaped incision:

Pitanguy [18]
Freeman and Wiemer [19] (called inverted Omega incision)

Vertical incision:

Matarasso [20]
Lee and Mustoe [21]
Akbaş [22]
Aly [23]

Vertical ellipse excision:

Thomas et al. [24]

The following are techniques that are similar in design and results but different in names:

1. U-shape, inverted Omega, V-shape
2. Inverted U-shape, inverted V-shape

10.2 Techniques

10.2.1 The Use of Various Flaps, Tissue Transfer, and Suturing Techniques

The use of various flaps, tissue transfer, and suturing techniques was used for the more difficult cases such as extensive malformation or loss of the umbilicus. Southwell-Keely [25] published his review of techniques for umbilicoplasty.

Some of the techniques that have been reported include:

Sabatier et al. [26] – crossbow.
Avelar [27] – three flaps.
Jamra [28] – double V–Y.
Hodgkinson [29] converting an "innie to an outie" by excising umbilical scar and using two flaps.
Ohana et al. [30] – hourglass with four flaps.
Hatoko and Harashina [31] – skin graft.
Matsuo [32] – conchal cartilage composite graft.
Ribeiro et al. [33] – four-pointed star and rotation of navel.
Itoh and Arai [34] – triangle flap and rhombic flap.
Miller and Balch [35] – four flaps and Iris technique.
De Lacerda et al. [36] – four flaps.
Marconi [37] –purse string.
Sugawara et al. [38] – triangular flap and conical flap.
Sawada [39] – two rhomboid flaps.
Onishi et al. [40] – lunch box with flaps.
Massiha [41] – purse-string suture of three flaps.
Baack et al. [42] – two circles and for stenosis double-opposing Z-plasty.
Yotsuyanagi et al. [43] – two twisted flaps.
Schoeller et al. [44] – purse-string suture.
Cannistrà and Pecorelli [45] – double Y.
Shinohara et al. [46] – inverted C-V flap.
Abenavoli et al. [47] – skin graft spiraled to form tortellini-shaped umbilicus.

Schoeller et al. [48] – three-suture technique
Masuda et al. [49] – reversed fan-shaped flap.
Meirer et al. [50] – purse string.
Ozbekand Ozcan [51] modified reversed fan-shaped flap.
Uraloğlu et al. [52] – C and U flaps.
Sevin et al. [53] – bilobed flap.
Kakudo et al. [54] used spindle island flap with depression rolled into a cone.
Castillo et al. [55] – skin flaps.
Rozen and Redet [56] – two dermal flaps.
Rogliani et al. [57] – Maltese cross.
Amud [58] – suture dermis to rectus fascia.
Barbosa et al. [59] – two triangle flaps.
Takasu and Watanabe [60] – three triangular skin flaps.
Gonçalves de Freitas et al. [61] – double V.
Mazzocchi et al. [62] – double Y elliptical vertical incision.
Cló and Nogueira [63] – four V-shaped flaps.
Arai et al. [64] – two rectangular pedicle flaps.
Gera and Henry [65] – double purse string.
Donnabella [66] – two rectangular flaps.

Morshed [67] reported a simple technique for neo-umbilicoplasty by excising a triangle of the skin and closing the defect in a manner that would reform the umbilicus.

There have been reports of repairs for umbilical hernias and umbilical stenosis, with or without the loss of the umbilicus as well as loss of the umbilicus from urachal pathology, abdominal wall scars, exstrophy, omphalocele, gastroschisis, and melanoma.

10.2.2 Umbilical Hernia

10.2.2.1 Classifications

Kajikawa et al. [68] devised a classification for umbilical hernia by the height and shape of protrusion (Table 10.1), while Kom et al. [69] devised a classification for huge umbilical hernias (HUH) (Table 10.2).

10.2.2.2 No Loss of Umbilicus

The presence of a small umbilical hernia when doing an abdominoplasty usually requires a repair to complete the procedure properly. The hernia can be repaired by an inferior or lateral approach so as not to disturb the vascularity of the umbilical stalk that will be released from the abdominal wall skin [70]. The large umbilical

Table 10.1 Modified classification of umbilical hernia [67]

Type 0: flat abdomen without excess skin for umbilicoplasty
Type I: small protrusion of the umbilicus with little surplus skin for umbilicoplasty
Type II: large protrusion with wide base (more than 15 mm) with significant surplus skin
Type III: large protrusion with narrow base and excess skin for umbilicoplasty
Type IV: small protrusion of the umbilicus with excess skin for umbilicoplasty

Table 10.2 Classification of huge umbilical hernia (HUH)

Using the basis of diameter:
Group 1: 3 cm<BD 5 cm or less
Group 2: 5 cm<BD under 7 cm
Group 3: BD>7 cm
Morphology of HUH:
Sessile
Pediculate
Hornlike HUH

hernia that distorts the umbilicus will require umbilical reconstruction after a repair of the hernia that transects the base of the umbilicus at the level of the linea alba leaving a scar in the abdominal wall skin.

Aaronson [71] describes the use of an incision at the bottom of the belly button; the protruding tissues, fluids, or organs are pushed back in place, and the weak spot is eliminated by suturing it closed. Aaronson [72] also stated that some plastic surgeons choose to overlay the fatty muscle on top of the area to cover the tissue or organ, while others use special patches to create less tension on the muscle surrounding it. These techniques are not described adequately.

Bruner et al. [73] reported that after the umbilicus is dissected from the anterior abdominal wall flap while maintaining blood supply from its underlying fascial attachment, a 3–4 cm midline longitudinal laparotomy incision is made through the primarily avascular linea alba inferior to the umbilical stalk. The fascial defect is identified and the hernia reduced from the undersurface of the umbilicus either in the preperitoneal or intraperitoneal space. The hernia is then repaired with interrupted monofilament sutures, and the midline laparotomy fascial incision closed with running suture. Plication of the rectus fascia is then performed.

Neinstein et al. [74] presented a series of umbilical hernia repairs in abdominoplasty patients using a minimal access incision by means of the rectus fascia and the Ventralex patch that is fast and reliable and preserves the blood supply to the umbilicus.

10.2.2.3 Loss of Umbilicus

The umbilicus may be lost because of a very large umbilical hernia where repair of the defect may be more important than trying to save the umbilicus:

Borges [75] used a quadrilateral segment of the skin that is excised on each side of the proposed navel. Both flaps are rotated and sutured.
Apfelberg et al. [76] described two types of umbilicoplasties for patients with absent umbilicus following umbilical hernia repair.
Reyna et al. [77].
Blanchard et al. [78] used a square cutaneous flap for neoumbilicus.
Billmire [79] designed an inferior skin flap that was tubularized to create a neoumbilicus.
Tamir and Kurzbart [80] devised a "lazy-M" and omega flaps.
el-Dessouki et al. [81] used a double half-cone flap.
Kaneko and Tsuda [82] described a four-triangular-skin-flap.
Ikeda et al. [83] developed two fan-shaped skin flaps.
Sankalé et al. [84] used a lateral left plasty and horseshoe plasty and umbilical graft.
Kajikawa et al. [68] inverted a pouch and V–Y advancement flap and pair of fan-style flaps.
Kom et al. [69] – two lateral flaps technique.

References

1. Vernon S. Umbilical transplantation upward and abdominal contouring in lipectomy. Am J Surg. 1957;94(3):490–2.
2. Lopez-Tallaj L, Gervain J. Restaurção umbilical naabdominoplastia: uma simples técnica rectangular. Rev Soc Bras Cir Plast. 2001;16(3):39–46.
3. Malic CC, Spyrou GE, Hough M, Fourie L. Patient satisfaction with two different methods of umbilicoplasty. Plast Reconstr Surg. 2007;119(1):357–61.
4. Ng JA. Abdominoplastias: neo-onfaloplastiasemcicatriz e semexcisão de gordura. Rev Bras Cir Plast. 2010;25(3):499–503.
5. Daher JC, Benedik A, CevaFaria CAD, Di Lamartine J, Neto JNR, Cosa OM, Cammarota MC. Umbilicoplastia: experiência com a técnica do minicirculo de pele. Rev Bras Cir Plast. 2011;26(2):302–5.
6. Baroudi R. Umbilicoplasty. Clin Plast Surg. 1975;2(3):431–85.
7. Shiffman MA. Reconstruction de l'ombilicdansl'abdominoplastie. Rev Chir Esthet Langue Franc. 1999;25(95):49.
8. Pallua N, Markowicz MP, Grosse F, Walter S. Aesthetically pleasant umbilicoplasty. Ann Plast Surg. 2010;64(6):722–5.
9. Lesavoy MA, Fan K, Guenther DA, Herrera F, Little JW. The inverted-v chevron umbilicoplasty for breast reconstruction and abdominoplasty. Aesthet Surg J. 2012;32(1):110–6.
10. Delerm A. Refinements in abdominoplasty with emphasis on reimplantation of the umbilicus. Plast Reconstr Surg. 1982;70(5):632–7.
11. Se B, van derLei B, Tan TL, Luijendijk RW, Stevens HPJD. "Scarless" umbilicoplasty: a new umbilicoplasty technique and a review of the English language literature. Ann Plast Surg. 2009;63(1):15–20.

12. Pitanguy I, Radwanski HN. Personal approach to aesthetic abdominal deformities. In: Shiffman MA, Mirrafati S, editors. Aesthetic surgery of the abdominal wall. Berlin: Springer; 2005. p. 102–14.
13. D'Assumpção EA. Técnica para umbilicoplastia, evitando-se un dos principaisestimas das abdominoplastias. Rev Bras Cir Plast. 2005;20(3):160–6.
14. Rish BB, Prado A. Umbilicoplasty in abdominoplasty: a demonstration. Am J Cosm Surg. 1999;16(4):311–3.
15. Ramirez OM. Abdominoplasty and abdominal wall rehabilitation: a comprehensive approach. Plast Reconstr Surg. 2000;105(1):425–35.
16. Regnault P, Daniel RK. Abdominoplasty. In: Regnault P, Daniel RK, editors. Aesthetic plastic surgery: principles and techniques. Boston: Little Brown and Company; 1984. p. 617–54.
17. Santanelli F, Mazzocchi M, Renzi L, Cigna E. Reconstruction of a natural-looking umbilicus. J Plast Surg Hand Surg. 2013;47(2):155–7.
18. Pitanguy I. Abdominal lipectomy. Clin Plast Surg. 1975;2(3):401–10.
19. Freeman BS, Wiemer DR. Abdominoplasty with special attention to construction of the umbilicus: technique and complications. Aesthetic Plast Surg. 1978;2(1):65–74. 41.
20. Matarasso A. Abdominoplasty. In: Guyuron B, editor. Plastic surgery: indications, operations, and outcomes. St. Louis: Mosby; 2000. p. 2783–821.
21. Lee MJ, Mustoe TA. Simplified technique for creating a youthful umbilicus in abdominoplasty. Plast Reconstr Surg. 2002;109(6):2136–40.
22. Akbaş H, Güneren E, Eroğlu L, Uysal OA. Natural-looking umbilicus as an important part of abdominoplasty. Aesthetic Plast Surg. 2003;27(2):139–42.
23. Aly A, Rotemberg SC, Cram A. Abdominoplasty. In: Guyuron B, Eriksson E, Persing JA, Chung KC, Dis JJ, Gosain AK, Kinney BM, Rubin JP, editors. Plastic surgery: indications and practice. Edinburgh: Saunders Elsevier; 2009. p. 1609–26.
24. Thomas M, DSilva JA, Menon H, Padubidri R. Deciding the position of neoumbilicus in abdominoplasty: a novel idea. Am J Cosm Surg. 2007;24(4):181–2.
25. Southwell-Keely JP, Berry MG. Umbilical reconstruction: a review of techniques. J Plast Reconstr Aesthet Surg. 2011;64(6):803–8.
26. Sabatier PH, Barray L, Picaud AJ. Une technique originale de refection de l'ombilic. Ann Chir Plast. 1978;23(4):245–8.
27. Avelar J. Abdominoplasty-Systematization of a technique without external umbilical scar. Aesthetic Plast Surg. 1978;2(1):141–51.
28. Jamra FA. Reconstruction of the umbilicus by a double V-Y procedure. Plast Reconstr Surg. 1979;64(1):106–7.
29. Hodgkinson DJ. Umbilicoplasty: conversion of "outie" to "innie". Aesthetic Plast Surg. 1983;7(4):221–2.
30. Ohana J, Illouz YG, Elbaz JS, Flageul G. New approach to abdominal plasties. Technical classification and surgical indications. Progress allowed by liposuction, neo-umbilicoplasty and use of biological glue. Ann Chir Plast Esthet. 1987;32(4):344–53.
31. Hatoko M, Harashina T. Reconstruction of the umbilicus using a full thickness skin grafting. Jpn J Plast Reconstr Surg. 1989;32:1279–82.
32. Matsuo K, Kondoh S, Hirose T. A simple technique for reconstruction of the umbilicus, using a conchal cartilage composite graft. Plast Reconstr Surg. 1990;86(1):149–51.
33. Ribeiro L, Muzy S, Accorsi A. Omphaloplasty. Ann Plast Surg. 1991;27(5):457–75.
34. Itoh Y, Arai K. Umbilical reconstruction using a cone-shaped flap. Ann Plast Surg. 1992;28(4):335–8.
35. Miller MJ, Balch CM. "Iris" technique for immediate umbilical reconstruction. Plast Reconstr Surg. 1993;92(4):754–6.
36. de Lacerda DJ, Martins DM, Marques A, Brenda E, de Moura Andrews J. Umbilicoplasty for the abdomen with a thin adipose layer. Br J Plast Surg. 1994;47(5):386–7.
37. Marconi F. Reconstruction of the umbilicus: a simple technique. Plast Reconstr Surg. 1995;95(6):1115–7.

38. Sugawara Y, Hirabayashi S, Asato H, Yoshimura K. Reconstruction of the umbilicus using a single triangular flap. Ann Plast Surg. 1995;34(1):78–80.
39. Sawada Y. An umbilical reconstruction using a subcutaneous pedicle flap. Eur J Plast Surg. 1995;18(4):185–8.
40. Onishi K, Yang YL, Maruyama Y. A new lunch box-type method in umbilical reconstruction. Ann Plast Surg. 1995;35(6):654–6.
41. Massiha H, Montegut W, Phillips R. A method of reconstructing a natural-looking umbilicus in abdominoplasty. Ann Plast Surg. 1997;38(3):228–31.
42. Baack BR, Anson G, Nachbar JM, White DJ. Umbilicoplasty: the construction of a new umbilicus and correction of umbilical stenosis without external scars. Plast Reconstr Surg. 1996;97(1):227–32.
43. Yotsuyanagi T, Nihei Y, Sawada Y. A simple technique for reconstruction of the umbilicus, using two twisted flaps. Plast Reconstr Surg. 1998;102(7):2444–6.
44. Schoeller T, Wechselberger G, Otto A, Rainer C, Schwabegger A, Lille S, Ninković M. New technique for scarless umbilical reinsertion in abdominoplasty procedures. Plast Reconstr Surg. 1998;102(5):1720–3.
45. Cannistrà C, Pecorelli E. Umbilical restoration in abdominal dermolipectomy: a simple double-Y, double M technique. Aesthetic Plast Surg. 1999;23(5):364–6.
46. Shinohara H, Matsuo K, Kikuchi N. Umbilical reconstruction with an inverted C-V flap. Plast Reconstr Surg. 2000;105(2):703–5.
47. Abenavoli FM, Cusano V, Cucchiara V, D'Amico C, Corvelli L. An idea for umbilicus reconstruction. Ann Plast Surg. 2001;46(2):194.
48. Schoeller T, Rainer C, Wechselberger G, Piza-Katzer H. Immediate navel reconstruction after total excision: a simple three-suture technique. Surgery. 2002;131(1):105–7.
49. Masuda R, Takeda A, Sugimoto T, Ishiguro M, Uchinuma E. Reconstruction of the umbilicus using a reverse fan-shaped flap. Aesthetic Plast Surg. 2003;27(5):349–53.
50. Meirer R, Wechselberger G, Schoeller T. Purse-string method for immediate umbilical reconstruction. Plast Reconstr Surg. 2004;114(3):831–2.
51. Ozbek S, Ozcan M. Umbilicus reconstruction with modified 'unfolded cylinder' technique. Br J Plast Surg. 2005;58(4):500–3.
52. Uraloğlu M, Tekin F, Orbay H, Unlü RE, Sensöz O. Simultaneous abdominoplasty and umbilical reconstruction using a modified C-V flap technique. Plast Reconstr Surg. 2006;117(7):2525–6.
53. Sevin A, Sevin K, Senen D, Erdogan B. A new method for umbilicus reconstruction: preliminary report. Aesthetic Plast Surg. 2006;30(5):589–91.
54. Kakudo N, Kusumoto K, Fujimori S, Shimotsuma A, Ogawa Y. Reconstruction of a natural-appearing umbilicus using an island flap: case report. J Plast Reconstr Aesthet Surg. 2006;59(9):999–1002.
55. Castillo PF, Sepúlveda CA, Prado AC, Troncoso AL, Villamán JJ. Umbilical reinsertion in abdominoplasty: technique using deepithelialized skin flaps. Aesthetic Plast Surg. 2007;31(5):519–20.
56. Rozen SM, Redett R. The two-dermal-flap umbilical transposition: a natural and aesthetic umbilicus after abdominoplasty. Plast Reconstr Surg. 2007;119(7):2255–62.
57. Rogliani M, Silvi E, Arpino A, Gentile P, Grimaldi M, Cervelli V. The Maltese cross technique: umbilical reconstruction after dermolipectomy. J Plast Reconstr Aesthet Surg. 2007;60(9):1036–8.
58. Amud RJM. Neo-onfaloplastiasemcicatriz. Rev Bras Cir Plast. 2008;23(1):37–40.
59. Barbosa MV, Nahas FX, SabiaNeto MA, Ferreira LM. Strategies in umbilical reconstruction. J Plast Reconstr Aesthet Surg. 2009;62(6):e147–50.
60. Takasu H, Watanabe Y. Umbilicoplasty with 3 triangular skin flaps and excised diamond-shaped skin flap. J Pediatr Surg. 2010;45(10):2041–4.
61. Gonçalves de Freitas JO, Guerreiro V, Sperli AE. Neo-onfaloplastiana dermolipectomia abdominal: técnica do duplo "V". Rev Bras Cir Plást. 2010;25(3):504–8.

62. Mazzocchi M, Trignano E, Armenti AF, Figus A, Dessy LA. Long-term results of a versatile technique for umbilicoplasty in abdominoplasty. Aesthetic Plast Surg. 2011;35(4):456–62.
63. Cló TC, Nogueira DS. A new umbilical reconstruction technique used for 306 consecutive abdominoplasties. Aesthetic Plast Surg. 2012;36(5):1009–14.
64. Arai K, Yamashita K, Suda T, Ikeda K, Yamauchi M, Yotsuyanagi T. Primary reconstruction of the umbilicus, using two rectangular subcutaneous pedicle flaps. J Plast Reconstr Aesthet Surg. 2012;65(1):132–4.
65. Gera P, Henry G. Double purse string makes a nice umbilical ring: a novel technique for umbilicoplasty. Eur J Pediatr Surg. 2013;23(2):164–6.
66. Donnabella A. Reconstrução anatômica da cicatriz umbilical. Rev Bras Cir Plast. 2013;28(1):119–23.
67. Morshed G. A simple new technique for neo-umbilicoplasty. Med J Cairo Univ. 2012;80(1):759–61.
68. Kajikawa A, Ueda K, Suzuki Y, Ohkouchi M. A new umbilicoplasty for children: creating a longitudinal deep umbilical depression. J Plast Surg. 2004;57(8):741–8.
69. Kom AN, Anani MA, Azanledji BM, Komlan A, Komla G, Hubert T. Umbilicoplasty in children with huge umbilical hernia. Afr J Paediatr Surg. 2014;11(3):256–60.
70. Shiffman MA. Umbilical hernia repair with abdominoplasty. Am J Cosm Surg. 2013;30(3):189–92.
71. Aaronson A: Tummy tuck can also repair your umbilical hernia. http://EzineArticles.com/?expert=A_Aaronson. Accessed 17 June 2011.
72. Aaronson A. Tummy tuck can also repair your umbilical hernia. http://www.articlesbase.com/diseases-and-conditions-articles/tummy-tuck-can-include-umbilical-hernia-repair-472821.html#ixzz1PjltCfPd Accessed 19 June 2011.
73. Bruner TW, Salazar-Reyes H, Friedman JD. Umbilical hernia repair in conjunction with abdominoplasty: a novel surgical technique to maintain umbilical blood supply. Aesthet Surg J. 2009;29(4):333–4.
74. Neinstein RM, Matarasso A, Abramson DL. Concomitant abdominoplasty and umbilical hernia repair using the ventralex hernia patch. Plast Reconstr Surg. 2015;135(4):1021–5.
75. Borges AF. Reconstruction of the umbilicus. Br J Plast Surg. 1975;28(1):75–6.
76. Apfelberg DB, Maser MR, Lash H. Two unusual umbilicoplasties. Plast Reconstr Surg. 1979;64(2):268–70.
77. Reyna TM, Hollis Jr HW, Smith SB. Surgical management of proboscoid herniae. J Pediatr Surg. 1987;22(10):911–2.
78. Blanchard H, St-Vil D, Carceller A, Bensoussan AL, Di Lorenzo M. Repair of the huge umbilical hernia in black children. J Pediatr Surg. 2000;35(5):696–8.
79. Billmire DF. A technique for the repair of giant umbilical hernia in children. J Am Coll Surg. 2002;194(5):677–80.
80. Tamir G, Kurzbart E. Umbilical reconstruction after repair of large umbilical hernia: the "lazy-M" and omega flaps. J Pediatr Surg. 2004;39(2):226–8.
81. el-Dessouki NI, Shehata SM, Torki AM, Hashish AA. Double half-cone flap umbilicoplasty: a new technique for the proboscoid umbilical hernia in children. Hernia. 2004;8(3):182–5.
82. Kaneko K, Tsuda M. Four-triangular-skin-flap approach to umbilical diseases and laparoscopic umbilical port. J Pediatr Surg. 2004;39(9):1404–7.
83. Ikeda H, Yamamoto H, Fujino J, Kisaki Y, Uchida H, Ishimaru Y, Hasumi T, Hamajima A. Umbilicoplasty for large protruding umbilicus accompanying umbilical hernia: a simple and effective technique. Pediatr Surg Int. 2004;20(2):105–7.
84. Sankalé AA, Ngom G, Fall I, Coulibaly NF, Ndoye M. Umbilical reconstruction in children. Prospective report of 77 cases. Ann Chir Plast Esthet. 2004;49(1):17–23.

Part IV
Techniques

Chapter 11
Pathological Umbilical Scar Management with 5-FU Injections

Guillermo Blugerman, Diego Schavelzon, Gabriel Wexler, and Marcelo Lotocky

11.1 Introduction

The surgeon's struggle against wound healing disorders also takes place in the umbilical region. The umbilicus is the only scar the surgeon has to reconstruct because this procedure will refine the outcomes of the abdominal surgery, and at the same time new scar development risk must be lowered to avoid the stigmata of surgery. Unfortunately many times the scarring process is overactive, producing deviations of the normal process resulting in hypertrophic scars and keloids.

Scar resulting from umbilical reconstruction or reimplantation is treated by physical or chemical methods. Hypertrophic scars and keloid formation may require some treatment to stop the growth of the scar tissue and to keep the natural appearance of the belly button.

Wound healing disorders can lead to the complete closure of the umbilicus. The prevention of umbilical stenosis lies in the operative techniques, pressotherapy, and adjuvant treatments.

Wound healing process has three phases:

1. Phase one or the inflammatory phase starts within the very few minutes after injury and lasts about 2 or 3 days (not complicated scenario). The objective is to

G. Blugerman, M.D. (✉) • D. Schavelzon
B & S Center of Excellence in Plastic Surgery, Laprida 1579, Buenos Aires, Argentina
e-mail: blugerman@centrosbys.com; drschavelzon@gmail.com; gabrielew555@hotmail.com; aliasmarce@hotmail.com

G. Wexler, M.D. • M. Lotocky, M.D.
B & S Center of Excellence in Plastic Surgery, Private Practice, Laprida 1579, Buenos Aires, Argentina

M.A. Shiffman (ed.), *Adult Umbilical Reconstruction*,
DOI 10.1007/978-3-319-43887-0_11

remove damaged tissue and strange bodies as well as to establish immunological control. Several mediators of the inflammatory response stimulate the production of collagen.
2. Phase two or the tissue proliferation phase starts about 72 h later after the injury and lasts about 3–6 weeks. The objective is to reestablish the integrity of the functional structure of the damaged tissue as soon as possible. Macrophages, fibroblasts, and capillary endothelial cells prevail.
3. Phase three or the remodeling phase is characterized by the replacement of collagen fibers deposited in an anarchical way in order to get a more organized structure. There is a prevalence of macrophages and fibroblasts, and this stage can last about 6–12 months.

11.2 Abnormal Wound Healing

11.2.1 Hypertrophic Scar

1. The overgrowth of scar tissue that typically does not expand beyond the boundaries of the initial injury. This growth occurs by pushing the margins of the scar outward rather than the invasion of the surrounding normal tissue.
2. It affects only humans.
3. No genetic predisposition demonstrated.
4. The occurrence of hypertrophic scars has equal sex, age, and race distribution.
5. Hypertrophic scars often develop in 2nd- and 3rd-degree burns.
6. Hypertrophic scarring develops in wounds at anatomic locations in all the body especially limbs and trunk.
7. The scars that cross joints in a right angle are more susceptible.
8. Remission can be spontaneous in 12–18 months.
9. It can be improved with surgery.

11.2.2 Characteristics of Keloids

Keloids are thick scars in human skin or cornea produced by an excessive amount of collagen synthesis over long periods of time. They can progressively invade surrounding tissue and produce benign dermal tumors with no malignant potential. It only affects humans.

Keloids may have a genetic component, but the way they are inherited is not yet clear:

1. More frequent in dark-skinned patients (high melanocytes content).
2. Genetically associated with HLA-B14, BW16, and blood group A.
3. They have equal sex distribution and may appear at any age; however, the peak age is 10–30 years.
4. They can occur even years after the injury.

5. The size of the scar is not related with the initial injury. The margins of the scar go beyond the initial injury.
6. Spontaneous remittance is uncommon.
7. Most sensitive areas are the presternal region, the back, and the nape, followed by the ears, the deltoid region, and the beard.

The clinical appearance of wounds varies from pedunculated and multilobular ones to those flat with regular margins. It is uncommon that keloids penetrate subcutaneous tissue. Keloids can invade surrounding skin from few millimeters to 2–3 cm, and they range in consistency from soft and elastic to rubbery and hard. They constantly itch, but they rarely send stinging pain through the skin. They can continue growing, cause muscle contraction, and hinder movement

11.3 Therapeutic Options for the Treatment of Hypertrophic Scars and Keloids

1. Surgery
2. Radiation therapy
3. Compression
4. Silicone gel sheets
5. Laser
6. Corticosteroid
7. Cryotherapy
8. Interferon

11.3.1 Other Pharmacological Agents

1. 5-FU intralesional
2. Topical retinoic acid
3. Topical putrescine
4. Injected verapamil
5. Imiquimod
6. Vancomycin

11.4 Combined Therapy

11.4.1 5-Fluorouracil

Since Fitzpatrick [1] published his work with 5-fluorouracil (5-FU) in 1999, the authors included it in the daily practice. The most frequent use of this drug is for the treatment and prevention of hypertrophic scars, keloids, and foreign body granulomas [2].

Fibroblast proliferation and migration play a major role in wound healing. Their main metabolic function is collagen, elastin, and proteoglycan synthesis. Fibroblast suppression in hypertrophic scars and keloids is essential since collagen synthesis is increased by 14 % and 20 %, respectively, compared to normal skin. Other studies show a higher amount of fibroblasts without significant increase in collagen synthesis, but with altered proportions between collagens I, III, and IV. These studies also show an increase in the production of fibronectin by fibroblasts. The local increase of collagenase inhibitors has also been reported.

Other subsequent studies have shown in vitro and in vivo that 5-FU modulates the fibroblast activity reducing and regulating collagen production, thus avoiding chaotic arrangement of collagen bundles, which is typical of hypertrophic scars and keloids

Local steroids have been the gold standard treatment for umbilical inflammatory and fibrotic processes for years, but its use has important side effects and complications. Triamcinolone usually generates different grades of skin atrophy and telangiectasia. Therefore, we prefer to use Fitzpatrick's formula: the combination of 0.1 mL of triamcinolone and 0.9 ml of 5FU per ml used for infiltration [3].

5-FU is a cytostatic antimetabolite drug, which inhibits cell proliferation by:

1. Inhibition of thymidylate synthase avoiding DNA synthesis
2. Incorporation in RNA and DNA altering its function
3. Interference with glycosyltransferases altering cell membranes

5-FU has been used for years in treatment of premalignant and malignant lesions of the skin and mucosa due to its selective toxicity for dysplastic epithelium and fibroblasts. The first application of 5-FU was as an antifibrotic to prevent fibrous scarring after glaucoma surgery and to avoid relapse in pterygium surgery in the 1960s [4–7]. In 1999 Fitzpatrick published his 7-year experience of over a thousand patients with 5-FU in hypertrophic scars and keloids. This magnificent work encouraged our team to include it in our office with positive results.

When performing umbilical surgery in patients with history of wound healing disorders, a gauze is soaked in 1 mL of 5 FU (50 mg/mL) and applied for 5 min in the surgical field. When the topical application is finished, the skin is closed. This protocol was adapted from hand surgeons that use 5-FU to repair tendons and avoid adhesion [8].

It has been proven in laboratory tests that 5-FU produces a slight reduction of collagen synthesis in normal fibroblasts but a drastic reduction in altered ones, as in Dupuytren's contracture [9]. Apparently it also inhibits the collagen synthesis stimulation effect of TGF1 (transforming growth factor).

Triamcinolone is a steroid; it diffuses through cell membranes binding with cytoplasmic receptors that are translocated to the nucleus generating the transcription of proteins that are responsible of their effects. It reduces tissue response to inflammation, reducing its symptoms without treating the specific cause. To do this it reduces the white blood cells (WBC) migration to the affected tissue.

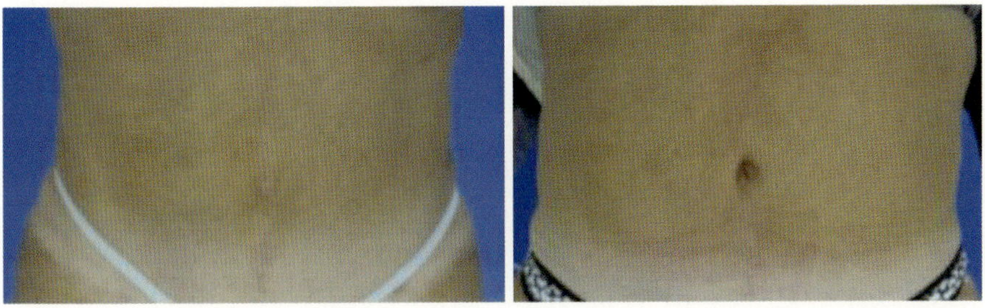

Fig. 11.1 (*Left*) Patient after abdominoplasty with umbilical transposition. Observe the umbilical stenosis created by scar contracture. (*Right*) After 3 sessions of 5-FU and external tutor

The most important effects are:

1. Inhibition of phagocytosis
2. Inhibition of liberation of lysosomal enzymes and inflammatory mediators
3. Reduction of capillary permeability and WBC adhesion to capillary endothelium
4. Reduction of blood concentration of T cells, eosinophils, and monocytes
5. Reduction of immunoglobulin binding with cellular receptors

For the past 16 years, the authors have been using a preparation of 5-FU and triamcinolone for the umbilical area, and we have not had the complications and side effects observed with steroid mono-treatment (Fig. 11.1 and 11.2).

Another possibility for the umbilicus surgery is the perioperative calcium channel antagonist therapy, which has been shown to be effective to stop hypertrophic scarring [10]. To avoid umbilical stenosis, a little glass ball (marble) can be used to exert even compression around the entire circumference of the umbilicus, thus keeping it dilated.

11.5 Technique

5-FU (fluorouracil-filaxis 500 mg) is presented commercially as ampules of 10 mL containing 50 mg per mL. Triamcinolone (Kenacort-A-BSM) is used in its acetonide form of 40 mg/mL and is commercialized in ampules of 1 mL (Fig. 11.3). For the application, a Luer Lock syringe and 30G needle are preferred. This allows a better dosage and correct plane of infiltration. We have never used more than 3 mL of the solution in the umbilicus per session. The infiltration is done with multiple punctures in the "heart" of the fibrotic lesion. The first month sessions are carried out weekly and then every 15 days. The improvement is evaluated with three parameters: hardening reduction, loss of volume, and reduction of cutaneous retraction. Positive changes are observed since the first session, not only in the above

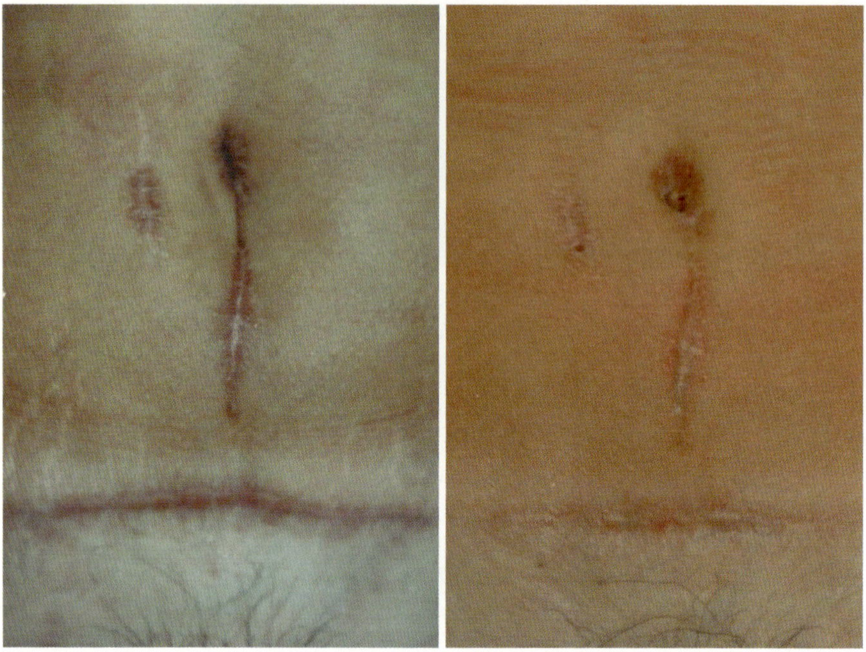

Fig. 11.2 (*Left*) Patient after combined gynecologic and abdominal wall surgery with hypertrophic scarring. (*Right*) After 3 sessions of 5-FU

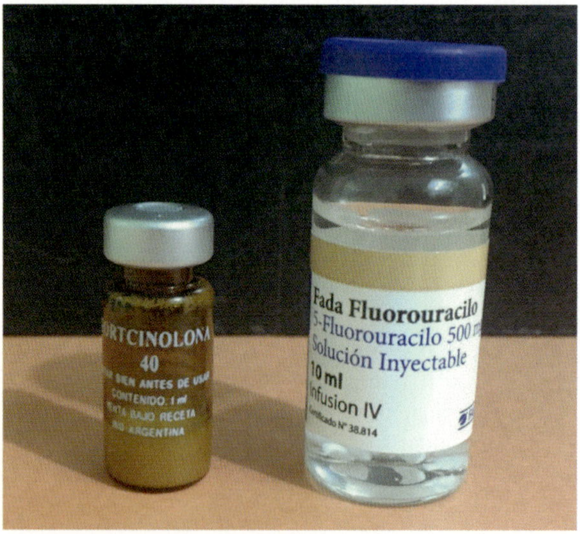

Fig. 11.3 Commercial presentation of 5-FU and triamcinolone

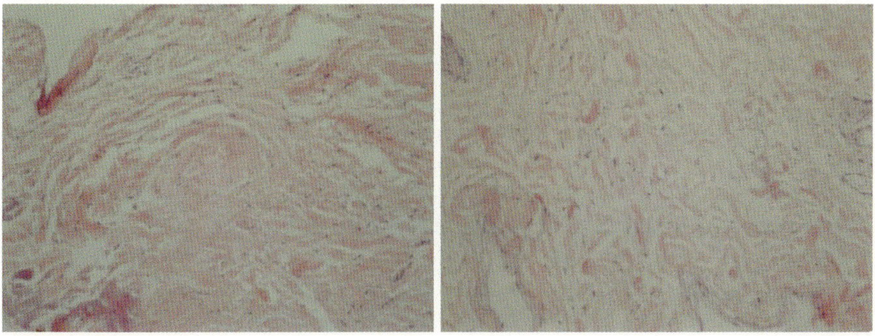

Fig. 11.4 Microscopic image of fibrosis without any infiltration treatment (*left*). Microscopic image of fibrosis after infiltration with 5-FU on the (*right*). Observe the organization of collagen fibers and fibroblasts

parameters but also in aesthetics and pain-itching symptomatology. Some cases are complemented with kinesiology treatment in order to obtain a better functional and cosmetic result.

11.6 Histopathology

If after finishing the treatment a surgical procedure was needed to improve the result, the surgical piece was sent to the pathologist and compared to non-treated scarring tissue resections. Results informed reduction of fibrosis and rearrangement of collagen tissue in the treated pieces (Fig. 11.4). These results are illustrated in the images. In the tissue of the right side of the scar, proliferation of fibrous tissue, great amount of fibroblasts, and collagen fiber-forming tangles are seen. In the tissue of the left, treated with 5-FU solution, there are fewer fibroblasts, and the collagen fibers adopt a parallel disposition.

11.7 Complications

The use of 5-FU solution, in young patients mostly, can cause tissue necrosis. This is relatively frequent in keloid treatment, resulting in ulcers or brown stains in the application spots. However in the umbilical region, we have not observed this complication, mainly because of the low dosage. In this way, by using progressive treatment instead of aggressive one, side effects are kept to a minimum.

11.8 Conclusions

Through this chapter, the authors have presented their experience in the treatment of scars, fibrosis, retractions, and deformities over the umbilical skin. The results of 16 years of experience with 5-FU solution (5-FU, triamcinolone) have histopathologically demonstrated the effectiveness of collagen fiber synthesis reduction and fiber rearrangement, thus explaining the positive clinical effect.

References

1. Fitzpatrick RE. Treatment of inflamed hypertrophic scars using intralesional 5-FU. Dermatol Surg. 1999;25(3):224–32.
2. Blugerman G. Keloids and Hypertrophic scars. Congreso de Cirugía Plástica del Cono Sur, Porto Alegre. Brasil: Mayo; 2001.
3. Blugerman G, Schavelzon D. Intralesional use of 5-FU in subcutaneous fibrosis. J Drugs Dermatol. 2003;2:169–71.
4. Yamamoto T, Varani J, Soong HK, Lichter PR. Effect of 5-fluorouracil and mitomycin on cultured rabbit subconjunctival fibroblast. Ophthalmology. 1990;97:1202–10.
5. Yeatts RP, Ford JG, Stanton CA, Reed JW. Topical 5-fluorouracil in the intra epithelial neoplasia of the conjuntiva and cornea. Ophthalmology. 1995;102:1388–44.
6. Lee DA, Shapourifar-Tehrani S, Kitada S. The effect of 5-fluorouracil and cytarabine on human fibroblasts from Tenon's capsule. Invest Ophthalmol Vis Sci. 1990;31:1848–55.
7. Schellini SA, Shiratori CN, Spirandelli PH, Shiratori CA, Padovani CR. Uso do 5-fluorouracil no intra-operatório da cirurgia do pterígio. Arq Bras Oftalmol. 2000;63(2):111–4.
8. Acali A, Khan U, Khaw PT, McGrouther AD. Decrease in adhesión formation by a single application of 5Fluorouracil after flexor tendon injury. Plast Reconstr Surg. 1999;103(1):151–8.
9. Jemec B, Linge C, Grobbelaar AO, Smith PJ, Sanders R, McGrouther DA. The effect of 5-fluorouracil on Dupuytren fibroblast proliferation and differentiation. Chir Main. 2000;19(1):15–22.
10. Viera MH, Amini S, Valins W, Berman B. Innovative therapies in the treatment of keloids and hypertrophic scars. J Clin Aesthet Dermatol. 2010;3(5):20–6.

Chapter 12
The Umbilicus

Charlotte W. Ying and Darryl J. Hodgkinson

12.1 Introduction

The umbilicus is the only natural scar in the body and marks the attachment site of the umbilical cord to the placenta. All placental mammals have a navel, and it is quite conspicuous in humans. Other animals' navels are smoother and flatter, often not more than a thin line, and are usually obscured by hair.

12.2 Anatomy

The umbilicus is a visual guide for the separation of the abdomen into quadrants, it being the "center" of the abdomen, and this position is relatively consistent among humans [1]. Even as early as the 15th century, Leonardo da Vinci recognized the navel as being the center of the circle enclosing the "spread-eagle" figure of his famous Vitruvian Man drawing. The nerve supply to the umbilicus is from the tenth thoracic dermatome (Fig. 12.1) [2]. The principle blood supply to the umbilicus is from the deep inferior epigastric arteries; the ligamentum teres and the median umbilical ligament vessels also contribute. Lymphatic drainage of the umbilicus can

C.W. Ying, MB.BCh (Hons); BAO (Hons); LRCP.SI (✉)
The Cosmetic and Restorative Surgery Clinic, Private Practice, 20 Manning Road, Double Bay, Sydney, NSW 2028, Australia
e-mail: cywing@gmail.com

D.J. Hodgkinson, MB.BS (Hons); FRCS (C);FACS;FACCS
Diplomat American Board of Plastic and Reconstructive Surgery, The Cosmetic and Restorative Surgery Clinic, 20 Manning Road, Double Bay, Sydney, NSW 2028, Australia
e-mail: djh@drhodgkinson.com

M.A. Shiffman (ed.), *Adult Umbilical Reconstruction*,
DOI 10.1007/978-3-319-43887-0_12

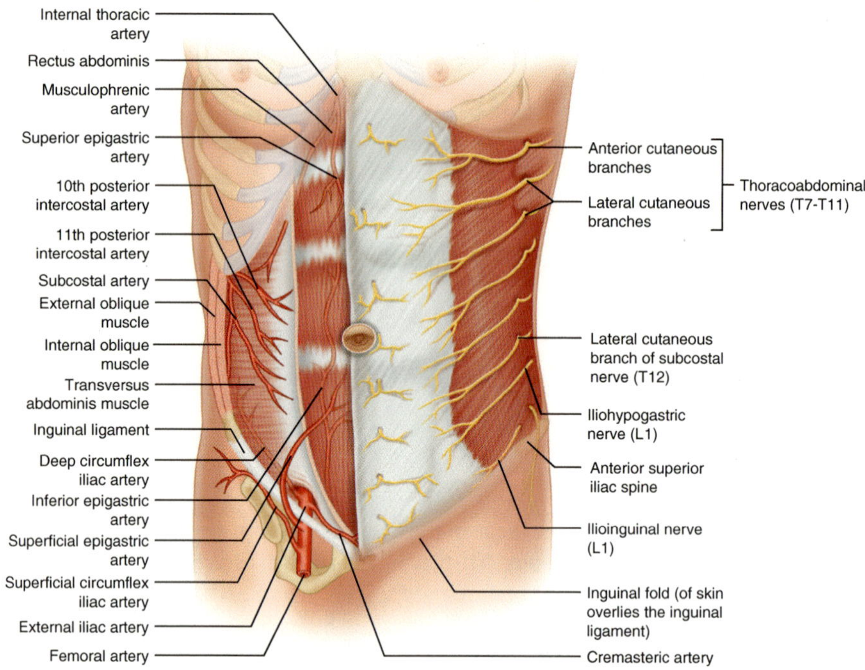

Fig. 12.1 Innervation and blood supply to the umbilicus [3]

be seen to be divided in a "quadrantic" manner, draining into the deep axillary and superficial inguinal nodes (Fig. 12.2) [3].

Surface anatomy of the umbilicus is typically at a vertical level corresponding to the level of the fibrocartilage between the third and fourth lumbar vertebrae, with a normal variation among people between L3 and L5 vertebrae. Anteriorly, it lies along the midline at the level of the superior iliac crests and is halfway between the xiphisternum and pubic symphysis [4].

12.3 Umbilicus Development

The umbilicus marks the location where the umbilical cord was attached. It is the point at which the lateral somatopleuric plates fused and thus shut off the intraembryonic coelom from the extraembryonic coelom, which is enclosed between the amnion and chorion. When the embryo is an inch (25.4 mm) long at 9-weeks' gestation, the primitive umbilicus, not having kept pace with body growth, remains comparatively small [5]. When the somatic layers gradually contract around the yolk sac and allantoic stalk, the umbilicus and umbilical cord are formed. The umbilical cord

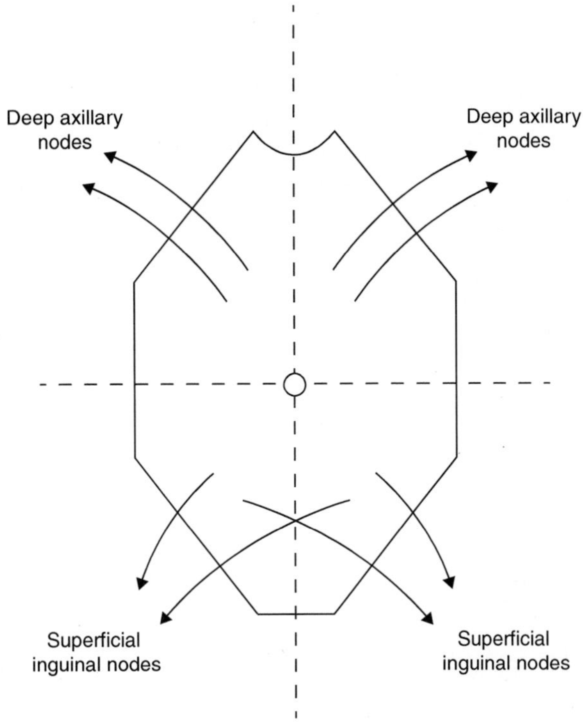

Fig. 12.2 Lymphatic drainage of the anterior abdominal wall [1]

continues to provide nutritional support to the fetus until birth [5]. After birth, the umbilical cord is clamped and the remnant desiccates over time, eventually detaches to reveal the umbilicus.

12.4 Cultural Influences

The exposure of the male and female midriff and bare navels was taboo and considered immodest or indecent in Western cultures [6]. This was even banned in some jurisdictions; however, public perceptions have changed, and exposure of female midriff and navel is widely accepted today [6]. While the West was relatively resistant to midriff-baring clothing until the 1980s, it has long been a fashion with the Asian and Indian cultures. The Japanese in particular have long had a special regard for the navel. During the early Jomon period (5000–2500 B.C.) in northern Japan, three "small balls" illustrating the umbilicus and breasts were pasted onto flat clay bodies to represent the female form. The navel was exaggerated in size, informed by the belief that it symbolizes the center of where life begins (Fig. 12.3) [7]. An interesting observation of their clay sculptures shows that the navels were all represented

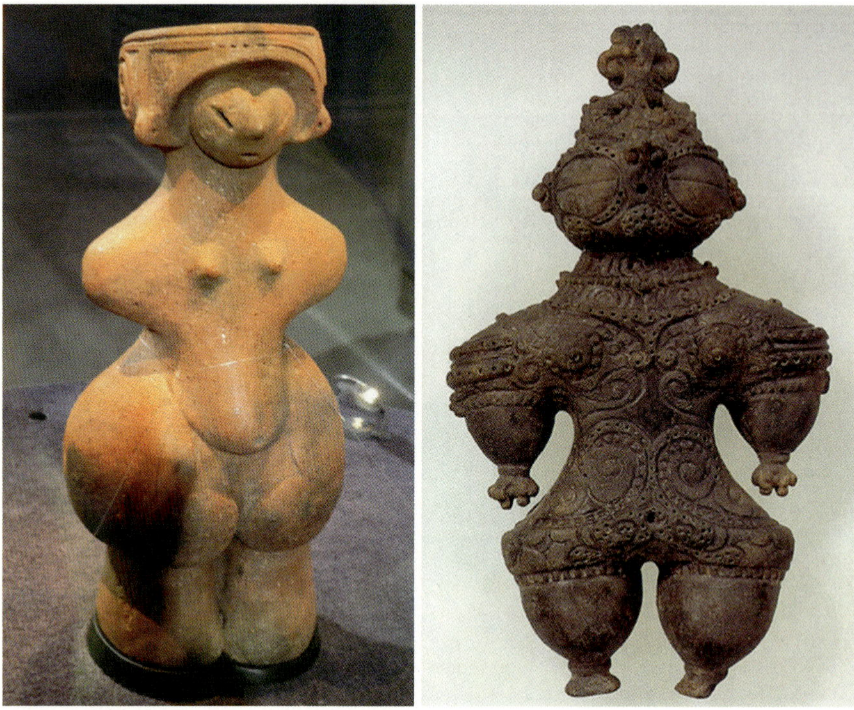

Fig. 12.3 Jomon period clay sculpture with the oval-shaped navel representing center of life [7] (Photographs a and b by Takuma-sa and Bigjap respectively, distributed under a CC-BY-SA 3.0 license. Cropped from originals)

as an "innie" and oval shaped, which corresponds to the modern-day aesthetic standards of a navel (see Sect. 12.5).

12.5 Shapes

The umbilicus is essential in contributing to a pleasant visual abdominal contour. It helps define the medial abdominal sulcus and provides a shapely curve for the inferior abdomen. Its absence leads to an unnatural abdominal appearance, and an abnormally shaped or misplaced umbilicus may draw undue attention to the central abdomen [8].

The umbilicus is a "depressed scar" surrounded by a natural skin fold that measures 15–20 mm in diameter. It is usually flat and vertically oriented in young individuals, and over time "hooding" develops with a deepening of the stalk as fat accumulates along the deep fat pocket that surrounds the umbilicus [9, 10]. A transverse orientation generally occurs after childbirth. Aging in combination with weight gain will contribute to a deeper umbilical stalk and an overall widened appearance [11].

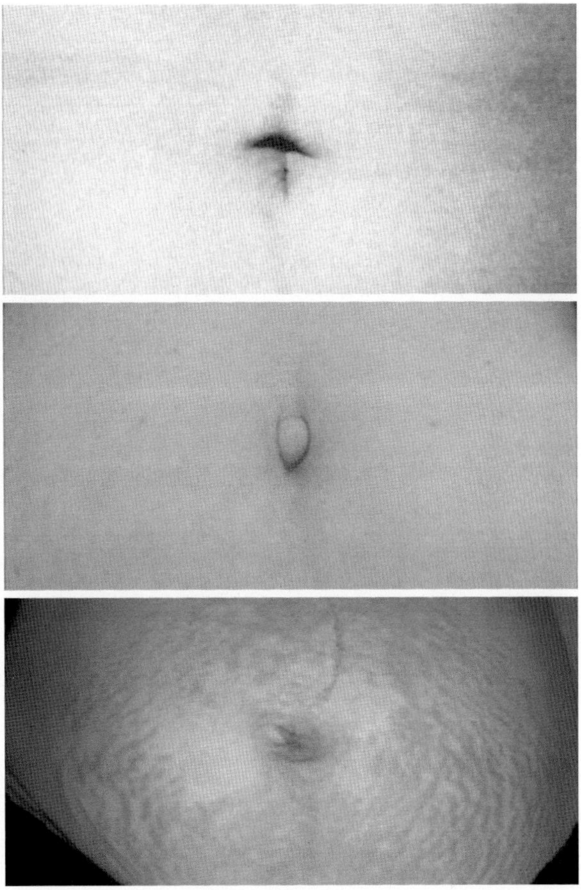

Fig. 12.4 (*Above*) Umbilical hooding characterized by a superior hood or shelf; (*center*) umbilical protrusion outside central concavity; and (*below*) an excessively large umbilicus [12]

A wide and deep umbilicus and an exceedingly small umbilicus are considered unattractive (Fig. 12.4). The presence of outward protrusion (an "outie") is also considered unappealing (Fig. 12.4) [12]. A "sad" umbilicus is when there is drooping of superior umbilical skin with "downward hooding". Characteristics thought to be appealing include a moderately small umbilical size with an overall vertical orientation. The presence of a subtle superior hood or shelf is also thought to add a youthful, more pleasing yet "mysterious" appearance to the abdomen.

Five main types of umbilical shapes were described by Craig et al. when they set out to search for the "ideal female umbilicus" (Fig. 12.5): T shaped, oval shaped, vertically shaped, horizontally shaped, and distorted shapes [13]. Other characteristics considered were umbilical hooding, protrusion, and size (Fig. 12.4). They summarized that "the most aesthetically pleasing umbilicus is small in size, T or vertical in shape, and possesses a superior hood or shelf." The unappealing characteristics are large, horizontal, or distorted shaped and the presence of a protrusion [13].

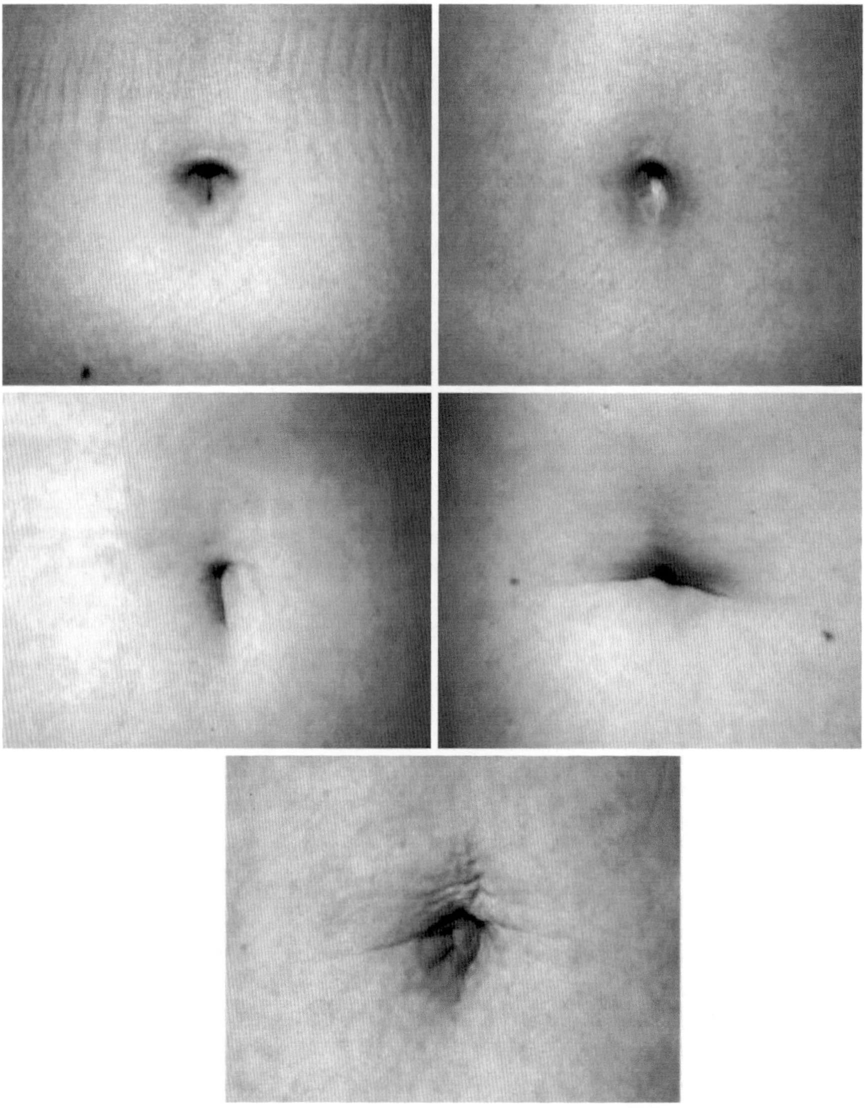

Fig. 12.5 The five main umbilical shapes. (*Above, left*) T shaped, (*above, right*) oval shaped, (*center, left*) vertical shaped, (*center, right*) horizontally shaped, (*below*) distorted shape [12]

12.6 Umbilical Pathology

Most pathology related to the umbilicus occurs during neonatal years. Among these, umbilical hernias are most prevalent, followed by iatrogenic causes in adults and obesity causing an aesthetically unpleasant appearance.

An umbilical hernia is a full-thickness protrusion of the umbilicus with an underlying fascial defect and may contain peritoneal fluid, pre-peritoneal fat, intestine, or omentum. Umbilical hernias are more frequent in premature, low birth weight infants. They also occur more often in children and adults with ascites and obesity and postpartum women with weakness of the rectus sheath and certain syndromes including Beckwith-Wiedemann, Down's, and Marfan's syndrome [14]. An umbilical hernia results when the umbilical ring fails to close. In children, umbilical hernias often resolve when the umbilical ring closes spontaneously. This usually occurs in small defects (<10 mm) rather than larger ones (>20 mm). The skin overlying an umbilical hernia may continue to stretch and result in a proboscoid umbilical hernia. Once the umbilical defect has spontaneously closed, the nipple-like umbilical skin may continue to flatten out during adolescence [15].

Iatrogenic causes include surgical complications, including necrosis following umbilicoplasty, infection, wound dehiscence, and scarring in laparotomy and/or endoscopic cases. An interesting patient-caused umbilical pathology in the New Age is umbilical piercings, which can lead to cysts and skin tears requiring repair and reconstruction.

Obesity with or without massive weight loss poses multiple health and aesthetic issues, one of which relating to this topic is the effect on the umbilicus. Obese patients generally have a large, "stretched-out" appearance of their umbilicus with an exaggerated and over-draping shelf to create a horizontal shape (Fig. 12.6).

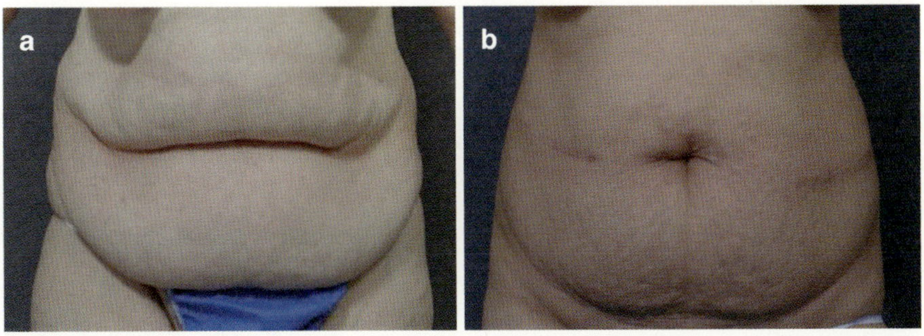

Fig. 12.6 (**a**, **b**) Effect of obesity on the umbilicus. Patients usually have a large and stretched-out umbilicus with over-draping

12.7 Umbilicoplasty in Plastic and Aesthetic Surgery

12.7.1 Hernia

Umbilical hernia repairs are almost always accompanied by umbilicoplasties due to stretching of skin to accommodate the hernial sac and therefore residual skin laxity after the repair (Fig. 12.7). The need of umbilicoplasty is dependent on the size of hernia and patient requests. As mentioned above, majority of umbilical hernias occur in neonates; however, it is common for plastic and cosmetic surgeons to encounter umbilical hernias in our patient group, mainly due to weak abdominal muscles and skin laxity. Surgical approach to umbilical hernia management is similar in both neonates and adults. The goal is to reduce the hernia and repair the fascial defect either by direct closure with nonabsorbable sutures or by using mesh repair for larger defects. Once the hernia is reduced, there are multiple methods described in the approach of umbilicoplasty, in which major differences lie in flap designs. Fan-shaped flaps of excess skin surrounding the umbilicus can be excised to reduce the diameter of the navel; superior or inferior skin flaps can also be considered, excess skin excised and redraped around the umbilicus. The umbilicus is then inverted and fixed caudally onto the fascia and skin [15–17].

12.7.2 "Outie" Umbilicus

An "outie" umbilicus is usually regarded as unattractive, and it is becoming increasingly common in the modern society for patients to consider umbilicoplasty as an aesthetic consideration. In 1983, Hodgkinson [18] described a surgical technique to convert "an outie to an innie" in a patient with scaring (Fig. 12.8). Superior and

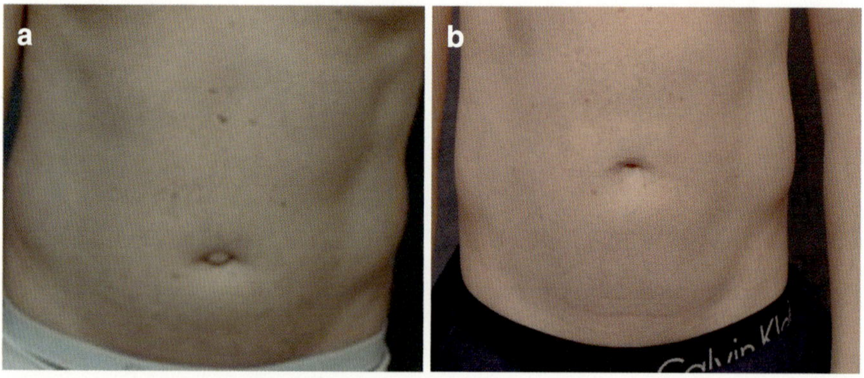

Fig. 12.7 (**a**) Preoperative. (**b**) Postoperative after umbilicoplasty with hernia repair. Excess supraumbilical skin was excised as an ellipse

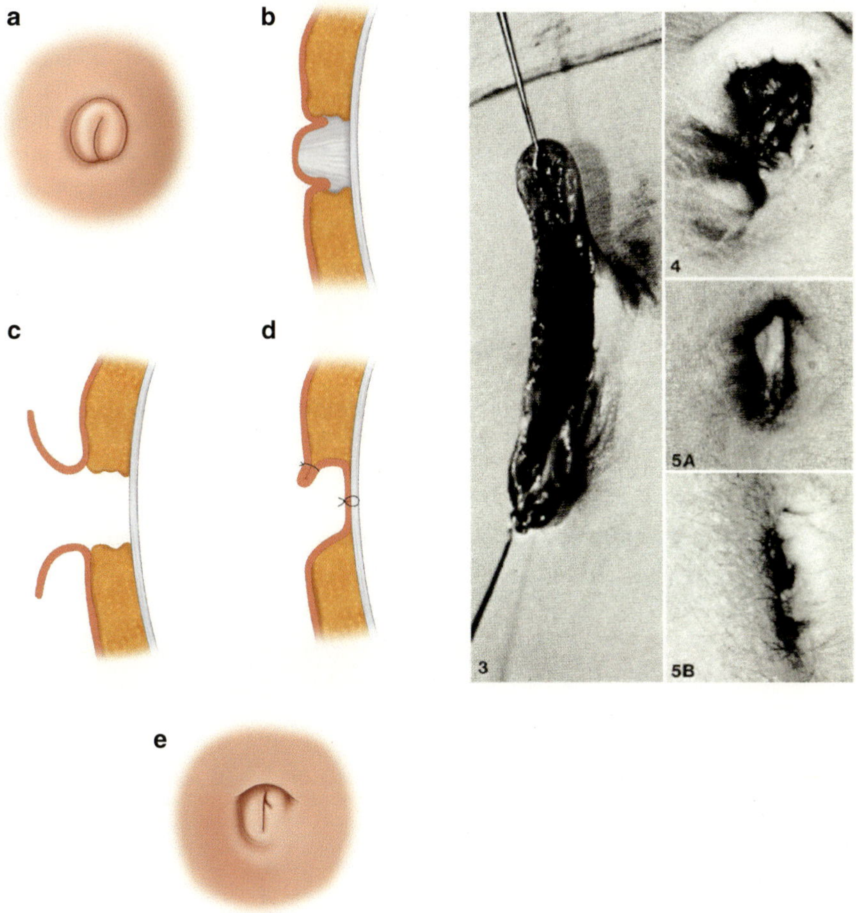

Fig. 12.8 Converting an outie to an innie. (*Left*) (**a–e**) Illustration of the surgical technique. (*Right*) Intraoperative technique with end result [17]

inferior skin flaps are elevated, the underlying scar is excised, and a hood is created by folding the superior flap upon itself. The inferior flap is then advanced into the neo-tube and sutured.

12.7.3 Abdominoplasty

Among the several mentioned situations in which a new neo-umbilicoplasty is required, the commonest reason for such is for an abdominoplasty procedure. Until the late 1950s, when Vernon advocated the preservation of the umbilicus, the umbilicus was routinely discarded during abdominoplasty, which led to unattractive results and caused problems such as omphalitis related to material accumulation [19, 20]. Since then there has been a continuing evolution in the performance of umbilical repositioning and reconstruction, which is now considered a crucial step in performing abdominoplasty. The goal in navel reinsertion is to create a natural-looking umbilicus at an appropriate depth, height, and midline position with minimal scarring (Figs. 12.9, 12.10, and 12.11). There are numerous techniques described to achieve an aesthetically acceptable navel, many authors have proposed the use of skin grafts, flaps, or even conchal cartilage composite grafts to create the anatomical shape of the umbilicus [12, 21–24].

There are three vital steps that comprise umbilical reconstruction in abdominoplasty: release of original umbilicus, reposition, and reinsertion with excess skin excision. The majority of the existing releasing procedures involve an elliptical vertical excision of the old umbilicus. Reinsertion techniques, however, differ greatly from surgeon to surgeon. Circular incision of the abdominal flap was popular until some authors reported a greater incidence of umbilical stenosis associated with this incision due to the tendency of scar contraction [24, 25]. Newer techniques then emerged to counter this problem, including the "Y"-shaped cutaneous

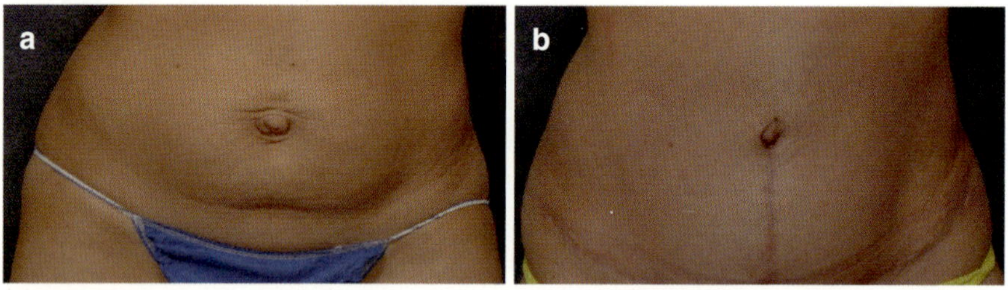

Fig. 12.9 Abdominoplasty with repair of umbilical hernia. (**a**) Preoperative. (**b**) Four months after surgery. Excess loose skin required to be excised with addition of central incision; this acts to simulate a linea alba

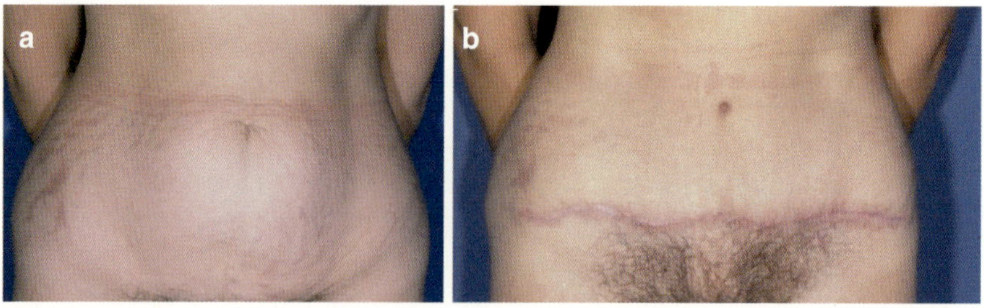

Fig. 12.10 (**a**) Preoperative (**b**) Three months postoperative following abdominoplasty with umbilicus repositioning and umbilicoplasty. Note scarring around umbilicus is much less than the horizontal low abdominoplasty scar

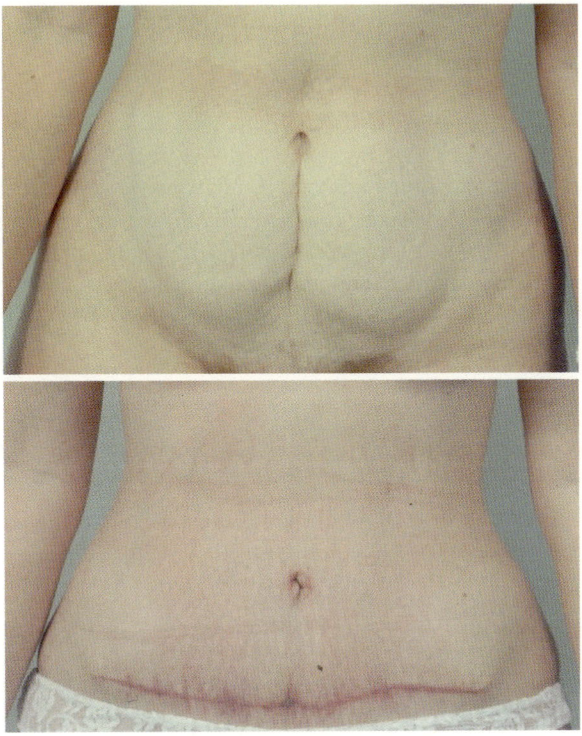

Fig. 12.11 Before and after: Abdominoplasty with umbilicus repositioning and umbilicoplasty with resection of old ventral laparotomy scar at three months

incision of the abdominal flap, with or without deepithelialization; small and multiple triangular flaps; dermal transposition flaps; etc. [23]. Scarless techniques were also described but necessitate removal of subcutaneous fat and purse-stringing of periumbilical skin, thereby risking the blood supply to the skin [22]. Umbilical stalk length and diameter are often altered to fit into the recipient abdominal site. To create gradual periumbilical concavity (the "crater" effect, which is also considered to be aesthetically pleasing), the umbilical dermis is attached to the abdominal rectus fascia with absorbable sutures. This technique eliminates the possibility of having a "floating" or "life-saver" umbilicus appearance with an overt scar [23].

In patients with umbilical hernias, the hernia should be repaired at the time of the abdominoplasty, which usually can be achieved during rectus sheath plication (Fig. 12.5). Without hernia repair, herniation through the designed natural "crater" will create an unpleasant "target"-like appearance [23]. It is vital to conduct a thorough physical examination to look for an umbilical hernia; an ultrasound scan may be necessary in patients who have increased BMIs due to the difficulty in detecting hernias in this patient group.

Naturally, no technique is perfect or fitting for all scenarios; therefore a surgeon needs to have a variety of techniques available.

12.8 Conclusions

The umbilicus was once regarded as small and insignificant by surgeons until Vernon [20] advocated the preservation of it in 1957. With this, together with evolving societal views on self-image, the umbilicus now plays an important role in defining abdominal contour. A relatively small, vertically shaped umbilicus with "hooding" represents youth; therefore, we as surgeons are constantly striving to recreate the same in patients with different umbilical pathologies presented to us or as a component of abdominal contour surgery.

References

1. Hackett R. Dunning's examination of torsos is a truly navel experience. Seattle Post-Intelligencer, Seattle, 30 May 2002.
2. Terfera D, Jegtvig S. Nerves, blood vessels, and lymphatics of the abdomen. New Jersey: Wiley; 2012. p. 110.
3. Auplish S, Hossain-Ibrahim MK. Extended matching questions for the MRCS. Cambridge: Cambridge University Press; 2001. p. 33.
4. Baburaj P. Hari's essentials of clinical medicine. New Delhi: Jaypee Brothers Publishers; 2008. p. 205.
5. Hill MA. Embryology book – human embryology and morphology 8. UNSW Cricos, Sydney, 2015. https://embryology.med.unsw.edu.au/embryology/index.php/Main_Page. Accessed 8 Feb 16.
6. Scarborough AD, Hunt-Hurst P. The making of an erogenous zone: the role of exoticism, dance, and the movies in midriff exposure, 1900–1946. Costume Soc Am. 2014;40:47–65.
7. Nelly N. First indications of symbolic expressions. Japanese prehistory: the material and spiritual culture of the Jomon period. Wiesbaden: Otto Harrassowitz Verlag; 2000. p. 114–6, 119–202.
8. Abhyankar SV, Rajguru GA, Patil AP. Anatomical localization of the umbilicus: an Indian study. Plast Reconstr Surg. 2006;117(4):1153–7.
9. Psillakis JM, Appiani E, de la Plaza R. Color atlas of aesthetic surgery of the abdomen. New York: Thieme Medical Publishers; 1991. p. 40–2, 57,61.
10. Markman B, Barton Jr FE. Anatomy of the subcutaneous tissue of the trunk and the lower extremity. Plast Reconstr Surg. 1987;80:248–54.
11. Teimourian B, Marefat S. Body contouring with suction-assisted lipectomy. Mastery Plast Reconstr Surg. 1994;3:2186–200.
12. Baroudi R. Umbilicoplasty. Clin Plast Surg. 1975;2:431–48.
13. Craig SB, Faller MS, Puckett CL. In search of the ideal female umbilicus. Plast Reconstr Surg. 2000;105(1):389–92.
14. Snyder CL. Current management of umbilical abnormalities and related anomalies. Semin Pediatr Surg. 2007;16:41–9.
15. Meier DE, OlaOlorun DA, Omodele RA, Nkor SK, Tarpley JL. Incidence of umbilical hernia in African children: redefinition of "normal" and reevaluation of indications for repair. World J Surg. 2001;25:645–8.
16. Takato T, Itoh M, Kamei M, Uchiyama K. Our method of umbilical reconstruction. JPN J Plast Reconstr Surg. 1989;32:133–6.
17. Apfelberg DB, Maser MR, Lash H. Two unusual umbilicoplasties. Plast Recontr Surg. 1979;64:268–70.

18. Hodgkinson DJ. Umbilicoplasty: conversion of 'outie' to 'innie'. Aesthetic Plast Surg. 1983;7:221–2.
19. Baack BR, Anson G, Nachbar JM, White DJ. Umbilicoplasty: the construction of a new umbilicus and correction of umbilical stenosis without external scars. Plast Reconstr Surg. 1996;97: 227–32.
20. Vernon S. Umbilical transplantation upward and abdominal contouring in lipectomy. Am J Surg. 1957;94(3):490–2.
21. Cannistra C, Pecorelli E. Umbilical restoration in abdominal dermolipectomy: a simple double-Y, double-M technique. Aesthetic Plast Surg. 1999;23:364–6.
22. Castillo PF. Umbilical reinsertion in abdominoplasty: technique using deepithelialized skin flaps. Aesthetic Plast Surg. 2007;31:519–20.
23. Rozen SM, Redett R. The two-dermal-flap umbilical transposition: a natural and aesthetic umbilicus after abdominoplasty. Plast Reconstr Surg. 2007;119:2255–62.
24. Schoeller T, Wechselberger G, Otto A, Rainer C, Schwabegger A, Lille S, Ninkovic M. New technique for scarless umbilical reinsertion in abdominoplasty procedures. Plast Reconstr Surg. 1998;102:1720–3.
25. De Lacerda DJ, Martins DM, Marques A, Brenda E, De Moura Andrews J. Umbilicoplasty for the abdomen with a thin adipose layer. Br J Plast Surg. 1994;47:386–7.

Chapter 13
Umbilical Repositioning to Correct Sad Umbilicus: Umbilicosliding

Guillermo Blugerman, Diego Schavelzon, Gabriel Wexler, and Marcelo Lotocky

13.1 Introduction

The umbilicus is an anatomical element that has interested many individuals since ancient times. Based on the eugenic patterns, the abdomen is perceived as a plain anatomic area interrupted by a single topographical feature, the umbilicus. The umbilicus is the only scar that must be restored and preserved to provide a natural outcome after surgery. It is also the only point of direct and firm adherence of the skin to the deep fascial planes around the body. Its presence aids in dividing the abdomen into supra- and infraumbilical areas. The skin in these two areas has anatomical, histological, and biomechanical differences that affect skin behavior during pregnancy and after abdominal liposuction. The upper abdominal skin is thicker and less elastic, and the lower abdomen is thinner, more elastic, and more likely to develop atrophic stretch marks.

G. Blugerman, M.D. • D. Schavelzon, M.D. (✉)
B & S Center of Excellence in Plastic Surgery, Laprida 1579, Buenos Aires, Argentina
e-mail: blugerman@centrosbys.com; drschavelzon@gmail.com; aliasmarce@hotmail.com

G. Wexler, M.D. • M. Lotocky, M.D.
B & S Center of Excellence in Plastic Surgery, Private Practice,
Laprida 1579, Buenos Aires, Argentina
e-mail: gabrielew555@hotmail.com

M.A. Shiffman (ed.), *Adult Umbilical Reconstruction*,
DOI 10.1007/978-3-319-43887-0_13

13.2 Anatomical Review

The umbilicus is a second intention healing scar. It occurs as a result of stump falling 5–6 days after birth. This scar may have different diseases ranging from different degree hernias to skin cancer. In the third month of intrauterine life, the umbilicus is represented by a small hole pierced by two umbilical arteries and the umbilical vein through which the fetus is attached to the placenta, surrounded by gelatinous layer of Wharton. After birth, once the cord is ligated, blood stops circulating through these vessels. The vessels collapse and obliterate and are gradually transformed into fibrous cords. The navel of the adult has a depression circumscribed by a sort of umbilical skinfold called umbilical roll. At the bottom of the depression, there is a small irregular eminence, the nipple, which has in its apex, the umbilicus scar, and it is separated from the umbilical roll by a circumferential groove, called the umbilical groove. The roll is made of umbilical skin and subcutaneous tissue and has various shapes.

13.3 Umbilicus Location

The umbilicus is located below the midpoint between the xiphoid and the pubic symphysis [1]. The umbilicus scar is from 18 to 23 cm over the vulvar commissure in women, with a range of 2–4 cm below the vulvar commissure connecting the anterior superior iliac spines. It has a circular or slightly oval vertical shape, a mean diameter of 1 cm, and a variable depth according to the thickness of the adipose tissue. This form undergoes changes throughout life. Factors that can influence the shape and position of the umbilicus include weight changes, pregnancy, abdominal surgery, and hernias. Anatomically, the navel is located at the height of the 3rd and 4th vertebral joint [2], but this localization method is not very helpful in surgical planning. We usually locate the umbilicus in the midline two fingers over a line that joins both anterior superior iliac spines.

13.4 The Shape of the Umbilicus

Vertical or T-shaped umbilicus has greater aesthetic appeal than other shapes (horizontal, protruding, distorted) [3]. Deep skin scar fixation to the fascia makes the upper abdomen skin usually thicker and less elastic than the lower abdomen, falling in front and sides of the umbilicus causing what is known as sad umbilicus. This problem can be primary or secondary after abdominal liposuction. To determine the appropriate treatment, we should note the umbilicus location in respect to the other structures in the abdomen and thus determine whether we are dealing with a high,

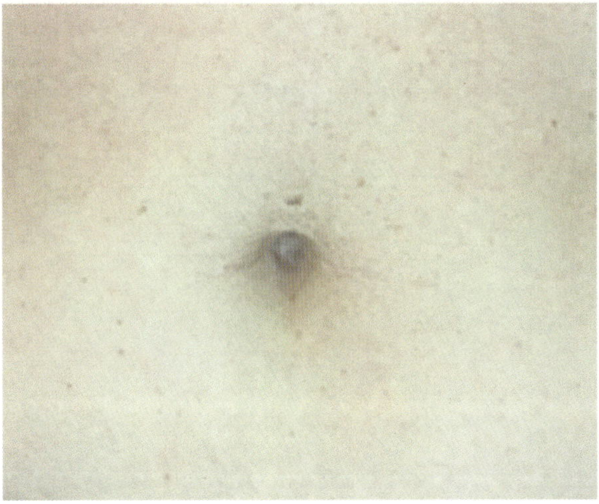

Fig. 13.1 Grade I is the umbilicus that loses the slightly vertically oval or round shape becoming an oval hole with maximum axis horizontal

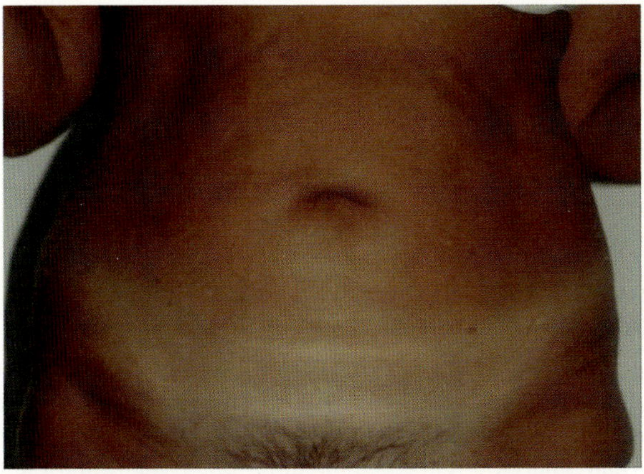

Fig. 13.2 Grade II is the umbilicus with upper abdomen skin falling over not covering it completely

normal, or low insertion umbilicus, referenced to the iliac crest. Based on the external appearance of the umbilicus when viewed from the front, we have classified the sad umbilicus into three grades. Grade I is the umbilicus that loses the slightly vertically oval or round shape becoming an oval hole with maximum axis horizontal (Fig. 13.1). Grade II is the umbilicus with upper abdomen skin falling over not covering it completely (Fig. 13.2). Grade III is the umbilicus that has become a slit

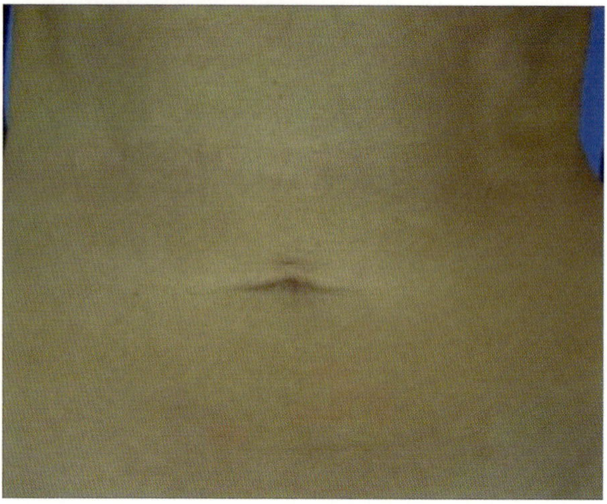

Fig. 13.3 Grade III is the umbilicus that has become a slit because the upper abdomen skin has covered it completely

because the upper abdomen skin has covered it completely (Fig. 13.3). In this stage the scar or depression is completely hidden.

13.5 Surgical Technique

Evaluation of the abdominal wall integrity is done before proceeding with the technique. Performing a physical examination with palpation at rest and during the Valsalva maneuver is fundamental to discern the umbilical hernia. If there is any uncertainty, abdominal wall ultrasound is requested. Before surgery, exhaustive umbilicus hygiene must be conducted, especially in cases of grade III of sad umbilicus, to avoid the risk of contamination of the surgical wound. Preoperative photographs are taken before surgery. The marking starts with the patient standing so that the most important anatomic points can be highlighted including the following: the midline from the xiphoid to the pubic symphysis, the anterior superior iliac spines, a "cross" in the bottom, and walls of the umbilicus to use it as a path for this surgical procedure (Fig. 13.4). The procedure could be performed under tumescent local anesthesia or general anesthesia.

In both cases the infiltration of the umbilical scar and subcutaneous tissue in a diameter of 10 cm around the umbilicus is important. Under tumescent anesthesia, the dilution is 800 mg of lidocaine per 500 mL of saline with the addition of 1 mL of 1:1,000,000 adrenaline.

After tumescent anesthesia infiltration, the bottom of the umbilicus is held with a Gillies hook [4], pulled up and cut in cross shape creating four triangular flaps. It is important not to leave skin or scarring tissue adherent to the aponeurosis to avoid inclusion cysts and long-term infections. Dissection proceeds in the aponeurotic

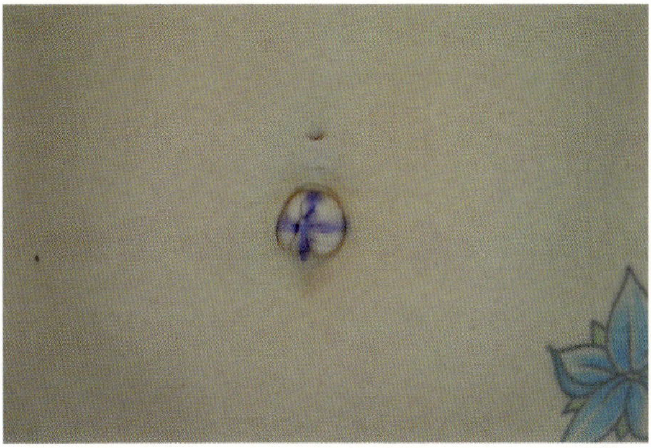

Fig. 13.4 With the patient standing, markings are made at the midline (from the xiphoid to the pubic symphysis), the anterior superior iliac spines, and a "cross" in the bottom and walls of the umbilicus

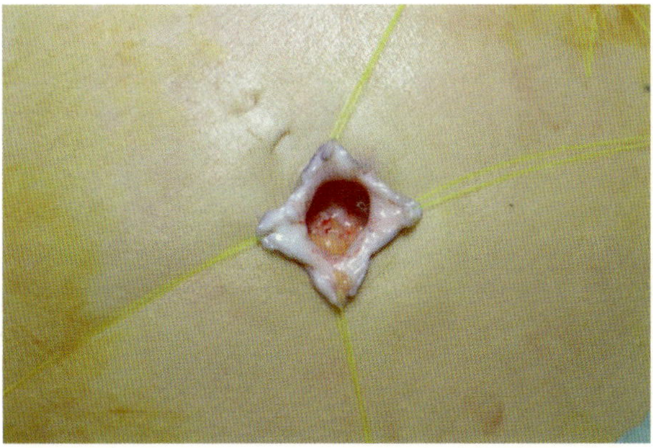

Fig. 13.5 Four triangular flaps are made

layer up and down on the alba line extending to both sides using blunt dissection technique to prevent damage to the perforating vessels (Fig. 13.5). To obtain enough mobilization, all fibrous adhesions found around the umbilicus must be dissected. Following previous skin markings, umbilicus is repositioned, usually about 2 cm below its previous location.

The first suture is a crisscross suture placed to close the aponeurotic defect after the umbilicus detachment with braided polyester 0. If there is a hernia, two or three sutures are required to plicate the rectus muscle and close the defect. The same suture that closed the aponeurotic defect is used to fix the supraumbilical skin in his new position, taking the subcutaneous tissue using it as a quilting suture proposed by Baroudi [5]. Once the upper abdominal skin is fixed without tension on the flaps, these are fixed to the aponeurotic layer, placing a suture from the inner base of each triangular flap to the fascia 1 cm away from the center of the new umbilicus. All the

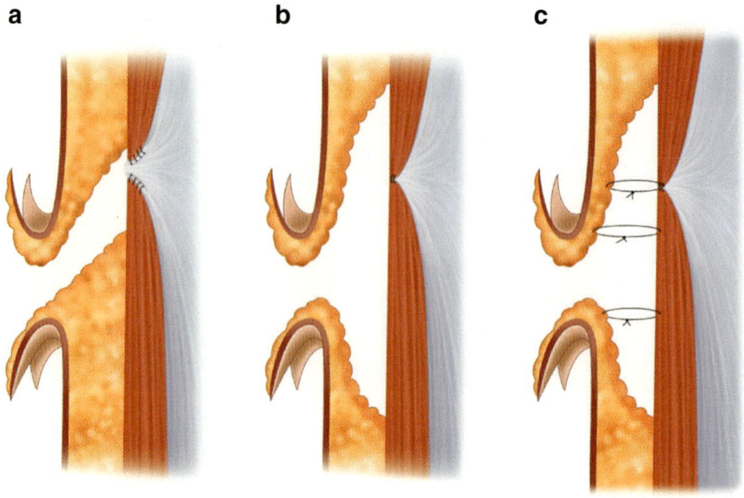

Fig. 13.6 (*Left*) Original position of umbilicus. (*Middle*) The umbilicus is repositioned, usually about 2 cm below its previous location. (*Right*) Once the upper abdominal skin is fixed without tension on the flaps, these are fixed to the aponeurotic layer

subcutaneous tissue and skin sutures are with Monocryl 3/0. The umbilicus fixation from the base to the fascia allows us to keep the depth and tubular appearance of the umbilicus and thereby natural shape (Fig. 13.6). Finally, a purse-string suture is performed connecting the four flap tips and anchoring them to the fascia in the center of the new umbilicus.

Antibiotic ointment-soaked gauze is placed in the neo-umbilicus to prevent skin damage. A girdle must be placed over the wound.

13.6 Results

We have used this technique in 32 patients, 28 females and 4 males. In 30 patients the reason was purely aesthetic, in two patients it was used to correct an umbilical hernia, and 1 of them underwent rectus abdominis muscle fascia plication through the incision. Of the 32 patients 22 were performed to correct a secondary sad umbilicus (post liposuction) and 10 for primary sad umbilicus, simultaneous to liposuction.

The scars were completely unable to be detected, inconspicuous from the month after the surgery (Figs. 13.7, 13.8, and 13.9).

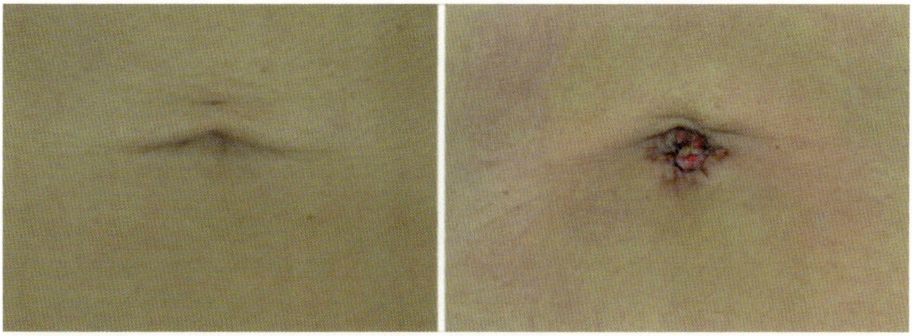

Fig. 13.7 (*Left*) Original position of umbilicus preoperatively. (*Right*) Postoperative after repositioning

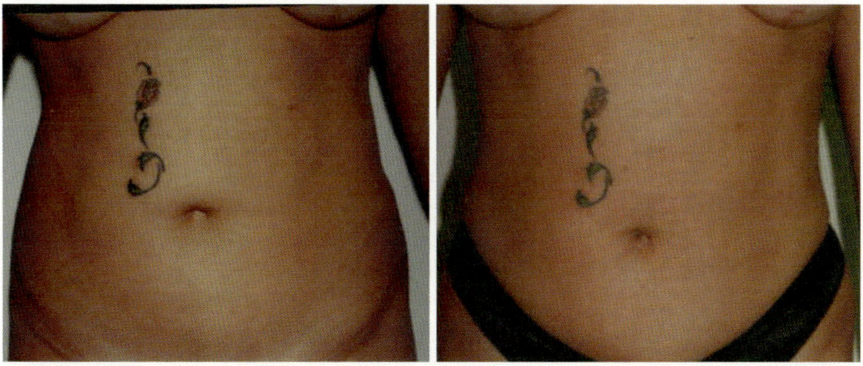

Fig. 13.8 (*Left*) Original position of umbilicus preoperatively. (*Right*) Postoperative after repositioning

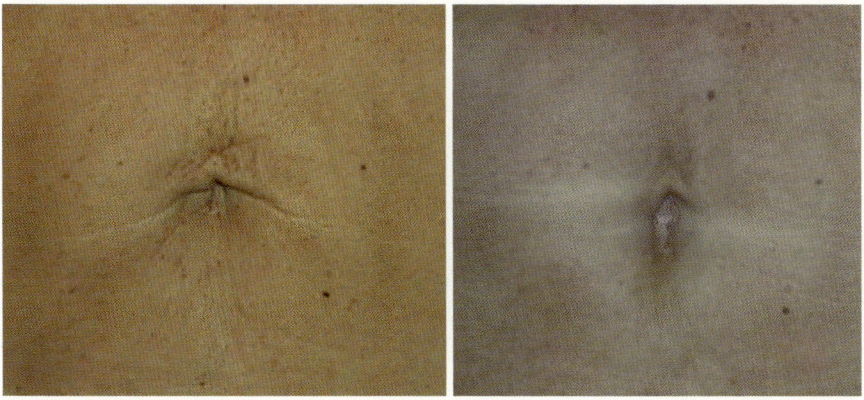

Fig. 13.9 (*Left*) Original position of umbilicus preoperatively. (*Right*) Postoperative after repositioning

13.7 Discussion

Previous authors proposed the mobilization and refixation of umbilical scar during a mini abdominoplasty process as Matarasso [6] using the terminology of floating umbilicus. In a large literature review, we could not find techniques for navel mobilization and reposition in patients without other concomitant surgery or with minimal scar surgery as liposuction. Because supra- and infraumbilical skin are anatomically different, the aging process, pregnancy, and even liposuction have different outcomes in both. The strong fixation of the umbilical scar to the fascia makes the upper abdominal skin excess redraping impossible, thus falling over the navel. Repositioning the umbilicus with or without concomitant liposuction is an interesting technique in mind of a cosmetic surgeon to enhance the abdominal area.

For patients' sad umbilicus, scar subcision and refixation without external scar were done for some months by the senior authors without promising results. With this minimal invasive technique, results were variable because the absence of a strong fixation to the fascia modifies the regular umbilical shape leaving superficial navels or funnel-shaped navels.

After learning from the work of Alexander that recreates the umbilicus suturing dermal flaps from inside the abdominoplasty flap to the fascia [7–11], we modified the subcision technique. An open minimal invasive procedure was designed to offer a better enhancement of the umbilical structures. This allowed reconstruction of the navel in the exact and correct anatomical shape.

The mobilization of the umbilical scar can be done simultaneously with the primary procedure of liposuction if the defect is present before surgery or in a second surgery when the sad umbilicus deformation is a secondary sequela. Post liposuction sad umbilicus can be caused by poor upper abdominal skin contraction or wrong preoperative diagnosis (upper abdominal skin excess). The first can be corrected by repositioning the navel. If upper abdominal skin excess is important, other techniques should be considered: abdominoplasty (traditional or inverted).

13.8 Conclusions

The sad umbilicus is an aesthetic deformation that can be primary or secondary. Correction can be performed as adjunctive of liposuction or separately. Overall aesthetic outcome is satisfactory as assessed by experienced specialists and patients. It is a simple technique and easy to reproduce by any surgeon who knows the abdominal area anatomy and possesses an aesthetic relation to it.

References

1. Dubou R, Ousterhout DK. Placement of the umbilicus in an abdominoplasty. Plast Reconstr Surg. 1978;61(2):291–3.
2. Baroudi R. Umbilicoplasty. Clin Plast Surg. 1975;2:431–48.
3. Craig SB, Faller MS, Puckett CL. In search of the ideal female umbilicus. Plast Reconstr Surg. 2000;105:389–92.
4. Sillitoe AT, Thornton DJ, Srinivasan J, Hart NB. Elevation of the umbilicus with skin hooks aids excision in abdominoplasty. Plast Reconstr Surg. 2005;115(1):349.
5. Baroudi R, Ferreira C. Seroma; how to avoid it and how to treat it. Aesthet Surg J. 1998;18:439–41.
6. Matarasso A. Abdominoplasty. In: Guyuron B, Achauer BM, Eriksson E, et al., editors. Plastic surgery: indications, operations, outcomes, vol. 4. Philadelphia: Mosby-Yearbook; 2000. p. 2783–821.
7. Abreu JA. Abdominoplastias: neo-onfaloplastia sem cicatriz e sem excisão de gordura. Abdominoplasty: neoomphaloplasty without scar or fat excision. Rev Bras Cir Plást. 2010;25(3):499–503.
8. Wechselberger G, Otto A, Rainer C, Schwabegger A, Lille S, et al. New technique for scarless umbilicul reinsertion in abdominoplasty procedures. Plast Reconstr Surg. 1998;102(5):1720–3.
9. Amud RJM. Neo-onfaloplastia sem cicatriz. Rev Bras Cir Plast. 2008;23(1):37–40.
10. Otto A, Wechselberger G, Schoeller T, Lille S. A method of reconstructing a natural-looking umbilicus in abdominoplasty. Ann Plast Surg. 1997;39(4):435.
11. Santanelli F, Mazzocchi M, Renzi L, Cigna E. Reconstruction of a natural-looking umbilicus. Scand J Plast Reconstr Surg Hand Surg. 2002;36:183–5.

Chapter 14
Low Scar Abdominoplasty with Inferior Positioning of the Umbilicus

Amy S. Colwell and Michael J. Frederick

14.1 Introduction

Abdominoplasty procedures are designed to resect variable amounts of excess fat and skin and correct musculoaponeurotic laxity. Multiple classification systems exist to define the degree of abdominal deformity and respective treatment [1, 2]. The traditional abdominoplasty classically removes the excess skin and fat of the abdomen with umbilical transposition resulting in a low transverse scar and a new position for the umbilicus. However, a subgroup of women do not have enough excess skin laxity to transpose the umbilicus and maintain a low transverse scar. An alternative to a high transverse scar or a low scar with a vertical component is the umbilical float procedure. In this technique, the umbilicus remains attached to the surrounding skin for vascularity and is disconnected from the abdominal base. This allows access for rectus diastasis correction and skin excision without a vertical component. Lowering of the artificially elevated umbilical position that occurs after pregnancy can correct minor to modest upper abdominal skin laxity. Technical details are discussed.

A.S. Colwell, M.D. (✉) • M.J. Frederick, M.D.
Division of Plastic Surgery, Harvard Medical School, Massachusetts General Hospital,
55 Fruit St. WACC 435, Boston, MA 02114, USA
e-mail: AColwell@mgh.harvard.edu; MFrederick1@partners.org

M.A. Shiffman (ed.), *Adult Umbilical Reconstruction*,
DOI 10.1007/978-3-319-43887-0_14

14.2 Technique

14.2.1 Marking

The inferior skin incision is marked 5–6 cm above the vulvar commissure with the skin on stretch and carried laterally just above the inguinal crease (Fig. 14.1). The superior incision is tentatively marked to give a scar to naval distance of around 8–9 cm (minimum 7 cm) on stretch. The final superior incision is not determined until the abdominal flap is undermined.

14.2.2 Procedure

Flank liposuction is performed in patients with excess fat in this region. The low transverse scar is incised and dissection proceeds superiorly taking care to leave some fat on the fascia to help prevent seroma formation. To transect the umbilicus, a finger is placed externally into the umbilicus to ensure transection proceeds below the skin base. The stalk is palpated to ensure no hernia exists. The stalk is then transected below the skin base using a Metzenbaum scissors, which typically leaves a fascial defect. The umbilical fascial defect is then closed with a 0-Ethibond figure of eight suture. This suture is left long to mark the original position of the umbilicus (Fig. 14.2). Abdominal undermining is performed to the rib cage, and the diastasis

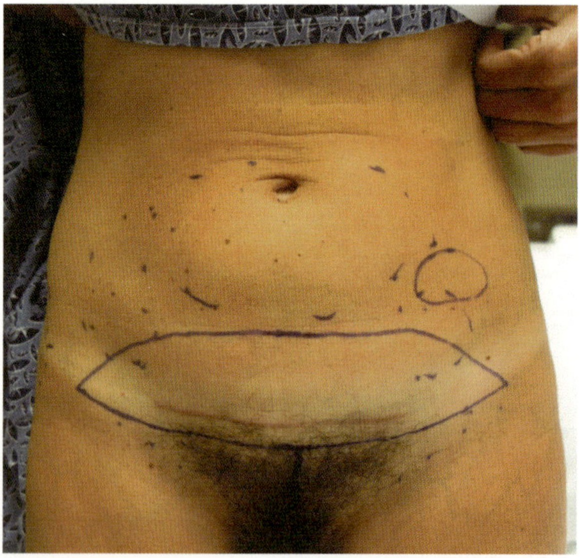

Fig. 14.1 Abdominoplasty marking centers on a low transverse incision approximately 5–6 cm from the vulvar commissure on stretch. The superior incision is marked to achieve a distance of at least 7 cm from the naval to the superior incision on stretch

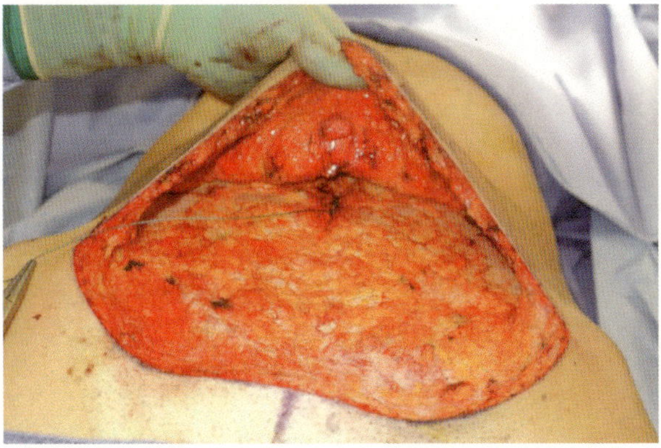

Fig. 14.2 The umbilicus is transected and the fascial defect closed with a 0-Ethibond figure-of-eight suture. One end of the suture is left long to mark the original umbilical position. Rectus diastasis is corrected

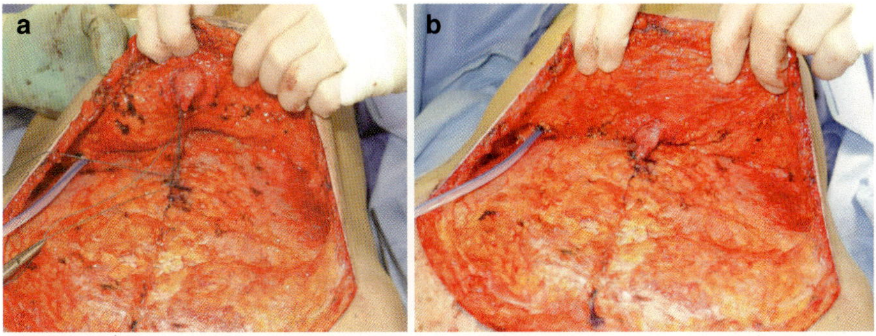

Fig. 14.3 (**a**) The new umbilical position is marked 1–6 cm from the original position and is determined after wide undermining and flexion of the patient. (**b**) The umbilicus is lowered as much as technically appropriate to correct upper abdominal skin laxity but to avoid an overly low umbilicus. An average distance from the umbilicus to the scar on stretch is approximately 8–9 cm. Less than 7 cm should be avoided

recti are closed from xiphoid to pubis with buried interrupted figure of eight 0-Ethibond sutures. The new position of the umbilicus is determined by flexing the patient and determining the skin excision. The umbilicus is typically lowered 1–6 cm, and its new position is secured by placing a single figure of eight 0-Ethibond suture from the umbilical base to the abdominal fascia (Fig. 14.3). A greater degree of umbilical lowering results in more upper abdominal skin laxity correction; however, a limit of lowering exists depending upon the height of the patient and the vertical height of the torso so that the umbilicus maintains a suitable distance superior to the low transverse incision. The transverse incision is closed with 2–0 polydioxanone sutures in Scarpa's fascia followed by 3–0 Monocryl deep dermal sutures and a running 3–0 Monocryl subcuticular stitch. Two 15 Bard drains are placed prior to closure approximately 1 cm from the end of the incision on both sides.

14.2.3 Postoperative Care

Incisions are dressed with either Steri-Strips or Dermabond and Tegaderm. Gauze and Tegaderm are placed over the umbilicus to help secure the new position for at least 2 weeks. An abdominal binder is kept in place for 6 weeks except when showering. If liposuction was performed with the procedure, Reston foam is used to decrease flank swelling and bruising. Drains are removed when the output is less than 30 mL/day for 2 days (Fig. 14.4)

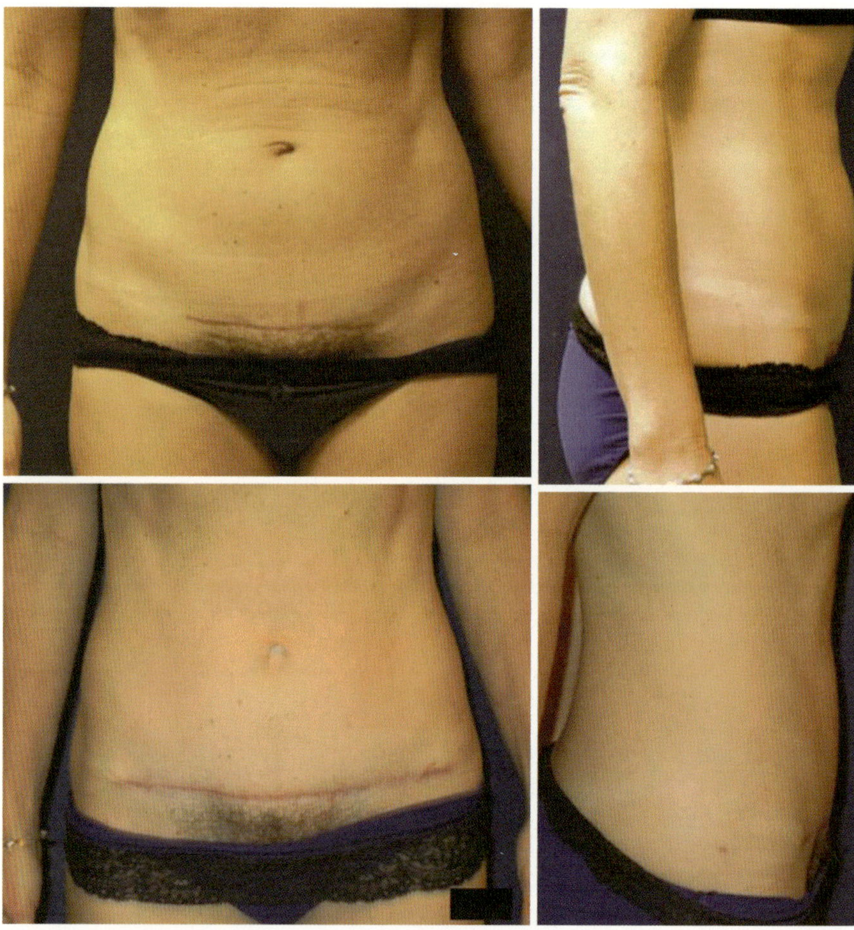

Fig. 14.4 (*Top*) Preoperative 48-year-old female and mother of two complained of rectus diastasis, excess fatty tissue around her umbilicus, and two areas of pain following her emergent C-section. (*Bottom*) Five months postoperative following abdominoplasty with umbilical float. No unusual findings related to the C-section were discovered

14.3 Discussion

With the growing trend toward more minimally invasive surgery, there has been increased enthusiasm toward the mini-abdominoplasty. This technique allows for infraumbilical tightening of the diastasis recti and skin and is often performed on an outpatient basis in patients with an abdominal deformity limited to the infraumbilical abdomen [3, 4]. However, excess supraumbilical skin and diastasis recti are not corrected. To address the supraumbilical area, some authors have advocated midline dissection around the umbilicus to the xiphoid with correction, but this is technically challenging if the umbilicus remains attached. Furthermore, this technique cannot address excess supraumbilical skin. Therefore, there remains a subgroup of patients with overall musculoaponeurotic laxity and minor to modest excess supraumbilical skin for whom there remains three surgical options: traditional abdominoplasty with a high transverse scar, traditional abdominoplasty with an anchor scar, or abdominoplasty with floating of the umbilicus.

A high transverse scar or vertical extension may be visible in many modern styles of clothing or swimsuits and thus not desirable. The technique of floating the umbilicus allows for a low scar, and we are placing our scar 5–6 cm above the vulvar commissure and within the mons pubis. A scar at this level is nearly always concealed, even with low-riding popular styles of clothing. A low incision also has the benefit of a mons reduction and lift, which most women desire and appreciate.

Although abdominoplasty with floating of the umbilicus was the subject of articles by Gradel [5] and Wilkinson [6] about 20 years ago, some reviews have eliminated it from the algorithm suggesting it may compromise the end abdominoplasty result with an abnormally low umbilical position [7]. However, there has been a recent resurgence in interest of umbilical positioning. Traditional abdominoplasty places the umbilicus at the location of the stalk or in relation to the bony landmarks such as the anterior superior iliac spine [1]. However, a recent review looking at ideal umbilical positioning suggests that the most aesthetic location of the umbilicus has no relation to the ASIS but correlates to a ratio of the xiphoid–umbilicus/umbilicus–abdominal mean crease of 1.62 [8]. In a separate study where plastic surgeons chose the ideal umbilical position on patient photographs with the umbilicus removed, the ideal umbilicus was placed on average 2.2 cm below its natural position following childbirth or weight loss and aging [9]. Furthermore, Rohrich et al. [10] looked at the transverse location of the umbilicus in 116 patients and found that it was rarely ever midline. Thus, there is no perfect "natural" location of the umbilicus that is generalizable, and each patient must be looked at individually to determine what is most ideal. In our experience, the ideal location is often just below the original position of the umbilicus, making the umbilical float a great option in many patients. We regularly position the umbilicus 1–6 cm below the original position of the stalk depending on the umbilical to vulvar commissure distance and the patient's height. The distance from the umbilicus to the scar must be at least 7 cm on stretch to appear natural, while concealing the scar with clothing and a distance of 8–9 cm is often chosen. For patients desiring the tightest abdomen without regard for scars, the traditional abdominoplasty with a vertical component better achieves those goals as the tightness of the abdominoplasty with umbilical float is often compromised to avoid an umbilical position that is too low.

The technical positioning of the umbilicus is relatively simple. After repairing the fascial defect with a figure of eight stitch, one end is left long as a frame of reference to the original umbilical position. After the tissue has been draped appropriately, the new site for the umbilicus is determined within 1–6 cm of the original location depending upon the degree of upper abdominal laxity, the vertical height of the torso and overall height, and the relation to the low abdominal incision. The stalk should then be attached to the fascia just above the final position of the umbilicus with the skin pulled down. This gives the appearance of a vertical oval navel with superior hooding, which many consider the most aesthetic appearance [8].

14.4 Conclusions

The low scar abdominoplasty with inferior positioning of the umbilicus at 1–6 cm is safe and provides excellent aesthetic results. Appropriate patient selection is the key to a successful outcome for this technique, and the postpartum woman with complete diastasis recti and minimal to moderate skin excess is the ideal candidate.

References

1. Bozola AR, Psillakis JM. Abdominoplasty: a new concept and classification for treatment. Plast Reconstr Surg. 1988;82:983–93.
2. Matarasso A. Abdominolipoplasty: a system of classification and treatment for combined abdominoplasty and suction-assisted lipectomy. Aesthetic Plast Surg. 1991;15:111–21.
3. Matarasso A, Smith D. Strategies for aesthetic reshaping of the postpartum patient. Plast Reconstr Surg. 2015;136(2):245–57.
4. Shestak KC. Marriage abdominoplasty expands the mini-abdominoplasty concept. Plast Reconstr Surg. 1999;103:1020–31.
5. Gradel J. Umbilical technical maneuvers to facilitate abdominoplasty with limited incisions. Aesthetic Plast Surg. 1991;15:251–6.
6. Wilkinson TS. Limited abdominoplasty techniques applied to complete abdominal repair. Aesthetic Plast Surg. 1994;18:49–55.
7. Sozer SO, Agullo FJ, Santillan AA, Wolf C. Decision making in abdominoplasty. Aesthetic Plast Surg. 2007;31(2):117–27.
8. Visconti G, Visconti E, Bonomo L, Salgarello M. Concepts in navel aesthetic: a comprehensive surface anatomy analysis. Aesthetic Plast Surg. 2015;39:43–50.
9. Colwell AS, Kpodzo D, Gallico 3rd G. Low scar abdominoplasty with inferior positioning of the umbilicus. Ann Plast Surg. 2010;64(5):639–44.
10. Rohrich RJ, Sorokin ES, Brown SA. Gibby DL Is the umbilicus truly midline? Clinical and medicolegal implications. Plast Reconstr Surg. 2003;112(1):259–63.

Chapter 15
Umbilicoplasty with Vertical Incision in Abdominoplasty

Amir Lebaschi

15.1 Introduction

The umbilicus occupies the central locus of the abdomen and is one of the most influential determinants of aesthetic outcome of abdominoplasty. Although umbilical issues could be the presenting complaint, most patients apparently request an abdominoplasty owing to non-umbilical complaints, implying that they are not appreciating or focusing on this key anatomic structure. However, their attention eventually will be drawn to the aesthetics of the umbilicus, and their accurate description of the umbilicus aesthetic outcome could well surprise the surgeon. As such, the surgeon should diligently and meticulously address the issue of umbilicus reconstruction as an integral part of abdominoplasty. It is imperative to seek and understand the patient's view on his/her current and ideal umbilicus.

15.2 Key Anatomy

The umbilicus is located in the midline at the level of superior iliac spines, 9–10 cm above the pubic hair line. As a rule of thumb, a ratio of upper to lower abdomen of 60–40 % exists when umbilicus at its correct location. The blood supply to the periumbilical area is supplied by branches from the subdermal plexus, from both deep inferior epigastric arteries, as well as a blood supply from the median umbilical ligament.

A. Lebaschi, MD
Department of Tissue Engineering, Repair, and Regeneration, Hospital for Special Surgery, 535 East 70th Street, New York, NY 10021, USA
e-mail: ah_lebaschi@yahoo.com

M.A. Shiffman (ed.), *Adult Umbilical Reconstruction*,
DOI 10.1007/978-3-319-43887-0_15

15.3 Characterization of a Beautiful Umbilicus

The aesthetically pleasing umbilicus is a small, fixed, vertical elliptoid structure with a superior depression (hooding) and inferior widening without any visible bulging or mass inside it. Every effort should be made to restore these features as much as possible in any abdominoplasty. Anatomical localization should be less variable than the size of the elliptoid, as patients have different preferences for umbilical size. Patients with larger bodies should also have slightly larger umbilicus.

15.4 Operative Technique

15.4.1 Release

There are two principle approaches for releasing the umbilicus in abdominoplasty.

15.4.2 Skin Incision with Fascial Attachment Preservation

This is the usual method of umbilical release and can be performed in almost all techniques of abdominoplasty. Initially, the umbilicus boundaries are tattooed at 12, 3, 6, and 9 o'clock locations. Using two hooks to stretch the umbilicus superiorly and inferiorly, the umbilicus is sharply cut in a vertical ellipse shape. It is possible to adjust the size of the future umbilicus at this stage by incorporating a variable amount of abdominal skin (to enlarge the umbilicus) or discarding a rim of umbilical skin (to make it smaller), but it is recommended to make the incision at umbilical-abdominal skin junction and adjust the final size of the umbilicus when the new opening in the abdominal flap is being made.

Making a clean and smooth incision at umbilical-abdominal skin junction can be a tricky task. A fresh, sharp blade should be used for this purpose and the skin should be cut by thrusting movements. Although pulling on the hooks at either ends of the umbilicus will stabilize the skin, considerable laxity may still be present especially when a large umbilicus is being dealt with.

Following skin incision, the fatty tissue around the stalk is cleared using sharp dissection down to the fascia, leaving a thin film of tissue attached to the stalk. It is important not to try to visualize the glistering fascia at this time as it could be difficult to control the bleeding in case of umbilical vessels transection due to limited visualization.

Following development of the abdominal flap, the tissues are cleared from around the umbilical stalk, and its fascial attachment and the perforating vessels are cauterized/ligated.

When performing myofascial plication, it is important to leave enough space around the stalk in order to prevent strangulation.

15.4.3 Umbilical Transposition

In this approach, the umbilical stalk is detached from the fascia and umbilical-abdominal skin junction is left untouched. The stalk is then transferred and affixed to a new location. This technique provides excellent cosmetic outcome which is almost indistinguishable from a native umbilicus. This approach is useful in mini abdominoplasty candidates with significant infraumbilical skin redundancy and an apparent high-riding umbilicus, leaving at least between 14 and 16 cm between umbilicus and symphysis pubis. Myofascial plication can be performed without any concern for stalk strangulation as the stalk is already detached and the umbilicus is not dependent upon perforating vessel for survival.

15.4.4 Relocation and Inset

In cases with fascial attachment preservation, a Pitanguy clamp is useful to determine the center of the new umbilical location, which should respect the anatomic localization rules (see above). There are two popular methods for creation of the new umbilical opening: vertical and inverted V (or omega) incisions. It is advocated that inverted V incision can provide the desired flattening at the lower end of the umbilicus. Author has not noticed a significant difference between these two incisions as the skin incision gapes all the same. Besides, flap defatting around the orifice is almost always performed which contributes substantially to restoration of superior hooding and inferior flattening. Regardless of the technique, it is advisable to keep the size of the incision relatively small, although overly small openings should be avoided as this may lead to umbilical stenosis. As a rule of thumb, incision between 1.5 and 2 cm should be suitable for most patients.

Circumferential defatting of the flap around the opening is then performed. Although some surgeons do not defat the flap, the author has found this maneuver effective. Care should be taken not to compromise the blood supply of the abdominal flap around the opening. More fatty tissue should be removed from the lower half than the upper half to help restore normal umbilical contour.

Although myofascial plication almost always shortens the stalk, it may still be necessary to shorten this structure in cases of an elongated stalk. Tacking sutures to the fascia can be performed at this time to reduce the length of the stalk.

A variety of methods have been advocated for insetting the umbilicus into the new opening. Author's preferred technique is using vertical mattress sutures at the previously tattooed locations incorporating the fascia adjacent to the stalk. Stalk rotation should be avoided, although this is a rare occurrence except in thin stalks. A running subcuticular suture will finish the insetting.

Restoration of umbilical aesthetic characteristics is more difficult in patients with fatty abdomens. A combination of effective liposuction, judicious subfascial excision, and artistic final asymmetric defatting is needed for this end. In cases of fascial attachment preservation, all that is needed is to secure the stalk to the fascia with nonabsorbable suture. Here the determination of the new level at which the umbilicus should be located depends heavily on the amount of abdominal skin excision. Stalk attachment has little effect in this regard and mainly serves to prevent umbilical floating.

15.4.5 Postoperative Care

In cases of stalk detachment, no specific wound care is necessary. A bolster is recommended to mildly press the stalk down to prevent traction on the new attachment site.

Vaseline-impregnated gauze is used for dressing the umbilicus in cases of stalk attachment preservation. A dressing is also recommended to mildly press the periumbilical skin to ease the tension off the umbilical edge.

15.5 Complications and Their Management

15.5.1 Necrosis

Necrosis (partial or complete) results from a variety of causes including excessive traction on the umbilical stalk, strangulation of the stalk owing to overly tight myofascial plication, and damage to blood vessels around the stalk as a result of excessive skeletonization. Umbilical necrosis almost invariably leads to residual deformity and will need revision surgery. Sometimes the umbilicus cannot be salvaged and a new umbilicus should be reconstructed.

15.5.2 Flattening

In conventional abdominoplasties where the stalk is not divided, flattening of the umbilicus is usually due to diminished subcutaneous fat. In these cases, a purse-string suture thrown on the fascia surrounding the stalk using nonabsorbable material is usually sufficient to increase the depth of the umbilicus. Flattening can also result from detachment of the stalk in cases where the stalk is divided and reaffixed to the fascia. Revision of the detachment will correct floating and flattening of the umbilicus.

15.5.3 Stenosis

Umbilical stenosis results from ischemia of the umbilicus or relative small size of the opening in the abdominal flap. If the latter is the cause the stenosis, the umbilical cavity will be intact and will accumulate debris and will lead to a foul smelling umbilicus. In case of ischemia, fibrosis may diminish residual umbilical volume, and patients may not have a hygiene issue and present solely for aesthetic reasons. Mild to moderate stenosis can be corrected by multiple small Z-plasties around the junction of the umbilicus and abdominal skin. This may increase the circumference of the umbilicus but will not correct possible underlying umbilical flattening. Therefore, in addressing umbilical stenosis, it is important to evaluate residual umbilical cavity volume. For moderate to severe stenosis, two-flap and slit technique is recommended to incorporate abdominal skin into the umbilicus. Author's experience with management of umbilical stenosis is that most cases of stenosis resulting from ischemia will require ultimate excision and reconstruction of a new umbilicus.

Chapter 16
Neo-umbilicus in Vertical Abdominoplasty

Fabio Neves da Silva and Everardo Abramo de Oliveira

16.1 Introduction

The navel is a scar. It follows from umbilical cord loosening that occurs between the first and second week after birth. Each scar that we have tells us a story. The umbilicus certainly has the most beautiful of all because it comes from the biological link that connects the mother to the child, expressing the relationship of dependency between one life and another. We are predestined to have it from conception. Thus, it is an integral part of the human form. Its position and shape are essential in the aesthetic appearance of the abdomen [1], and the presence of protrusions, distortion, or change in the vertical axis will harm its beauty.

Obesity is a worldwide epidemic. Since the mid-1990s, bariatric surgery came acquiring world leadership. According to the American Society for Metabolic and Bariatric Surgery (ASMBS), in 2013, 179,000 bariatric surgeries were held in the USA. Brazil comes second with 72,000 surgeries done in 2012 (75 % by video laparoscopy). Those techniques produce substantial weight loss, which often represents more than 50 % of the patient's original weight. So, plastic surgeons had to adapt themselves to this new reality, developing and improving the techniques to correct the intense sagging created in different body areas. In the last decade, several techniques have been described for the treatment of excess skin on the face, neck, breasts, arms, back, abdomen, buttocks, and lower limbs for post-bariatric patients. This represented a huge advance in the surgical treatment with better results. Thus, the purely reconstructive goal is giving way to a demand for more and more aesthetic results.

F.N. da Silva, M.D., M.S., Ph.D. (✉)
Department of Plastic Surgery, Hospital Federal de Ipanema,
Rua Almirante Saddock de Sá 7/1004, Ipanema, Rio de Janeiro, Brazil, 22411-040
e-mail: contato@fabioneves.com.br

E.A. de Oliveira, M.D.
Private Practice, Leblon, Rio de Janeiro, Brazil
e-mail: everardoabramo@hotmail.com

M.A. Shiffman (ed.), *Adult Umbilical Reconstruction*,
DOI 10.1007/978-3-319-43887-0_16

As the patients' abdominal skin will not retract enough to allow it to accompany such reduction in fat content, the authors needed a technique based on vertical and horizontal skin resection. Resection of a horizontal skin band, even when performed circumferentially, does not correct the excess flabbiness, as there is no reduction in the perimeter. The authors needed to combine it to a vertical skin resection extensive enough to properly envelop the new body. The vertical abdominoplasty technique, also known as "anchor" or "fleur-de-lys," courses with a better composition of body contouring. More often the navel is held in position. The meeting of the navel with a vertical incision generates a surrounding scar with the risk, of course, to all sorts of unaesthetic results as hypertrophy, stenosis, unnatural shapes, scars from sutures, and other distortions.

In 1951, two Argentine authors, Fernandes and Correa-Iturraspe [2, 3], devised the making of a new navel from two rectangular skin flaps with a lateral base in vertical abdominoplasties without the horizontal component (Fig. 16.1). These flaps avoid the presence of a circular scar around the umbilicus and, depending on how

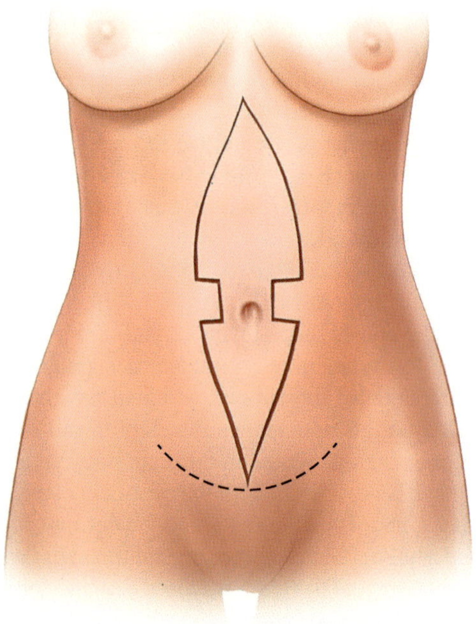

Fig. 16.1 Neo-umbilicoplasty with rectangular dermal-epidermal flaps described by Fernandes and Iturraspe in 1951 [2]

they are designed, create an aesthetically appealing and natural navel. Like other authors, we started to use this technique in repairing cases where the form or viability of the umbilicus was compromised (moderate or large umbilical hernias, median scarring sequel with deformation of the navel, or severe abdominal wall defects, as in laparotomy) [1, 4, 5]. The neo-umbilicus created by lateral skin flaps provided a great aesthetic result that we proposed to use it routinely, indicating it on all vertical abdominoplasties since 2008 [6].

En bloc resection of the abdominal flap with amputation of the original umbilicus after previous marking is mandatory in this case. There should be no skin undermining. It reduces the surgical time, minimizes the occurrence of complications such as hematomas or seromas, and provides better symmetry in results. When using the en bloc resection, the flaps must be drawn before the resection and traction. The correct position and shape are essential for a cosmetic appearance of the abdomen [7, 8]. So, how do we position the new navel exactly where the original was without any margin of error? At the beginning of our experience, we directly draw the umbilical flaps. In some cases, we noted that the new navel stood at slightly cranial or caudal position to its original location. Although these small changes (<2 cm) did not cause unsightly effects, it was reason enough for us to develop a way to avoid it. In this way we create the dermal-epidermal safety strip, a 10 cm wide skin band on which we mark the flaps only after tractioning and advancing the sutures. This is a simple tactic that creates results with a precise positioning.

16.2 Preoperative Preparation

Post-weight-loss patients represent the vast majority of current indications of vertical abdominoplasty. The procedure is indicated only after weight is stable for at least 6 months and close to the ideal. The BMI must be at least under 30 kg/m^2 and ideally under 25 kg/m^2. Physical examination should look for hernias in the midline, especially in patients who underwent open surgery. Ultrasound examination of the abdomen and abdominal wall is essential in the preoperative evaluation, as with the classic technique. Cholelithiasis is not an uncommon pathology in patients undergoing gastroplasty and must be corrected in advance. In case of large incisional hernias, we indicate the use of compression garments preoperatively to reduce respiratory disorders. As a consequence of low absorption of nutrients, protein deficit and anemia are frequent and must be given special attention. The risk of deep vein thrombosis is also elevated in these patients. The use of elastic stockings and pneumatic compressors of the lower limbs starts with the arrival of the patient in the operating room and is only removed on the next day when they begin walking. Anticoagulants are used only in high-risk patients.

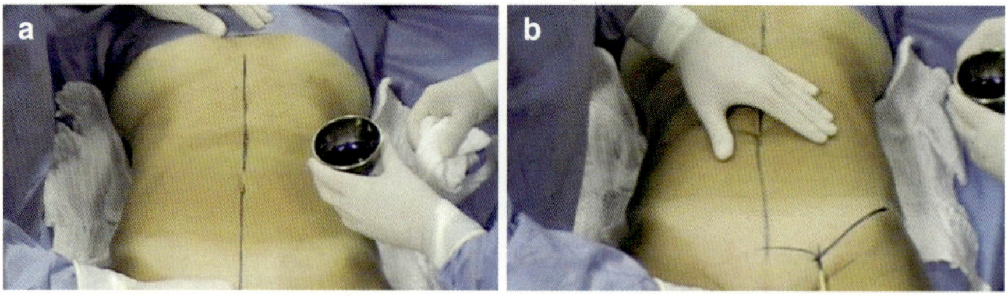

Fig. 16.2 Marking (**a**) vertical and (**b**) horizontal lines

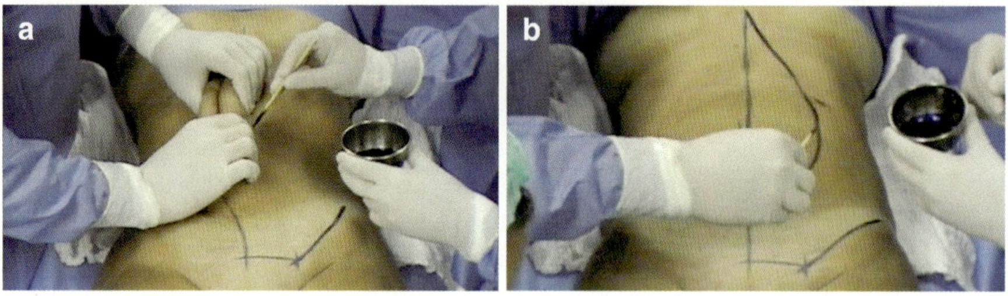

Fig. 16.3 (**a**, **b**) Marking the curved lateral line

16.3 Technique

16.3.1 Marking

The markings are done with the patient anesthetized in supine position. We strongly believe that this favors symmetry. We initially mark the abdominal midline and the 10–15 cm length horizontal inferior line, positioned 3 cm above the pubic symphysis with a light cranial traction of the abdominal skin. From the end point, we draw an oblique line toward the anterior superior iliac spine (Fig. 16.2).

The final appearance is similar to a bicycle handlebar. Using a clamping maneuver, with both hands, we estimate the width of the vertical flap, drawing a point (W point) at the level of the iliac crease. A large curved line is then drawn from the xiphoid appendix to the pubic symphysis passing through the point marked before (Fig. 16.3). It is very important to go medially while drawing after reaching the W point to avoid excess tension at the pubic area. The caudal end of the vertical incision is marked by pulling the curved line toward the pubic area without tension (Fig. 16.4).

Now it is time to estimate the location of the neo-umbilicus measuring the distance between the xiphoid process and the original navel (to be amputated). This distance is transferred to the curved line while keeping its traction toward the pubis, thus approximating the point where to position the side flaps for the new navel (Fig. 16.5).

For more accurate fixation of the neo-umbilicus to the point where the original navel is, the authors conceived skin bands (safety strip) measuring 10 × 3 cm where the flaps for the new navel will be drawn after abdominal traction. Each band

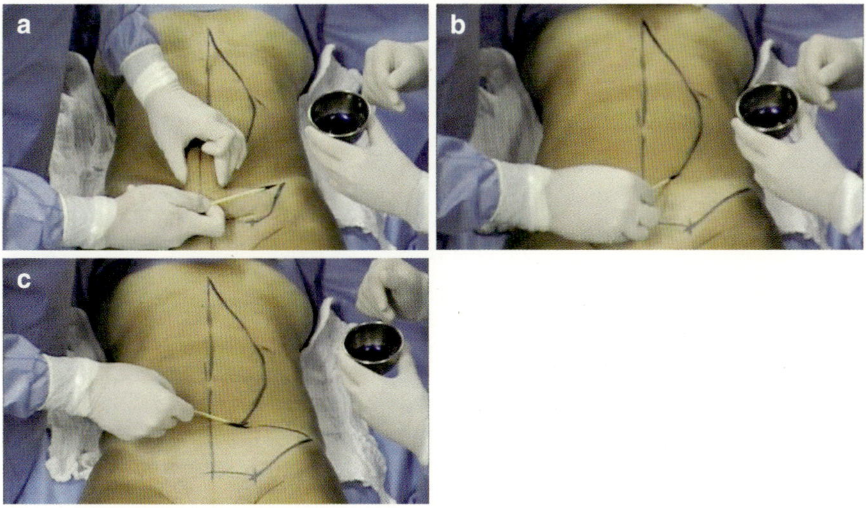

Fig. 16.4 (**a–c**) Marking the inferior limit of the curved line

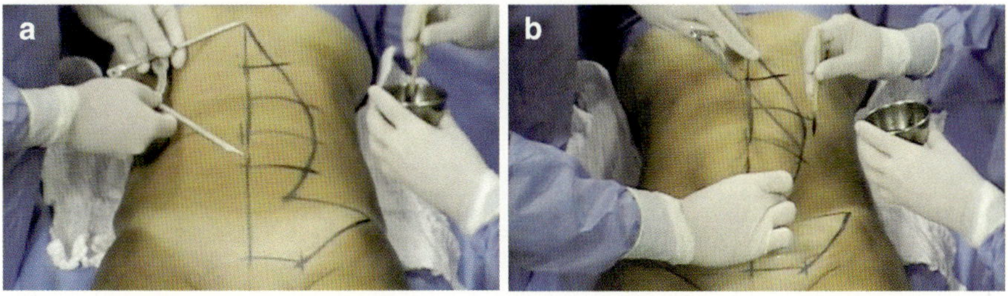

Fig. 16.5 (**a**, **b**) Estimating the new navel position

extends from 5 cm above to 5 cm below the point marked before on the curved line. This tactic prevents possible positioning errors. Symmetrical points are marked with methylene blue on both sides of the line, as well as across the base of the safety strip. At this time one side is copied to the other with the aid of a compass, and this completes the marking (Fig. 16.6).

16.3.2 Surgery

After the infiltration of markings subcutaneously (saline with epinephrine 1:500,000), the incisions are performed to the aponeurotic level. The detachment of the whole segment is carried out in the supra-aponeurotic plane. No lateral dissection is necessary. When the navel is reached, it is amputated at its base, and its hole is sutured with mononylon 3-0. The thread is cut long to mark the original site of the umbilicus (Fig. 16.7).

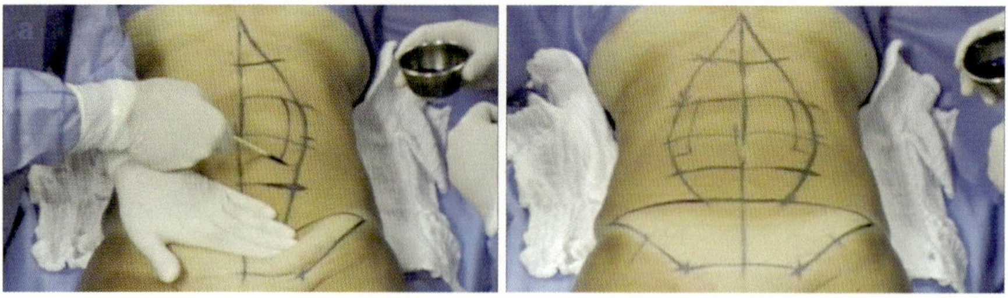

Fig. 16.6 (**a**, **b**) Marking the safety strip

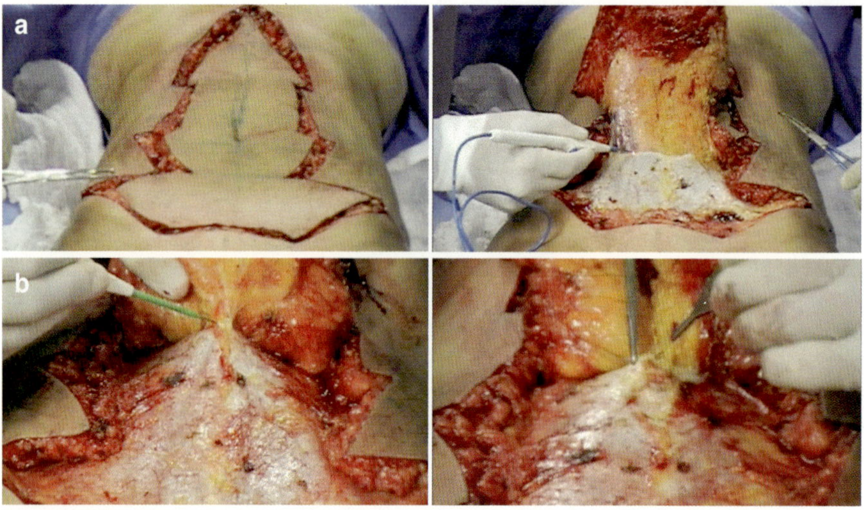

Fig. 16.7 (**a**) Detachment. (**b**) Umbilical disinsertion

At this time the final hemostasis is performed. The marking and preparation of plication of the rectus abdominals are held 3 cm lateral to the inner edge of these muscles. Polypropylene thread 0 is used at points "X" and then a continuous suture. The long thread of the original navel marking is maintained (Fig. 16.8).

The skin starts to be closed. To avoid the presence of dog-ears in the cranial portion of the incision, the skin should be strongly pulled medially and caudally in the epigastric region. This maneuver is very important. At this time the aponeurosis is joined at midline to the edges of the fascia of Scarpa with separate sutures. This prevents the presence of dead space and abolishes the need for active drainage (Fig. 16.9).

Only after fixing these tissues and this advance in skin closure, the flaps are designed that will result in the new navel. This umbilicoplasty technique consists of the union in the midline of two small trapezoidal side-based flaps that are joined to each other until their base, resulting in a tubular appearance. The marking is done at the safety strip using the long thread to mark the navel position. The flap has a

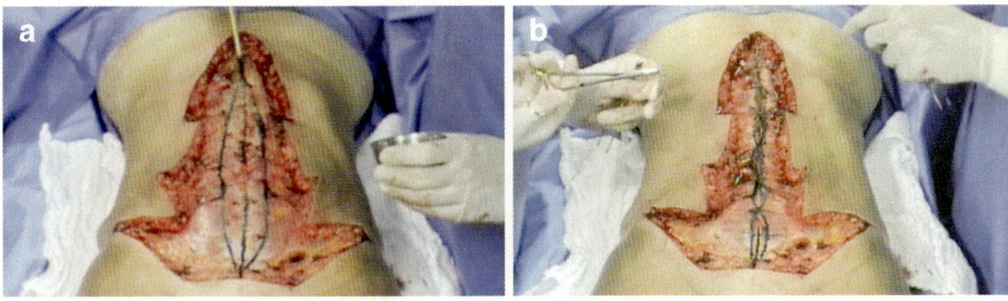

Fig. 16.8 (**a**) Marking muscle for plication. (**b**) Muscular plication

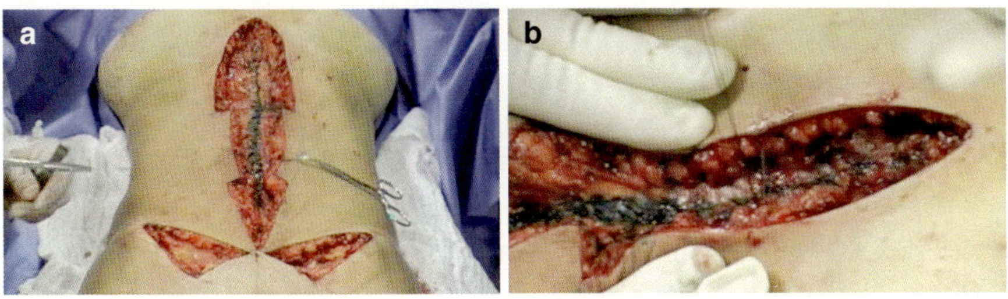

Fig. 16.9 (**a**, **b**) Skin approximation

3.5–4.0 cm base and 2.5–3.0 cm at the top with a 2.0–2.5 cm height. This results in a trapezoidal shape. The authors want to create an elongated navel, with a top shelf. The caudal margin needs to superficialize smoothly without the presence of a lower shelf. For this, an arched line is designed from the top of the flap to its base. The height of the flap will vary with the thickness of the adipose tissue (Fig. 16.10).

The remainder of the safety strip is excised and the umbilical flaps defatted. The flaps are joined together at the midline aponeurosis with three separate sutures using mononylon 3-0. They are joined together with dermal sutures using mononylon 4-0, creating a tubular aspect (Fig. 16.11).

The surgery is completed with the remainder of the suture and wound dressing. Drains are not used (Fig. 16.12).

16.4 Discussion

Abdominoplasty is among the most frequently performed cosmetic surgeries in the world. In almost every case, there is an intervention in the navel, changing its shape and/or location. To rebuild or improve the appearance of the navel, the ideal shape must be known [1]. In contrast to the large number of umbilicoplasty techniques described in literature [4, 5, 7, 9–13], we do not find lots of papers on the standards of appearance of an aesthetically attractive umbilicus [1, 7, 8]. In Craig's paper [1], 147 women had their navels photographed and classified with scores 1–10

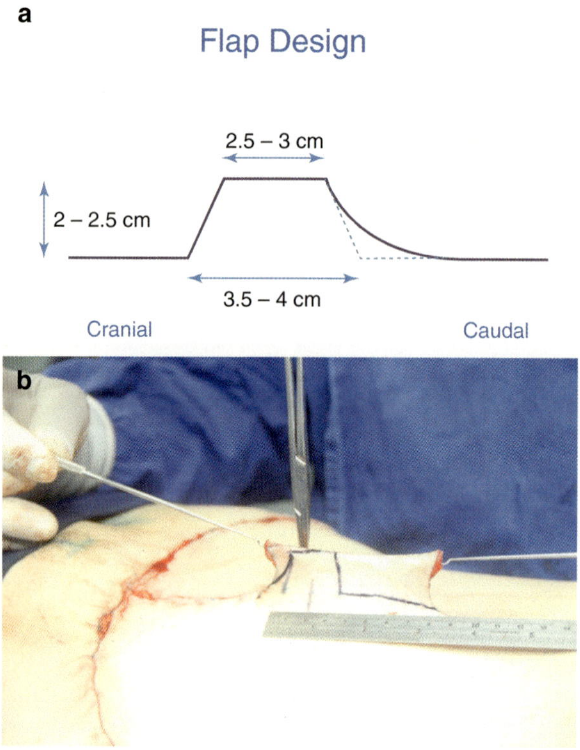

Fig. 16.10 (**a**) Optimal measures of the flap. (**b**) Marking. Note the importance of the safety strip. The exact point of fixation was not in the middle of the safety strip, but 3 cm lower

according to their attractive characteristics by a team of 21 professionals. The shallow, small, T-shaped or vertically oriented navels obtained the best scores on the aesthetic appeal. In contrast, the broad ones, with protrusions or horizontally orientated navels received the worst grades. According with this observation, Santana's paper demonstrates a tactic to prevent or treat this occurrence [14]. While Craig's work prioritized the study of the ideal shape of the navel, the paper of Abhyankar [8] was based on the most frequent location of the umbilicus, obtained through measurements and proportions between the navel and fixed points as the pubic symphysis, the xiphoid process, and the anterior superior iliac spines. One of his results demonstrated that the ideal relationship between the distance between the xiphoid process and the navel and between the navel and the pubic symphysis is 1.6:1. Chang and Baroudi [15] also use the side flaps technique in vertical tummy tuck. The upper margin of the iliac crest is the anatomical reference, for them, to position the new navel. Pallua developed, in Germany, a study that covers both the characteristics (shape and position) [7]. The oval shape obtained the best scores. The greatest motivation is to create an aesthetically attractive navel, elongated vertically, small, and with no externally visible scars. Furthermore, after a few months, the reduction

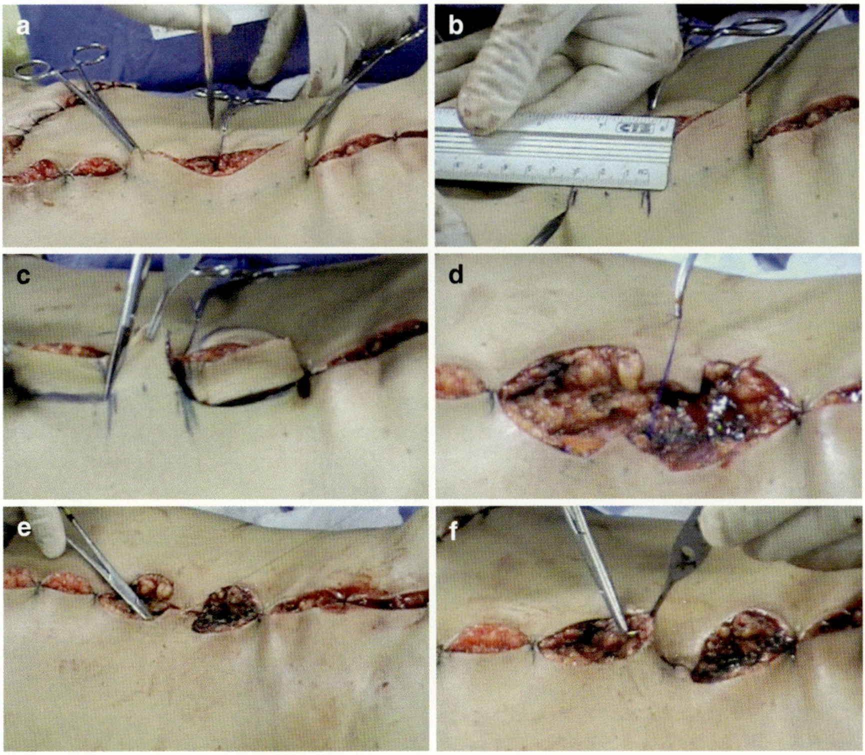

Fig. 16.11 Neo-umbilicus. (**a**) Safety flap marked. (**b**) Measuring flap for neo-umbilicus. (**c**) Incision and defatting of the flap for neo-umbilicus. (**b**) Flap defatted and positioned at the exact point of the surgical suture (original umbilicus point). (**c**) Excision of excess flap. (**d**) Excision completed. (**e**) Fixation of the flaps at the midline aponeurosis. (**f**) Suturing the flaps together creating the tubular effect

of skin tension naturally developed a mild upper shelf at the cranial edge of the navels, providing even more natural results.

The use of two side flaps U-shaped vertical abdominoplasty was first described by the Argentines Fernandes and Correa-Iturraspe in 1951 [2, 3]. This technique propitiated natural navels in only vertical resection. In Brazil, we highlight the dissemination of the use of these flaps in the work of Franco et al. [5]. Franco indicated this technique for patients with a median scar with umbilical distortion after bariatric surgery or not. The same flaps are used in various abdominoplasty techniques [15, 16]. It includes post-bariatric cases and special situations like moderate or large umbilical hernias or severe abdominal wall defects as in laparotomy. At the time the authors published the first work (2010) [6], it was unknown who used the same techniques in all cases of vertical tummy tuck, even when there was no median scar. Other authors also perform the neo-umbilicoplasty routinely, but with different purposes and techniques [17, 18].

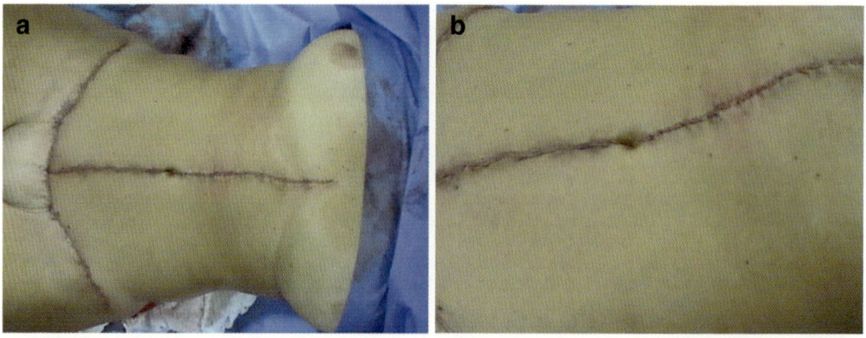

Fig. 16.12 (**a**, **b**) Immediately postoperative

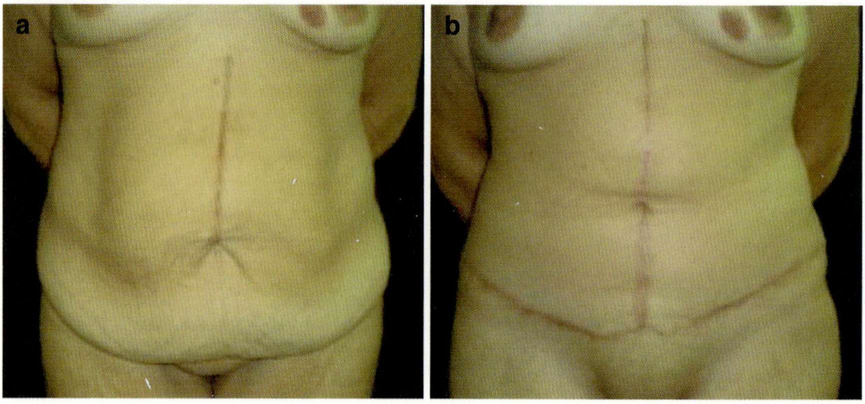

Fig. 16.13 (**a**) Preoperative. (**b**) Six months postoperative

To avoid cranial or caudal malposition of the new navel, it is prudent to use the 10 cm safety strip. Since starting this tactic, there have been no more problems in fixating the neo-umbilicus at the exact original place.

Some of the patients had concomitant midline hernias. While surgery is harder, there is no contraindication to this technique even though the use of a polypropylene mesh is required. Although some of them had bulky hernias, the release of muscle compartments was not required for enhanced mobilization of the abdominal wall as described by Barbosa et al. [19].This work is performed as en bloc resection of the abdominal flap in all cases as done for the classic abdominoplasty. This tactic is recommended by Pontes [20] to minimize asymmetry. Drains are not used because there are no side detachments. The deep sutures avoid the creation of dead spaces as the fascia of Scarpa is fixed to the aponeurosis in the midline.

The positive results of this technique stimulated us to standardize it, making it reproducible, including by the residents in our department who perform it today with the same predictable results (Figs. 16.13, 16.14, 16.15, 16.16, and 16.17). The positive assessment by patients encourages us to follow this line and try to improve.

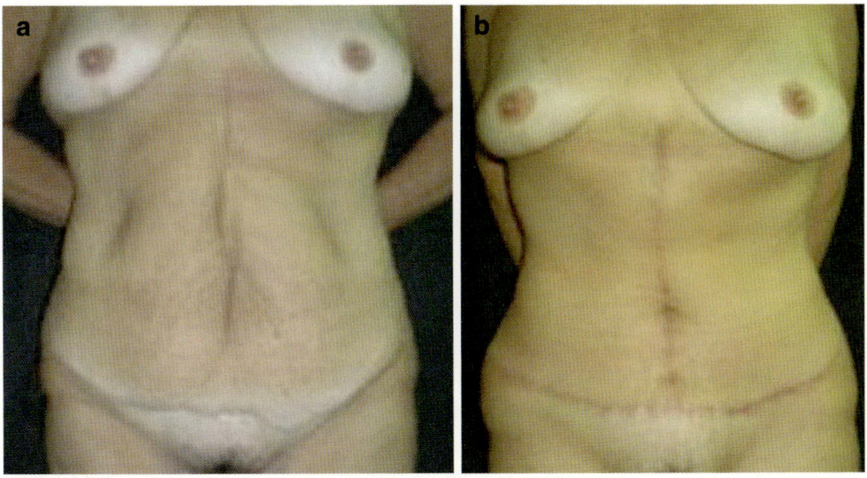

Fig. 16.14 (**a**) Preoperative. (**b**) Six months postoperative

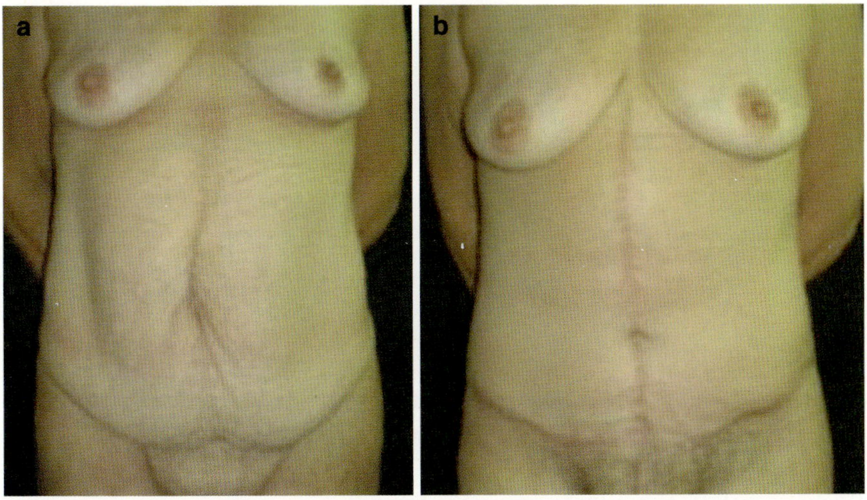

Fig. 16.15 (**a**) Preoperative. (**b**) Six months postoperative

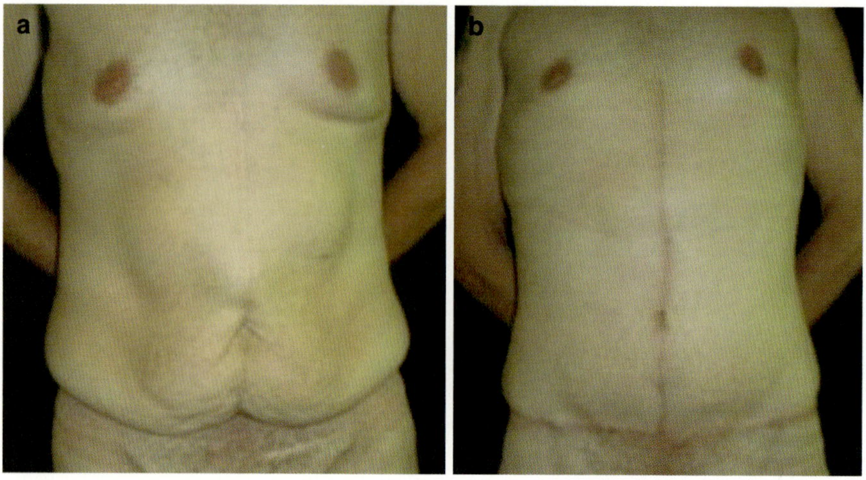

Fig. 16.16 (**a**) Preoperative. (**b**) Six months postoperative

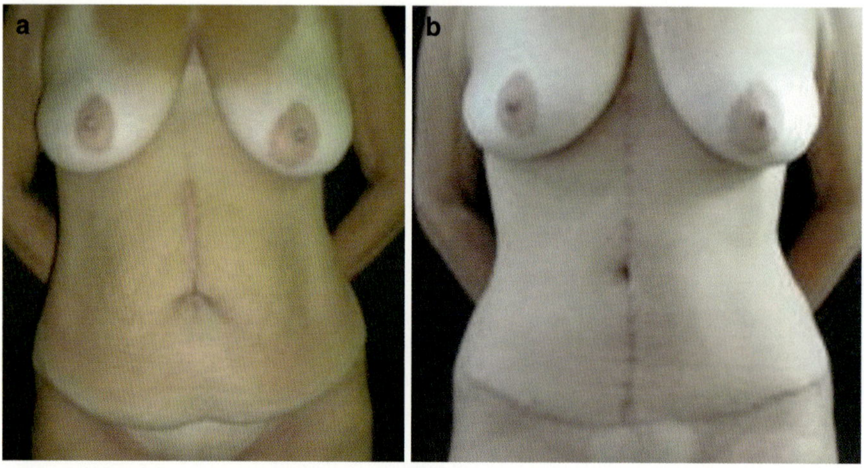

Fig. 16.17 (**a**) Preoperative. (**b**) Six months postoperative

16.5 Conclusions

The neo-umbilicoplasty technique with vertical flaps is a procedure easy to perform, reproducible, and with low incidence of complications. The aesthetic result is superior to the traditional vertical tummy tuck technique that advocates maintaining the umbilical stump. The design of the safety strip allows the precise placement of neonavel in the location of the original navel. This technique can be used not only for vertical tummy tuck but also to rebuild the navel after scarring sequel, laparotomy, or voluminous hernias that compromised its shape.

References

1. Craig SB, Faller MS, Puckett CL. In search of the ideal female umbilicus. Plast Reconstr Surg. 2000;105:389–92.
2. Fernades JC, Correa-Iturraspe M. Dermolipectomia vertical en el delantal grasoso. El Dia Medico. 1951;23:1483.
3. Sinder R. Cirurgia Plástica do Abdome. Rio de Janeiro: R. Niteroi; 1979.
4. Dogan T. Umbilicoplasty in abdominoplasty: a new approach. Ann Plast Surg. 2010;64(6):718–21.
5. Franco D, Medeiros J, Farias C, Franco T. Umbilical reconstruction for patients with a midline scar. Aesthetic Plast Surg. 2006;30:595–8.
6. Silva FN, Oliveira EA. Neo-onfaloplastia na abdominoplastia vertical. Rev Bras Cir Plást. 2010;25(2):330–6.
7. Pallua N, Markowicz MP, Grosse F, Walter S. Aesthetically pleasant umbilicoplasty. Ann Plast Surg. 2010;64(6):722–5.
8. Abhyankar SV, Rajguru AG. Anatomic localization of the umbilicus: An Indian study. Plastic Reconst Surg. 2006;117(4):1153–7.
9. Bruekers SE, van der Lei B, Tan TL, Luijendijk RW, Stevens HP. "Scarless" umbilicoplasty: a new umbilicoplasty technique and a review of the English language literature. Ann Plast Surg. 2009;63(1):15–20.
10. Mazzocchi M, Trignano E, Armenti AF, Figus A, Dessy LA. Long-term results of a versatile technique for umbilicoplasty in abdominoplasty. Aesthetic Plast Surg. 2011;35(4):456–62.
11. Baack BR, Anson G, Nachbar JM, White DJ. Umbilicoplasty: the construction of a New umbilicus and correction of umbilical stenosis without external scars. Plastic Reconst Surg. 1996;97(1):227–32.
12. Southwell-Keely JP, Berry MG. Umbilical reconstruction: a review of techniques. J Plast Reconstr Aesthet Surg. 2011;64(6):803–8.
13. Massiha H, Montegut W, Phillips R. A method of reconstructing a natural-looking umbilicus in abdominoplasty. Ann Plast Surg. 1997;38(3):228–31.
14. Santana KP, Pereira LH, Sterodimas A. Sad umbilicus: prevention and treatment. Aesthetic Plast Surg. 2009;33:471–2.
15. Chang TN, Baroudi R. Abdominoplasty techniques. In: Mathes SJ, editor. Plastic surgery. 2nd ed. Philadelphia: Saunders; 2006. p. 168–70.
16. Rozen SM, Redett R. The two-dermal-flap umbilical transposition: a natural and aesthetic umbilicus after abdominoplasty. PlastReconstr Surg. 2007;119(7):2255–62.
17. Nogueira DSC. Neo-onfaloplastia de rotina em abdominoplastias. Rev Bras Cir Plást. 2008;23(3):207–13.
18. Amud RJM. Neo-onfaloplastia sem cicatriz. Rev Bras Cir Plast. 2008;23(1):37–40.
19. Barbosa MVJ, Nahas FX, Ferreira LM. Hernioplastia incisional associada a abdominoplastia. Rev Bras Cir Plást. 2010;25(Suppl):1–102.
20. Pontes R. Abdominoplastia: ressecção em bloco e sua aplicação em lifting de coxa e torsoplastia. Rio de Janeiro: Revinter; 2004. p. 119–38.

Chapter 17
Inverted U-Shaped Umbilical Reconstruction in Abdominoplasty

Melvin A. Shiffman

17.1 Introduction

There are a variety of incisions for reconstructing the umbilicus during abdominoplasty. Many of them have similar results. These include the U-shape, inverted U-shape, V-shape, inverted V-shape, and even the omega-shape. Each of these breaks the circle of the umbilicus and prevents stenosis.

17.2 Inverted U-Shaped Umbilicoplasty in Abdominoplasty

Producing a normal-appearing umbilicus during abdominoplasty is best achieved with the inverted U-shaped umbilicoplasty. If done properly, the umbilicus is hooded superiorly, has a central opening, and proceeds slightly superiorly as it approaches the abdominal wall fascia.

17.3 Technique

Preoperatively a line is marked from the xiphoid to the mid-umbilicus and at the pubis where the hairs diverge to show the midline. This establishes the center of the abdominal wall at the time of closure. After elevation of the flap from the fascia overlying the muscles from the pubis to the umbilicus, the umbilical stalk is separated from the surrounding fat and the skin incised around the umbilical opening

M.A. Shiffman, M.D., J.D.
Private Practice, 17501 Chatham Drive, Tustin, CA 92780, USA
e-mail: shiffmanmdjd@gmail.com

M.A. Shiffman (ed.), *Adult Umbilical Reconstruction*,
DOI 10.1007/978-3-319-43887-0_17

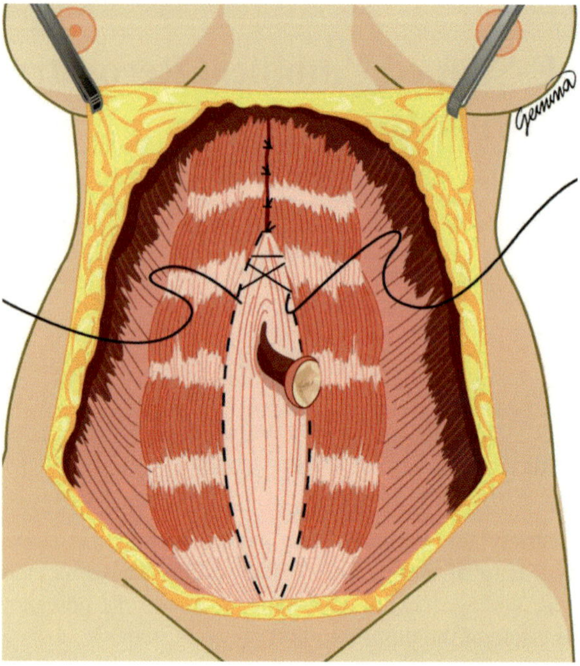

Fig. 17.1 The umbilical stalk base is identified and used as the level for the new umbilicus and the fascia of the rectus muscles closed around the linea alba

leaving about 1 cm of skin on the stalk. The dissection then proceeds on top of the fascia from the umbilicus to the xiphoid process and lowest portion of the ribs. The umbilical stalk base is identified and used as the level for the new umbilicus and the fascia of the rectus muscles closed around the linea alba (Fig. 17.1). A U- or V-shaped excision of the inferior portion of the umbilical stalk is carried out, 2 cm wide at the top and narrowing down to near the base of the umbilical pedicle (Fig. 17.2). The umbilical pedicle is shortened by suturing, with 3–0 nonabsorbable sutures, from a few millimeters below the top of the pedicle to the linea alba and rectus muscle fascia in four places equally spaced (Fig. 17.3). This reestablishes the original orientation of the umbilicus and is a stable deep suture site to invert the superficial skin of the abdominal wall. Usually, a 4–0 nonabsorbable suture is inserted through the lowest part of the V- or U-shaped excised area grasping the stalk of the umbilicus and leaving the needle intact. Another convenient suture is inserted through the edge of the superior part of the umbilical stalk leaving the needle attached. Without cutting the threads, a tonsil hemostat is placed on the ends of the threads (one hemostat for the two ends of each suture) in order to pass them through the opening in the abdominal wall for the umbilicus. This makes it easier to suture the remaining umbilical stalk to the abdominal wall skin after the flap is sutured in the midline of the pubis. The center of the superior flap overlapping the inferior flap is incised until it reaches the transverse pubic lower flap at which time

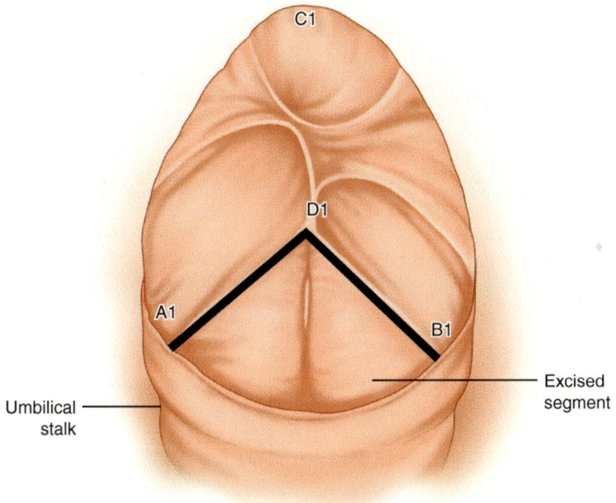

Fig. 17.2 A U- or V-shaped excision (*D1* to *A1* to *B1*) of the inferior portion of the umbilical stalk is carried out, 2 cm wide at the top and narrowing down to near the base of the umbilical pedicle. *C1* is the superior part of the umbilical stalk

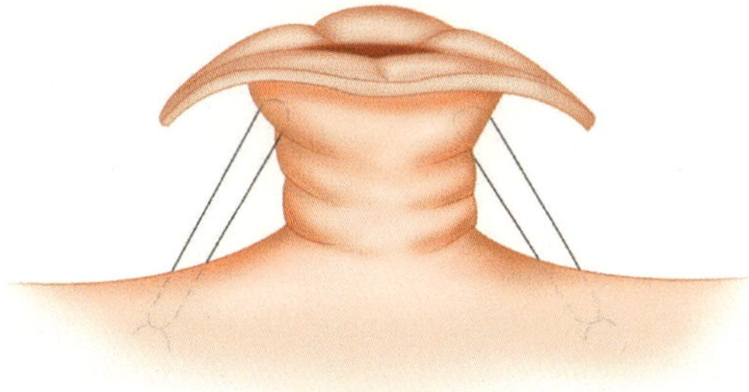

Fig. 17.3 The umbilical pedicle is shortened by suturing, with 3–0 nonabsorbable sutures, from a few millimeters below the top of the pedicle to the linea alba and rectus muscle fascia in four places equally spaced

the center point is sutured with a temporary holding suture of 2–0 nylon to the center of the lower flap determined by the diversion of hairs at the pubis.

The abdominal wall flap is incised superiorly from the center of the flap until the incised portion of the flap meets the pubis with tension. The center of the flap is then sutured to the center of the marked pubis with a subcuticular 2–0 chromic suture. The abdominal wall is then marked to indicate the position of the new umbilicus by

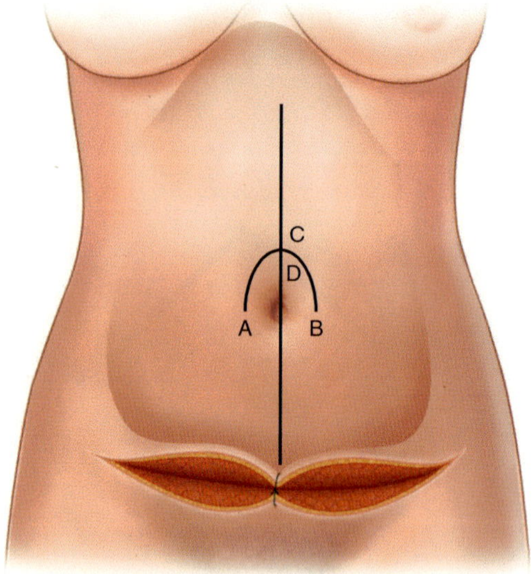

Fig. 17.4 The inverted U has points *A* and *B* each 1.3 cm from the midline. The top of the U (*C* is abdominal wall, *D* is flap) is 2 cm superior to *A*,*B*

using a tonsil hemostat on the umbilical stalk center with the tip pointing toward the skin. An inverted U-shape is marked so that the tip of the inverted U-flap is 1.0 cm below this point. The inverted U-shape is 2.6 cm wide at the base, and the flap is 2 cm in length (Fig. 17.4). The inverted U-shaped flap is incised, and the dissection proceeds through the fat. The hemostats holding the sutures in the umbilical stalk are passed through the opening and grasped from the outside. The umbilical stalk (A1, C1, B1, D1) is sutured to the skin (A,B,C) and U-flap (A,B,D) (Fig. 17.5). The excess skin of the abdominoplasty flap is excised and the wound closed.

By placing the center of the marked inverted U-shape 1.0 cm inferior to the level of the umbilical base, the suturing of the wounds results in an umbilical opening with the canal of the umbilicus oriented superiorly and forcing the superior portion of the opening to appear hooded (Fig. 17.6).

17.4 Discussion

The reason for the excision of tissue from the umbilical stalk is because the lack of excision results in excess tissue of the skin end of the pedicle that on closure tends to pleat (ripple). This will usually improve over 6 months but sometimes does not completely disappear.

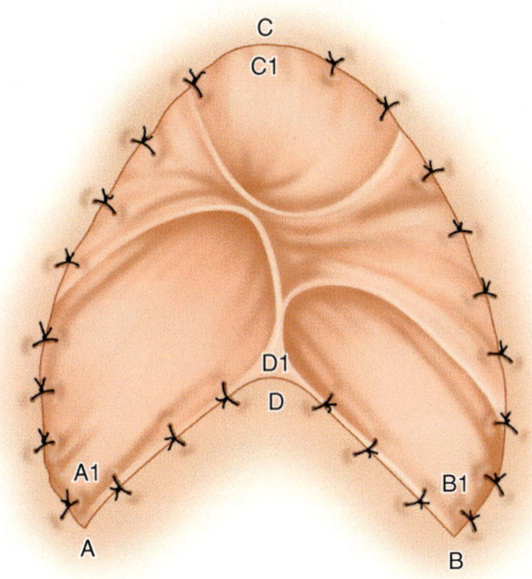

Fig. 17.5 The umbilical stalk (*A1*, *C1*, *B1*, *D1*) is sutured to the skin (*A*,*B*,*C*) and U-flap (*A*,*B*,*D*)

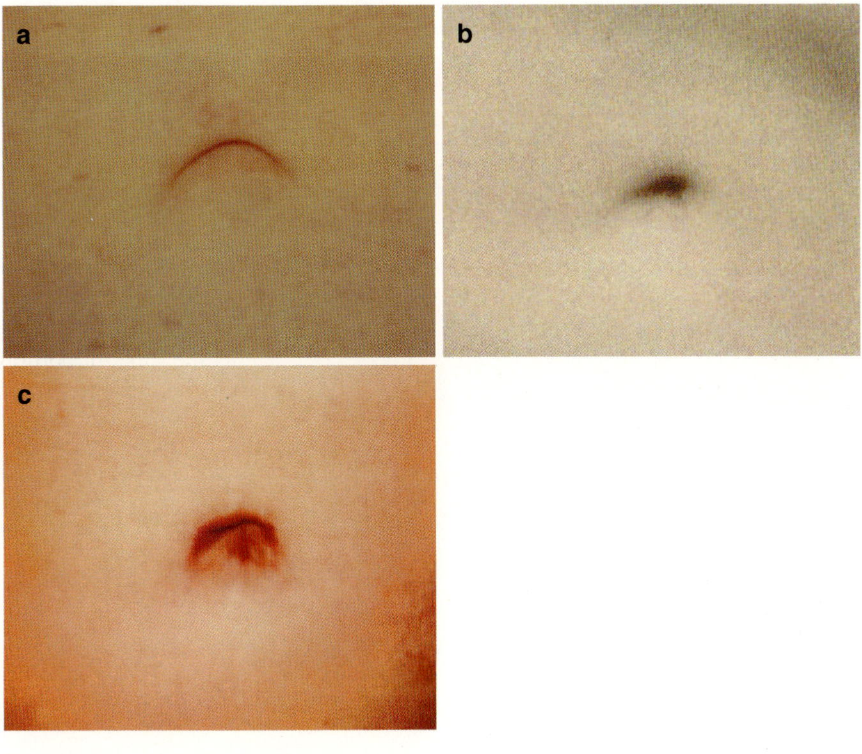

Fig. 17.6 **(a–c)** Postsurgical umbilicuses

Some of the closures with circular excision and transverse or vertical incisions have a tendency for occasional stenosis of the umbilicus. The inverted U-shape breaks the circle that tends to become stenotic that occurs with these other procedures. Stenosis is not aesthetic pleasing and repair is frequently necessary. Stenosis can be treated with the inverted U-shaped incision with good success.

Chapter 18
Umbilicoplasties Postabdominal Free Flap Harvest

Joey Corkum, Joshua A. Gillis, Ammar Al-Dhamin, and Steven F. Morris

18.1 Introduction

The umbilical cord supplies the developing fetus with oxygenated blood while in vitro. It forms during the fourth to eighth week, as the embryo enlarges relative to a ventral open area, resulting in a tubular structure enclosing the omphalomesenteric duct, allantois, and fetal blood vessels. The umbilical cord is truncated following birth, and any remainder falls off approximately 10 days after, leaving only the umbilicus; it is therefore a normal scar.

Ultimately four fibrous cords are responsible for the shape of the umbilicus [1]. The obliterated left umbilical vein runs upward as the round ligament of the liver. The remaining three structures are the obliterated urachus centrally and the obliterated umbilical arteries, which run caudally as the medial umbilical ligaments. The resultant force vector is typically inward and upward, creating the characteristic superior hooding. The umbilicus measures approximately 1.5–2 cm in diameter and is midline at the level of the superior iliac crest or 10–12 cm above the pubic hairline

J. Corkum, B.Sc., M.D.
Private Practice, 4443-1796 Summer Street, Halifax, NS B3H 2A7, Canada
e-mail: joeycorkum@gmail.com

J.A. Gillis, B.Sc., M.D.
Department of Surgery, Section of Plastic Surgery, Dalhousie University,
1339 Brenton Street, Halifax, NS B3J2K5, Canada
e-mail: jgillis@dal.ca

A. Al-Dhamin, M.B.Ch.B., M.R.C.S.
Tawam Hospital, P.O. Box 15258, Al Ain, United Arab Emirates
e-mail: dr.aldhamin@gmail.com

S.F. Morris, M.Sc., M.D. (✉)
Division of Plastic Surgery, Dalhousie University,
4443-1796 Summer Street, Halifax, NS B3H 2A7, Canada
e-mail: sfmorris1@gmail.com

M.A. Shiffman (ed.), *Adult Umbilical Reconstruction*,
DOI 10.1007/978-3-319-43887-0_18

[2]. Depending on the scarring of the fibrous cords, the shape is variable between round and oval. It is flat early in life but then develops hooding and deepens as fat accumulates circumferentially. Aging and weight gain contribute to a more transverse orientation. Pregnancy, herniation, and scarring can alter the shape of the umbilicus [2]. In an obese person, there is the adipose tissue and skin surrounding the umbilicus proper, which may not be seen secondary to excess adiposity. In thinner patients, the umbilicus is more shallow, and the base of the umbilicus can be identified [3].

As far back as 129–199 AD, it was recognized that the umbilicus represents an important physiologic and aesthetic feature of the abdomen [4]. Until the 1950s, the umbilicus was routinely excised following abdominoplasty, but Vernon et al. [5] advocated for its reconstruction. This was due to an inability to produce an aesthetically pleasing umbilicus that leads to stenosis and omphalitis. Attention to umbilicus aesthetics has since been of increasing importance. The umbilicus now plays a prominent role in everyday society that is accentuated by advertisements and the fashion industry. The umbilicus represents a natural reference point, and the lack of one has been described as unsettling [6]. This is supported by statistics from the American Society for Aesthetic Plastic Surgery that shows an increase in umbilicoplasty by 57 % from 2003 to 2004 [7].

Using autologous abdominal tissue for reconstruction obviates the need for creating a neoumbilicus similar to that of an abdominoplasty procedure. The ideal umbilicoplasty produces an aesthetically pleasing umbilicus with minimal visible scarring and risk for stenosis or ischemia. We aim for a vertical orientation of the umbilicus with superior hooding and central depression, which represents the majority of patient's preoperative umbilicus and has been shown to be the most appealing [8].

18.2 **Technique** (Figs. 18.1 and 18.2)

The umbilicus is marked, along with the autologous flap markings. With the deep inferior epigastric artery perforator (DIEP) or superficial inferior epigastric artery (SIEA) flap, the superior marking is typically at the superior aspect of the iliac crest, approximately one centimeter above the umbilicus, but can be at the umbilicus if there are concerns regarding primary closure of the donor site. The umbilicus is marked with a vertically oriented oval just outside of its margins. If the flap incision is at the umbilicus, the area of the umbilical incision will remain as a small vertical scar in the central portion of the raised abdominal flap once the donor site is closed.

The initial periumbilical incision is performed with the help of skin hooks in the superior and inferior aspects of the umbilicus to keep tension, ensuring to leave a small skin island on the umbilicus. The umbilical stalk is dissected subcutaneously with Metzenbaum scissors to remove significant subcutaneous tissue and fat and to ensure that an umbilical hernia is not entered. If a bilateral autologous free flap is planned, the skin paddles may be split in half to complete dissection of the umbilical

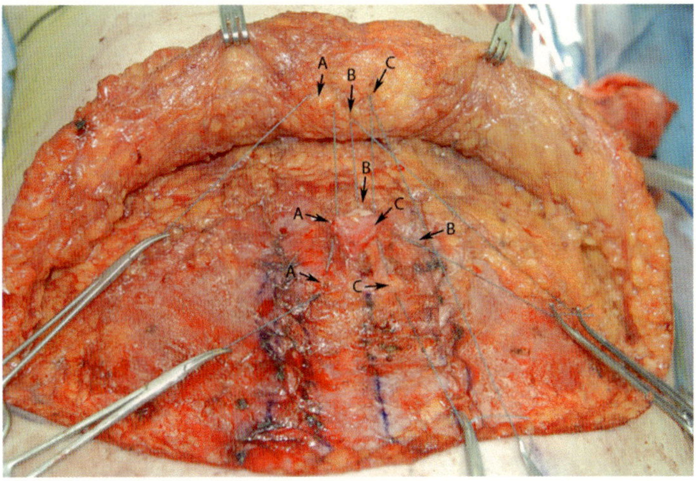

Fig. 18.1 To create a central depression of the umbilicus, the stalk is sutured to the anterior rectus fascia at the 12 o'clock, 4 o'clock, and 8 o'clock (*B*, *C*, and *A*, respectively) aspects of the umbilicus

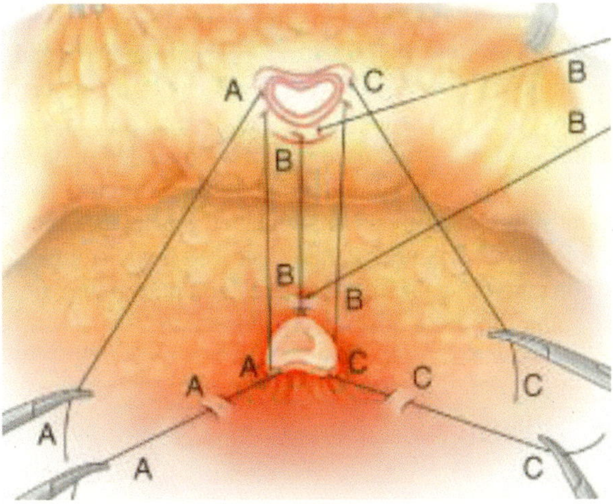

Fig. 18.2 Suturing the neoumbilicus to the abdominal rectus fascia

stalk down to the anterior rectus fascia. Once the autologous flap is raised, the umbilical stalk is sutured at the 3, 6, and 9 o'clock position to the anterior rectus fascia. This ensures the umbilicus maintains an appropriate depression or "crater" once sutured to the superior abdominal flap. When performing the fascial plication or repairing the fascial defect of the harvested pedicle, care must be taken to not move the umbilicus too far laterally in one direction. If a unilateral flap is raised, repair of the fascia will pull the umbilical stalk laterally, and a contralateral fascial plication should be performed. In a bilateral flap, the bilateral fascial repairs keep the umbilicus midline in relation to the xiphoid. Central rectus diastasis is typically plicated as well, using nonabsorbable 2–0 polyester sutures or an absorbable polydioxanone suture (PDS) (Ethicon, Somerville, NJ). Care must be taken to not bury the umbilical stalk while repairing the rectus diastasis, unless it is long, where burying a portion of it may be advantageous in a thinner patient to obtain appropriate umbilical depression.

Once the superior abdominal flap is dissected, it is brought midline of the pubic area and partially closed to ensure proper placement of the umbilicus. An inferiorly based inverted U-shaped flap is marked at the level of the umbilical stalk using digital palpation from both underneath and atop of the abdominal flap. The inverted U-shaped flap should have a base of approximately 2.5–3 cm and a height of 1.5–2 cm. This flap is developed, and the abdominal flap is thinned of subcutaneous fat in a 2 cm area surrounding the incision, making sure not to interrupt the blood supply of the skin. This helps to produce periumbilical concavity necessary for a smooth transition from the abdomen to umbilicus [9]. A caudal wedge is removed from the umbilicus at the 6 o'clock position, where the U-flap will insert. To create a central depression of the umbilicus, the stalk is then sutured to the anterior rectus fascia at the 12 o'clock, 4 o'clock, and 8 o'clock aspects of the umbilicus. The 2–0 polyester sutures should be placed from the rectus sheath to the dermal portion of the umbilical edges then to the corresponding dermal aspect of the neoumbilicus. The sutures should be secured well to ensure proper symmetry and prevent extrusion. Using one suture to both secures the umbilicus to the rectus fascia, and the abdominal flap will decrease the amount of suture material present. A nonabsorbable monofilament suture is then used for the remainder of the dermal sutures between the umbilicus and the abdominal flap, with a running 4–0 or 5–0 absorbable monofilament suture in a subcuticular manner. The inverted U-shaped flap may be trimmed to gain proper fit into the umbilical wedge incision without excess tissue. A piece of nonadherent gauze is then rolled and placed into the umbilicus with dry gauze placed over top, for a postoperative dressing.

18.3 Discussion

Umbilical placement following an abdominoplasty or abdominal wall donor site closure may appear to be a minor component of the procedure, but it is in fact integral to a good aesthetic outcome. The ideal umbilicus has been studied previously. Craig et al. [8] evaluated 147 female abdomens to identify the ideal umbilical shape. They identified five primary shapes – "T," vertical, oval, horizontal, and distorted. The "T"- shaped umbilici scored highest aesthetically among the group and, along with vertical and oval, were significantly more appealing than horizontal or distorted. Of note, over 70 % of the study population had a hooded umbilicus.

Typically the umbilicoplasty procedure involves excising the existing umbilicus. The skin is then undermined. The rectus abdominis muscle is usually plicated vertically from xiphoid to pubis. Some will then attach the umbilicus to the rectus fascia or linea alba to create the dimpled effect of the area surrounding the umbilicus. Suturing the stalk to the skin without fixating it to deeper fascia will increase the chance of scar visibility. By plicating it to the fascia, the scar is hidden deeper in the umbilicus, and umbilical depth is recreated. It is important to consider the length of the umbilicus stalk at this stage, which will depend on the size of the patient. The correct place for the umbilicus on the abdomen must then be established. The position is generally midline and between the superior iliac crests. Rohrich et al. [10] showed that the umbilicus is rarely midline in patients preoperatively, and this should be discussed with the patient. In a study of 100 nonobese patients, Dubou and Ousterhout [11] found the umbilicus to be at the level of the superior iliac crest in 96 % of cases, regardless of sex, age, or race. Templates have been invented for consistent placement relative to the abdominoplasty [12–14]. Many surgeons, however, decide on the placement of the umbilicus based on the natural position of the umbilical stalk, which they determine using a hand on the abdominal wall and one hand on top of the flap.

Many techniques of designing the neoumbilicus have been described. Pitanguy originally described a horizontal technique in 1967, and early on a number of horizontal techniques followed [15–17]. This technique fell out of favor because of the circular contraction and hypertrophic scarring common in circular incisions, which make the umbilicus less appealing and narrow [18]. To mitigate this effect, different shapes have been implemented to disrupt the circular scar. Massiha et al. [3] presented a triangular shaped "Y" incision in the abdominal flap. They described the importance of suturing the umbilical stalk to the rectus fascia to create a "crater" and hide the umbilical scar. Different modifications of "V" and "Y" incisions of the abdominal flap have been described [19–24]. Ramirez [19] described a circular incision with a superiorly or inferiorly based "V" based on patient's preference. The "V" is designed to avoid the concentric scar of a complete circle [16].

Franco and Franco [20] described a neoumbilicoplasty technique in which they create a "Y" flap sutured to the rectus fascia in which the base of the cavity is allowed to heal secondarily to simulate the sloughing off of the umbilicus after birth. This is used if the umbilical stalk needs to be resected due to incisional or umbilical hernia or absence from previous surgery. Baack et al. [25] used a similar technique using an inferiorly based inverted "U"-shaped flap with lateral extensions that was sutured to the fascia to create the central crater. The superior abdominal flap was then closed and sutured to the abdominal fascia with a vertical dog-ear at the superior rim of the navel rim to simulate umbilical hooding. De Lacerda et al. [26] described a four-flap technique along with a similar procedure of deepithelialization and fixation to the abdominal wall. Pardo et al. [27] outlined another flap technique but used three separate flaps and a purse-string-type suturing technique to tether the neoumbilicus to the aponeurotic plane. Choudhary et al. [28] revisited the circular design and made recommendations about "umbilicosculpting."

Akbas et al. [29], Dogan [30], Lee and Mustoe [31], Santanelli et al. [32], and later others demonstrated their design using a vertically oriented elliptical incision to inset the umbilical stalk after abdominoplasty. Akbas et al. [29] performed a vertical elliptical incision around the umbilicus, then sutured it to the abdominal fascia and buried the stalk within the plication. A vertical incision was made in the abdominal flap and sutured to the rectus fascia surrounding the umbilicus. They found that all of their 15 study patients were satisfied with their outcome when asked retrospectively. Rozen et al. [9] followed with a similar technique with similarly good results in 20 patients and described the importance of suturing the abdominal flap to the fascia to decrease the tension on the umbilical skin closure and thus reducing cicatricial scarring. Both Rozen and Akbas reported favorable rates of minor complications, at 5 % and 7 %, respectively. Malic et al. [33] compared two new techniques with good results in 25 patients. They compared an inverted "U" shape and a round shape and found that the "U" shape was preferred more frequently by patients.

In 2011, Mazzocchi et al. [2] reported on their long-term outcomes in 111 consecutive cases using a vertically oriented double-opposing "Y" technique and found no significant change in shape, depth, or dimension when comparing results at one and five years. Of the 111 patients, four patients experienced partial deepithelialization, and five patients had cicatricial umbilical stenosis. Lesavoy et al. [6] presented the inverted-V chevron umbilicoplasty with good results. They purported that the design prevented circumferential scar contraction and created a natural-appearing superior hood. This is the basis of our umbilicoplasty, as we have found the superior hooding and vertical orientation to be the most pleasing. We use a suture to capture the abdominal fascia, dermis of the abdominal flap, and dermis of the umbilical stalk to obtain further dimpling of the umbilicus and prefer an inverted "U" to prevent tip necrosis. Undermining the subcutaneous tissue surrounding the flap is important for creating the contour transition between the abdominal flap and umbilicus, especially in an obese patient.

18.4 Conclusions

The ideal umbilicoplasty technique should have a low rate of umbilical stenosis and cicatricial scarring, producing an aesthetically pleasing, depressed, vertically oriented umbilicus with superior hooding and periumbilical concavity. The inferiorly based inverted "U"-shaped umbilicoplasty technique with plication of the abdominal flap to fascia and the umbilical dermis has produced excellent results postabdominal flap reconstruction.

References

1. Dick ET. Umbilicoplasty as a treatment for persistent umbilical infection. Aust N Z J Surg. 1970;39(4):380–3.
2. Mazzocchi M, Trignano E, Armenti AF, Figus A, Dessy LA. Long-term results of a versatile technique for umbilicoplasty in abdominoplasty. Aesthetic Plast Surg. 2011;35(4):456–62.

3. Massiha H, Montegut W, Phillips R. A method of reconstructing a natural-looking umbilicus in abdominoplasty. Ann Plast Surg. 1997;38(3):228–31.
4. Niranjan NS, Staiano JJ. An anatomical method for re-siting the umbilicus. Plast Reconstr Surg. 2004;113(7):2194–8.
5. Vernon S. Umbilical transplantation upward and abdominal contouring in lipectomy. Am J Surg. 1957;94(3):490–2.
6. Lesavoy MA, Fan K, Guenther DA, Herrera F, Little JW. The inverted-v chevron umbilicoplasty for breast reconstruction and abdominoplasty. Aesthet Surg J. 2012;32(1):110–6.
7. Surgery ASFAP. Cosmetic Surgery National Data Bank: Statistics. 2004.
8. Craig SB, Faller MS, Puckett CL. In search of the ideal female umbilicus. Plast Reconstr Surg. 2000;105(1):389–92.
9. Rozen SM, Redett R. The two-dermal-flap umbilical transposition: a natural and aesthetic umbilicus after abdominoplasty. Plast Reconstr Surg. 2007;119(7):2255–62.
10. Rohrich RJ, Sorokin ES, Brown SA, Gibby DL. Is the umbilicus truly midline? Clinical and medicolegal implications. Plast Reconstr Surg. 2003;112(1):259–63.
11. Dubou R, Ousterhout DK. Placement of the umbilicus in an abdominoplasty. Plast Reconstr Surg. 1978;61(2):291–3.
12. Avelar J. Abdominoplasty-Systematization of a technique without external umbilical scar. Aesthetic Plast Surg. 1978;2(1):141–51.
13. Hoffman S. A simple technique for locating the umbilicus in abdominoplasty. Plast Reconstr Surg. 1989;83(3):537–8.
14. Kurul S, Uzunismail A. A simple technique to determine the future location of the umbilicus in abdominoplasty. Plast Reconstr Surg. 1997;100(3):753–4.
15. Delerm A. Refinements in abdominoplasty with emphasis on reimplantation of the umbilicus. Plast Reconstr Surg. 1982;70(5):632–7.
16. Pitanguy I. Abdominal plastic surgery. Hospital. 1967;71(6):1541–56.
17. Otto A, Wechselberger G, Schoeller T, Lille S. A method of reconstructing a natural-looking umbilicus in abdominoplasty. Ann Plast Surg. 1997;39(4):435.
18. Grazer FM, Goldwyn RM. Abdominoplasty assessed by survey, with emphasis on complications. Plast Reconstr Surg. 1977;59(4):513–7.
19. Ramirez OM. Abdominoplasty and abdominal wall rehabilitation: a comprehensive approach. Plast Reconstr Surg. 2000;105(1):425–35.
20. Franco T, Franco D. Neoomphaloplasty: an old and new technique. Aesthetic Plast Surg. 1999;23(2):151–4.
21. Cannistra C, Pecorelli E. Umbilical restoration in abdominal dermolipectomy: a simple double-Y, double-M technique. Aesthetic Plast Surg. 1999;23(5):364–6.
22. Castillo PF, Sepulveda CA, Prado AC, Troncoso AL, Villaman JJ. Umbilical reinsertion in abdominoplasty: technique using deepithelialized skin flaps. Aesthetic Plast Surg. 2007;31(5):519–20.
23. Sugawara Y, Hirabayashi S, Asato H, Yoshimura K. Reconstruction of the umbilicus using a single triangular flap. Ann Plast Surg. 1995;34(1):78–80.
24. Masuda R, Takeda A, Sugimoto T, Ishiguro M, Uchinuma E. Reconstruction of the umbilicus using a reverse fan-shaped flap. Aesthetic Plast Surg. 2003;27(5):349–53.
25. Baack BR, Anson G, Nachbar JM, White DJ. Umbilicoplasty: the construction of a new umbilicus and correction of umbilical stenosis without external scars. Plast Reconstr Surg. 1996;97(1):227–32.
26. de Lacerda DJ, Martins DM, Marques A, Brenda E, de Moura Andrews J. Umbilicoplasty for the abdomen with a thin adipose layer. Br J Plast Surg. 1994;47(5):386–7.
27. Pardo Mateu L, Chamorro Hernandez JJ. Neoumbilicoplasty through a purse-string suture of three defatted flaps. Aesthetic Plast Surg. 1997;21(5):349–51.
28. Choudhary S, Taams KO. Umbilicosculpture: a concept revisited. Br J Plast Surg. 1998;51(7):538–41.
29. Akbas H, Guneren E, Eroglu L, Uysal OA. Natural-looking umbilicus as an important part of abdominoplasty. Aesthetic Plast Surg. 2003;27(2):139–42.

30. Dogan T. Umbilicoplasty in abdominoplasty: a new approach. Ann Plast Surg. 2010;64(6):718–21.
31. Lee MJ, Mustoe TA. Simplified technique for creating a youthful umbilicus in abdominoplasty. Plast Reconstr Surg. 2002;109(6):2136–40.
32. Santanelli F, Mazzocchi M, Renzi L, Cigna E. Reconstruction of a natural-looking umbilicus. Scand J Plast Reconstr Surg Hand Surg. 2002;36(3):183–5.
33. Malic CC, Spyrou GE, Hough M, Fourie L. Patient satisfaction with two different methods of umbilicoplasty. Plast Reconstr Surg. 2007;119(1):357–61.

Chapter 19
A Simple New Technique for Umbilical Reconstruction

Ghada Morshed

19.1 Introduction

McMillan in 1955 [1] first reported umbilical reconstruction after umbilical herniorrhaphy. Nowadays it can be done in many cases like congenital absence (omphalocele, bladder exstrophy, cloacal exstrophy and gastroschisis) or after loss (destruction by inflammation, e.g. umbilical sepsis, periumbilical necrotizing fasciitis) or by surgical procedures (abdominoplasty, umbilical herniorrhaphy, laparotomy) or excision due to skin cancer.

Different techniques to reconstruct the umbilicus, like a number of techniques, describe the use of a small piece of skin or may use a pedicled flap creating the basis of the umbilicus with its attachment to the abdominal fascia [2–6]. This may be accompanied with a skin or cartilaginous graft [7].

Other techniques may use the skin of the abdominal wall for creating a depression of the umbilicus [8–15]. Also, secondary healing may be used for the creation of the umbilical bottom [16].

The aim of this study is to describe a new and simple technique for umbilical reconstruction.

G. Morshed, M.D., M.R.C.S.
Department of Surgery, Fayoum University,
9 Said Zo El Fokkar-Manyal, Cairo, El Fayoum City, Al Fayyum, Egypt
e-mail: ghadamorshed@yahoo.com

M.A. Shiffman (ed.), *Adult Umbilical Reconstruction*,
DOI 10.1007/978-3-319-43887-0_19

19.2 Material and Methods

The study included 20 cases in whom abdominoplasty was performed from July 2013 to March 2014, and a new simple technique was performed for neo-umbilicoplasty in 13 cases.

19.3 Surgical Technique

A triangular skin flap is excised at the site of the new umbilicus, each border of the triangle measures about 4 cm (Fig. 19.1), and after excision of the triangular flap, defatting is performed to the edges, and then purse-string sutures with 2–0 PROLENE are placed on the three borders of the remaining triangular cavity. Then each corner of the remaining triangular cavity is fixed to the underlying rectus

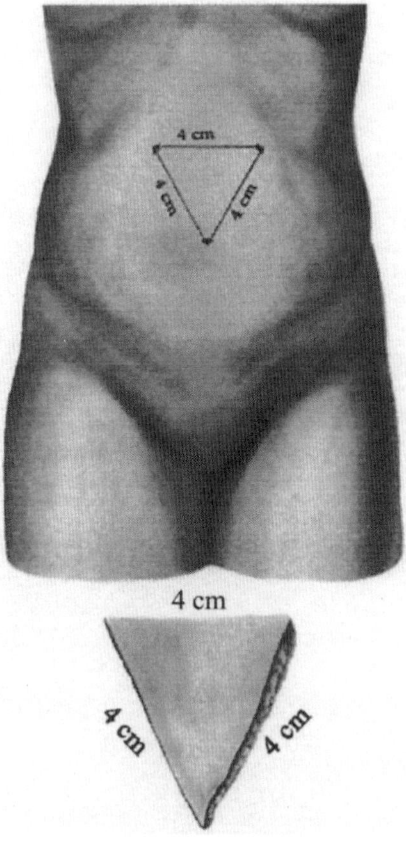

Fig. 19.1 Showing the excised flap

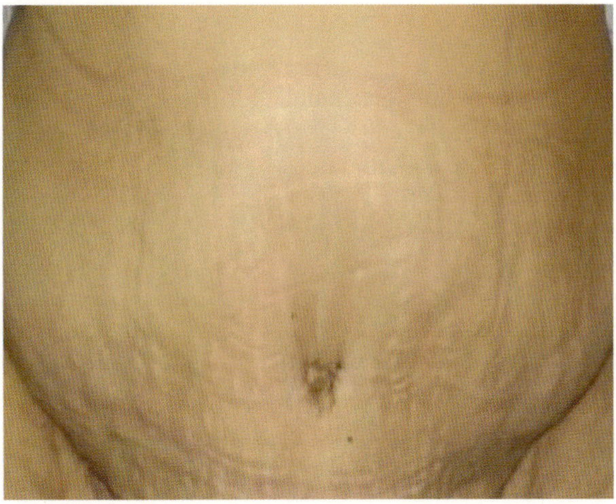

Fig. 19.2 A case of neo-umbilicus

sheath (after repairing of the rectus diastasis). After firm attachment of the three corners to the rectus sheath, the purse string is tightened (Fig. 19.2).

19.4 Results

Over 20 cases of abdominoplasty using a neo-umbilicoplasty were performed with a new and simple technique for 13 cases; follow-up for 1 year revealed the success of the neo-umbilicus without complications.

19.5 Discussion

Neo-umbilicus construction is usually needed postabdominoplasty. There are different techniques; in some techniques, the umbilicus needs resection after repeated abdominoplasty. In other techniques, after the remaining deformed umbilicus is excised and circumumbilical skin resected, the skin is tightened with a purse string [1, 10, 16]. Following hernia surgery, patients consult for neo-umbilicus, and more exceptional indications like umbilical hypogenesis [2, 17] and bladder exstrophy were recorded [11, 18].

The neo-umbilicus must have a prominent depression, a natural morphology without causing many additional scars. It should be placed above the superior iliac spine by about 3 cm [19, 20]. Some studies have described the purse-string methods [4, 21, 22].

In this study, this is a simple technique for the creation of a harmonious umbilicus, with a natural shape without complications with 1 year follow up. I consider this new technique as the preference technique postabdominoplasty.

19.6 Conclusions

This study describes a new simple technique for neo-umbilicoplasty without complications. Long-term results over 1 year revealed a successful natural appearance and harmonious shape of the neo-umbilicus.

References

1. McMillan WM. Surgery of umbilical hernia with reconstruction of an artificial umbilicus. Q Bull Northwest Univ Med Sch. 1955;29(4):379–82.
2. Iida N, Ohsumi N. Reconstruction of umbilical hypogenesis accompanied by a longitudinal scar. Plast Reconstr Surg. 2003;111:322–5.
3. Itoh Y, Arai K. Umbilical reconstruction using a cone-shaped flap. Ann Plast Surg. 1992;28:335–8.
4. Marconi F. Reconstruction of the umbilicus: a simple technique. Plast Reconstr Surg. 1995;95:1115–7.
5. Shinohara H, Matsuo K, Kikuchi N. Umbilical reconstruction with an inverted C-V flap. Piast Reconstr Surg. 2000;105:703–5.
6. Yotsuyanagi T, Nihei Y, Sawada Y. A simple technique for reconstruction of the umbilicus, using two twisted flaps. Plast Reconstr Surg. 1998;102:2444–6.
7. Matsuo K, Kondoh S, Hirose T. A simple technique for reconstruction of the umbilicus, using a conchal cartilage composite graft. Plast Reconstr Surg. 1990;86:149–51.
8. Lee SL, DuBois JJ, Greenbolz SK, Huffman SG. Advancement flap umbilicoplasty after abdominal wall closure: postoperative results compared with normal umbilical anatomy. J Pediatr Surg. 2001;36:1168–70.
9. Borges AF. Reconstruction of the umbilicus. Br J Plast Surg. 1975;28:75–6.
10. Miller MJ, Balch CM. 'Iris' technique for immediate umbilical reconstruction. Plast Reconstr Surg. 1993;92:754–6.
11. Feyaerts A, Mure PY, Jules JA, Morel-Journel N, Mouriquand P. Umbilical reconstruction in patients with exstrophy: the kangaroo pouch technique. J Urol. 2001;165:2026–7.
12. Sugawara Y, Hirabayashi S, Asato H, Yoshimura K. Reconstruction of the umbilicus using a single triangular flap. Ann Plast Surg. 1995;34:78–80.
13. Baack BR, Anson G, Nachbar JM, White DJ. Umbilicoplasty: the construction of a new umbilicus and correction of umbilical stenosis without external scars. Plast Reconstr Surg. 1996;97:227–32.
14. Jamra FA. Reconstruction of the umbilicus by a double V-Y procedure. Plast Reconstr Surg. 1979;64:106–7.
15. Onishi K, Yang YL, Maruyama Y. A new lunch box-type method in umbilical reconstruction. Ann Plast Surg. 1995;35:654–6.
16. Santanelli F, Mazzocchi M, Renzi L, Cigna E. Reconstruction of a natural-looking umbilicus. Scand J Plast Reconstr Surg Hand Surg. 2002;36:183–5.
17. Krummel TM, Sieber WK. Closure of congenital abdominal wall defects with umbilicoplasty. Surg Gynecol Obstet. 1987;165:168–9.
18. Pinto PA, Stock JA, Hanna MK. Results of umbilicoplasty for bladder exstrophy. J Urol. 2000;164:2055–7.
19. Koshy CE, Taams KO. Umbilicoplasty. Plast Reconstr Surg. 1999;104:1203.
20. Dubou R, Ousterhout DK. Placement of the umbilicus in an abdominoplasty. Plast Reconstr Surg. 1978;61:291–3.
21. Bartsich SA, Schwartz MH. Purse-string method for immediate umbilical reconstruction. Plast Reconstr Surg. 2003;112:1652–5.
22. Ghada M. Simple new technique for neo-umbilicoplasty. Med J Cairo Univ. 2012;80:759–61.

Chapter 20
Bilobed Flap for Umbilicus Reconstruction

Asuman Sevin, Durdane Keskin, Ibrahim Orgun Deren, and Kutlu Sevin

20.1 Introduction

The umbilicus is located at the intersection of the vertical line joining the xiphoid and midpubis and the horizontal line joining the superior iliac crests. It is usually located approximately 9–12 cm above the superior margin of the mons pubis and is an important aesthetic unit of the abdominal wall. The shape is elliptical in vertical direction or T-shaped with the long axis lying vertically in the midline. The umbilical diameter averages 1.5–2 cm [1], with a conical depression whose apex is tethered to the anterior muscular wall.

The umbilicus may be absent because of some congenital anomalies such as gastroschisis, bladder exstrophy, cloacal exstrophy, or omphalocele; inflammatory conditions such as necrotizing fasciitis and umbilical sepsis; and surgical causes such as umbilical herniorrhaphy, skin cancer ablation surgery and also after abdominoplasty, and breast reconstruction using abdominal tissues (Table 20.1). The goal

A. Sevin, M.D. (✉)
Ankara Koru Hospital, Kizilirmak District, 1450 Str., 13, Cukurambar, Ankara, Turkey
e-mail: basevin@gmail.com

D. Keskin, M.D.
Plastic Surgery Department, Ataturk Training and Research Hospital,
PK: 06800, Cankaya, Ankara, Turkey
e-mail: durdaneergun@gmail.com

I.O. Deren, M.D.
Plastic Surgery Department, Near East University, PK: 99138, Lefkosa, Turkey
e-mail: orgunderen@yahoo.com

K. Sevin, M.D.
Plastic Surgery Department, Cayyolu Guven Medical Center, Alacaatli Str. No:15 PK: 06810
Cayyolu, Ankara, Turkey
e-mail: basevin@gmail.com

M.A. Shiffman (ed.), *Adult Umbilical Reconstruction*,
DOI 10.1007/978-3-319-43887-0_20

Table 20.1 Etiology of absent umbilicus

Congenital	Inflammatory	Iatrogenic
Gastroschisis	Necrotizing fasciitis	Umbilical herniorrhaphy
Bladder exstrophy	Umbilical sepsis	Skin cancer ablation
Cloacal exstrophy		Abdominoplasty
Omphalocele		Breast reconstruction with abdominal flaps

of any reconstructive procedure should be an aesthetically pleasing umbilicus with a natural look and permanent depth [2].

Various methods have been employed in order to reconstruct the umbilicus, including the purse-string method [3], the use of several local flaps [4–10], and the use of an ear conchal cartilage graft [11]. Thomas et al. [12] reported a new technique for reconstruction of the nipple using a local cutaneous flap in the design of an unfolded cylinder. Ozbek and Ozcan [2] modified this method and formed a flap designed as an unfolded horizontal cylinder. We modified these methods and formed a vertical bilobed flap, which is simpler in design. Our method leaves a vertical scar, which is more acceptable, and results in sufficient and permanent depth.

20.2 Technique

The procedure was performed with the patient under general anesthesia. Before surgical cleaning, the locations of the new umbilicus and the flap were drawn on the abdominal skin (Figs. 20.1, 20.2, and 20.3). A small portion of the skin opposite to the flap pedicle was marked for removal. The pedicle length of the bilobed flap had to be equal to one-third of the vertical flap length. The horizontal length of the flap had to equal the length of the pedicle. The length of the flap pedicle was planned to be 1.5 times the vertical diameter of the neoumbilicus. The flap pedicle would form half of the neoumbilicus circle. The other half would be formed by one of the bilobed flap lobes.

After surgical cleaning and draping, the edges of the bilobed flap were cut through the subcutaneous adipose layer. The skin flap was elevated enough to permit the formation of a cylinder. After meticulous hemostasis, flaps x and y were sutured together (Fig. 20.1). The base of the cylinder was also sutured. The cylinder then was embedded in its place and fixed to the bottom with 4–0 nonabsorbable sutures. The donor site was closed by separated sutures (Fig. 20.4). The neoumbilicus was filled with a piece of moisture gauze, and the operation site was dressed. After ten days, all sutures were removed. There were no complications such as wound disruption, flap necrosis, hematoma, or infection. After 1 year, sufficient and permanent depth was observed, and the patient was satisfied (Fig. 20.5).

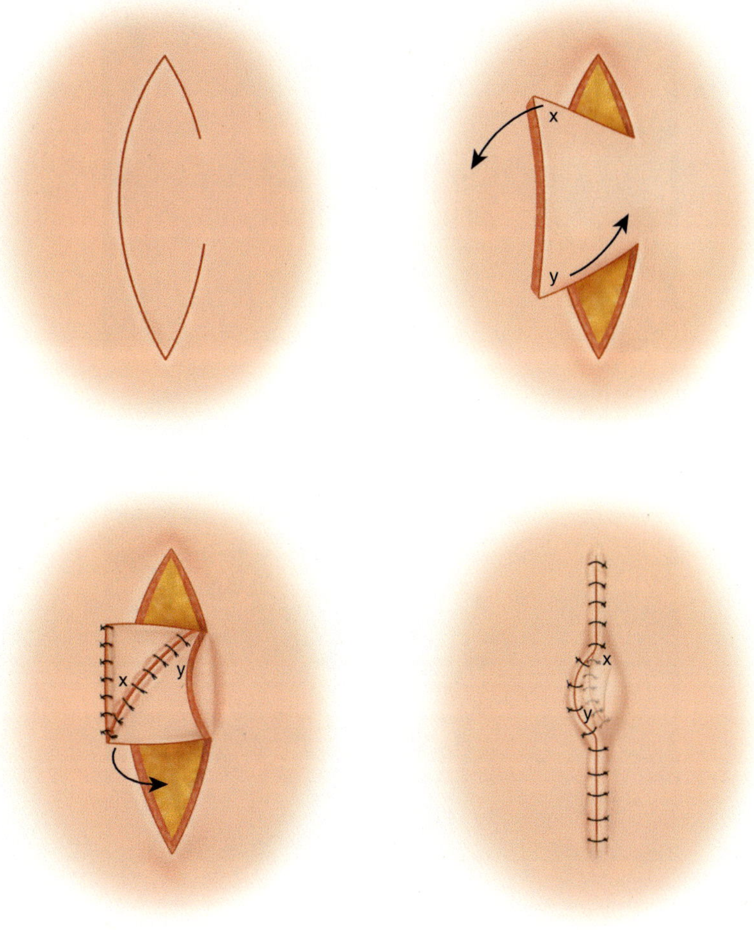

Fig. 20.1 (**a**) Umbilical bilobed flap design. (**b**) Bilobed flap x and y elevated. (**c**) Flap x and y sutured together to create a cylinder formation. Flap x is fixed to the deep fascia to form the bottom of the umbilicus. Lateral side of the flap y forms the umbilical circle. (**d**) The donor site defect closed by separate sutures

20.3 Discussion

Reconstruction of a neoumbilicus is often required after a previous abdominoplasty [8, 11]. The neoumbilicus should have a natural look as well as a sufficient and permanent depth without too many additional scars [8]. The neoumbilicus should be placed 3 cm above the superior iliac spine or at the highest level of the iliac crest [1, 13]. Shinohara [14] described that an umbilicus with a natural appearance consists

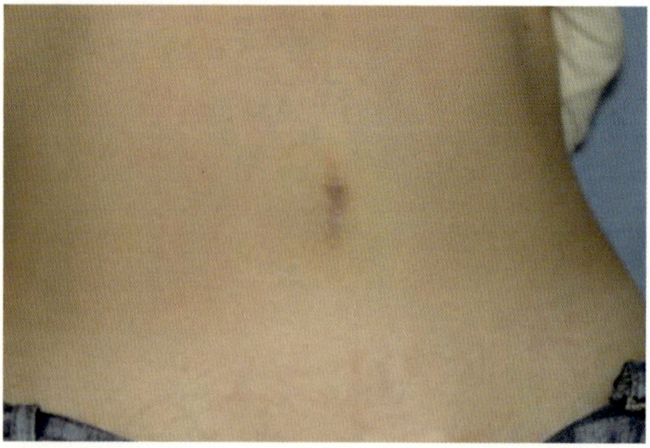

Fig. 20.2 Preoperative patient

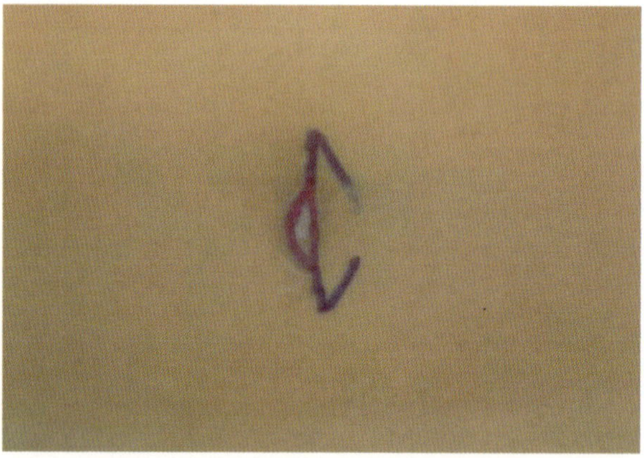

Fig. 20.3 Preoperative planning of the flap on the abdominal skin

of a ring, a tubular wall, a sulcus, and a bottom, without any excess skin that would interfere with the aesthetic aspect of the umbilicus. Marconi [6], and later Bartisch and Schwartz [3], described purse-string methods. Although this is a simple method, this technique requires thorough wound care for an extended period, and long-term results have not been described. Borges reported reconstruction by lateral skin excisions and a rotation of two small paramedian flaps [15]. Jamra [4] reconstructed the umbilicus with flaps on a double V-Y pattern. An elliptical skin island with fat excisions underneath and depression created through a purse-string suture was reported by Marconi [6]. Mateu and Hernandez [7] described their technique of depressing three triangular flaps by suturing their vertices to the aponeurotic plane, similar to Kirianoff's technique, and constructing the inner walls of the neoumbilicus through tightening of a pure-string suture [5].

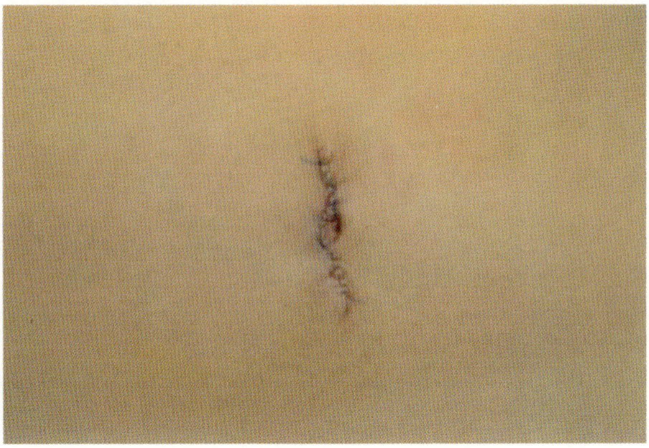

Fig. 20.4 Postoperative

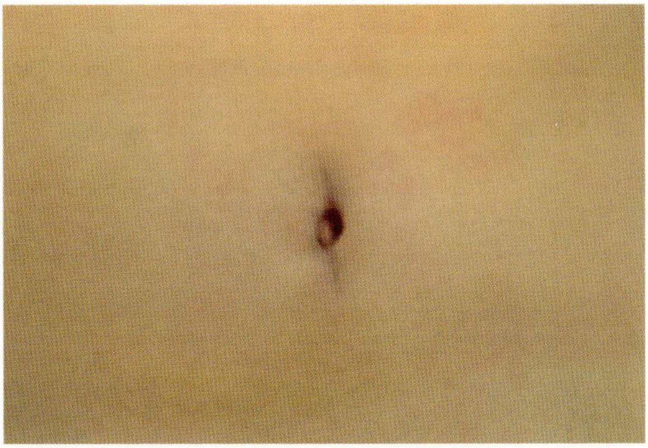

Fig. 20.5 One year postoperative

All the aforementioned techniques may create an umbilicus-like depression, but some have used distant donor sites. Using most of these techniques, the umbilical depth is maintained by the use of a long-term stent. In practice, this is a challenging task for slim patients and pediatric patients. However, with our technique, flap survival is secured, and there is no need for a stent after 2 weeks. The flaps are not under tension if correctly planned. Because the incision lines of the flap lie under minimal tension lines, the final scar also is satisfactory.

In the presented case, there was vertical scar tissue on the midline, which resulted from a previous umbilicus necrosis after abdominoplasty. The bilobed flap was planned laterally to this scar. We believe that removal of some skin portion opposite the flap pedicle helped to centralize the umbilicus. We did not see any lateral displacement after 1 year. We think that for cases in which there is no such vertical or horizontal bad scar, the bilobed flap should be planned with a vertical axis passing from the midline to avoid lateral displacement of the umbilicus. There is no need for a tissue removal.

20.4 Conclusions

Technically the procedure gives many advantages; being simple and stable, resulting in an acceptable scar, there is no need to use stent. Considering these advantages and the fact that it leads to aesthetically satisfactory results, this technique is widely employed as a useful neoumbilicoplasty technique in patients suffering from an absent or disfigured umbilicus.

References

1. Dubou R, Ousterout DK. Placement of the umbilicus in an abdominoplasty. Plast Reconstr Surg. 1978;61:291–3.
2. Ozbek S, Ozcan M. Umbilicus reconstruction with modified unfolded cylinder technique. Br J Plast Surg. 2005;58:500–3.
3. Bartisch SA, Schwartz MH. Purse-string method for immediate umbilical reconstruction. Plast Reconstr Surg. 2003;112:1652–5.
4. Jamra FA. Reconstruction of the umbilicus by a double V-Y procedure. Plast Reconstr Surg. 1978;64:106.
5. Kirianoff TG. Making a neoumbilicus when none exist. Plast Reconstr Surg. 1978;61:603.
6. Marconi F. Reconstruction of the umbilicus: a simple technique. Plast Reconstr Surg. 1995;95:1115–7.
7. Mateu LP, Hernandez C. Neoumbilicoplasty through a purse-string suture of three defatted flaps. Aesthetic Plast Surg. 1997;21:349.
8. Pfulg M, Sijpe KV, Blondeel P. A simple new technique for neoumbilicoplasty. Br J Plast Surg. 2005;58:688–91.
9. Miller MJ, Balch CM. "Iris" technique for immediate umbilical reconstruction. Plast Reconstr Surg. 1993;92:754–6.
10. Matsuo K, Kondoh S, Hirose T. A simple technique for reconstruction of the umbilicus, using a conchal cartilage composite graft. Plast Reconstr Surg. 1990;86:149–51.
11. Friedland JA, Maffi TR. Abdominoplasty. Plast Reconstr Surg. 2008;121:1–11.
12. Thomas SV, Gellis MB, Pool R. Nipple reconstruction with a new local tissue flap. Plast Reconstr Surg. 1996;97:1053.
13. Koshy CE, Taams KO. Umbilicoplasty. Plast Reconstr Surg. 1999;104:1203–4.
14. Shinohara H, Matsuo K, Kikuchi N. Umbilical reconstruction with an inverted C-V flap. Plast Reconstr Surg. 2000;105:703–5.
15. Borges AF. Reconstruction of the umbilicus. Br J Plast Surg. 1975;28:75–6.

Chapter 21
Restoration of the Umbilicus After Abdominal Surgery: Versatility of Double-M Double-Y Technique

Claudio Cannistrà

21.1 Introduction

The repositioning and the restructuring of the umbilicus is the important goal when you perform surgery of the abdominal wall. Every time the umbilicus is in the center of the abdominal wall and it is the first area that is observed when the woman is partially or totally undressed. The umbilicus presents a focus for sexuality in women. Arabic people prefer decorating the umbilicus with precious stones to excite the sexuality of this area [1, 2].

Now, during abdominal surgery, this remarkable importance of the umbilicus is not considered, the scars are made on the umbilicus with deformation of its shape, and the remarkable signature of the surgeon is printed at the center of the abdominal wall. Normally, the umbilicus is a neonatal invisible scar which is localized on the white line and which is associated to the abdominal skin retraction [3]. The aesthetic umbilicus is an abdominal skin depression with a small scar at the bottom. This depression is perpendicular at 12 o'clock and more oblique at 6 o'clock.

When the surgeon corrects deformation of the abdominal skin, different techniques are used to mark a circular or elliptic scar around the external edge of the umbilicus [4–11].

Finally, the visible scar is present in the center of the abdomen (Fig. 21.1). After this analysis of the natural aspect of the umbilicus and the problems secondary to the umbilicus surgery, the author proposes a simple procedure to restore the umbilicus when performing dermolipectomy or correcting congenital or secondary deformation of the umbilicus.

C. Cannistrà, M.D., Ph.D.
Praticien Hôspitalier, Unity of Plastic Surgery, Centre Hôspitalier Universitaire Bichat Claude Bernard, 48 rue Henry Huchard, 75018 Paris, France
e-mail: Cla.cannistra@gmail.com

M.A. Shiffman (ed.), *Adult Umbilical Reconstruction*,
DOI 10.1007/978-3-319-43887-0_21

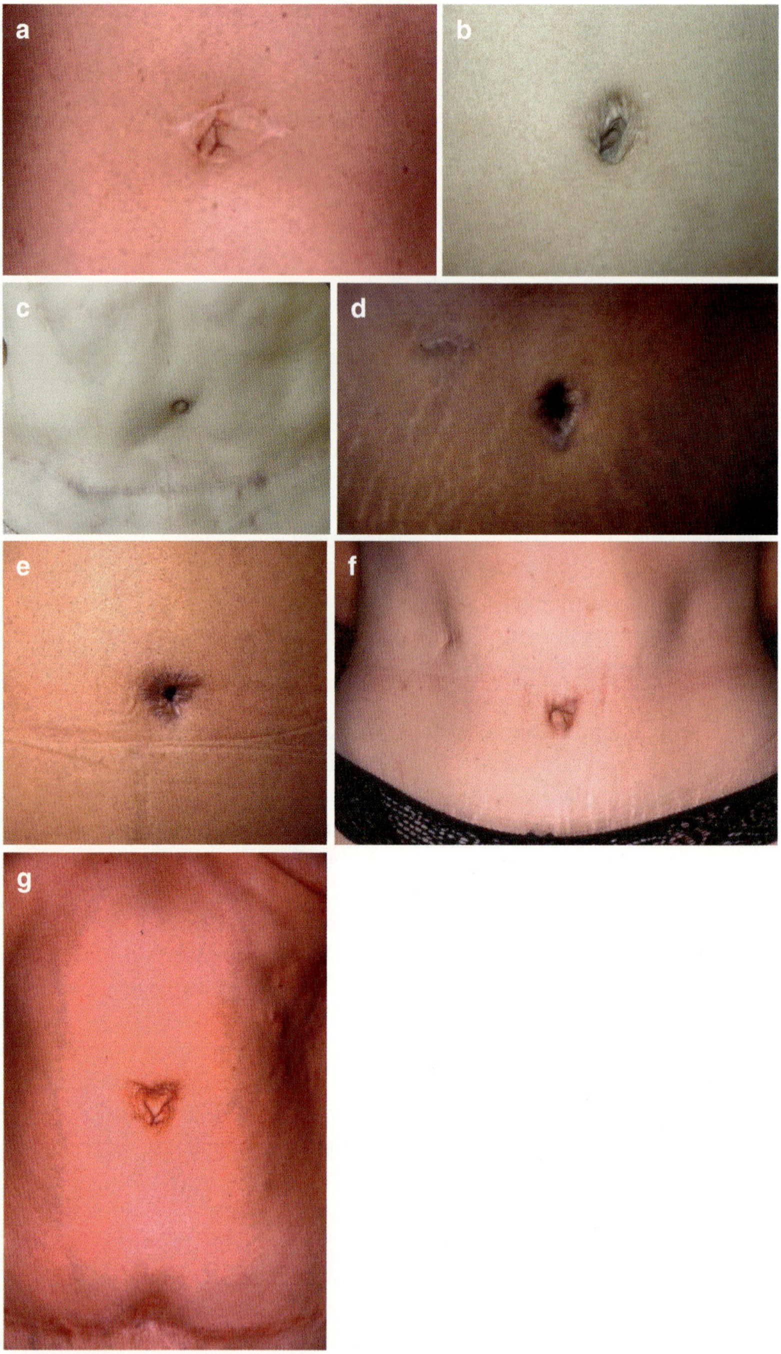

Fig. 21.1 (**a**) Elliptic scar around the umbilicus. (**b**) Circular scar around the umbilicus with excess of depth. (**c**) Circular scar around the umbilicus complicated by stenosis. (**d**) Circular scar around the umbilicus complicated by keloid. (**e**) Circular scar around the umbilicus complicated by severe stenosis. (**f**) Distorted umbilicus. (**g**) Triangular deformation

21.2 Surgical Technique

First, the marking on the bottom of the old umbilicus is performed. The incision form is a double M where point 1 and point 2 of the M are positioned at 12 o'clock and 6 o'clock and the distance between point 3 and point 4 should not exceed 10 mm (Fig. 21.2). Two Gillies hooks are positioned at the bottom of the umbilicus at points 1 and 2. Upward traction of the hooks allows the cone of the umbilicus to be turned outward (Fig. 21.3).

The cutaneous incision is begun, and the superficial skin is detached from the lowest level releasing the umbilicus until the muscular aponeurosis (Fig. 21.4). After resection of the abdominal skin excess, the repositioning of the neo-umbilicus

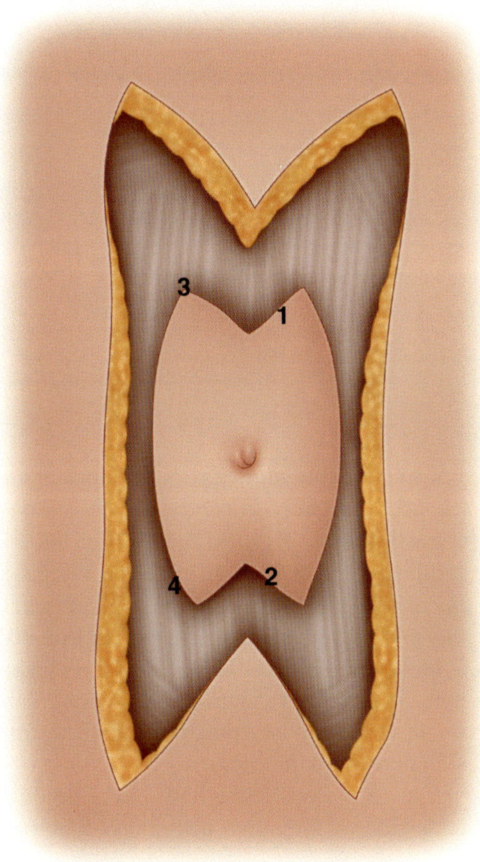

Fig. 21.2 (*1–4*) Design of the umbilical incision

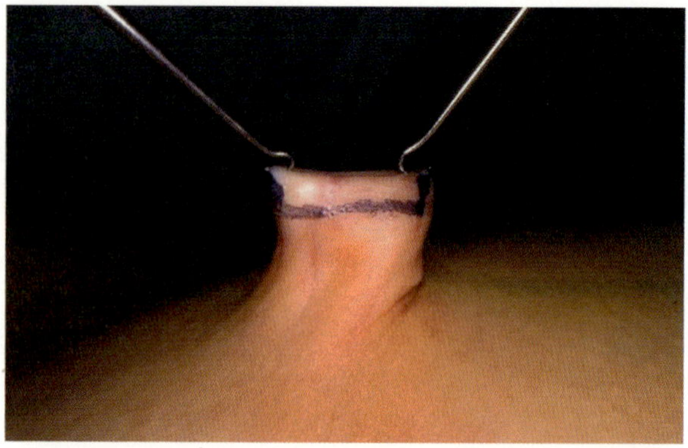

Fig. 21.3 Traction of the umbilicus before incision

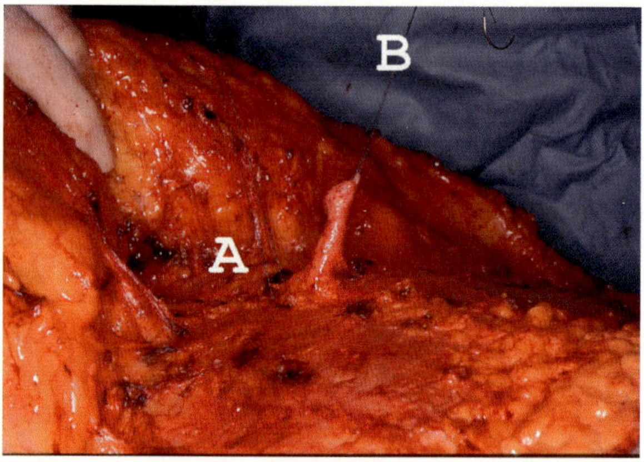

Fig. 21.4 Releasing of the umbilicus. (**a**) Thread on the umbilical basis. (**b**) Thread for umbilical traction

can start. The position of a resorbable suture is at 12 o'clock at the level of the base of the umbilicus. A second suture is positioned at 6 o'clock on the marge of the umbilicus affecting its traction (Fig. 21.4). At the level of the abdominal skin, the position of the neo-umbilicus is marked at 10 cm from the pubic hairs; it is very important to control this new position that is on the line between the iliac crests.

Then, a double-Y line is traced (Fig. 21.5). Four small skin flaps are created (G, I, H, L). Points A, B, C, and D are placed at 11, 1, 5, and 7 o'clock, respectively. The length of the line E-F must not exceed 0.5 mm and B-C 1 cm. The subcutaneous fat is removed at the level of the neo-umbilical position with the form of a large lozenge to restore the natural skin depression in this area.

The suture positioned at 12 o'clock at the base of the umbilicus is fixed at the dermis level on the underside of the small abdominal flap 1 cm from the apex (Figs. 21.6 and 21.7).

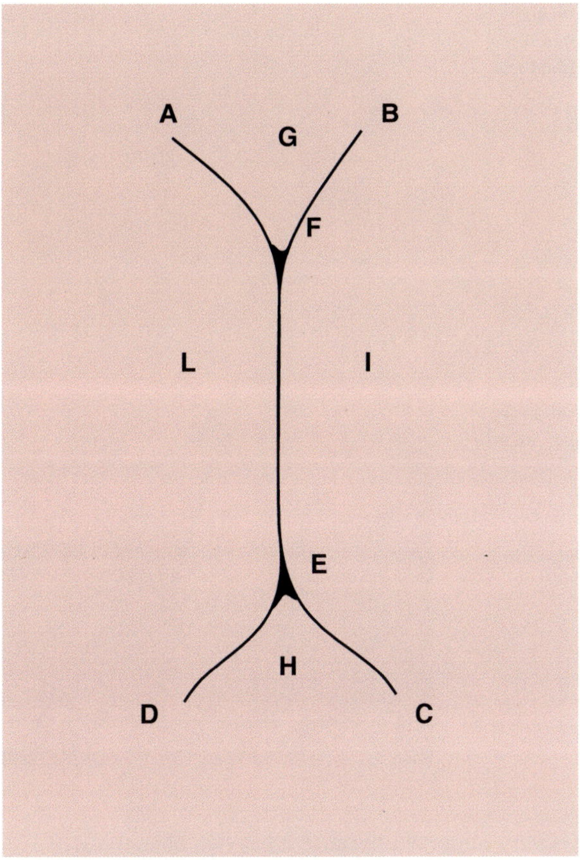

Fig. 21.5 (*A–I, L*) Double-Y incision of the abdominal skin

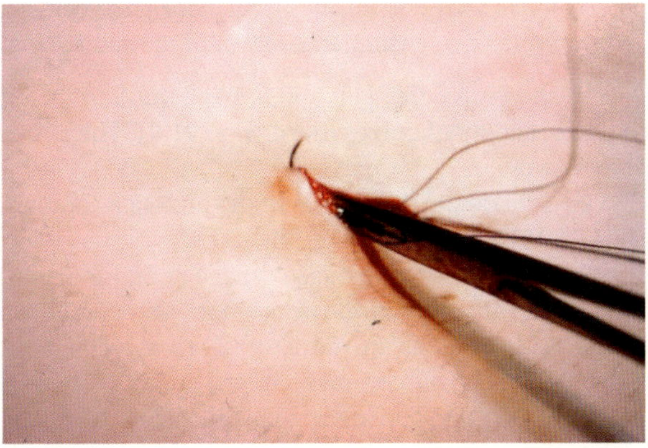

Fig. 21.6 Suture at 12 o'clock

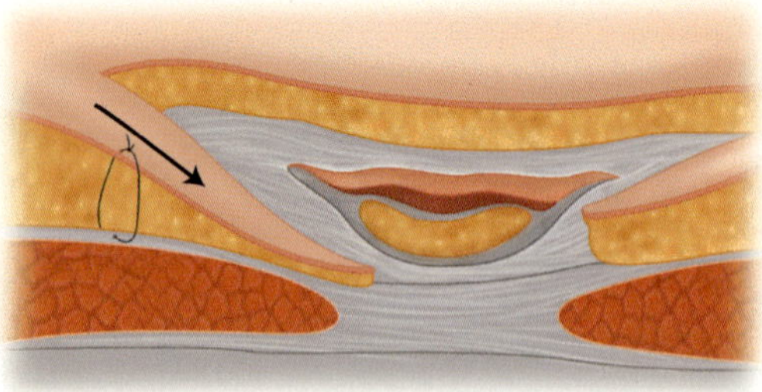

Fig. 21.7 Fixation and pushback (*arrow*) of the skin to the abdominal wall

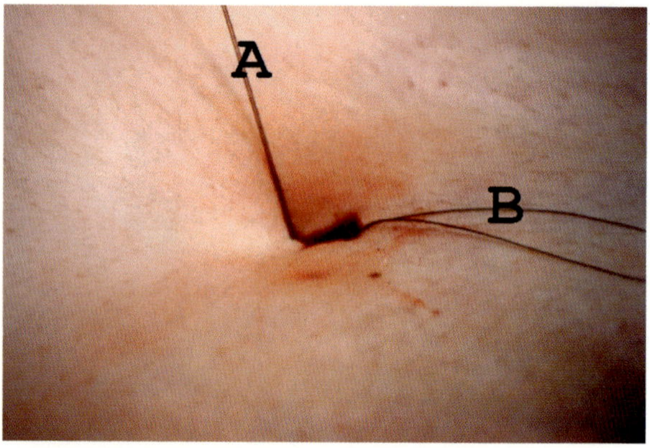

Fig. 21.8 Suture at 12 o'clock. (**a**) Thread on the umbilical base. (**b**) Thread for umbilical traction

This suture is very important because it has two objectives:

1. Recreate the skin depression of the umbilicus.
2. Absorb some of the cutaneous tension created at the level of the xipho-pubic line and reduce the possibility of cutaneous necrosis on the pubic suture caused by excessive skin tension at the level of the suture (Fig. 21.8).

The abdominal flap H is sutured to point 2 of the umbilical double M, the flap I to line 3, and the flap L to line 4 (Fig. 21.9). The author prefers using rapid resorbable sutures.

The skin around the bottom of the umbilicus is sutured by the resorbable threads (Fig. 21.10).

When the umbilicus cutaneous cone is very long, different techniques suggest its folding and fixation on the white line. The complication is the stagnation of the cutaneous secretions in the excessive cavity and the secondary infection with omphalitis. To avoid this problem, the author prefers resecting more portions of the umbilical skin and leaving a small cutaneous island at the bottom of the umbilicus at the level of the old embryological scar.

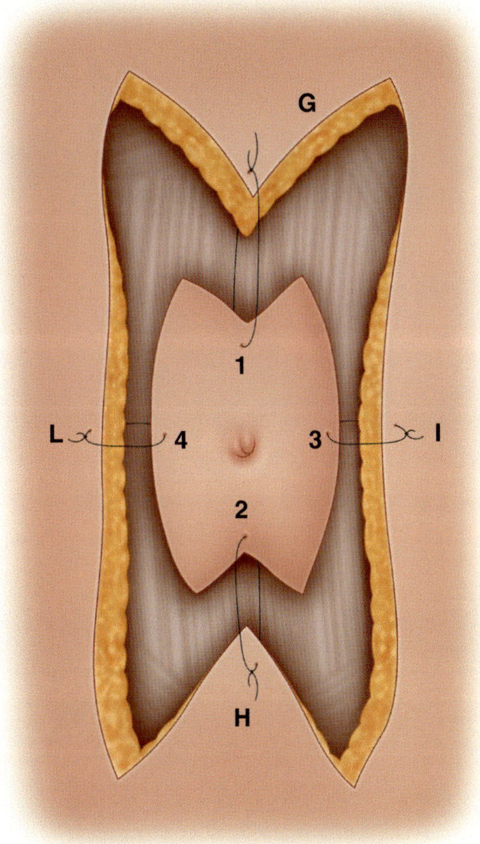

Fig. 21.9 (*G–I, L*) Umbilical fixation

21.3 Surgical Technique During a Dermolipectomy with Umbilical Hernia

When correcting a significant umbilical hernia during dermolipectomy, sometimes it is necessary to remove the old umbilicus completely (Fig. 21.11). In these cases, after the repair of the abdominal wall, it is possible to use one modification of this technique to reshape the umbilicus.

One thread is positioned along the vertical line between the xiphoid and the middle pubis (Fig. 21.12). After having identified the natural position of the umbilicus

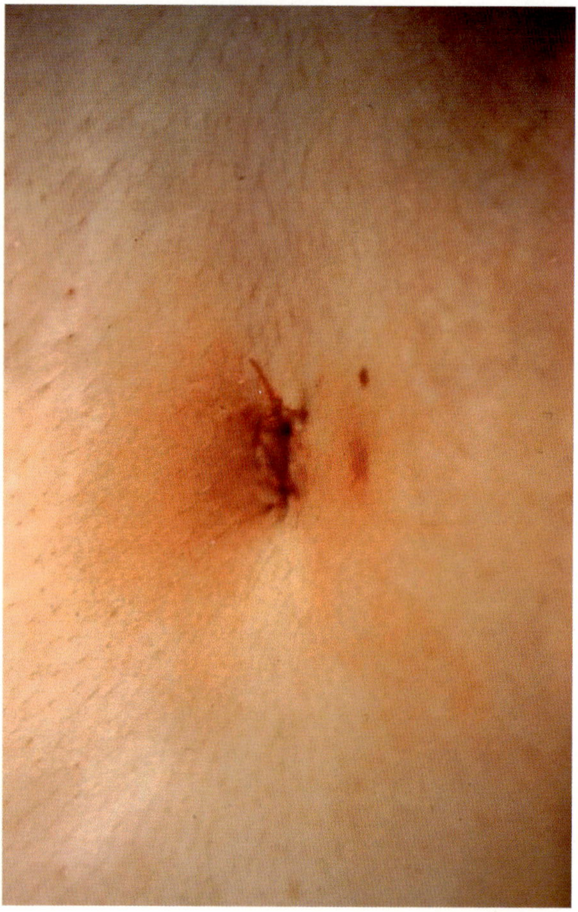

Fig. 21.10 Final result

on the abdominal white line, one line is traced between the anterior iliac crests (10 cm from the pubic hairs). Then, four sutures are positioned on the abdominal muscular aponeurosis at the level of the four cardinal points around the position of the umbilicus (Figs. 21.12, 21.13, and 21.14).

The abdominal skin is repositioned on the muscular wall. The new position of the umbilicus is identified on the abdominal skin. The skin is incised after marking a double Y (Fig. 21.13).

The small four skin flaps (G, I, H, L) are fixed with the four threads on the abdominal wall; the threads remain long (Figs. 21.14, 21.15, 21.16, and 21.17).

The small skin graft is molded and positioned on the bottom of the new umbilicus (Fig. 21.18). The gauzes with Vaseline are positioned on the bottom of the new umbilicus to compress; the skin graft and the threads are positioned around the gauzes to make a parachute dressing (Fig. 21.19). This dressing is removed after 5 days (Fig. 21.20).

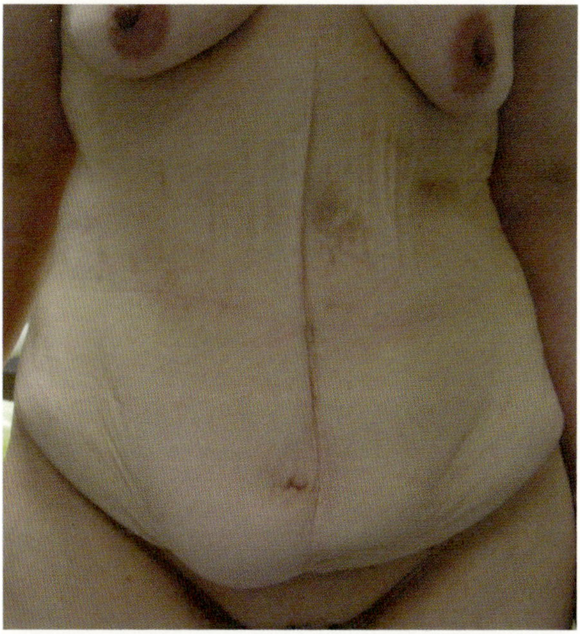

Fig. 21.11 Patient after weight loss of 50 kg. Damage of the umbilicus during old surgical treatment. Resection of the abdominal skin by the Fleur de Lis technique

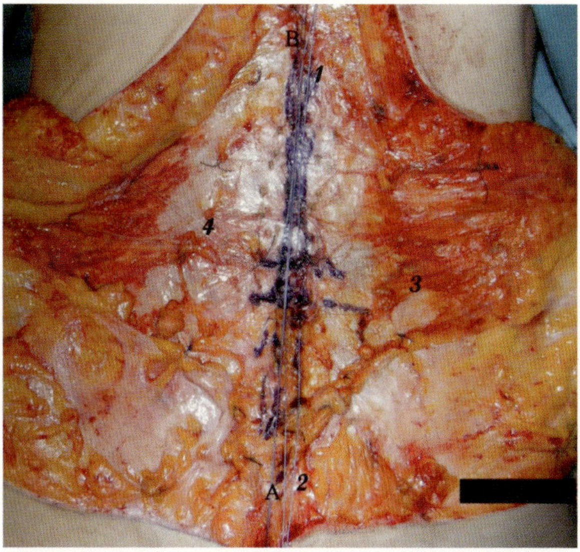

Fig. 21.12 Position of the threads 1-2-3-4- for reconstruction of the umbilicus. A and B thread positioned between the xiphoid and the pubis to localize the position of the umbilicus along the white line

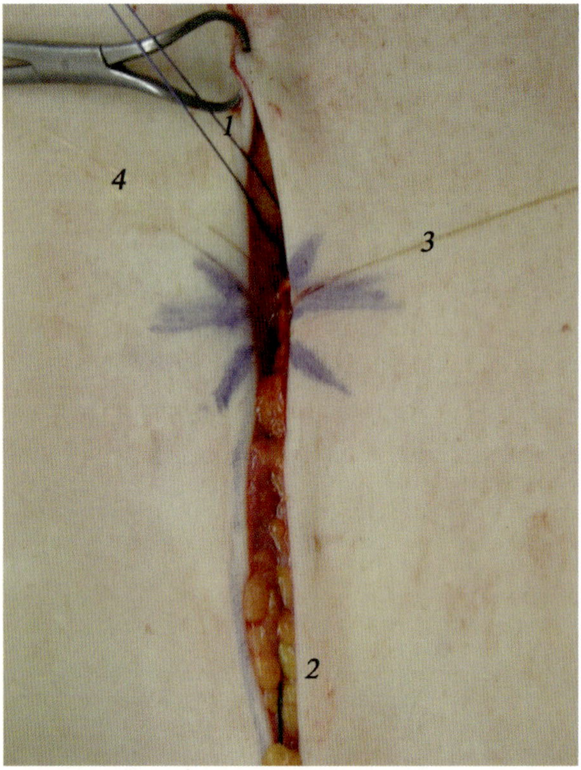

Fig. 21.13 (*1–4*) Four threads and double Y marked on the skin

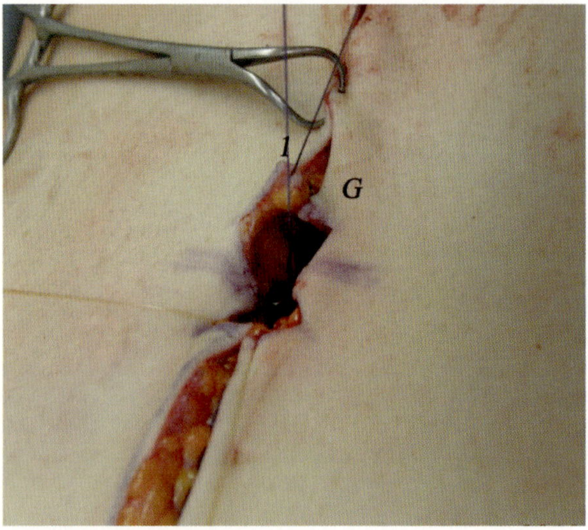

Fig. 21.14 Thread 1 fixed to G point at 12 o'clock

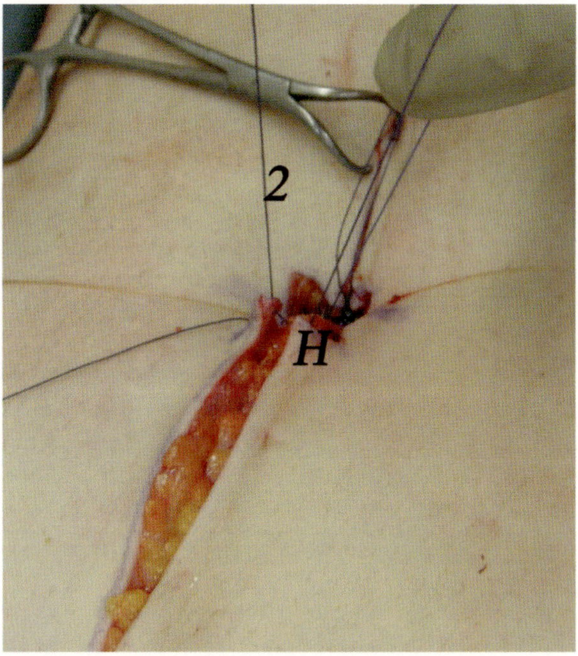

Fig. 21.15 Thread 2 fixed to H point at 6 o'clock

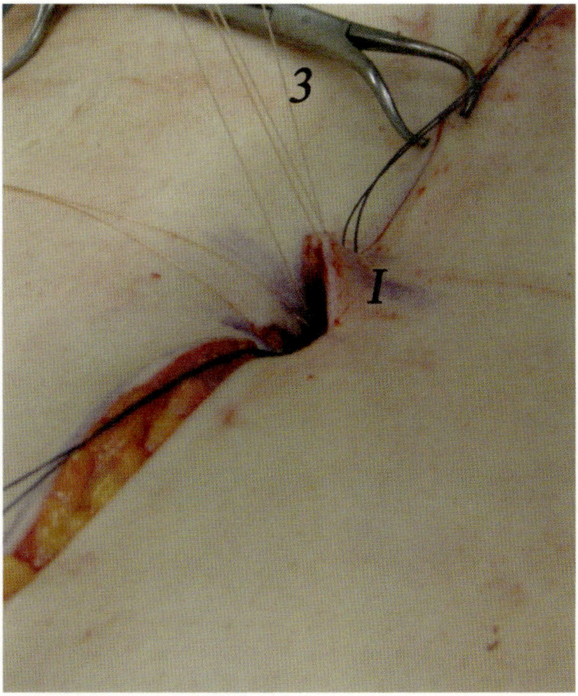

Fig. 21.16 Thread 3 fixed to I point at 3 o'clock

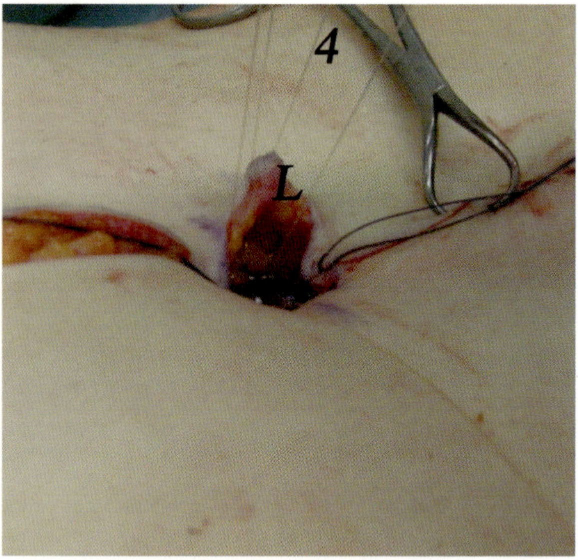

Fig. 21.17 Thread 4 fixed to L point at 9 o'clock

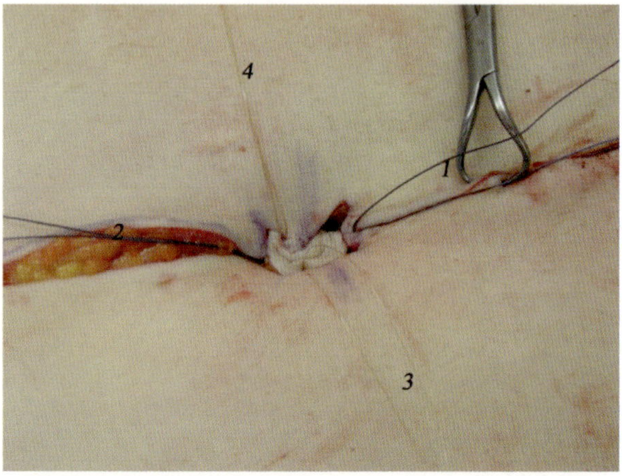

Fig. 21.18 Skin graft on the bottom of new umbilicus fixed with four sutures (1–4)

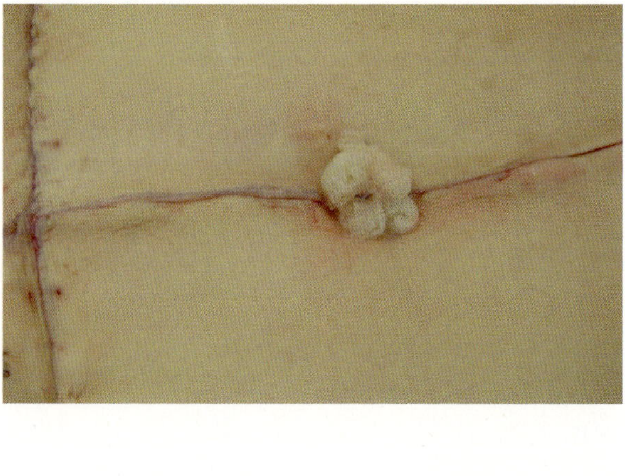

Fig. 21.19 Parachute dressing fixed by 1–4 threads

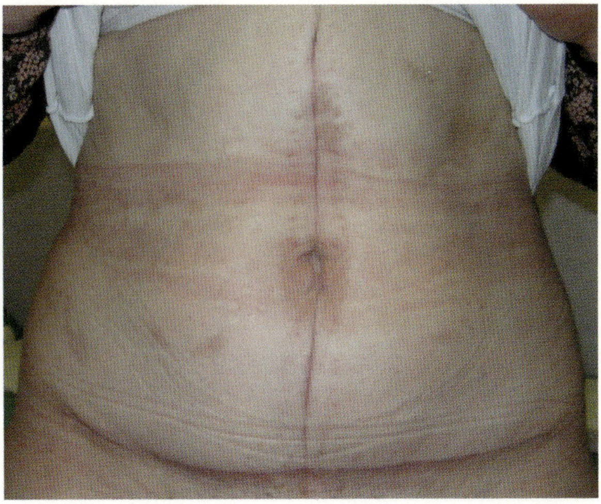

Fig. 21.20 Result after 3 months

21.4 The Procedure During Surgical Reparation of the Umbilical Hernia

This technique has benefit when you need to remove the umbilicus because it is deformed by hernia (Fig. 21.21) or it is secondary to a pathologic localization (endometriosis of the umbilicus or cancer).

Marking of the umbilicus a double M and, after incision, undermining the tissues until the muscular aponeurosis. Every time, when you have an umbilical hernia, it is necessary to make a dissection along the muscular abdominal aponeurosis along the white line cephalically and caudally to expose the muscular diastasis. After removing the umbilicus and suturing the abdominal wall, it is possible to restore the umbilicus with the same technique previously explained.

Four threads are positioned at the level of the four cardinal points in localization of the new umbilicus. Then, the sutures are fixed on the dermal face of the four skin flaps (G, I, H, L) of the abdominal skin. The fixation of the sutures restores the depression of the umbilicus. The sutures have to remain long because it is necessary to fix the umbilicus with a parachute shape dressing.

The small absence of the skin in the bottom of the umbilicus is restored by a small skin graft located in this area and fixed by a dressing with Vaseline. This dressing is fixed by the sutures knotted in parachute shape. After 3 days, the dressing is removed and replaced, after cleansing the scar, by a simple Vaseline dressing for 10 days.

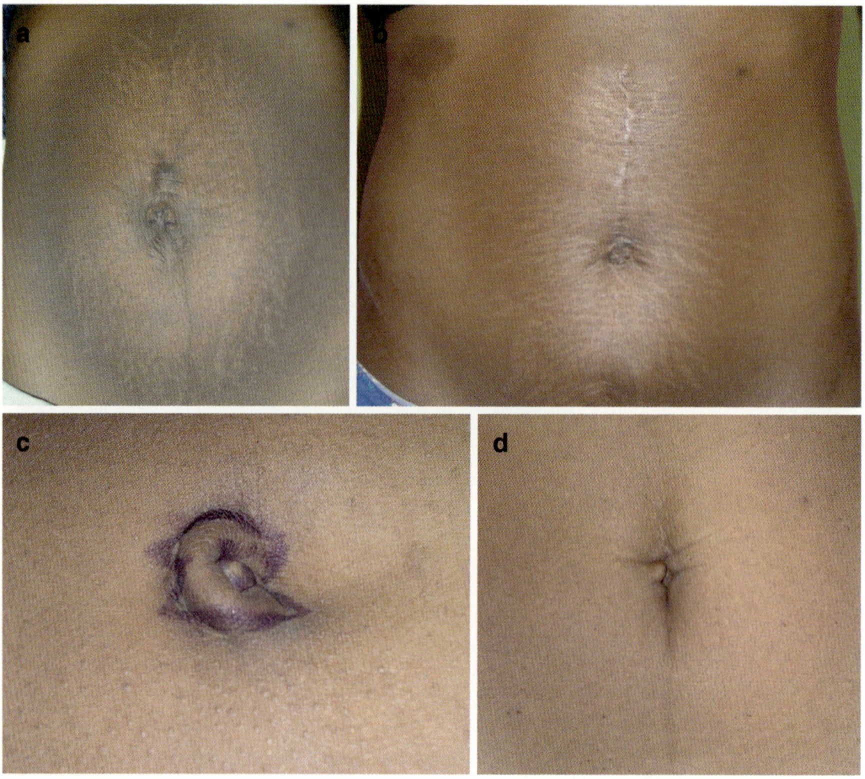

Fig. 21.21 (**a**) Diastasis of the abdominal muscles with umbilical hernia after pregnancy. (**b**) Postoperative control after resection of the abdominal skin, correction of the muscular diastasis by suture of the muscles, and reconstruction of the umbilicus with double-M double-Y technique. (**c**) Scar with deformation of the umbilicus after surgery to correct umbilical hernia. Aesthetic bad result. (**d**) Result after resection of the excess umbilical skin and restoration of the umbilicus by double-M double-Y technique

21.5 Discussion

The reconstruction of the umbilicus shape is the object of different techniques. Some authors have proposed the use of different types of cutaneous incisions to improve the shape of the umbilicus and to disguise the periumbilical scar [4–13]. Other ones have advised the use of a cartilaginous graft taken from the auricular concha to recreate the anatomical shape of the umbilicus [14].

The majority of the techniques propose the linear periumbilical incision. These incisions shape a circular or elliptical scar that, with its retraction, cause stenosis of the umbilicus. All these techniques forget that:

1. The umbilical depression is produced by retraction of the embryological scar positioned at the bottom of the umbilical cone.
2. The circular scar is complicated every time by stenosis.

Then, the author's technique is performed to restore the umbilical natural depression with localization of the scar on the bottom of the umbilicus [15, 16]. The central part of the abdomen, important reference for sexuality and maternity, must be seen without scar if it is possible.

21.6 Conclusions

This procedure is easy and safe with an optimal aesthetic result. It is possible to use this procedure during the reparation of the umbilical hernia (Fig. 23.21) [16]. The complications are very rare.

When you make a skin graft, a delayed scar can occur. The problem encountered most frequently, in 2 % of cases, is the loss of the depth of the depression caused by the umbilical suture at 12 o'clock breaking prematurely. Normally the patients are always satisfied with the result.

References

1. Brown ES. The umbilicus as sexual focus. Int J Psychoanal. 1997;28:577.
2. Craig S, Faller MS, Puckett CL. In search of the ideal female umbilicus. Plast Reconstr Surg. 2000;105(1):389–92.
3. Testut L, Jacob O. Trattato di anatomia topografica, vol. II. Torino, Italy: Utet; 1995. p. 391.
4. Baroudi R. Umbilicoplasty. Clin Plast Surg. 1975;2:431–4.
5. Borges A. Reconstruction of the umbilicus by double V-Y procedure. Br J Plast Surg. 1975;28:75–9.
6. Jamra FA. Reconstruction of the umbilicus by double V-Y procedure. Plast Reconstr Surg. 1979;64:106–9.
7. Itoh Y, Arai K. Umbilical reconstruction using a cone-shaped flap. Ann Plast Surg. 1992;28:335–9.
8. Massiha H, Montegut W, Phillips R. A method of reconstructing a natural looking umbilicus in abdominoplasty. Ann Plast Surg. 1997;38:228–30.
9. Marconi F. Reconstruction of the umbilicus: a simple technique. Plast Reconstr Surg. 1995;95:1115–8.
10. Sugawara Y, Hirabayashi S, Asato H, Yoshimura K. Reconstruction of the umbilicus using a single triangular flap. Ann Plast Surg. 1995;34(1):78–80.
11. Shinohara H, Matsuo K, Kikuchi N. Umbilical reconstruction with an inverted C-V flap. Plast Reconstr Surg. 2000;105(2):703–5.
12. Bruekers SE, Van der Lei B, Tan TL, Luijendijk RW, Stevens H. "Scarless" Umbilicoplasty. A new umbilicoplasty technique and a review of the English language literature. Ann Plast Surg. 2009;63(1):15–20.
13. Mazzocchi M, Trignano E, Armenti AF, Figus A, Dessy LA. Long term result of a versatile technique for umbilicoplasty in abdominoplasty. Aesthetic Plast Surg. 2011;35:456–62.
14. Matuo K, Kondoh S, Hirose T. A simple technique for reconstruction of the umbilicus using a conchal cartilage composite graft. Plast Reconstr Surg. 1990;86:1990–3.
15. Cannistrà C, Pecorelli E. Umbilical restoration in abdominal dermolipectomy: a simple double Y double M technique. Aesthetic Plast Surg. 1999;23:364–6.
16. Cannistrà C, Marmuse JP, Madelenat P. Hernie ombilicale. Tecnique nouvelle de reparation avec cicatrice a minima. Gynec Obstetr Fertil. 2003;31:471–5.

Chapter 22
Reconstructing a Natural-Looking Umbilicus

Ron Hazani, Ron Israeli, and Randall S. Feingold

22.1 Introduction

A youthful umbilicus is essential to the aesthetic appearance of the abdomen. It defines the midline abdominal sulcus and adds to a shapely abdominal curvature. The physical characteristics that contribute to an ideal umbilicus include size, shape, and location in the abdomen [1, 2]. A desirable goal in umbilical reconstruction is to create a small, vertically oriented umbilicus with the addition of a superior hood [2]. A concealed scar is also a necessary component of an appealing neo-umbilicus [3]. The multitude of methods to recreate an umbilicus [4–15] is testimony to the continued search for a more pleasing result.

The following details an innovative technique of umbilical reconstruction producing a natural appearing navel despite the ease with which it is created. Our method avoids the need for an existing umbilicus while producing minimal scarring on the abdomen. Indications for reconstructing a new umbilicus include cases in which the umbilical stalk is lost while harvesting a transverse rectus abdominis myocutaneous (TRAM) flap or during abdominoplasty, particularly in patients with a history of a prior umbilical hernia.

R. Hazani, M.D. (✉)
Private Practice, Hazani Plastic Surgery,
436 N. Bedford Dr. #308, Beverly Hills, CA 90210, USA
e-mail: ronmdsurg@hotmail.com

R. Israeli, M.D. • R.S. Feingold, M.D.
Private Practice, Aesthetic Plastic Surgery, P.C.,
833 Northern Blvd, Suite 160, Great Neck, NY, USA
e-mail: Risraeli@nybra.com; Risraeli@bodyplasticsurgery.com; Rfeingold@nybra.com

M.A. Shiffman (ed.), *Adult Umbilical Reconstruction*,
DOI 10.1007/978-3-319-43887-0_22

22.2 Surgical Technique

The site of the new umbilicus is marked on the abdomen (Fig. 22.1). The superior edge of the iliac crest determined the vertical height of the new umbilicus at the midline. Using a semicircular incision, an inferiorly based small flap of abdominal wall skin is elevated, and a core of subcutaneous tissue is excised. The flap is transposed deeply and secured with a buried 0-Vicryl suture to the level of fascia. The remaining wound is repaired with a full-thickness skin graft to complete the creation of a superior hood (Fig. 22.2).

A skin graft is harvested from the lateral edge of the previously healed abdominoplasty or TRAM donor site. The skin graft is cut to size, pie crusted, and applied to the remaining wound within the new umbilicus. It is secured with multiple 2–0 silk sutures and multiple interrupted 4–0 plain gut sutures. Bacitracin, Xeroform, and cotton are utilized to create a bolster stent-type dressing, secured with the previously placed 2–0 silk sutures.

22.3 Results

We achieved an aesthetically pleasing umbilicus with no complications of contracture, skin flap necrosis, or skin-graft loss (Figs. 22.3 and 22.4) in all patients ($n = 22$).

22.4 Discussion

The umbilicus is a unique aesthetic component of the abdominal wall. Features of an attractive umbilicus include a central sulcus, vertical orientation, and a superior hood [2]. Previous attempts to reconstruct a new umbilicus fall short of

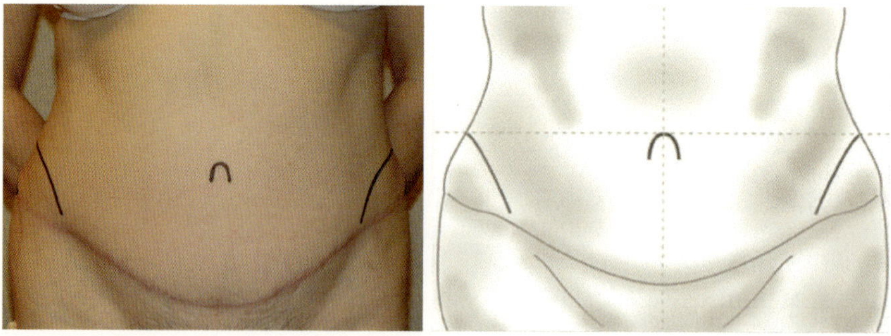

Fig. 22.1 (*Left* and *right*) positioning of the neo-umbilicus in the abdomen. The preoperative marking of the abdomen is based on the height of the iliac crest

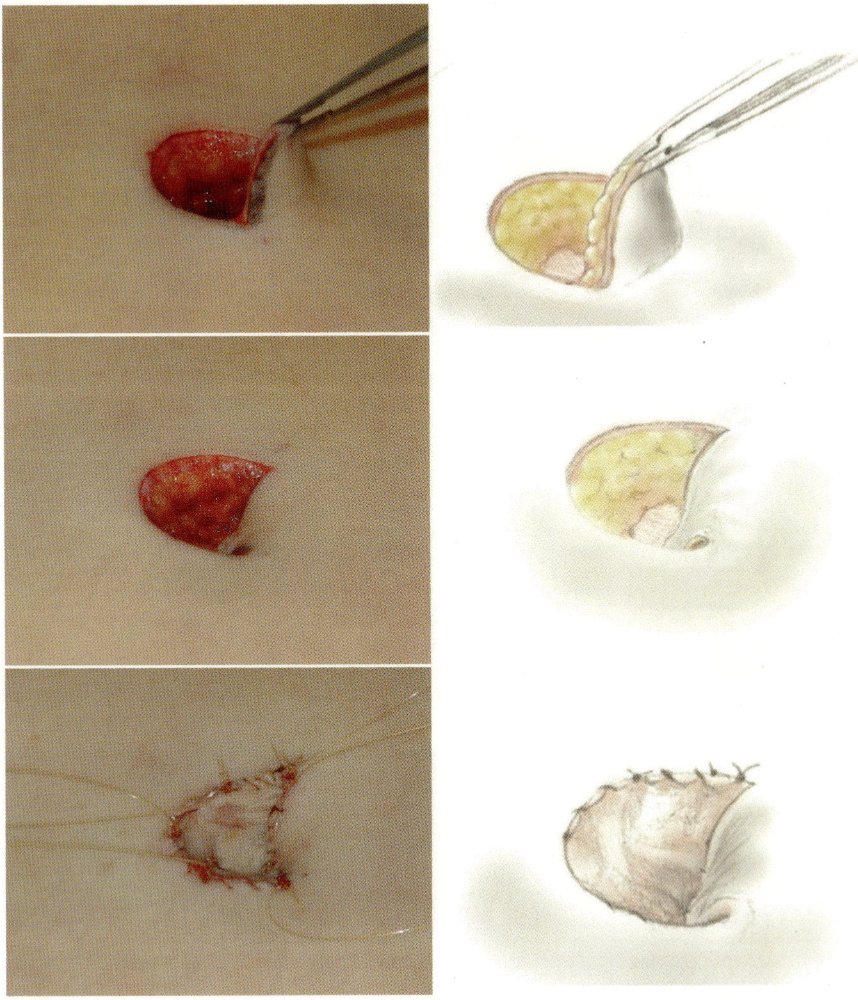

Fig. 22.2 Surgical technique. (*Top*) elevation of an inferiorly based skin flap. (*Middle*) transposition of skin flap to the abdominal wall fascia. (*Bottom*) creation of a superior hood with a skin graft

creating an ideal navel because of the need for a periumbilical scar [4–8]. Patients with umbilical hypogenesis or a postoperative abdominal scar may benefit from a procedure that incorporates the existing scar into the reconstructed umbilicus [9, 10].

Other techniques rely on the purse-string method or simply allow the umbilical wound to heal by secondary intention [11–14]. Refinements to the purse-string method aim at creating a more "innie" umbilicus by excising the subcutaneous fat and by shortening the umbilical stalk [11, 12]. A circular, contracted scar remains the pitfall of the purse-string technique unless a split at the 6 o'clock position is placed from the rim of the existing umbilicus along the neck

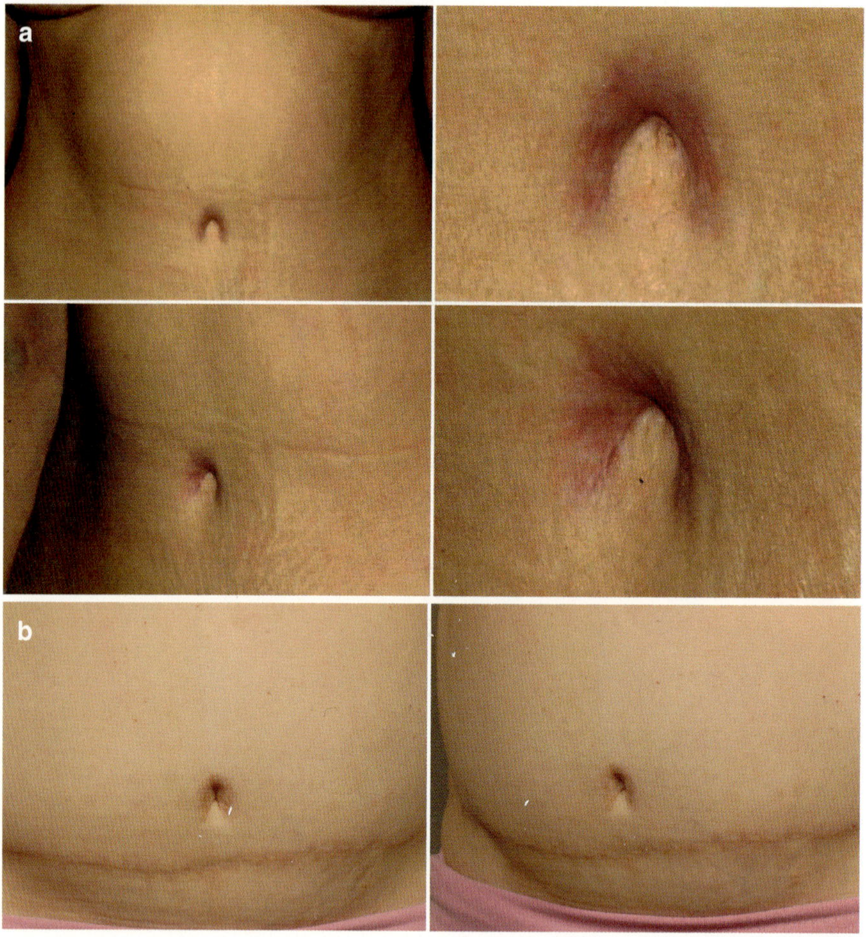

Fig. 22.3 (**a**) Six-month follow-up. (*Top* and *bottom*) abdomen following umbilical restoration. (**b**) One-year follow-up

down to the fascia [13]. This further incision retracts from the final result by forming an additional scar.

To circumvent these potential shortcomings, we report this new technique as a simple and reliable method of umbilical restoration. It avoids the need for external scars and allows for achieving an attractive, natural umbilicus. A major concern in umbilical reconstruction is whether the structure is likely to flatten with time [12]. Long-term follow-up of our patients demonstrates the durability of this technique with maintenance of vertical orientation and preservation of the depth of the restored navel [16].

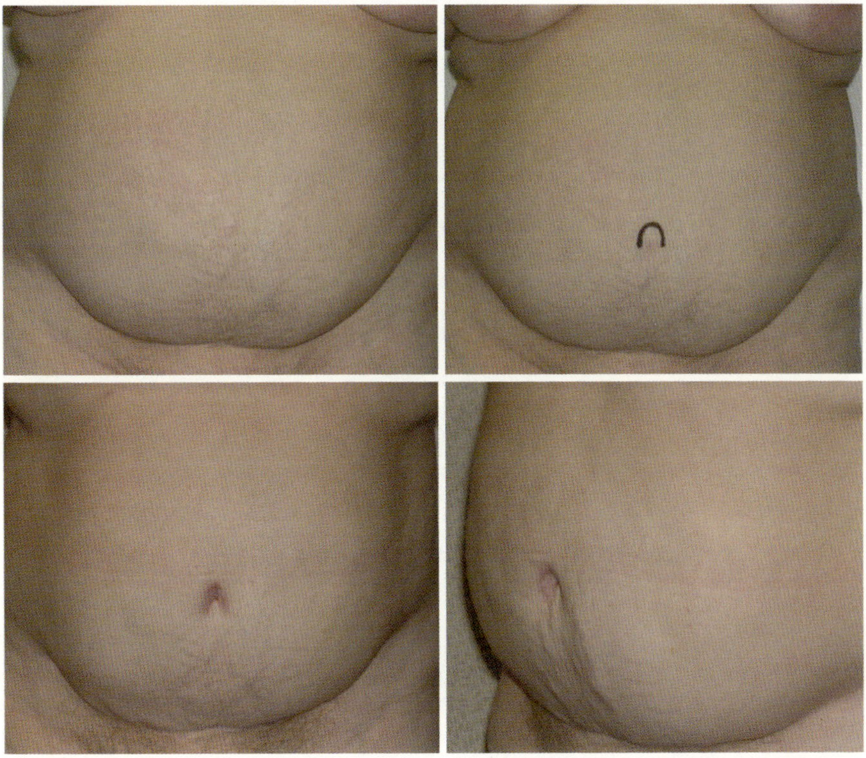

Fig. 22.4 A 52-year-old female with history of morbid obesity, BMI=40, underwent a bladder suspension procedure, umbilical hernia repair, and panniculectomy in July 2003. Subsequently, the patient underwent umbilical reconstruction in December 2004. Above (*left*), preoperative abdomen prior to reconstruction. Above (*right*), marking of the abdomen. (*Below*) postoperative at 6 months

22.5 Conclusions

The absence of an umbilicus distracts from the aesthetic appearance of the abdominal wall. Loss of the umbilicus during a procedure is unfortunate, but in some difficult cases, inevitable. We suggest a one-stage procedure for umbilical restoration, which produces cosmetic results while avoiding external scarring.

References

1. Massiha H. Superior positioning of the ptotic umbilicus in abdominoplasties and TRAM Flaps. Ann Plast Surg. 2002;48(5):508–10.
2. Craig SB, Faller MS, Puckett CL. In search of the ideal female umbilicus. Plast Reconstr Surg. 2000;105(1):389–92.

3. Choudhary S, Taams KO. Umbilicosculpture: a concept revisited. Br J Plast Surg. 1998;51(7):538–41.
4. Shinohara H, Matsuo K, Kikuchi N. Umbilical reconstruction with an inverted C-V flap. Plast Reconstr Surg. 2000;105(2):703–5.
5. Delerm A. Refinements in abdominoplasty with emphasis on reimplantation of the umbilicus. Plast Reconstr Surg. 1982;70(5):632–7.
6. Itoh Y, Arai K. Umbilical reconstruction using a cone-shaped flap. Ann Plast Surg. 1992;28(4):335–8.
7. Onishi K, Yang YL, Maruyama Y. A new lunch box-type method in umbilical reconstruction. Ann Plast Surg. 1995;35(6):654–6.
8. Yotsuyanagi T, Nihei Y, Sawada Y. A simple technique for reconstruction of the umbilicus, using two twisted flaps. Plast Reconstr Surg. 1998;102(7):2444–6.
9. Iida N, Ohsumi N. Reconstruction of umbilical hypogenesis accompanied by a longitudinal scar. Plast Reconstr Surg. 2003;111(1):322–5.
10. Abenavoli FM, Cusano V, Cucchiara V, D'Amico C, Corvelli L. An idea for umbilical reconstruction. Ann Plast Surg. 2001;46(2):194.
11. Marconi F. Reconstruction of the umbilicus: a simple technique. Plast Reconstr Surg. 1995;95(6):1115–7.
12. Bartsich S, Schwartz MH. Purse-string method for immediate umbilical reconstruction. Plast Reconstr Surg. 2003;112(6):1652–5.
13. Schoeller T, Wechselberger G, Otto A, Rainer C, Schwabegger A, Lille S, Ninković M. New technique for scarless umbilical reinsertion in abdominoplasty procedures. Plast Reconstr Surg. 1998;102(5):1720–3.
14. Santanelli F, Mazzocchi M, Renzi L, Cigna E. Reconstruction of a natural-looking umbilicus. Scand J Plast Reconstr Surg Hand Surg. 2002;36(3):183–5.
15. Malic CC, Spyrou GE, Hough M. Patient satisfaction with two different methods of umbilicoplasty. Plast Reconstr Surg. 2007;119(1):357–61.
16. Hazani R, Israeli R, Feingold RS. Reconstructing a natural looking umbilicus: a new technique. Ann Plast Surg. 2009;63(4):358–60.

Chapter 23
Umbilicoplasty in Abdominoplasty: Double "V" Technique with Hidden Scars

Vidal Guerreiro

23.1 Introduction

A natural-looking umbilicus is an essential component to the beauty of an abdomen after abdominoplasty. Apparent periumbilical scars are undesirable and can compromise the final outcome of this surgery. Weinhold [1] was the first to worry about preserving the umbilicus in the abdominal dermolipectomy in 1909, as well as Prudente [2] in 1943, and Andrews [3] turning it into a skin cylinder, in 1956. Pontes [4] and Lintillac and Tichadou [5] advocated the reconstruction of the umbilicus. Barraya and Deleuze [6] and Barraya and Nakpane [7] in 1967 made an anchor scar in the umbilicus. Callia [8, 9] improves the way to see the tummy tuck and therefore is the best way to prepare the umbilicus pedicle flap, culminating in Pitanguy [10, 11] and later Avelar [12], with his umbilicoplasty technique restoring the concept of the natural-looking umbilicus.

In recent years, several authors have published the most varied geometrical shapes in making the umbilicus: Star of "Mercedes," diamonds, ellipses, crosses, clovers, rectangles, shell, infinity symbol, double "V," etc. [3–16]. Based on the concept that the umbilicus is due to a process of healing by secondary intention, there are still those who amputate its pedicle and suture the abdominal flap edges directly on the abdominal rectus fascia, leaving healing by secondary intention [17]. Marconi [18], Onishi [19], and Franco and Franco [20] follow the line of neoonfaloplasty with minimal scars.

In the classical double "V" umbilicoplasty technique [15], the umbilical stump is made with a height corresponding to half the thickness of the abdominal flap, and the abdominal skin suture is made directly on it. This creates a certain tension on the

V. Guerreiro, M.D.
Department Plastic Surgery, Federal University of Mato Grosso,
Rua Buenos Aires, 579 Jardim das Américas, Cuiaba, MT, Brazil, CEP 78.060-634
e-mail: vidalguerreiro@yahoo.com.br

M.A. Shiffman (ed.), *Adult Umbilical Reconstruction*,
DOI 10.1007/978-3-319-43887-0_23

suture and eventually pulls the scars close to the surface of the abdomen. To avoid this some tactical changes were made to the original technique. The aim of this study is to describe in detail the double "V" umbilicoplasty technique with hidden scars, a variant of double "V" technique.

23.2 Technique

The first step is to isolate the umbilicus through a circular incision in the skin at the beginning of abdominoplasty. It is not necessary to preserve fat in the umbilical pedicle. After the abdominal flap detachment and the abdominal musculofascial plication, the umbilicoplasty begins. The umbilical stump is marked in a "V" shape with no more than 1.5 cm long on each side. It is intended to shape and decrease the size and depth of the umbilicus (Figs. 23.1 and 23.2). The umbilical dermis is attached to the abdominal rectus fascia superiorly, inferiorly, and on both the lateral sides with nonabsorbable sutures (nylon 4/0) (Figs. 23.3 and 23.4), aiming a flat and shallow umbilicus with a height of about 2–3 mm (Figs. 23.5 and 23.6). The correct position of the new umbilicus is determined, and a "V"-shaped cutaneous mark is made at this point with 1.5 cm (maximum 2 cm) long in each side, and vasoconstrictor solution is infiltrated (Fig. 23.7).

After the skin incision, the underlying fat tissue is removed through the "V" incision (Figs. 23.8 and 23.9) and from the inner aspect of the abdominal flap (Figs. 23.10 and 23.11) to obtain an inverted cone shape (Fig. 23.12). The next step is the attachment of the abdominal flap to the abdominal rectus fascia through four nonabsorbable sutures (nylon 3/0). It begins by the cranial portion (Figs. 23.13, 23.14, 23.15, 23.16, and 23.17) followed by the lateral and caudau sutures (Fig. 23.18). The suture bite is placed between the dermis of the abdominal flap and the abdominal rectus fascia, and it is done about 2 mm lateral to the umbilical stump edge in order

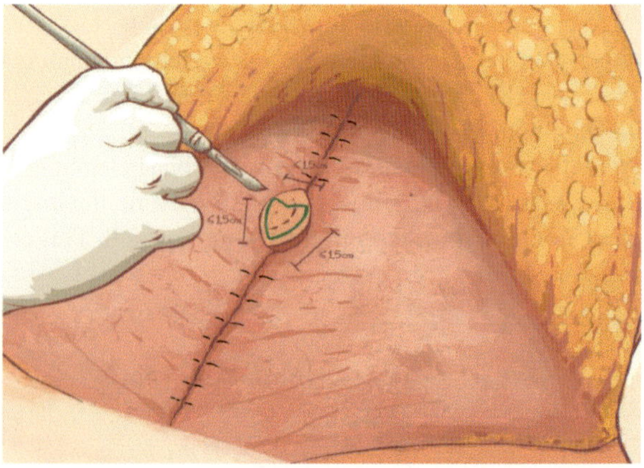

Fig. 23.1 The V-shaped umbilical mark. Each side of the incision is 1.5 cm in length maximum

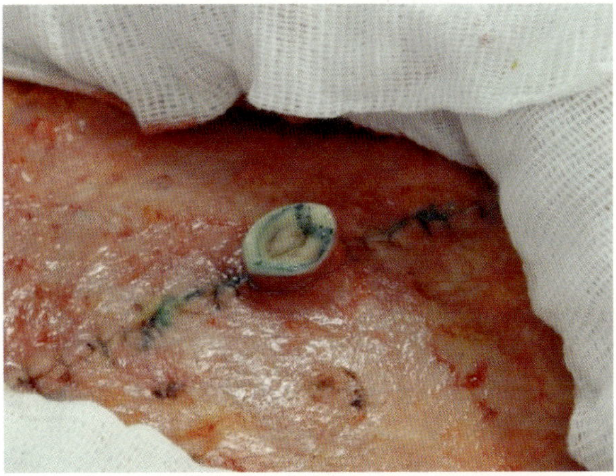

Fig. 23.2 V-shaped umbilical marking

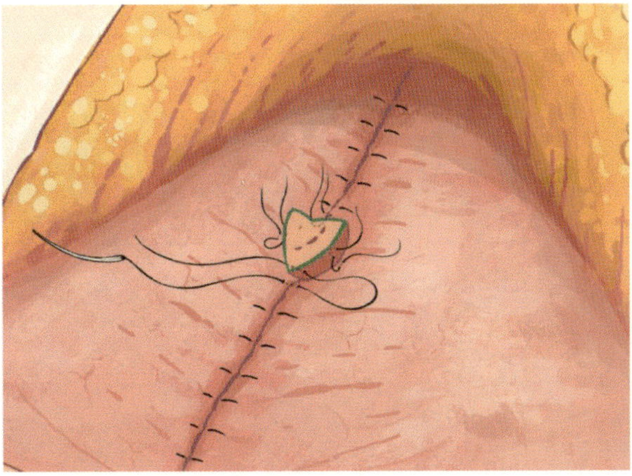

Fig. 23.3 The umbilical dermis is attached to the abdominal rectus fascia superiorly, inferiorly, and on both lateral sides with nylon 4/0 sutures

to prevent the neoumbilicus from becoming small (Figs. 23.19 and 23.20). The final suture is done with nonabsorbable sutures (nylon 5/0). The umbilicus now features a triangular shape and with the scars placed at its deepest point (Figs. 23.21, 23.22, 23.23, 23.24, 23.25, 23.26, 23.27, 23.28, and 23.29).

The patient is instructed to clean the umbilicus once a day and hold a dry gauze in place.

23.3 Discussion

This technique has been used universally, including in secondary cases (with loss of the umbilical stump) and when there is umbilical hernia. In these cases, the technique is done in the usual manner after the hernia repair, and the possible

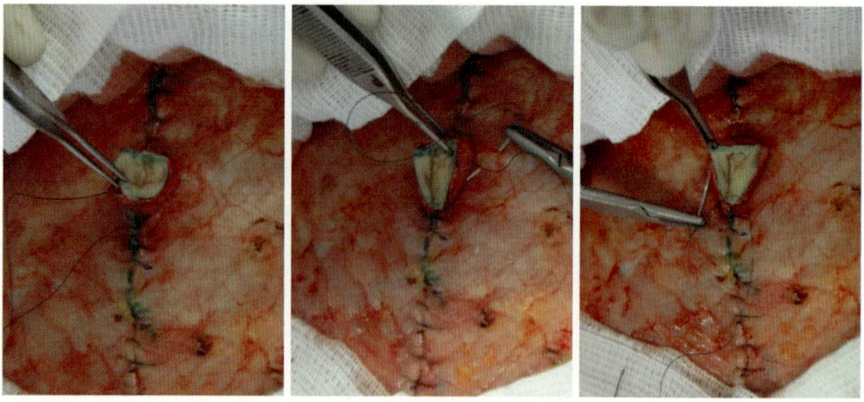

Fig. 23.4 (*Left*, *middle*, *right*) umbilical dermis attachment to the abdominal rectus fascia

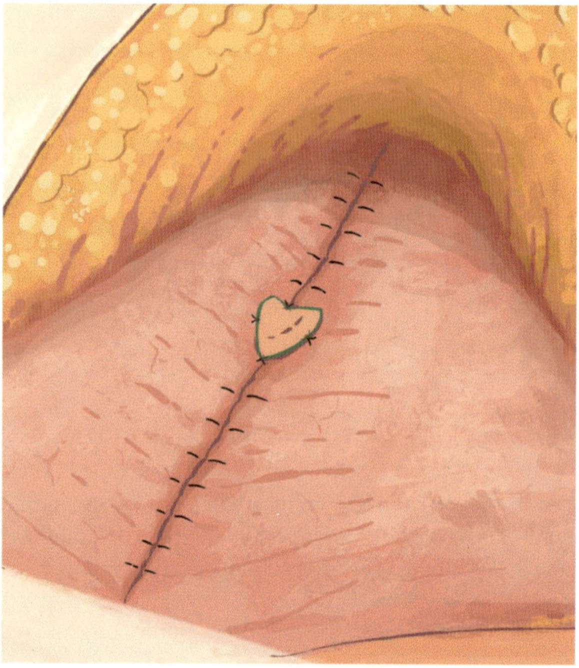

Fig. 23.5 The umbilical stump is already attached to the abdominal rectus fascia. It is now about a 2–3 mm height

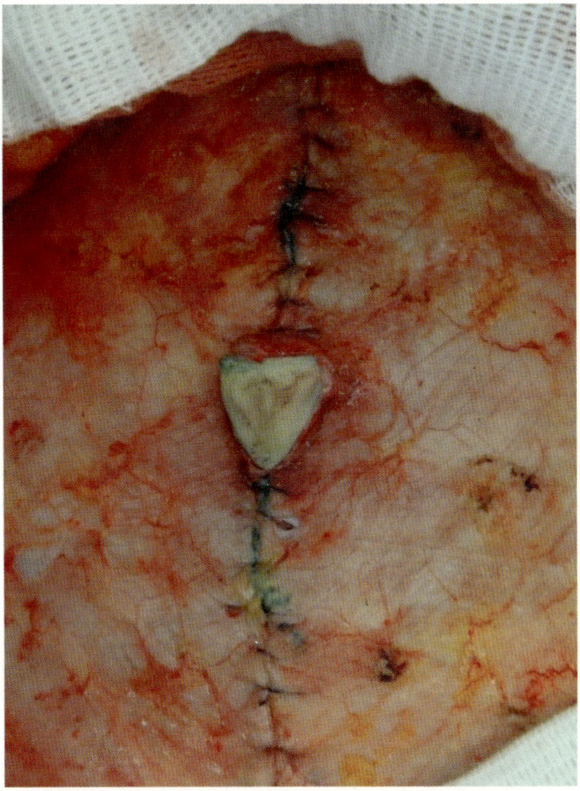

Fig. 23.6 Final aspect of the umbilical stump attachment

complications range from darkening to necrosis of the umbilical stump. Even then the aesthetic result is still good, since the scar remains in depth close to the aponeurosis. Umbilical stenosis has not been observed with this technique, so it is not our routine indicate silicone orthoses or any other material in order to prevent its constriction. It is important to note that the abdominal flap attachment should be done about 2 mm lateral to the umbilicus edge in order to prevent the umbilicus from becoming small. The umbilical stump swelling is common in the early postoperative period.

We recommend the use of silicone orthosis only when it is significant or enough to worry the patient. It is important to understand that the umbilical stump is only the base of the neoumbilicus. It must be shallow and small with no more than 1.5 cm long on each side, otherwise it will be redundant and protruding. The depth of the neoumbilicus is determined by the attachment of abdominal flap in the abdominal rectus fascia and is directly related to the thickness of abdominal fat tissue. Thus, in thin patients with thin fat tissue in the abdominal flap, the neoumbilicus will not be too deep and the scars may appear.

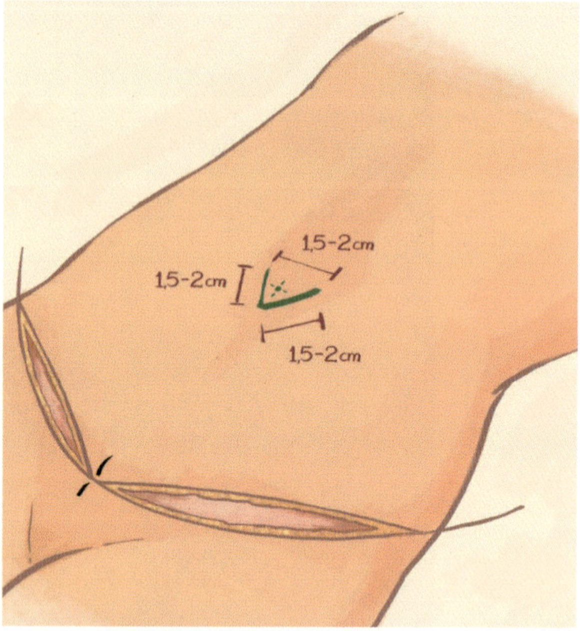

Fig. 23.7 The limbs of the V-shaped incision are 1.5–2 cm on each side, separated by the same 1.5–2 cm at the base (*equilateral triangle*)

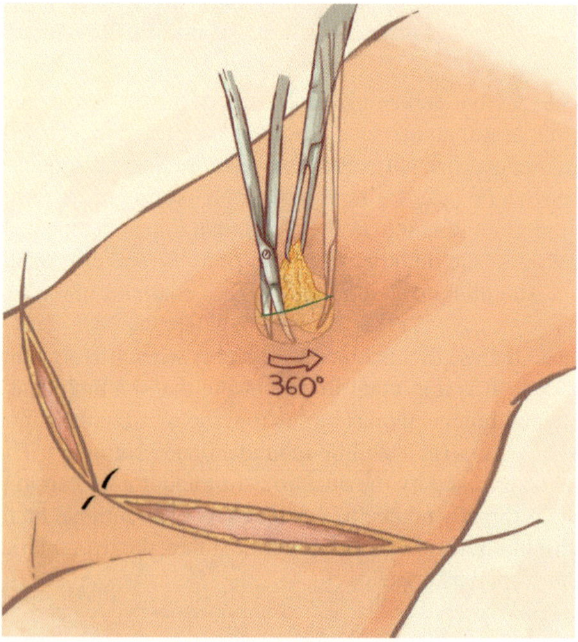

Fig. 23.8 Removal of underlying fat tissue through the "V" incision

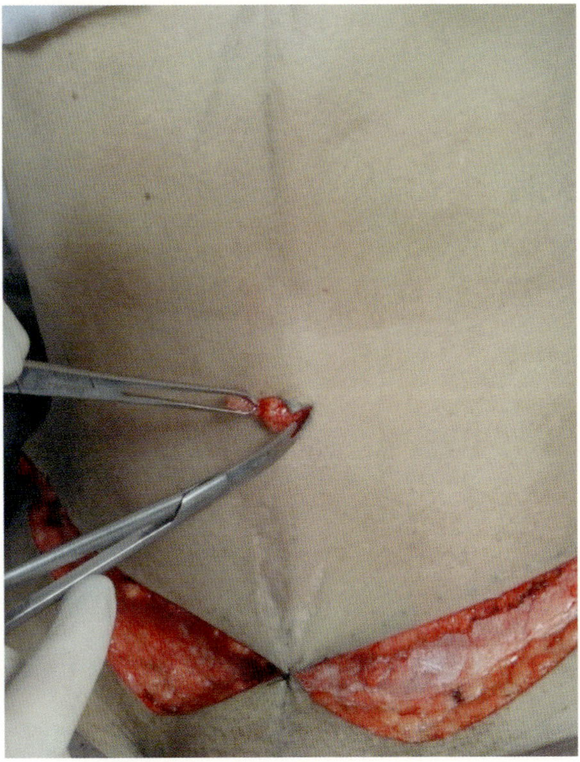

Fig. 23.9 Fat removal through the "V" incision

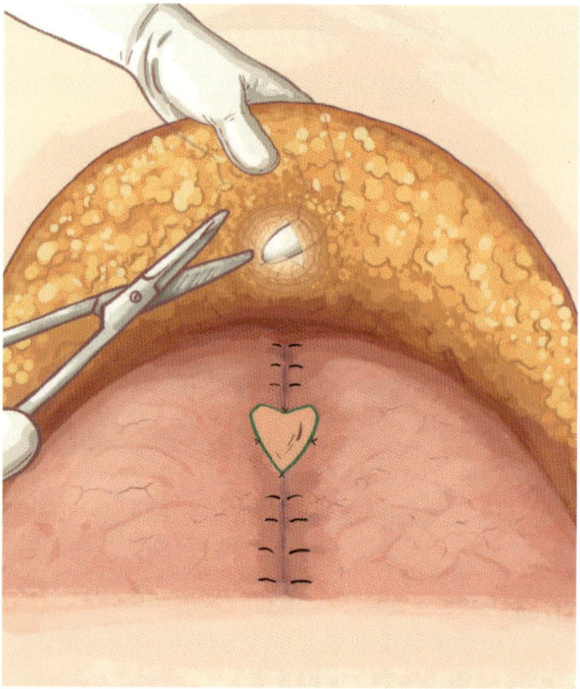

Fig 23.10 Defatting is also performed from the inner aspect of the abdominal flap in order to achieve an inverted cone shape. Internal aspect of the new umbilical site in the abdominal flap after defatting

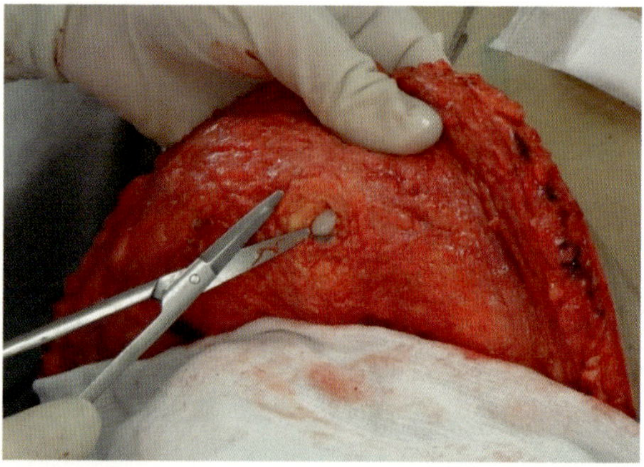

Fig. 23.11 Fat removal from the inner aspect of the abdominal flap

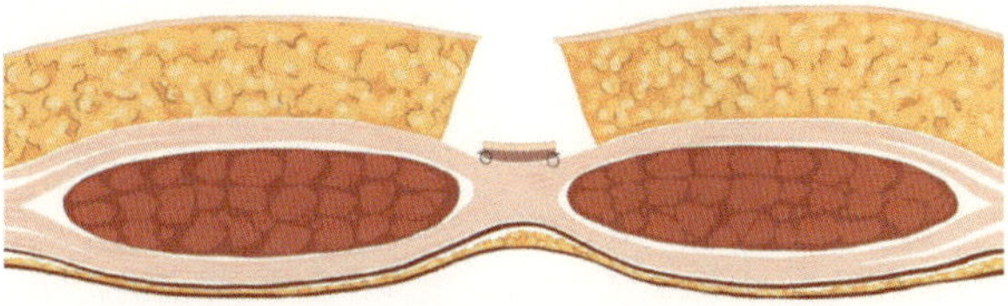

Fig. 23.12 Defatting final aspect showing the inverted cone shape

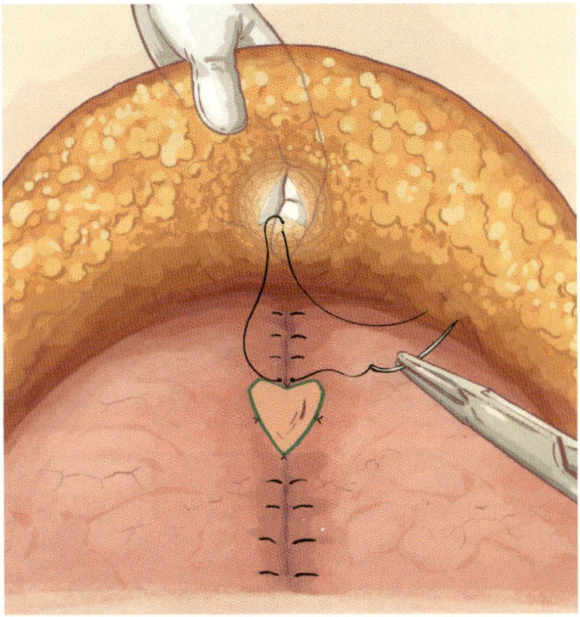

Fig. 23.13 First attachment suture of the abdominal flap (nylon 3/0). The suture bite between the dermis of the abdominal flap and the abdominal rectus fascia

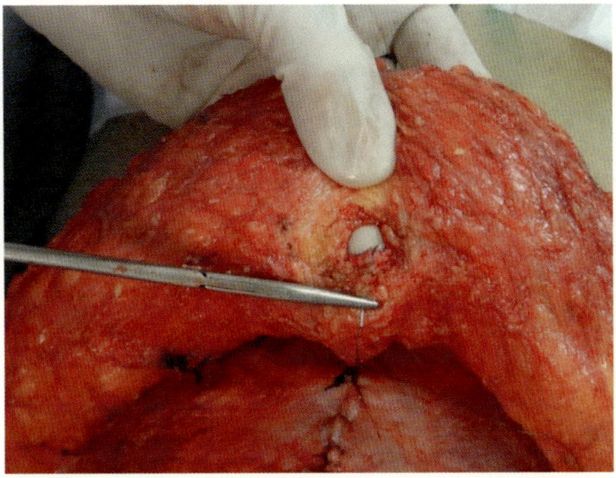

Fig. 23.14 Using the middle finger to steady the abdominal flap when we bite the dermis. This facilitates the suture and ensures to have caught a good amount of tissue

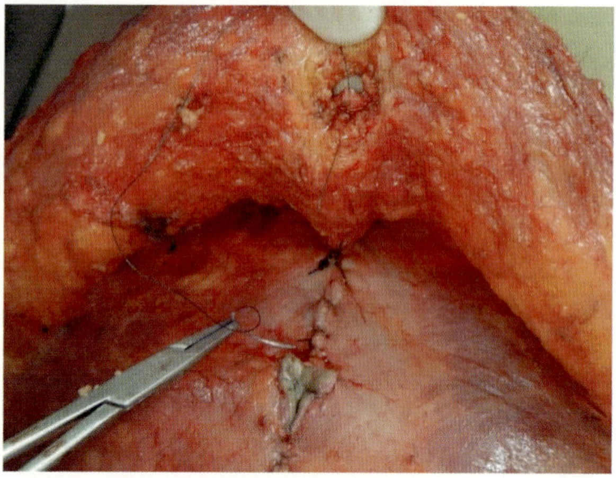

Fig. 23.15 First attachment suture of the abdominal flap

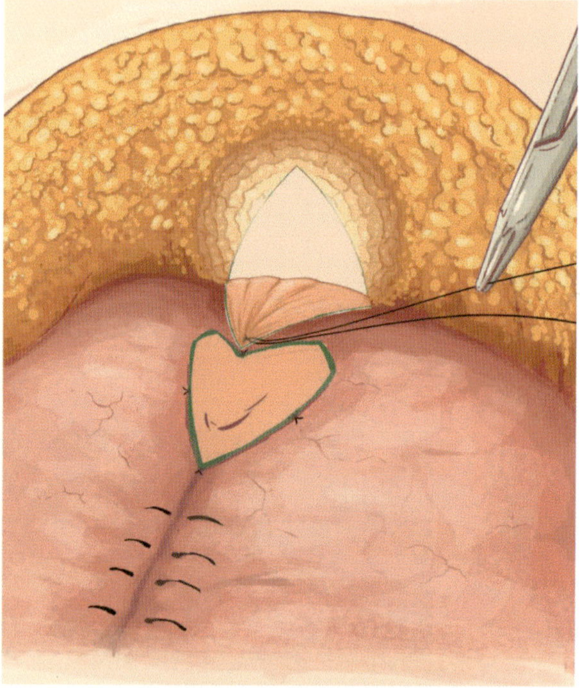

Fig. 23.16 First attachment suture of the abdominal flap – tied suture

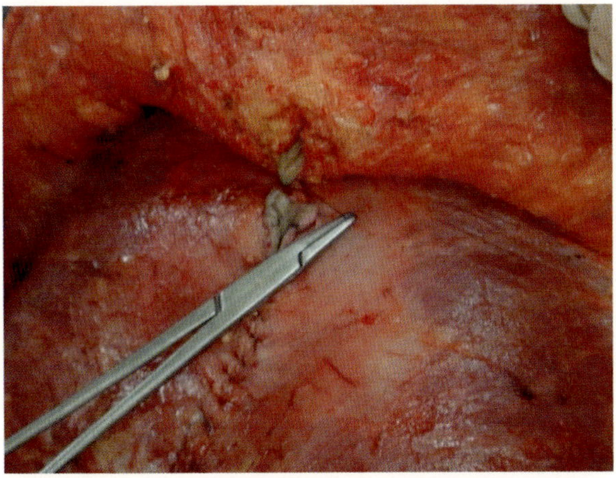

Fig. 23.17 First attachment suture of the abdominal flap – tied suture

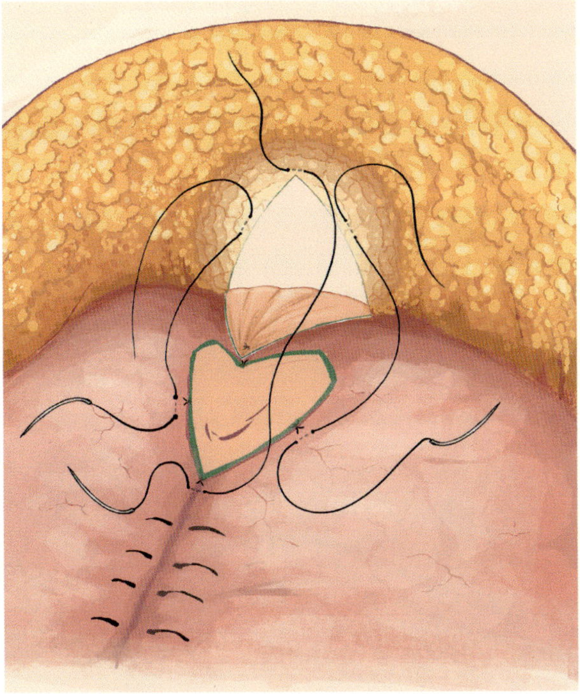

Fig. 23.18 Lateral and caudau attachment sutures of the abdominal flap (nylon 3/0). Note that the fixation is done about 2 mm lateral to the umbilical stump edge in order to prevent the neoumbilicus becoming small

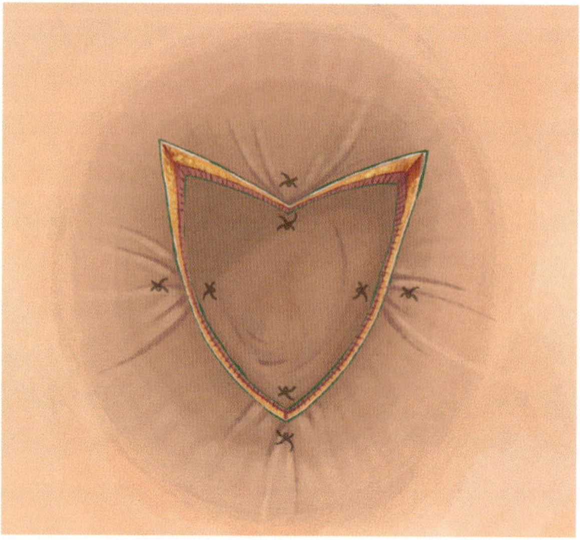

Fig. 23.19 Neoumbilicus attachment sutures (attachment suture on transparency)

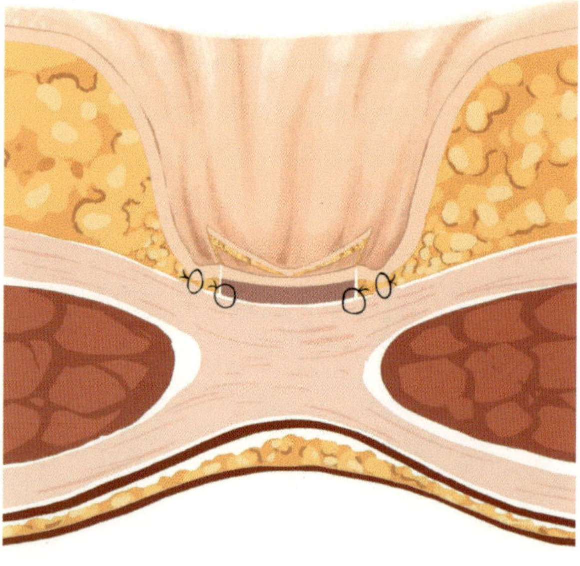

Fig. 23.20 Neoumbilicus attachment sutures

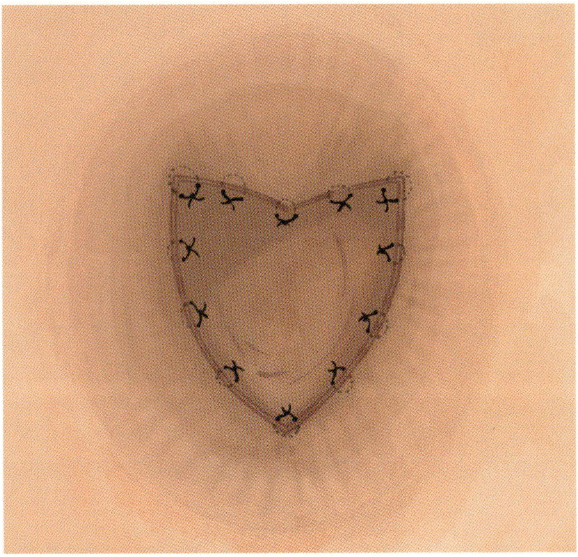

Fig. 23.21 Neoumbilicus final suture (nylon 5/0)

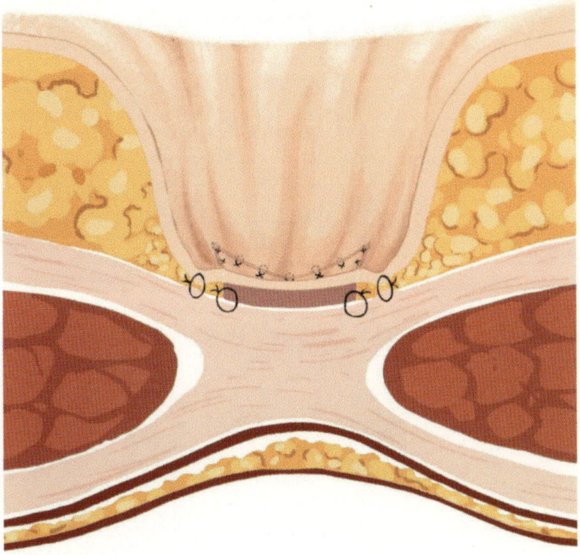

Fig. 23.22 Neoumbilicus final suture. Note that the scars are deep and the sidewall of the neoumbilicus is formed by invagination of the skin of the abdominal flap

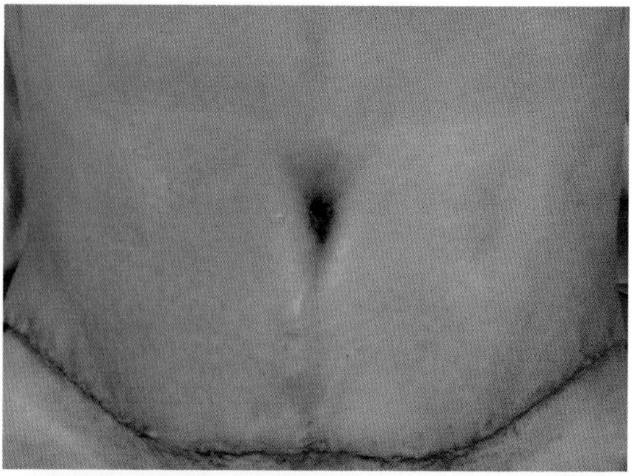

Fig. 23.23 Neoumbilicus final aspect (intraoperative)

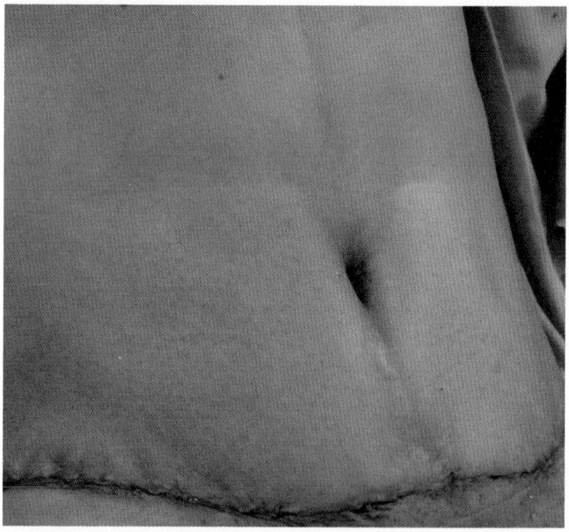

Fig. 23.24 Neoumbilicus final aspect (intraoperative)

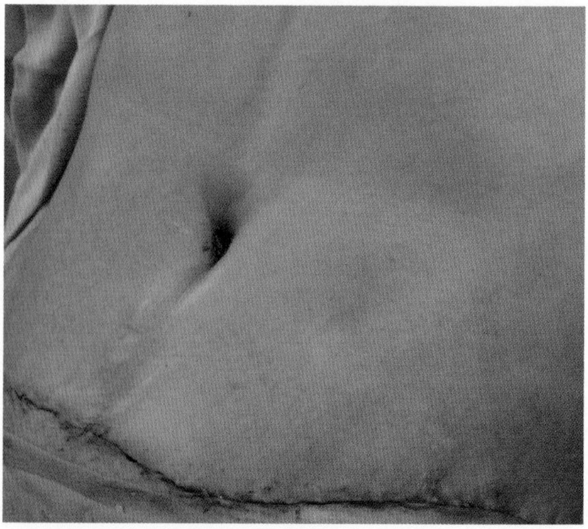

Fig. 23.25 Neoumbilicus final aspect (intraoperative)

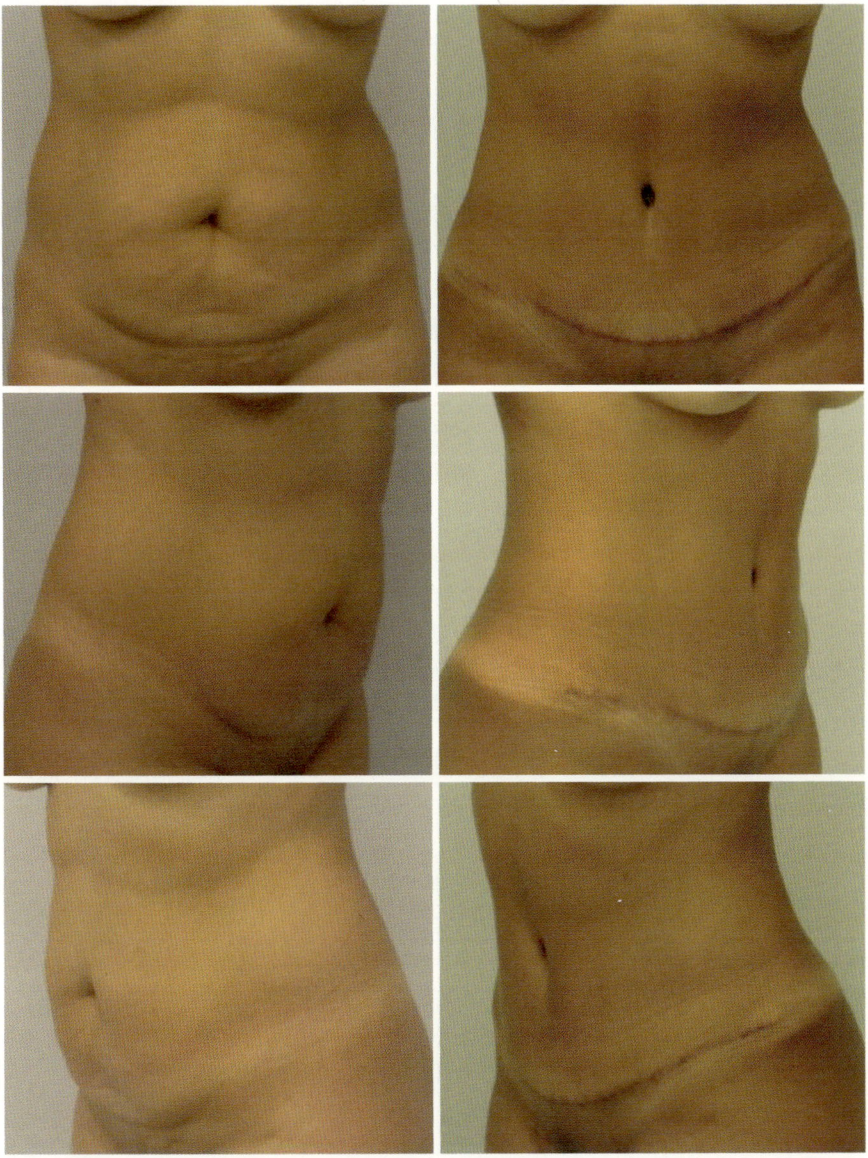

Fig. 23.26 (*Left*) preoperative. (*Right*) six months postsurgery

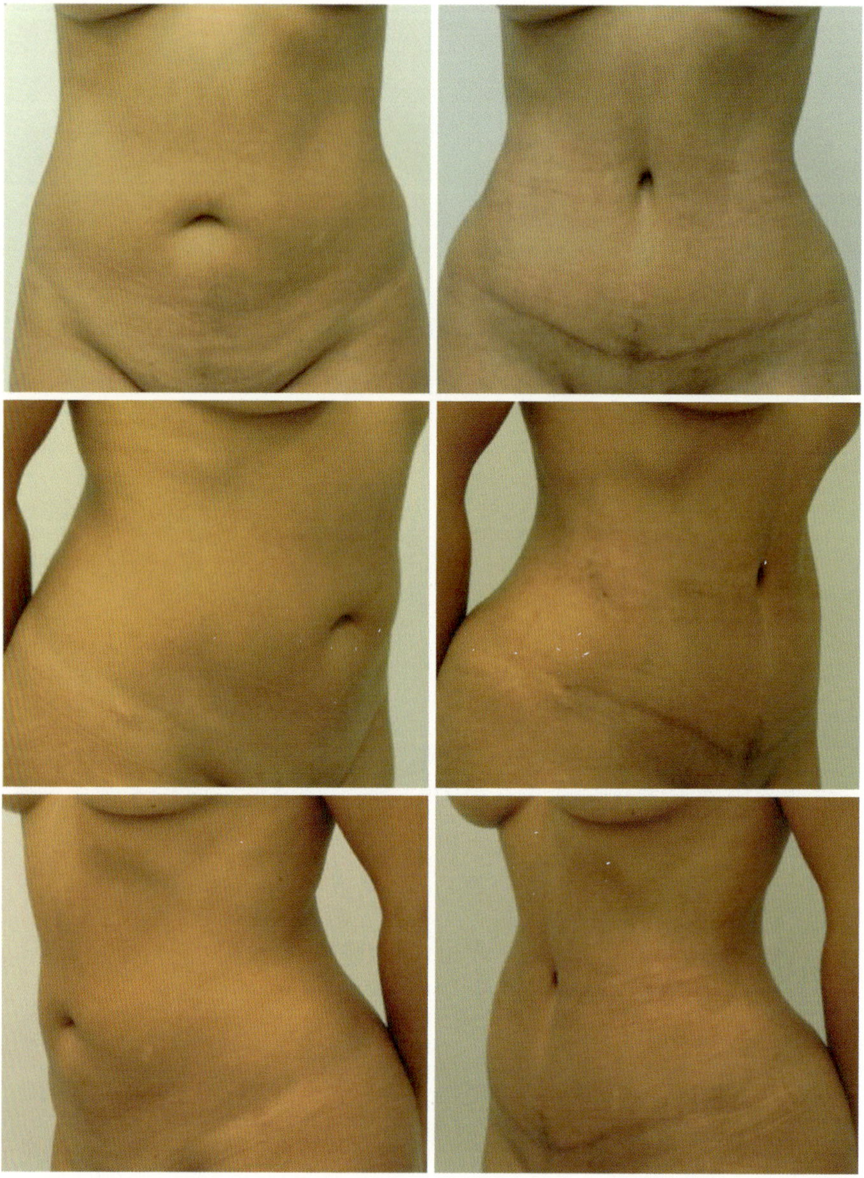

Fig. 23.27 (*Left*) preoperative. (*Right*) six months postsurgery

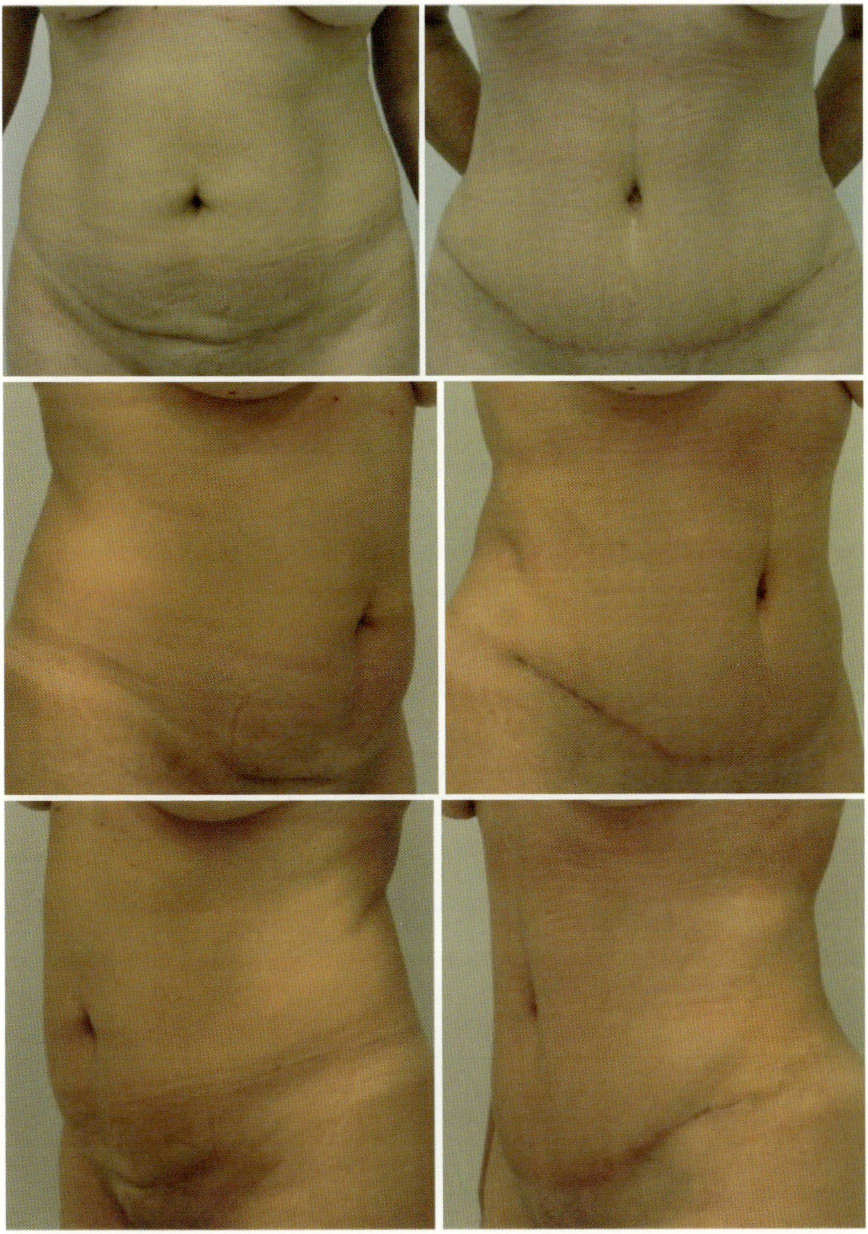

Fig. 23.28 (*Left*) preoperative. (*Right*) six months postsurgery

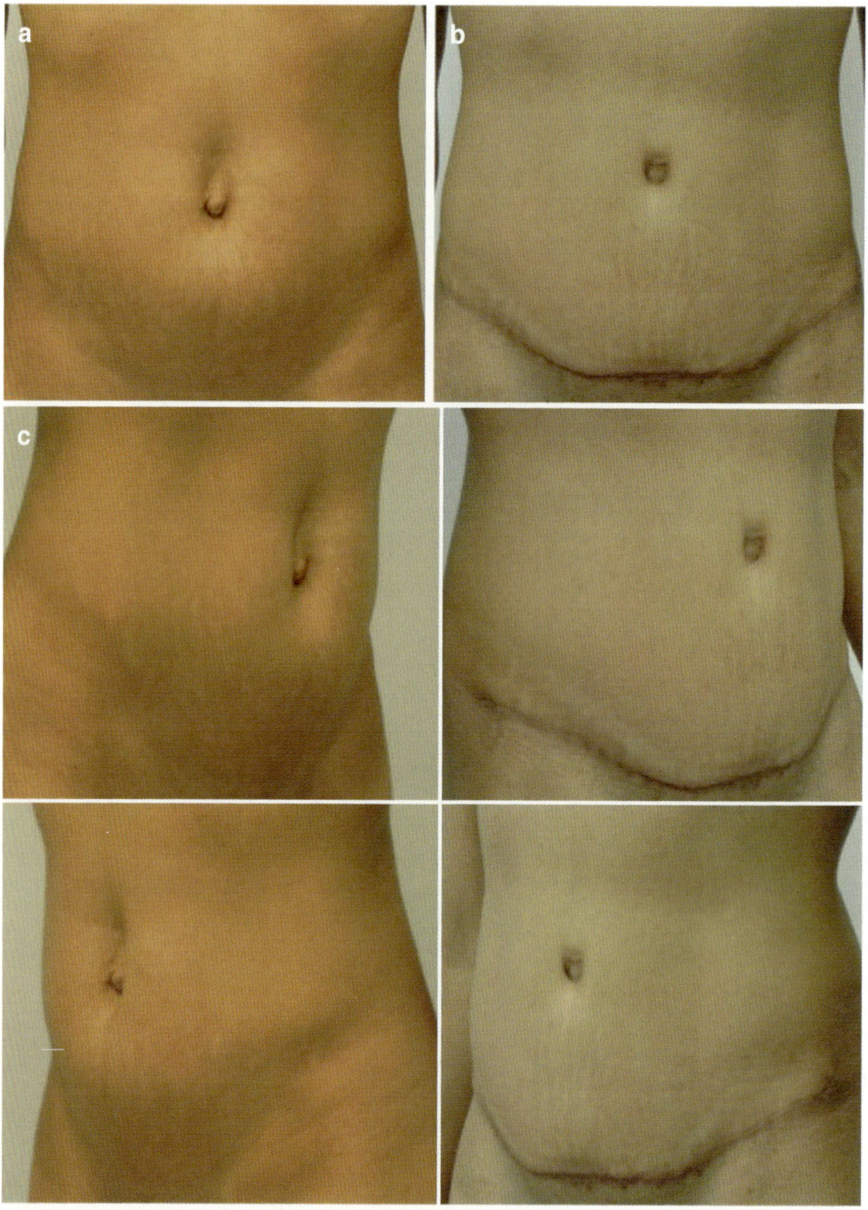

Fig. 23.29 (**a**) Preoperative patient with thin abdominal flap and umbilical hernia. (**b**) Six months postoperative. (**c**) (*Left*) preoperative. (**c**) (*Right*) six months postoperative. Note that even with hypertrophic scar in abdominoplasty, the neoumbilicus has good aesthetic results

23.4 Conclusions

This is another proposal to minimize the stigma of abdominoplasty with umbilical visible scars. It is an easy learning technique that allows us to build a natural-looking neoumbilicus with practically unapparent scars. Furthermore, it is very safe and has predictable results, because even when there are complications, such as necrosis of the umbilical stump by the umbilical hernia correction, the aesthetic result is still satisfactory.

References

1. Weinhold K, Zentrab F. Gynäk. 1901;38:1332. In: Thorek M, editor. Plastic surgery of the breast and abdominal wall. Springfield: Charles C. Thomas; 1942.
2. Prudente A. Dermolipectomia abdominal com conservação da cicatriz umbilical. Anais do II Congresso Latino-Americano de Cirurgia Plástica. Buenos Aires: Guilherme Karast; 1943. p. 468.
3. Andrews JM. Nova técnica de lipectomia abdominal e onfaloplastia. Cuba: Memória do 8o Congresso Latino-Americano de Cirurgia Plástica; 1956.
4. Pontes R. Plástica abdominal, importância de sua associação à correção das hérnias incisionais. Rev Bras de Cirurg. 1996;53:85–92.5.
5. Lintilhac JP, Tichadou M. The umbilicus in plastic surgery of the abdomen. Transposition or reconstruction. Maroc Med. 1966;45(490):266–71.
6. Barraya L, Deleuze J. Chirurgie abdominale, reparations parietales et dermolipectomies. Nouvel ombilic Mem Acad Chir. 1967;93(15/16):473–9.
7. Barraya L, Nakpane ET. Abdomen musculum abdomen pendulum. Reparations nouvel ombilic. La Prense Med. 1968;76(48):2287–9.
8. Callia W. Contribuição para o estudo da correção cirúrgica do abdome pêndulo e globoso. Técnica original. [Disertação]. São Paulo: Faculdade de Medicina da Universidade de São Paulo; 1963.
9. Callia W. Uma plástica para cirurgia geral. Med Hosp (São Paulo). 1967;1:40–1.
10. Pitanguy I. Abdominoplastias. Junho: O Hospital; 1967.
11. Pitanguy I. Abdominal lipectomy: an approach to it through an analysis of 300 consecutive cases. Plast Reconstr Surg. 1967;40(4):384–91.
12. Avelar JM. Abdominoplasty: systematization of a technique without external umbilical scar. Aesthetic Plast Surg. 1978;2:141–51.
13. Tavares Filho JM, Oliveira DF, Franco TR. Umbilico e neoumbilicoplastias. In: Lima Júnior EM, editor. Tratado de Cirurgia Plástica após Grandes Perdas Ponderais. São Paulo: Atheneu; 2010.
14. Bozola AR. Abdominoplastia: novos conceitos e tratamentos na mesma classificação de 25 anos. In: Mélega JM, Viterbo F, Mendes FH, editors. Cirurgia Plástica: Princípios e Atualidades. Rio de Janeiro: Guanabara Koogan; 2011.
15. Freitas JO, Guerreiro V, Sperli AE. Neo-onfaloplastia na dermolipectomia abdominal: técnica do duplo "V". Rev Bras Cir Plast. 2010;25(3):504–8.
16. Furtado IR. Onfaloplastia: técnica do infinito. Rev Bras Cir Plast. 2011;26(2):298–301.
17. Santanelli F, Mazzocchi M, Renzi C, Cigna E. Reconstruction of a natural-looking umbilicus. Scand J Plast Reconstr Surg Hand Surg. 2002;36(3):183–5.

18. Marconi F. Reconstruction of the umbilicus: a simple technique. Plast Reconstr Surg. 1995;95(6):1115–7.
19. Onishi K, Yang YL, Maruyama Y. A new lunch box-type method in umbilical reconstruction. Ann Plast Surg. 1995;35(6):654–6.
20. Franco T, Franco D. Neoomphaloplasty: an old and new technique. Aesthetic Plast Surg. 1999;23(2):151–4.

Chapter 24
Umbilical Reconstruction with the "Heart-Shaped Incision"

Oscar M. Ramirez

24.1 Introduction

Throughout history females have enchanted males changing exposures of their erotic zones. The female abdomen, although not erotic by itself, has always been the point of attention because of the close proximity to the primary sexual zone that lies beneath. Modern female fashion has followed the so-called law of shifting erogenous zones [1]. Following this law in the late 1990s in the Western world, there was a change in fashion for exposing the abdomen by wearing low-cut jeans combined with very short tops. That has changed the focus of attention to the navel because that became available for ready inspection. Women started decorating their navels with ring piercing and tattoos. Wearers and observers became more aware of the beauty of the navel, its shape, and position. Despite that, there are scant publications dealing with the aesthetics of the navel. However there are many publications dealing with surgical techniques to reconstruct the navel during an abdominoplasty or to reconstruct a new umbilicus following an unfavorable surgical outcome from the original abdominoplasty or in the presence of large umbilical hernia. This is probably a reflection that there is not an ideal method for its reconstruction. The aim of this chapter is to describe my personal approach to reconstruct the umbilicus during abdominoplasty.

O.M. Ramirez, M.D.
Ramirez Plastic Surgery, Elite Surgical & Aesthetic Center,
2665 Executive Park Dr., Weston, FL 33331, USA
e-mail: RamirezMDPS@gmail.com

M.A. Shiffman (ed.), *Adult Umbilical Reconstruction*,
DOI 10.1007/978-3-319-43887-0_24

24.2 Aesthetics of the Navel

The navel is the only scar in the body that has aesthetic and sensual attractiveness. Their look is of significant concern to prospective patients and surgeons due to its visible location and exposure in the center of the abdomen. Age, weight, pregnancies, and hernias influence its shape and size. It breaks the monotony of the abdominal surface and contributes to its identity and beauty. In some cultures, it is considered philosophically speaking the center of the body. In other cultures where the woman's face is covered, the abdomen and the navel represent the face of the soul. Therefore, a summary of the available information on the navel position, distance from classic landmarks, and shape is in order.

The navel is not located in a central midline as we traditionally thought. Studies by Rohrich et al. found out that the navel rarely is in the midline [2]. The position in the longitudinal axis has been subject of many personal opinions and during surgery placement of the navel used different reference anatomical landmarks. Vernon, the pioneer of the modern abdominoplasty, suggested placing it 4 cm below the waistline [3]. Baroudi [4] and Pitanguy [5] positioned at the level of the umbilical stalk in a neutral position. Hinderer [6] advised placing it 3 cm above the anterior iliac crest. Subsequently Baroudi advised to place the umbilicus 17 cm from the anterior vulvar commissure. Dubois and Ousterhout in their study found out that the navel was located at the level of the uppermost point of the iliac crest [7]. A more mathematical approach to locate the navel were the studies of Abhyankar et al. [8]. Their studies suggested that the navel should be located in a position that is in accordance with the golden ratio: Xipho-sternum-umbilicus distance/umbilicus-pubic symphysis distance ratio of approximately 1.6/1. Visconti et al. [9] used the abdominal crease as the lower limit of the umbilicus-pubic distance, and their findings on the location of the umbilicus were even closer to the golden ratio (i.e., 1.618).

Regardless of the shape, the most desirable navel should be small, should have a moderate hooding, and should be deep (an "innie"). The most desirable shape of the navel according to some studies is a vertical oval (1.5 cm or less vertical distance and 0.5 cm or less horizontal distance). A horizontally oriented navel with excess hooding is an aged navel and does not look athletic. Round, triangular, slit-shaped, and moderate large navels are of intermediate likeness. The less desirable is a navel with two or more of the following features: large navel, lack of hooding, horizontally oriented, and has an outie. The most beautiful navel has the following combination: small, vertical oval has an innie and a smooth skin hooding. In addition the beautiful navel should be the end of an aesthetically pleasing xipho-umbilical depression (Fig. 24.1).

24.3 The Consultation

During consultation for abdominoplasty, I spend a good amount of time dealing with the aesthetics and surgical technique of the navel. Among the undesirable aesthetic sequelae following an abdominoplasty, problems with the navel are the most

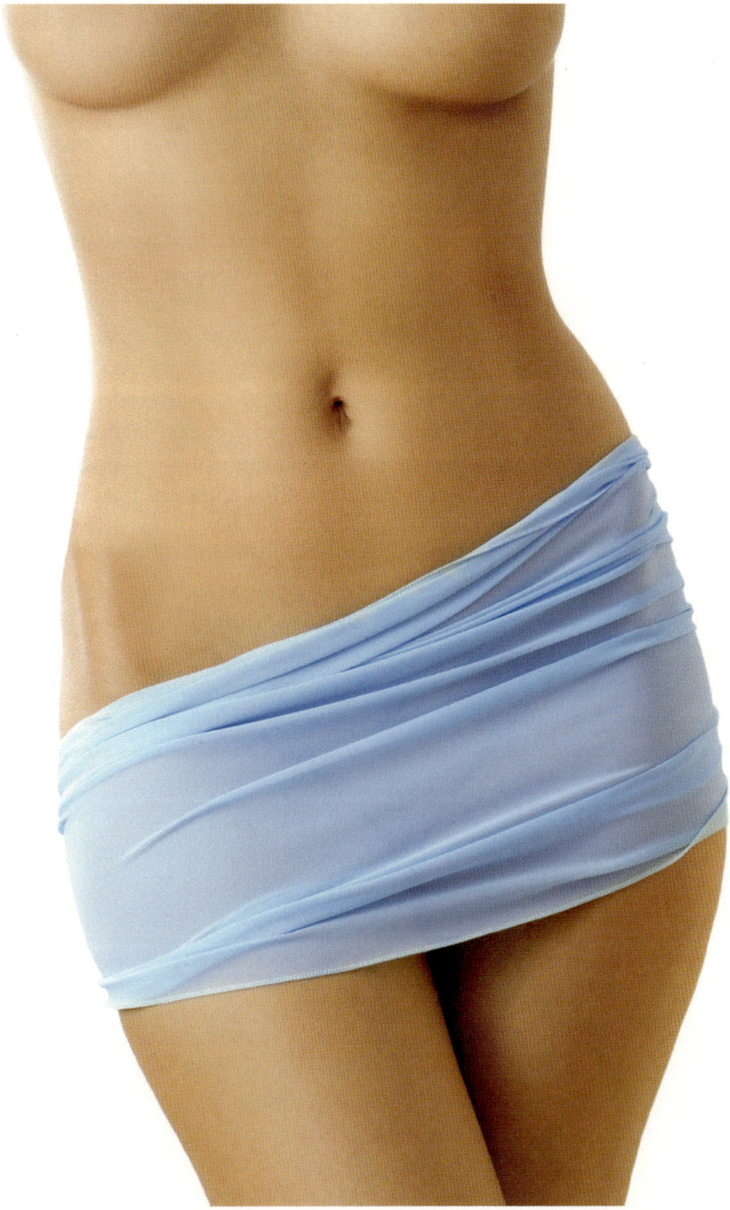

Fig. 24.1 A beautiful abdomen has as its central piece the navel located at 1.6/1 relationship between the xiphoid and the suprapubic crease. The navel is vertically oriented, is small, has a delicate hooding, and is located at the end of a xipho-umbilical depression. Credit: KMNPhoto/Shutterstock.com

distressful to patients. Since the navel is rarely in the midline, I make a point to the patient about her navel position and how much off is from the midline. This will prevent potential medicolegal claims. I discuss the options of navel transposition on the abdominal skin vs. navel floating. This will obviously depend of the original pubis-umbilicus distance and the vertical extent of the dermolipectomy needed to obtain a good aesthetic result. If the patient is not a candidate for the "floating abdominoplasty," I discuss the vertical extent of the abdominal skin resection, i.e., above or below the umbilicus. If the resection is going to be below the umbilicus, there will be a vertical scar from the closure of the navel defect. The patient has to be fully aware of this. Sometimes the decision of making a vertically short flap resection (with its resultant long umbilicus/suprapubic scar) will depend of the horizontal abdominal skin flap resection. This will be determined by the logistics of not having enough laxity in the upper abdomen to stretch the skin all the way down to the suprapubic/anterior hipline of closure. Some other times may be patient's choice, whom may elect not to have a long lower abdominoplasty scar. Basically, the length of the lower abdominoplasty scar is determined by the size of the ellipse of the skin/pannus that needs to be removed. In that context it is a patient's decision between having a shorter lower abdominal scar and a vertical scar or having a longer lower scar and no vertical scar. In my experience most patients elect to have a longer lower abdominal scar if that entails avoiding a vertical scar and maximizing the amount of panniculectomy.

Specific problems that need to be addressed beforehand are the presence of a large ventral or umbilical hernia. Hernia repair may require sacrifice of the blood supply to the umbilical stalk. If that is the case, the patient and surgeons should be prepared to create a new umbilicus with some of the techniques described in this book. Some patients regard their navel a highly erotic function. Sacrifice of the sensory input may be a sequel that needs to be informed. This is most likely to happen after a total amputation of the navel.

24.4 Surgical Technique

The technique about to be described has several considerations. Most navels particularly in overweight and obese patients have a long stalk. These umbilici need to the shortened, telescoped, or both. Standard rectus dehiscence repair may not tighten enough the abdominal muscles, and it will not give enough room to accommodate these long navels. Therefore the resultant reconstructed navel may not present an innie after surgery and will be located over an abdominal prominence (Fig. 24.2). It may become flat and sometimes will develop an outie (Fig. 24.3). Hooding is a difficult proposition to achieve because the abdominal flap that for necessity is placed under tension will transmit that tension to the navel, producing flattening of the navel. Absorbable braided sutures produce more inflammatory reaction than non-braided absorbable sutures. Absorbable sutures in general produce more inflammation than nonabsorbable material. On the other hand, braided materials being absorbable or permanent may harbor bacterial biofilm. Monofilament

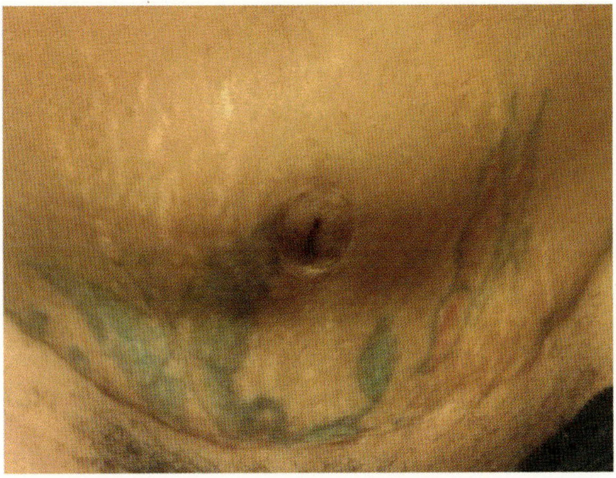

Fig. 24.2 Poorly executed umbilicoplasty. This is located too low near the suprapubic incision, the muscle repair is incomplete with a convexity, the navel is too large and flat

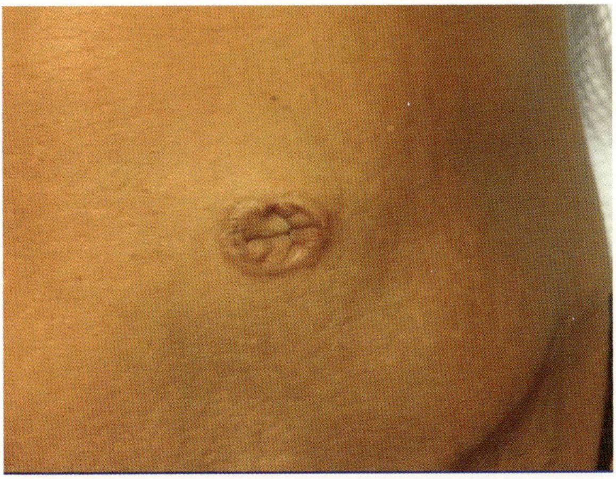

Fig. 24.3 Large navel with an "outie." Observe the redundant skin in the center of the navel

nonabsorbable sutures are the least reactive. Inflammation has a direct relationship with hypertrophic or keloid scarring (Fig. 24.4). Tension is another causation for hypertrophic scars. So to obtain the best scars, I use monofilament nonabsorbable suture material for the deep dermis and skin and avoid excessive tension during closure at the skin level.

The traditional method of coring out the umbilicus for transposition is through a circular incision. The recipient incision on the abdominal skin is also circular or a vertical or horizontal slit. Regardless of the abdominal skin incision, the circular incision on the navel upon healing will tend to produce a constricting scar usually associated with hypertrophy at the borders. The constriction may progress to a

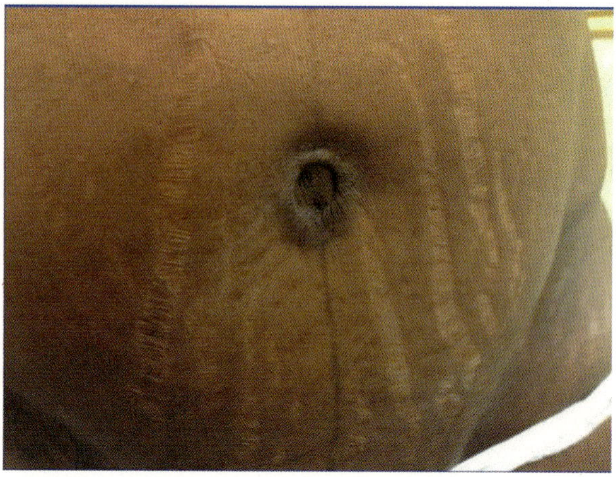

Fig. 24.4 Hypertrophic scarring will occur due to tension, poor skin border approximation, or the use of braided absorbable sutures

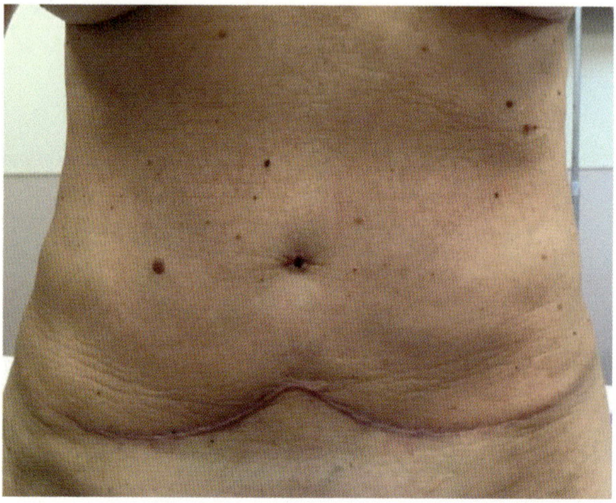

Fig. 24.5 Constricting scar around the navel. This is due to a small circumferential incision to fit the navel

pinhole entrance that may complicate hygiene and in some cases may even produce infection (Figs. 24.5 and 24.6). To avoid this problem, the umbilical separation from the abdominal skin is making an incision on the navel that has a heart shape. This implies to include in the resection a triangular flap in the meridian of the navel either at 12 o'clock position (superior triangle) or at 6 o'clock position (inferior triangle). I prefer resection of the superior triangle because at the time of the transposition and insetting in its new position, I could create a hooding of the new navel with the reciprocal triangular flap of the recipient. The triangular flap that is resected has a superior base and its apex is located at the very depth of the navel. This separation

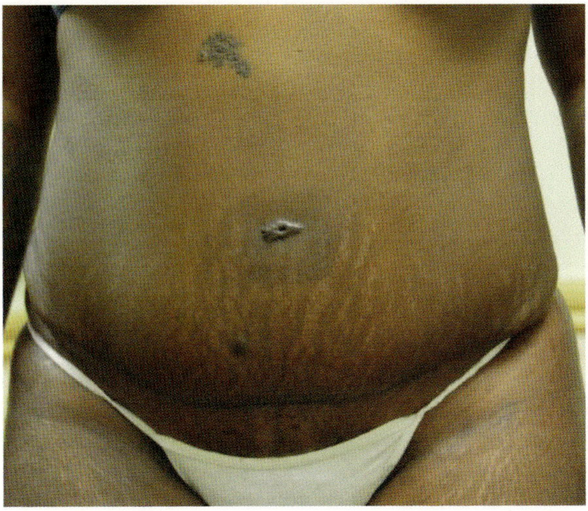

Fig. 24.6 Observe the pinhole navel with hypertrophic scarring

is done at the beginning of the surgery or when the abdominal flap elevation is about 5 cm below the umbilicus. Anterior-posterior circumferential dissection around the umbilicus is done down to the rectus fascia plane. This will isolate the navel from the abdominal flap. This is done to prevent accidental transection of the navel that may occur particularly when the panniculus is thick and the navel base attachment to the fascia is tenuous as may happen in cases of hernias or wide rectus diastasis. I have known of young plastic surgeons or trainees suddenly surprised with the presence of the navel in the elevated abdominal flap. After the skin-fat layer elevation usually up to the xiphoid process in the center and the costal margins or lower laterally the decision to plicate the rectus fascia is made at this point.

If you have a navel with a long umbilical stalk, there are two maneuvers to make it short. One is to cut the skin portion and the other is to telescope it or bury it in the muscle abdominal wall. Skin resection is limited because you need the skin component of the navel to create a natural-looking structure. You cannot cut the stalk unless you are prepared to create a neo-umbilicus. Telescoping along without pushing the stalk backwards is limited because this structure is too rigid to be compressed on itself. So the only option is to hide the stalk in the abdominal wall muscle plane. Standard rectus plication has also limited ability to hide the long stalk. I have found that the rectus partitioning and repair that I use in my abdominoplasty technique hides very well even the very long stalk [10, 11]. This technique also makes very good navel "innie."

The rectus fascia partitioning technique is outlined as follows. The borders of the rectus diastasis are marked with ink. A large ellipse outside the previous marking from xiphoid to pubis is marked with the widest portion about 3 cm above the navel or at the level of floating ribs. This is typically at the junction of the middle with the inner third of the width of the recti muscle. It can be less if the laxity of the abdomen in not significant. It can be more if there is no rectus diastasis and patient has

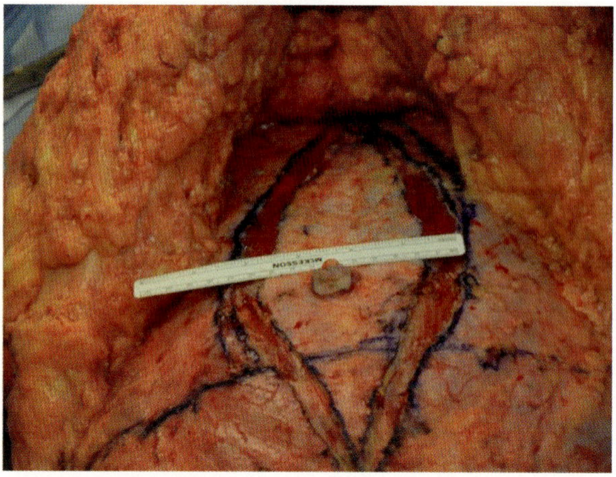

Fig. 24.7 The rectus partition has been completed. This is done well outside the recti border. The horizontal blue line indicates the projection of the iliac crests. Eleven cm of separation is very easy to correct with this technique even in the absence of rectus diastasis as in this patient. The widest portion is at the upper margins of the waistline

abdominal wall laxity. The rectus fascia splitting is done following the lines of the ellipse (Fig. 24.7). This is easily done making several perforations in the fascia with the electrocautery (every 2–3 cm) and introducing a curved hemostat underneath the fascia. The fascial bridges are cut with the electrocautery. Some musculocutaneous perforators are sometimes encountered. These are suture ligated. Prior to the fascia-muscle advancement, the navel stalk is tagged with a suture. The imbricating effect of the repair is so powerful that the navel can be lost in the depths of the advanced muscle so the navel is easily retrieved with the suture. The rectus fascia and muscle is advanced from the lateral border of the split with several interrupted sutures (Figs. 24.8 and 24.9). I prefer 1-0 monofilament nylon. The long navel stalk allows us to adjust its final position by 1–2 cm in a vertical or horizontal direction (Fig. 24.9).

This is anchored to the fascia at the line of closure with 3-0 nylon. This is done 3 mm below the navel dermis (Figs. 24.10 and 24.11).

The recipient location on the caudally advanced abdominal skin is done using the Pitanguy umbilical demarcator (Fig. 24.12). The location is checked against the aesthetic pleasing distances described in the section of aesthetics of the navel. The navel position on the abdominal wall can be changed to more superior or inferior, more to the left or to the right because the stalk is large and the space created by the muscle imbrication gives a lot of room for this. After the marking using the umbilical demarcator is done, a triangular incision on the abdominal skin is done. The triangle is superiorly based and measures about 8 mm at the base and 12 mm of length. This incision after traction of the abdominal flap for closure will have a reciprocal heart-shaped space to receive a similarly shaped navel (Fig. 24.13). From this incision in an anterior to posterior direction (vertical in the surgical position), a core of fat is removed to accommodate the navel and recreate the periumbilical valley (Fig. 24.14).

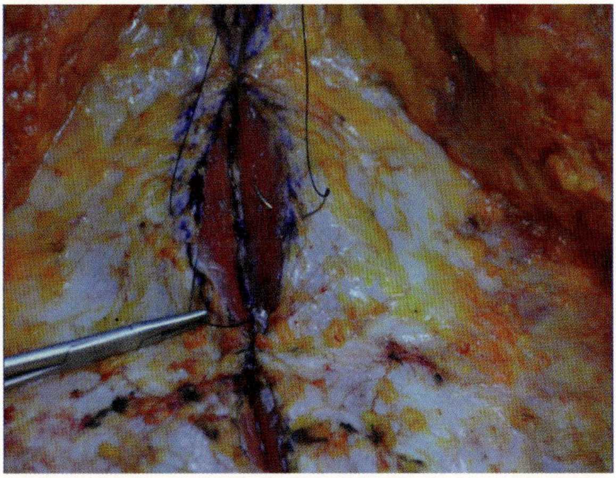

Fig. 24.8 Observe the easy approximation of the recti muscles. The medial border of the split fascia is down deep now

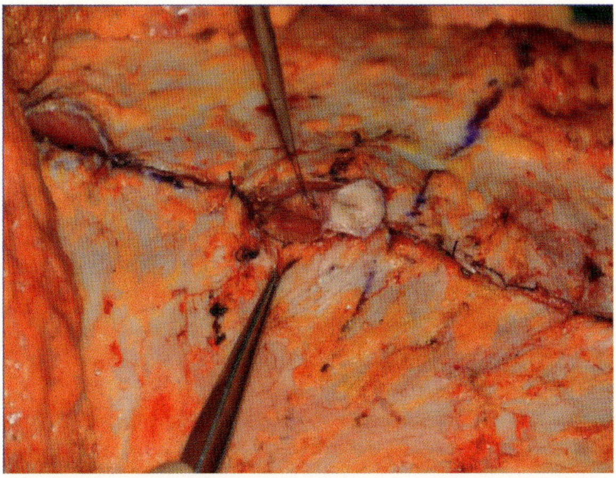

Fig. 24.9 The length of the umbilical stalk allows its repositioning in the vertical or horizontal dimension to fit the aesthetic distance guidelines

Prior to insetting of the navel, the next step is to create the xipho-umbilical depression that is an aesthetic landmark of a young and beautiful abdomen. As described in my abdominoplasty technique, this is done with a superficial liposuction toward the xiphoid starting from the recipient navel defect created.

An important addition to my umbilicoplasty technique is the recreation of the hooding. This is done by advancing the central supraumbilical portion of the abdominal flap with several quilting sutures from the xiphoid to near the umbilicus. I use 2-0 Nylon sutures for this. These sutures hold the deep dermis or the Scarpa's fascia to the muscle fascia at the midline repair. These will recruit several mm of

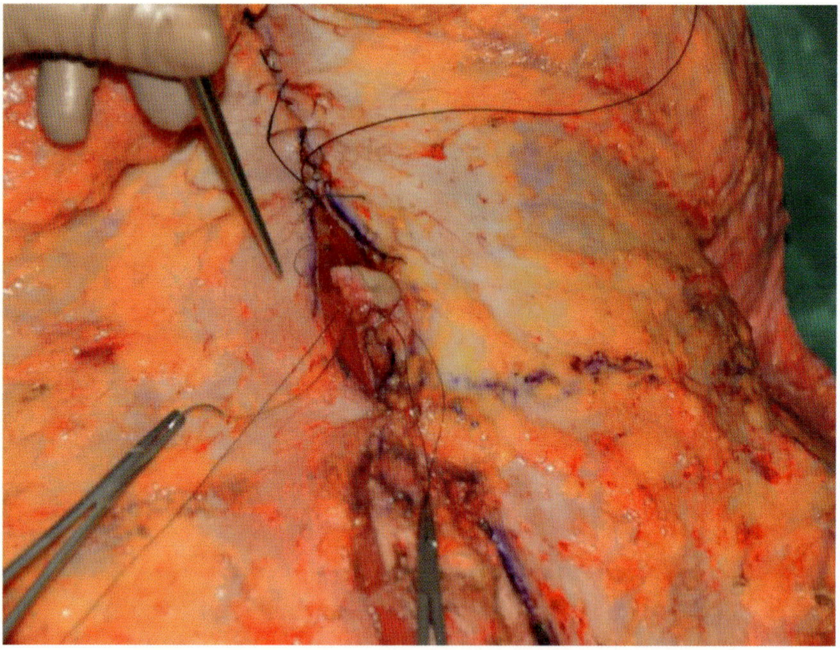

Fig. 24.10 The deep dermis of the navel is sutured to the borders of the fascia. The midline repair is almost completed, the navel stalk is down, and the navel is leveled to the fascia. The vertical position of the navel has been adjusted to the level of the iliac crests for better aesthetics

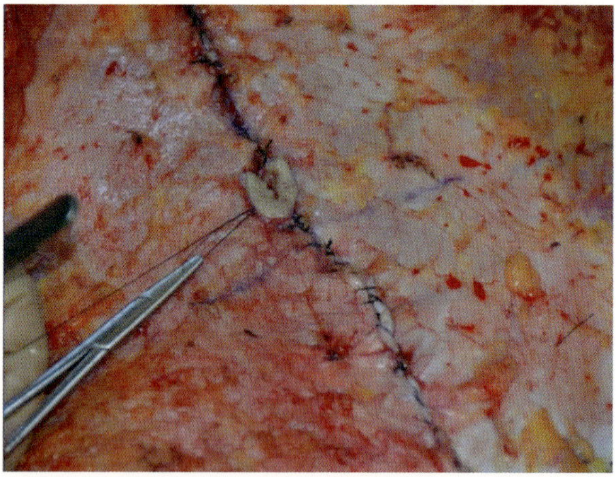

Fig. 24.11 The navel has been stabilized on the midline. It has the original heart shape. It is ready for the skin insetting

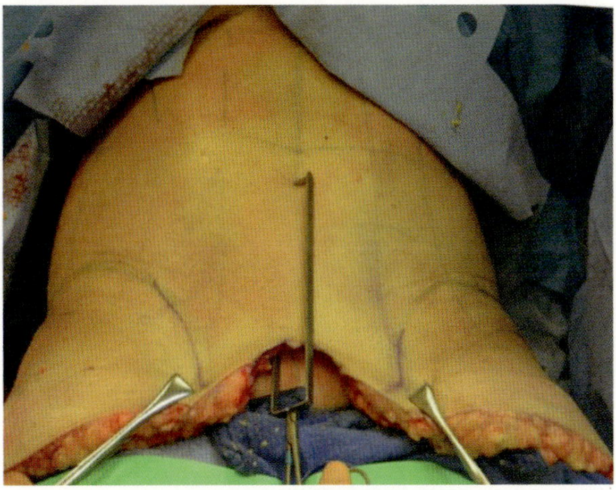

Fig. 24.12 The location of navel on the recipient skin is done with Pitanguy umbilical demarcator

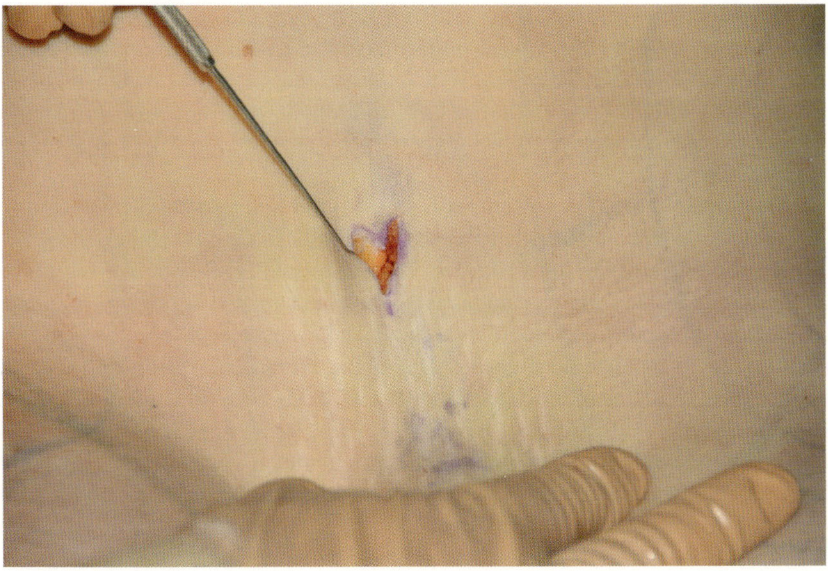

Fig. 24.13 The triangular incision at the recipient site

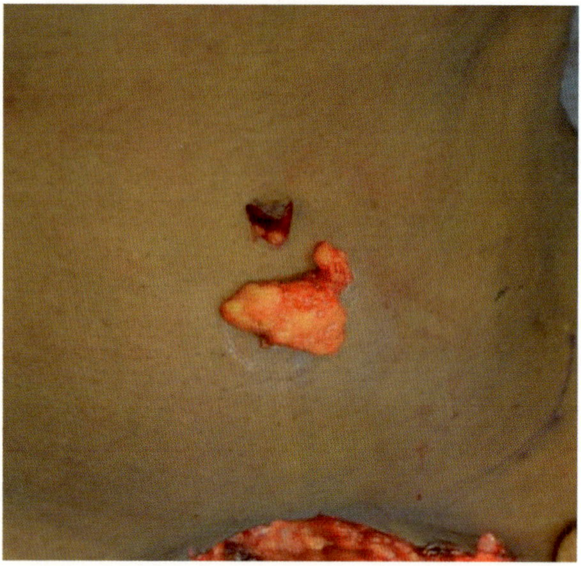

Fig. 24.14 The triangle now has a heart shape and the core of fat removed is shown

skin to recreate the hooding. This technique has several additional purposes: defines more the xipho-umbilical depression and decreases the tension on the lower abdominal flap. This will also prevent in the short and long term postoperative tension on the navel that otherwise will flatten the navel after a well-executed abdominoplasty.

The shortened navel has a 6 mm horizontal and 8 mm vertical diameters at the skin borders and its depth is usually 6 mm. This will usually fit well into the recipient site. Insetting is done in two layers. The subdermal layer is closed with interrupted inverted 3-0 or 4-0 nylon sutures and the skin with 4-0 or 5-0 Nylon sutures. Size of sutures depends on the thickness and how delicate the navel tissues are. Insetting starts from underneath the abdominal flap with anchoring the dermis of the tip of the triangular flap to the deepest portion of the dermis of the triangular defect of the navel (12 o'clock position) (Fig. 24.15). Next sutures are at the angles of the corresponding circular borders with the triangle (about 10 and 2 o'clock positions) (Fig. 24.16). The next suture is at the six o'clock position. The additional dermal sutures are placed at nine and three o'clock positions from the outside after the abdominal flap is turned over; the skin closure is done with interrupted nylon sutures (Fig. 24.17). The rest of the abdominoplasty closure is completed (Fig. 24.18). At the end you will notice a bit of redundancy and folding of the recipient triangular

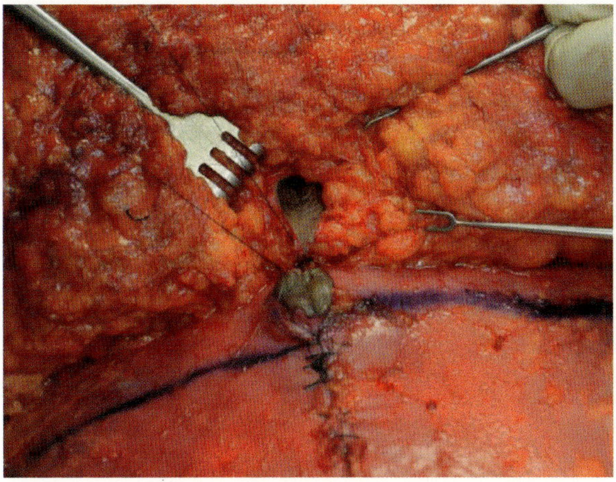

Fig. 24.15 The first insetting suture is done from underneath the abdominal flap at the tip of the reciprocal triangles

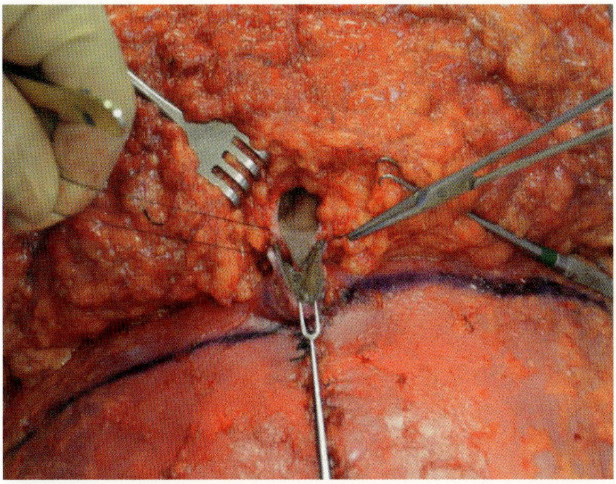

Fig. 24.16 The reciprocal angles are sutured next

flap. This is the hooding created with this technique. You will also notice the navel valley and "innie" as well as the xipho-umbilical depression (Fig. 24.19). These features are maintained over many years (Fig. 24.20). Figures 24.21 and 24.22 illustrate some aspects of the procedure.

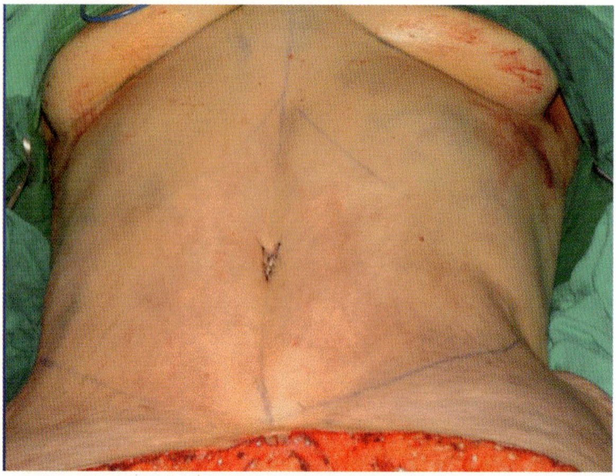

Fig. 24.17 The vertical heart-shaped reconstructed navel

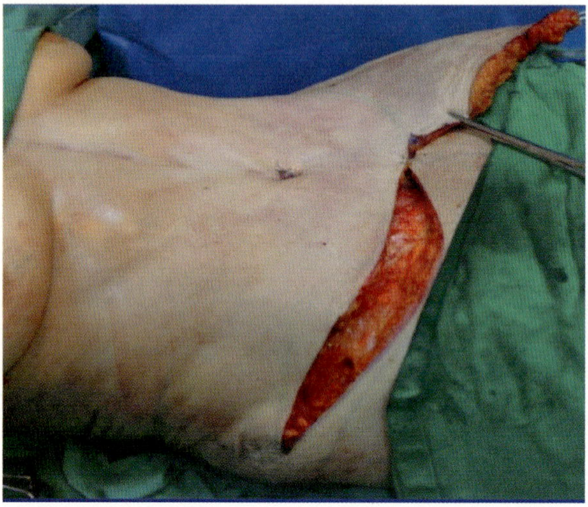

Fig. 24.18 After the navel is inset, the rest of the abdominoplasty is concluded. The panniculus was resected up to above the old navel level. Observe the new navel valley and the xipho-umbilical depression

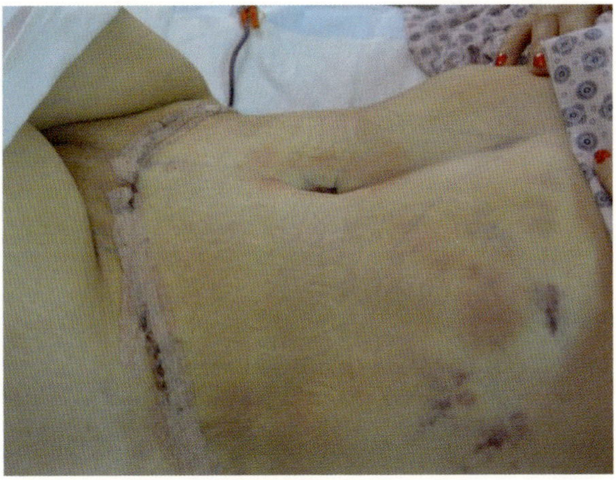

Fig. 24.19 Two days after surgery. Observe the navel position, navel valley, and xipho-umbilical depression

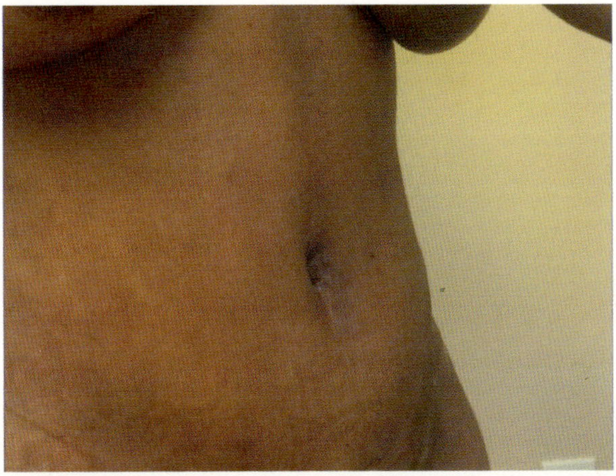

Fig. 24.20 Several years later the xipho-umbilical depression and navel "innie" are maintained. Also observe the navel hooding

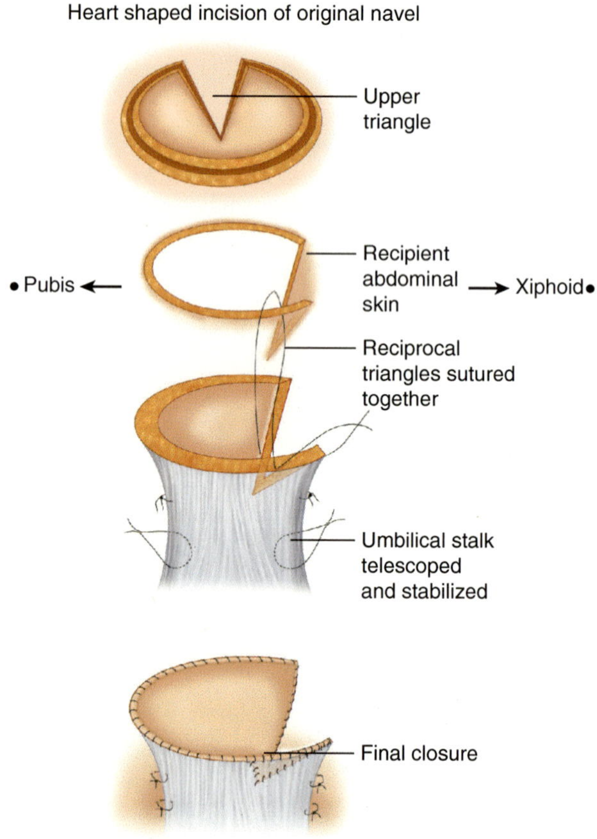

Fig. 24.21 Steps of the umbilical reconstruction

24.5 Postoperative Care

The navel is covered with a Xeroform dressing and circular conforming dry gauze sponges of 3–4 cm diameter around the navel. This helps to define better the navel concavity at and around the navel. Sutures are removed at around 7 days and the skin border protected with ¼ inch Steri-Strips applied radially. These are changed every 4–5 days and used for several weeks.

24.6 Clinical Experience

Since my original description of the umbilicoplasty was described within a larger paper dealing with a comprehensive abdominoplasty, many changes have been made [10, 11]. I do not use anymore the inferior triangle. My preference is

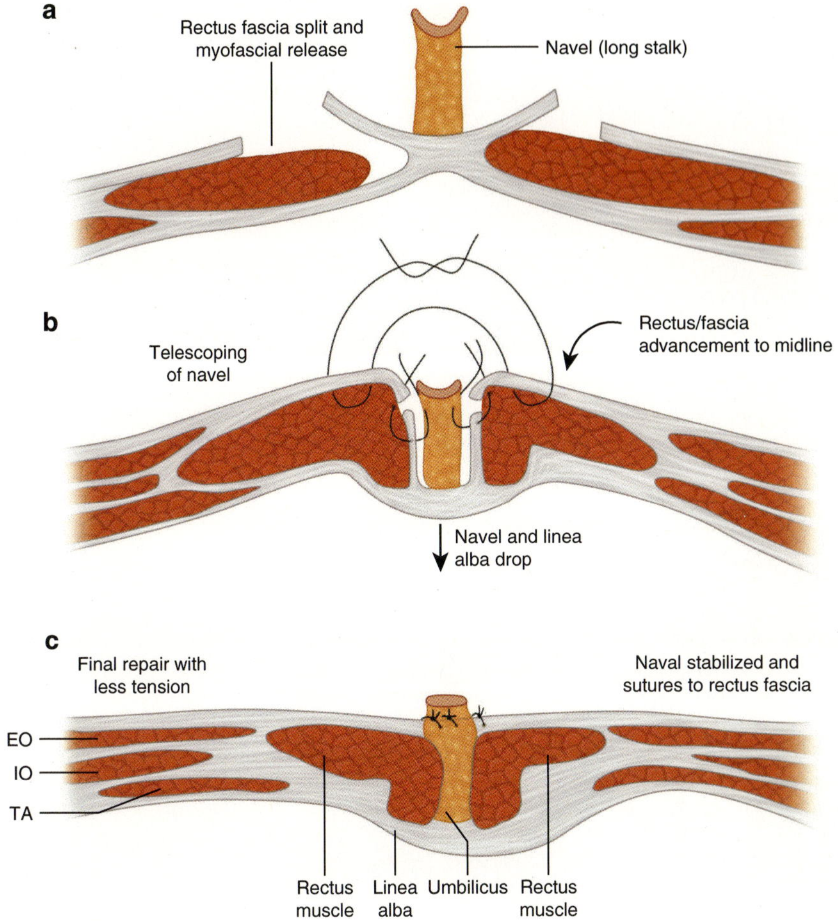

Fig. 24.22 Rectus fascia partitioning, burying of the umbilical stalk, new midline repair, and navel stabilization on the abdominal wall

for the superior triangle. The quilting sutures at the supraumbilical midline with simultaneous advancement of the flap emphasize the midline depression and recruits skin to create the hooding. The addition of this technique prevents tension and potential elongation and flattening of the navel. I still use the rectus partitioning and repair that decreases tension at the midline repair and creates a depth to accommodate the long umbilical stalk. I have applied some or all of these maneuvers to my umbilicoplasty with a high rate of success in several hundreds of abdominoplasty procedures since the early 1990s (Figs. 24.23, 24.24, 24.25, and 24.26).

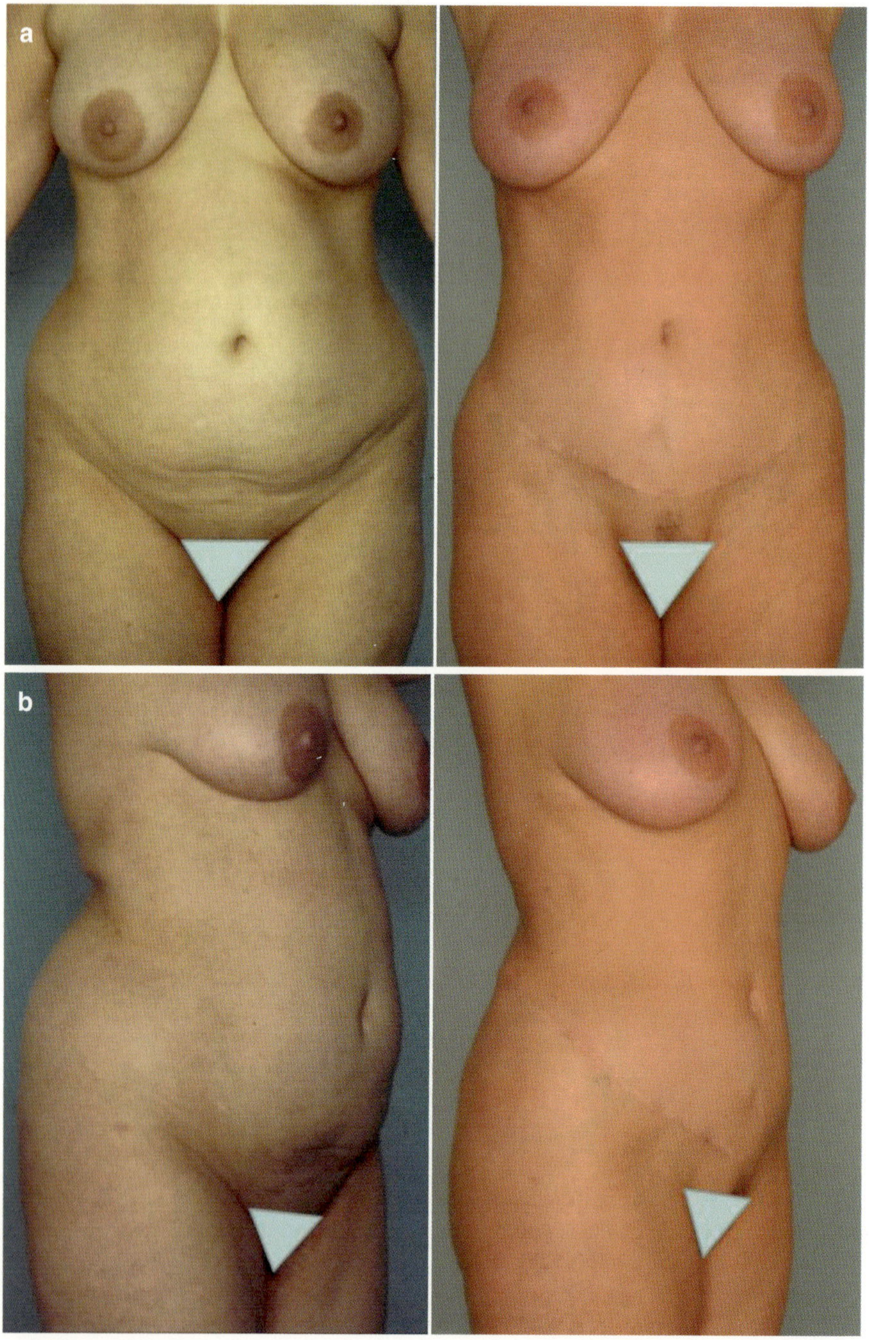

Fig. 24.23 (**a**) Preoperative. (**b**) Postoperative after using the described techniques minus recreation of the hooding with the upper flap advancement. Observe the vertical navel and the recreation of the "innie"

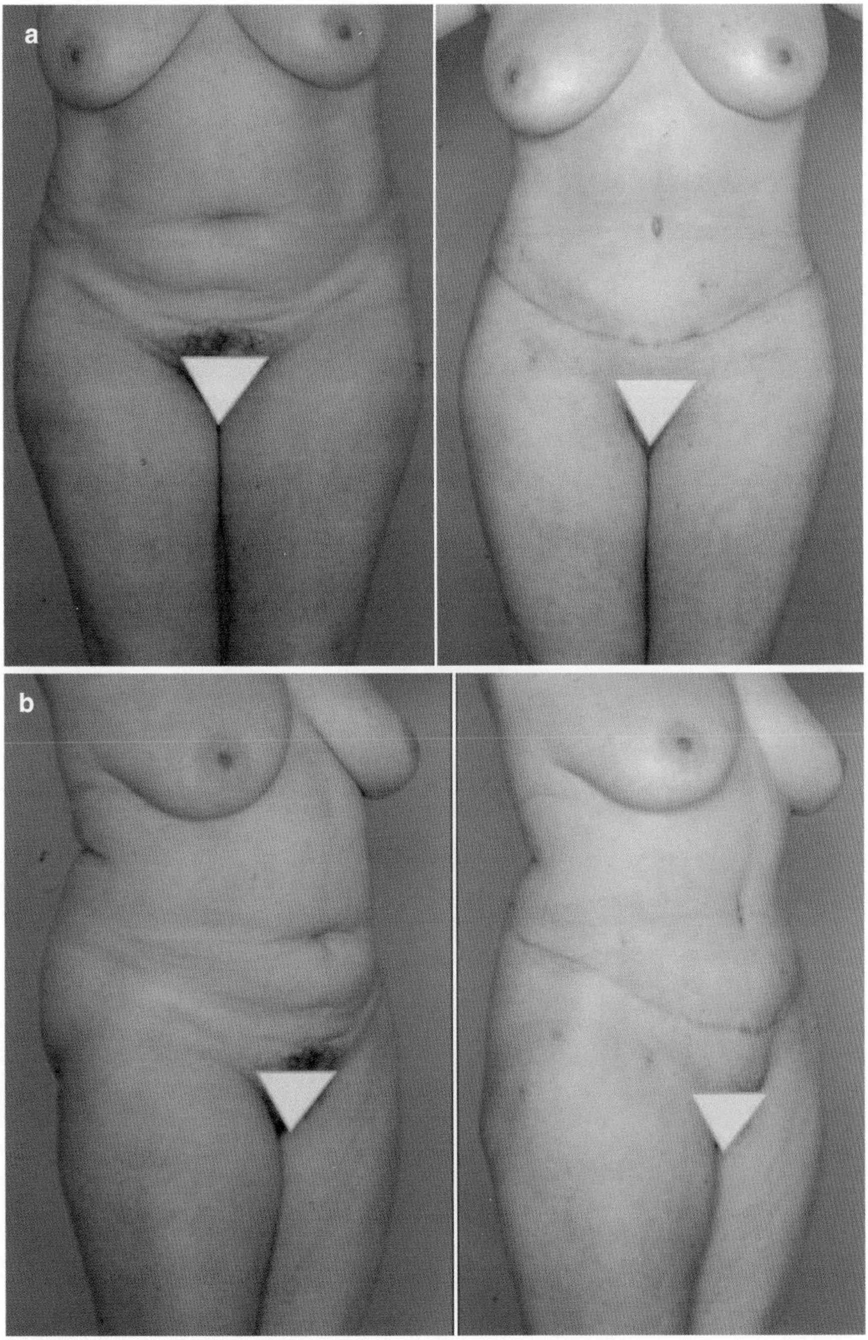

Fig. 24.24 (**a**, **b**) (*Left*) preoperative. (**b**) Postoperative after using the described techniques minus recreation of the hooding with the upper flap advancement. Observe the vertical navel and the recreation of the "innie"

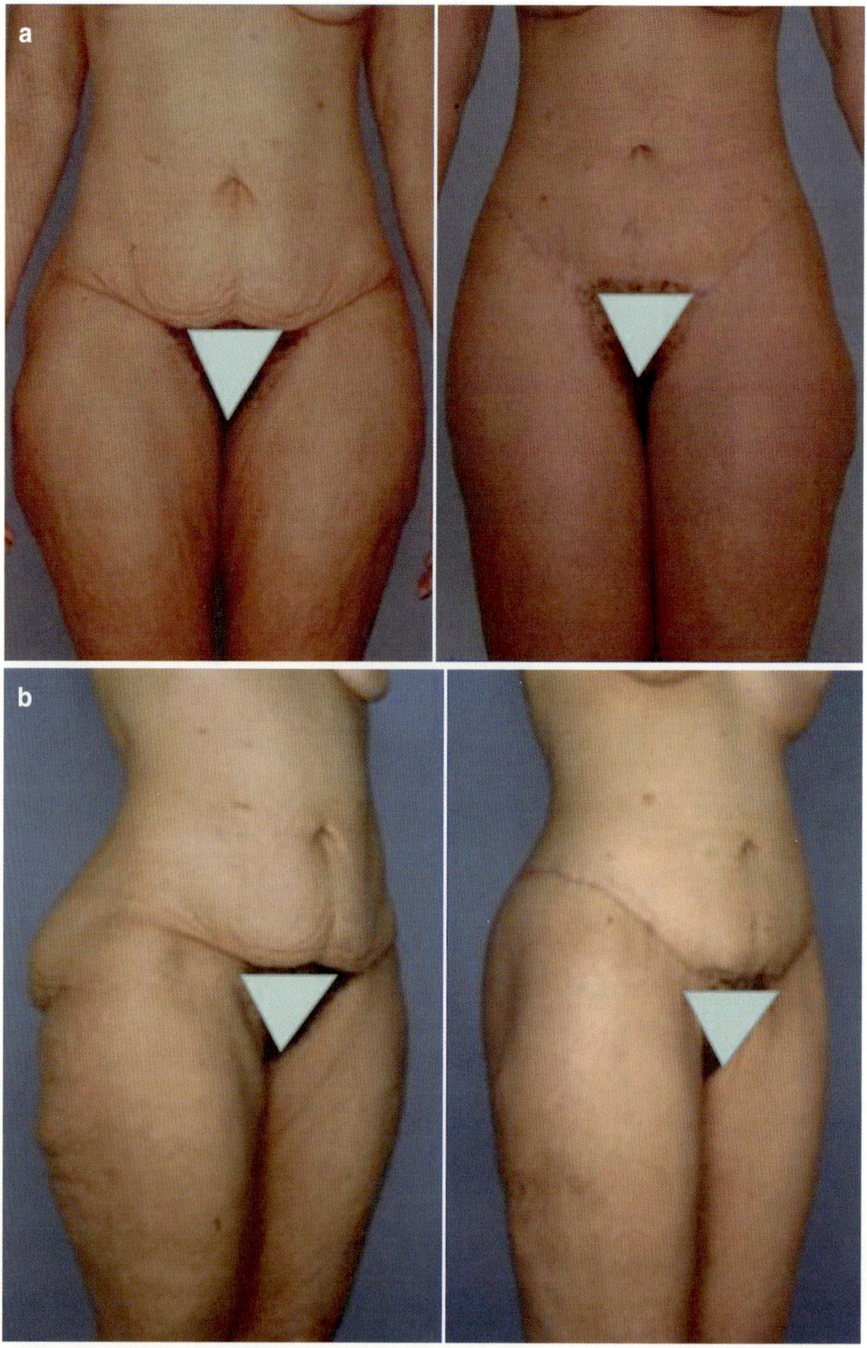

Fig. 24.25 (**a**, **b**) (*Left*) preoperative. (**b**) Postoperative where patient had in addition recreation of hooding

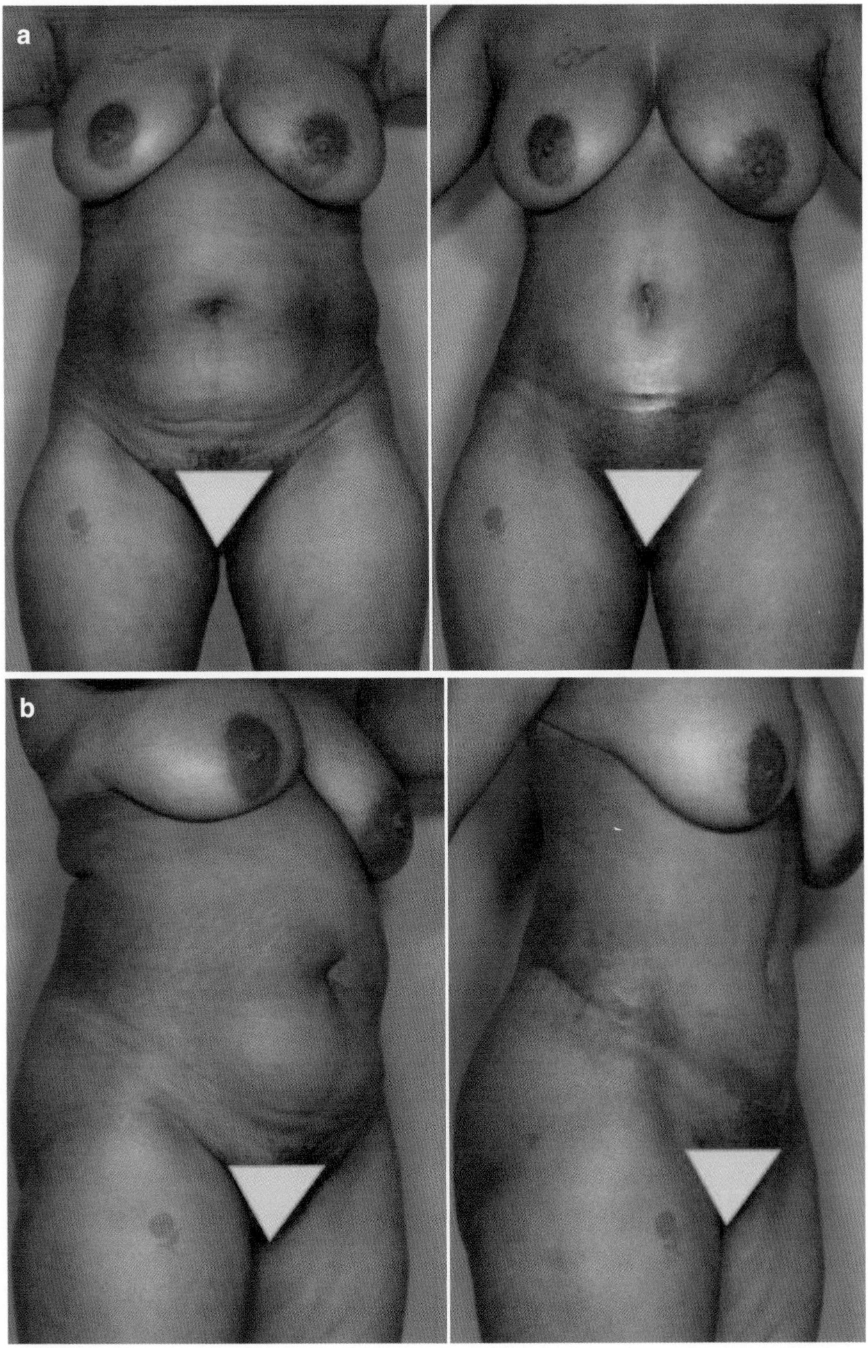

Fig. 24.26 (**a**, **b**) (*Left*) preoperative. (**b**) Postoperative where patient had in addition recreation of hooding. Observe the xypho-umbilical depression, vertically shaped navel and the periumbilical valley

24.7 Conclusions

Navel reconstruction after an abdominoplasty is not as simple as may be perceived. It does not simply entail to make a hole on the recipient skin to fit a similar circularly amputated navel. It requires a more careful assessment of the preoperative condition to determine horizontal midline and vertical position and where it will be the final placement on the abdomen. The rest of the planned abdominoplasty has direct impact on the navel aesthetics. The umbilicoplasty is integrated in the abdominoplasty technique taking into consideration the length of the umbilical stalk, thickness of the abdominal pannus, and laxity of the abdominal wall, and careful navel recreation to fit the aesthetic guidelines described at the beginning of this chapter is paramount. If the patient qualifies for a "floating" abdominoplasty or has a large umbilical hernia, the surgical and aesthetic strategy will be completely different. For the umbilical transposition in an overweight or obese patient or for those with abdominal deformities post childbearing, the technique described here provides a comprehensive approach to an aesthetically pleasing umbilicoplasty.

References

1. James L. Modesty in dress. London: Heinemann; 1969.
2. Rohrich RJ, Sorokin ES, Brown SA, Gibby DL. Is the umbilicus truly midline? Clinical and medicolegal implications. Plast Reconstr Surg. 2003;112(1):259–63.
3. Vernon S. Umbilical transplantation upward and abdominal contouring in lipectomy. Am J Surg. 1957;94(3):490–2.
4. Baroudi R. Umbilicoplasty. Clin Plast Surg. 1975;2:431.
5. Pitanguy I. Abdominal lipectomy. Clin Plast Surg. 1975;2(3):401–10.
6. Hinderer UT. The dermolipectomy approach for augmentation mammaplasty. Clin Plast Surg. 1975;2(3):359–69.
7. Dubou R, Ousterhout DK. Placement of the umbilicus in an abdominoplasty. Plast Reconstr Surg. 1978;61(2):291–3.
8. Abhyankar SV, Rajguru AG, Patel PA. Anatomical localization of the umbilicus: an Indian study. Plast Reconstr Surg. 2006;117(4):1153–7.
9. Visconti G, Visconti E, Bonomo L, Salparello M. Concepts in navel aesthetics: a comprehensive surface anatomy analysis. Aesthetic Plast Surg. 2015;39:43–50.
10. Ramirez OM. Abdominoplasty and abdominal wall rehabilitation: a comprehensive approach. Plast Reconstr Surg. 2000;105:425–35.
11. Ramirez OM. The U-M Dermolipectomy and Myofascial Release in Abdominoplasty. Oper Tech Plast Reconstr Surg. 2002;8(1):40–52.

Chapter 25
The Inverted-V Chevron Umbilicoplasty for Abdominoplasty

Malcolm A. Lesavoy and Erwin A. Kruger

25.1 Introduction

The umbilicus is a unique, conspicuous scar of the central abdomen whose anatomic position makes it aesthetically essential. Any deformities or absence is immediately recognizable. The aesthetically pleasing umbilicus in thin females tends to be small, shallow, and vertically oriented, with superior hooding and shadow, inferior retraction and slope, and positioning at the level of the anterior superior iliac crest (Fig. 25.1) [1–3]. An umbilicus is typically no wider than 1.5–2 cm, nor longer than 3 cm, and its size is proportionally decreased in smaller and thinner patients [3, 4]. The umbilicus will deepen and widen with age and weight gain, and it is a consequence to note when evaluating a patient prior to procedures involving umbilicoplasty [5].

Repositioning of the umbilicus in the setting of abdominoplasty or abdominal wall donor-site closure in autologous breast reconstruction, e.g., deep inferior epigastric perforator (DIEP) and transverse rectus abdominis myocutaneous (TRAM) flaps, should be treated with appropriate focus on aesthetic results. Many techniques have been described for achieving aesthetic repositioning through horizontal incisions [6], vertical incisions [1, 7], Scarpa's fascia [8], deep suture lines [9–11], single flaps [5, 12, 13], multiple flaps [14–16], deepithelialized flaps [4, 17], dermabrasion [18], and neo-umbilical creation [19–22]. In designing an approach to

M.A. Lesavoy, M.D. (✉)
Department of Surgery, Division of Plastic & Reconstructive Surgery, David Geffen School of Medicine at UCLA, Los Angeles, CA 90095, USA
e-mail: drlesavoy@aol.com

E.A. Kruger, M.D.
Division of Plastic Surgery, David Geffen School of Medicine at UCLA, Los Angeles, CA, USA
e-mail: EKruger@mednet.ucla.ed

M.A. Shiffman (ed.), *Adult Umbilical Reconstruction*,
DOI 10.1007/978-3-319-43887-0_25

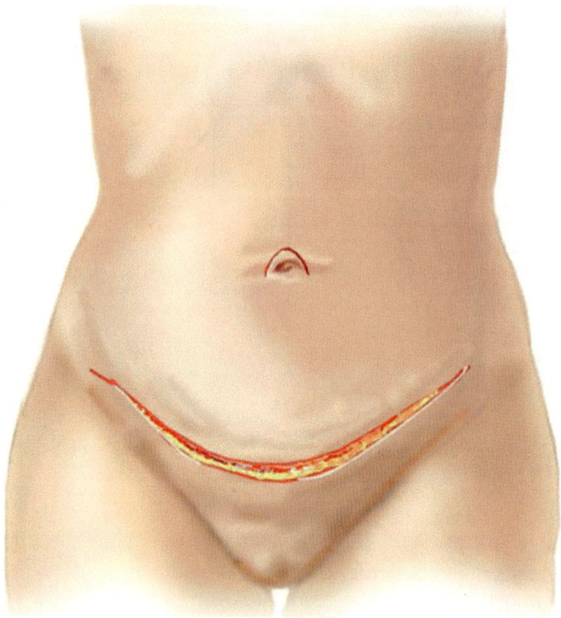

Fig. 25.1 The ideal umbilicus should rest in line with the uppermost edge of the iliac crests

umbilicoplasty, malposition, scarring, cicatricial ring formation, and poor shape or form should be avoided to maximize outcomes and patient satisfaction.

We have previously described the inverted-V chevron umbilicoplasty [23], which addresses the aesthetic concerns of umbilicoplasty and is the preferred method of the senior author (M.A.L.). Nuances of the procedure are described, and outcomes are based on the senior author's clinical experience of more than 35 years with this technique. This is an excellent method at restoring a consistent, youthful umbilicus in the clinical setting of abdominoplasty or autologous DIEP/TRAM breast reconstruction.

25.2 Surgical Technique and Outcomes

The inverted-V chevron umbilicoplasty is performed in conjunction with an abdominoplasty or autologous DIEP/TRAM breast reconstruction, under general anesthesia, with the patient in the supine position. After the abdominal flaps are dissected cephalad, the operating table is flexed so that proper assessment of skin resection can be performed. After the excess skin is resected, partial closure of the abdominoplasty incision is performed, and proper marking of the umbilicoplasty can proceed using the iliac crests as landmarks. The inverted-V chevron is marked with limbs of 1.5–2 cm, separated by 3 cm at the base (Fig. 25.2).

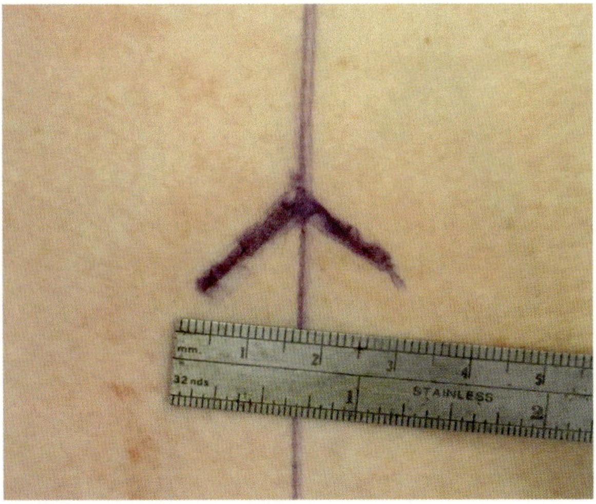

Fig. 25.2 The limbs of the V-shaped incision are at least 1.5–2 cm on each side separated by a 3 cm base. This can be adjusted to patient's body habitus

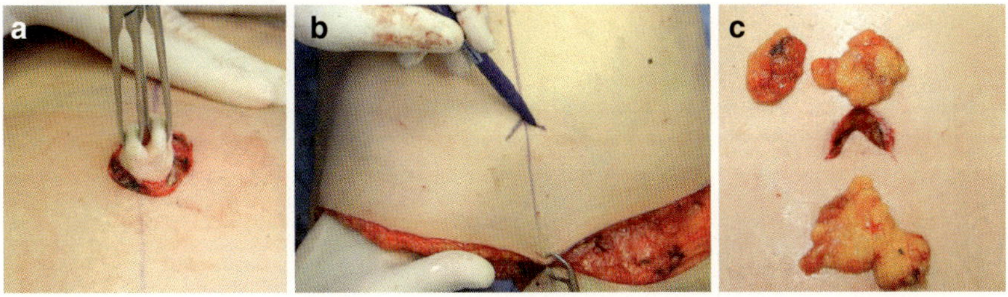

Fig. 25.3 (**a**) The original umbilicus is sharply circumscribed and separated from the native abdominal flap. (**b**) The transposition of the umbilicus is performed by palpating the native umbilicus under the abdominal flap, usually at the midline at the highest level of the iliac crest. (**c**) The chevron incision is made and core of abdominal fat removed for inset of neo-umbilicus. Avoid aggressive defatting that can lead to skin necrosis

The umbilicus is sharply circumscribed and separated from the abdominal flap (Fig. 25.3). Following the abdominoplasty or DIEP/TRAM harvest, the point of the new umbilical center is marked on the abdominal wall by placing the surgeon's hand beneath the abdominal flap to determine where the native umbilicus is to be positioned, using the iliac crests as landmarks. The limbs and base of the inverted-V are designed and limb incisions made. An inverted-V chevron-shaped skin flap is raised, and a core of abdominal fat is removed beneath the chevron abdominal flap to allow inset. The native umbilicus is exteriorized and incised vertically from its central bud to the 6 o'clock position, into which the inverted-V chevron-shaped skin flap is sutured (Fig. 25.4). Closure is performed in two circumferential layers (Fig. 25.5). The first layer captures the following: (1) the edge

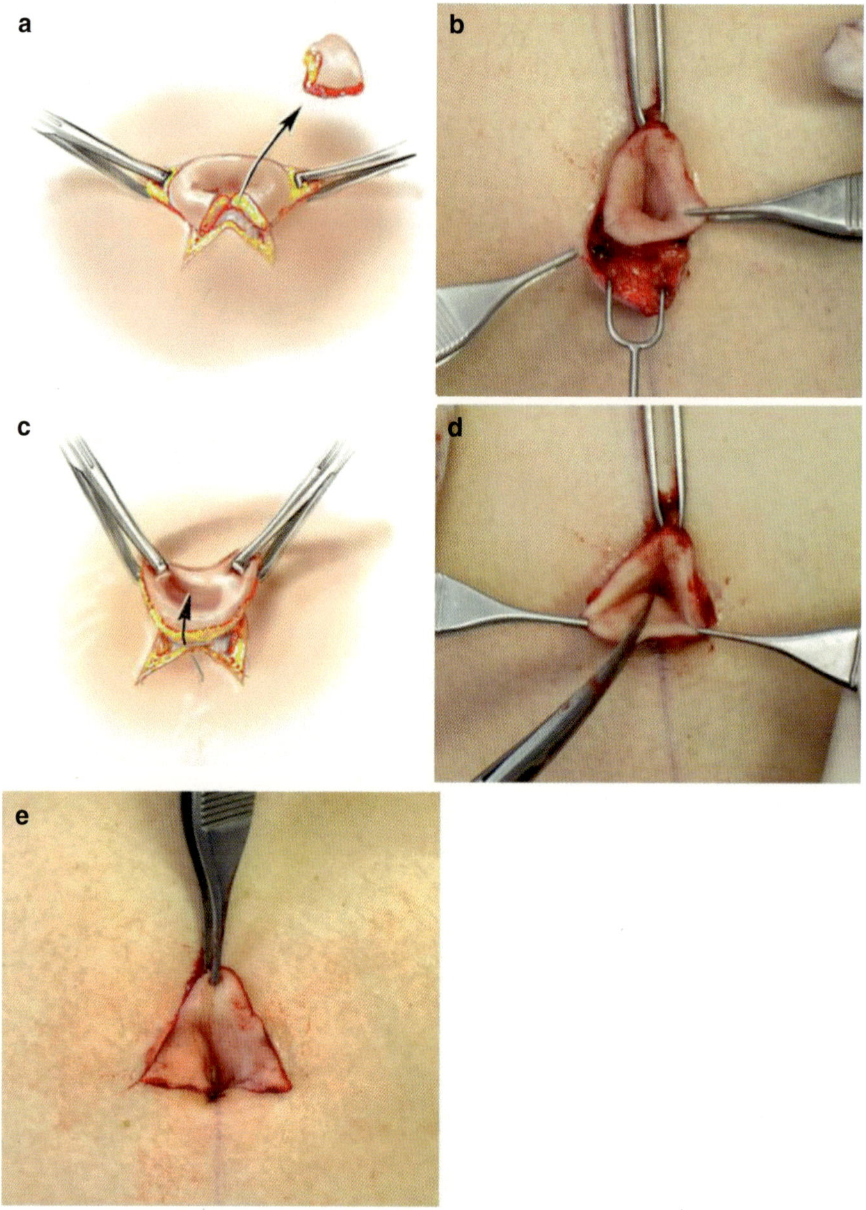

Fig. 25.4 (a–d) Exteriorization of the umbilicus is performed and incised at the 6 o'clock position and chevron-shaped skin flap inset. (e) Final inset recreates the natural retrusion and cranial fold of an aesthetic umbilicus

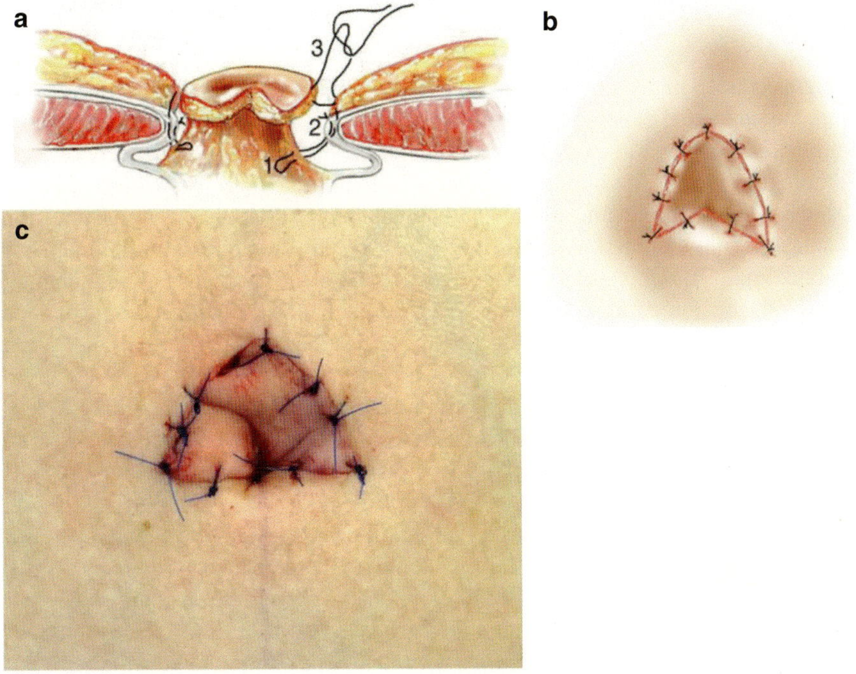

Fig. 25.5 Closure is achieved in two layers. (**a**) Absorbable sutures capture (*1*) the edge of the abdominal flap, (*2*) Scarpa's fascia, and (*3*) the umbilical stalk to recreate natural dimpling around the umbilicus. (**b**, **c**) The skin inset is closed with interrupted permanent sutures

of the abdominal flap skin, (2) Scarpa's fascia, and (3) the umbilical stalk. Tying these sutures down effectively restores the dimpling of the abdominal skin around the umbilicus. The superior tip of the inverted-V chevron skin flap is then inset into the central bud of the native umbilicus, and the skin flap and incisions are closed with interrupted permanent sutures. The umbilicus is dressed with petroleum gauze or Xeroform (Covidien, Mansfield, Massachusetts). After the inferiorly based chevron inverted-V flap is cut, the remaining portion of the abdominoplasty incision is closed.

With this technique, the surgeon can minimize cases of "misplaced umbilicus" or poor blood supply and necrosis of the umbilicus—complications which have not been seen in the senior author's clinical practice. Care should be taken if a patient's umbilicus has an unusually long stalk or pedicle (e.g., massive weight loss patients), since it is possible that the stalk could be telescoped, constricted, and vascularity compromised. In 35 years of clinical experience, approximately 3–5 % of inverted-V chevron umbilicoplasty patients have shown mildly hypertrophied postoperative scarring, which can be addressed with steroid injections or scar revisions [23].

25.3 Discussion

There have been many surgical techniques reported for umbilicoplasty; however all share the same goal of achieving a natural, aesthetic umbilicus. Historically, the first umbilical transposition performed during an abdominoplasty was reported by Vernon in 1957 [24], involving a circular excision of the umbilicus with reinsertion through a circular incision on the abdominal flap. Although the round incision remains the most common inset shape [13, 18], the literature on umbilicoplasty includes many modifications and designs, such as the superior-based triangular flaps [12], the three cutaneous flaps [25], vertical incision with tethering of the umbilical stalk [7], purse string [18, 26], dermal flaps [4], V-Y flaps [27], and U-shaped incisions [5]. Some reports, such as Ohana et al. [28], have even advocated complete excision of the umbilicus and creation of a neo-umbilicus.

The inverted-V chevron umbilicoplasty technique has several advantages from other techniques in the literature. First, the discontinuous incision design prevents circumferential scar contraction. Secondly, the inverted-V chevron inset achieves an arrowhead-shaped design of the original umbilicus that encourages natural retrusion, inferior slope, and a cranial fold. The inverted V-shaped chevron incision creates the appearance of small umbilicus with an appropriate opening that other incisions fail to recreate. Also, to avoid tethering sensation seen when the umbilicus is sutured to the abdominal fascia, we suture to Scarpa's fascia to allow mobility of the umbilical stalk while still achieving a natural contour [4, 8]. Removal of fat from the surrounding abdominal area creates depth by accommodating the horizontal dimension of the umbilicus, hiding the scar toward the base [5, 14].

Several technical issues should be avoided during navel transposition. First, malposition is avoided by placement of the umbilicus at the highest level of the iliac crest, which is the position seen in 96 % of nonobese individuals [3]. Interestingly, even though Rohrich et al. [29] identified only 1.7 % of the umbilicus is actually in the midline, we recommend midline placement. Next, a common result of umbilical reconstruction through a round, uninterrupted incision is a tight, cicatricial ring and hypertrophic scar, which cause flattening and umbilical stenosis [4, 19, 30]. Such established stenosis may be corrected secondarily [31]. As a precaution, we suggest conservative removal of abdominal fat from the V-shaped skin flap, since overzealous thinning can result in skin necrosis [8].

25.4 Conclusions

Aesthetic reconstruction of the umbilicus during abdominoplasty or autologous breast reconstruction is essential. It is often the only visible cue that an abdominoplasty has been performed. The inverted-V umbilicoplasty restores a natural, youthful umbilicus with minimal scarring (Fig. 25.6). A superior hood, natural retrusion, and inferior retraction and slope are achieved, while avoiding umbilical stenosis

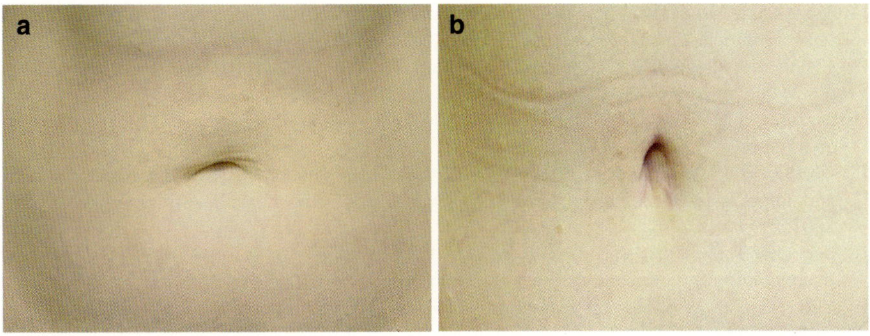

Fig. 25.6 (**a**) Preoperative 39-year-old female with excess abdominal laxity and subcutaneous fat with transverse opening of the umbilicus (**b**) Following abdominoplasty, the inverted-V chevron umbilicoplasty restores superior hooding and shadow, natural retrusion with inferior retraction and slope

with discontinuous incision. It is the authors' umbilicoplasty technique of choice during both for abdominoplasty and closure following TRAM/DIEP flap harvest.

References

1. Akbas H, Guneren E, Eroglu L, Uysal OA. Natural-looking umbilicus as an important part of abdominoplasty. Aesthetic Plast Surg. 2003;27:139–42.
2. Craig SB, Faller MS, Puckett CL. In search of the ideal female umbilicus. Plast Reconstr Surg. 2000;105:389–92.
3. Dubou R, Ousterhout DK. Placement of the umbilicus in an abdominoplasty. Plast Reconstr Surg. 1978;61:291–3.
4. Rozen SM, Redett R. The two-dermal-flap umbilical transposition: a natural and aesthetic umbilicus after abdominoplasty. Plast Reconstr Surg. 2007;119:2255–62.
5. Malic CC, Spyrou GE, Hough M, Fourie L. Patient satisfaction with two different methods of umbilicoplasty. Plast Reconstr Surg. 2007;119:357–61.
6. Baroudi R. Umbilicoplasty. Clin Plast Surg. 1975;2:431–48.
7. Lee MJ, Mustoe TA. Simplified technique for creating a youthful umbilicus in abdominoplasty. Plast Reconstr Surg. 2002;109:2136–40.
8. Niranjan NS, Staiano JJ. An anatomical method for re-siting the umbilicus. Plast Reconstr Surg. 2004;113:2194–8.
9. Choudhary S, Taams KO. Umbilicosculpture: a concept revisited. Br J Plast Surg. 1998;51:538–41.
10. Nahas FX. How to deal with the umbilical stalk during abdominoplasty. Plast Reconstr Surg. 2000;106:1220–1.
11. Bruekers SE, van der Lei B, Tan TL, Luijendijk RW, Stevens HP. "Scarless" umbilicoplasty: a new umbilicoplasty technique and a review of the English language literature. Ann Plast Surg. 2009;63:15–20.
12. Juri J, Juri C, Raiden G. Reconstruction of the umbilicus in abdominoplasty. Plast Reconstr Surg. 1979;63:580–2.
13. Delerm A. Refinements in abdominoplasty with emphasis on reimplantation of the umbilicus. Plast Reconstr Surg. 1982;70:632–7.

14. Massiha H, Montegut W, Phillips R. A method of reconstructing a natural-looking umbilicus in abdominoplasty. Ann Plast Surg. 1997;38:228–31.
15. Cannistra C, Pecorelli E. Umbilical restoration in abdominal dermolipectomy: a simple double-Y, double-M technique. Aesthetic Plast Surg. 1999;23:364–6.
16. Mazzocchi M, Dessy LA, Figus A. A versatile technique for repositioning of the umbilicus in abdominoplasty. Plast Reconstr Surg. 2008;121:357e–8.
17. Castillo PF, Sepulveda CA, Prado AC, Troncoso AL, Villaman JJ. Umbilical reinsertion in abdominoplasty: technique using deepithelialized skin flaps. Aesthetic Plast Surg. 2007;31:519–20.
18. Schoeller T, Wechselberger G, Otto A, et al. New technique for scarless umbilical reinsertion in abdominoplasty procedures. Plast Reconstr Surg. 1998;102:1720–3.
19. Lim TC, Tan WT. Managing the umbilicus during abdominoplasty. Plast Reconstr Surg. 1996;98:1113.
20. Santanelli F, Mazzocchi M, Renzi L, Cigna E. Reconstruction of a natural-looking umbilicus. Scand J Plast Reconstr Surg Hand Surg. 2002;36:183–5.
21. Ehrlich RM, Lesavoy MA, Fine RN. Total abdominal wall reconstruction in the prune belly syndrome. J Urol. 1986;136(Pt 2):282–5.
22. Ehrlich RM, Lesavoy MA. Umbilicus preservation with total abdominal wall reconstruction in prune-belly syndrome. Urology. 1993;41:231–2.
23. Lesavoy MA, Fan K, Guenther DA, Herrera F, Little JW. The inverted-v chevron umbilicoplasty for breast reconstruction and abdominoplasty. Aesthet Surg J. 2012;32(1):110–6.
24. Vernon S. Umbilical transplantation upward and abdominal contouring in lipectomy. Am J Surg. 1957;94:490–2.
25. Avelar J. Abdominoplasty systematization of a technique without external umbilical scar. Aesthetic Plast Surg. 1978;2:141–51.
26. Bartsich SA, Schwartz MH. Purse-string method for immediate umbilical reconstruction. Plast Reconstr Surg. 2003;112:1652–5.
27. Jamra FA. Reconstruction of the umbilicus by a double V—Y procedure. Plast Reconstr Surg. 1979;64:106–7.
28. Ohana J, Illouz YG, Elbaz JS, Flageul G. New approach to abdominal plasties. Technical classification and surgical indications. Progress allowed by liposuction, neoumbilicoplasty and use of biological glue. Ann Chir Plast Esthet. 1987;32:344–53.
29. Rohrich RJ, Sorokin ES, Brown SA, Gibby DL. Is the umbilicus truly midline? Clinical and medicolegal implications. Plast Reconstr Surg. 2003;112:259–63.
30. Pfulg M, Van de Sijpe K, Blondeel P. A simple new technique for neo-umbilicoplasty. Br J Plast Surg. 2005;58:688–91.
31. Baack BR, Anson G, Nachbar JM, White DJ. Umbilicoplasty: the construction of a new umbilicus and correction of umbilical stenosis without external scars. Plast Reconstr Surg. 1996;97:227–32.

Chapter 26
Rabbit-Head-Shaped Scar Flap Umbilicoplasty for a Secondary Umbilical Defect After Abdominoplasty

Koichi Watanabe and Kensuke Kiyokawa

26.1 Introduction

Herein is described a procedure that was reported in 2009 as an umbilical reconstruction method for secondary umbilical defects after abdominoplasty [1]. There are some differences between umbilicoplasty after omphalocele repair and that for addressing umbilical protrusion, or hernia. One difference is the existence of an abdominal midline scar after abdominoplasty, which makes it difficult to design the umbilicoplasty. Another is the presence of high skin tension caused by the abdominal plication. Finally, there is little subcutaneous fat tissue, which could also be due to abdominal plication, among other causes. These factors cause the reconstructed umbilicus to flatten. Thus, reconstruction with a natural look of sufficient depth has been difficult using conventional methods [2–10]. A completely original method was developed to avoid these unfavorable results. The unique features of our procedure are as follows:

1. Each wall of the umbilical depression is reconstructed by folding a single skin flap.
2. Using two "dog ears" in the flap folding process makes the cranial depression deeper.

K. Watanabe, M.D., Ph.D. (✉)
Section of Gross Anatomy and Clinical Anatomy, Department of Anatomy, Kurume University School of Medicine, 67 Asahi-machi, Kurume-shi, Fukuoka-ken 830-0011, Japan
e-mail: koichiwatanabeprs@gmail.com

K. Kiyokawa, M.D., Ph.D.
Department of Plastic and Reconstructive Surgery, and Maxillofacial Surgery, Kurume University School of Medicine, Kurume-shi, Fukuoka-ken, Japan
e-mail: prsmf@med.kurume-u.ac.jp

M.A. Shiffman (ed.), *Adult Umbilical Reconstruction*,
DOI 10.1007/978-3-319-43887-0_26

3. Moving the subcutaneous pedicle caudally heightens the lateral walls of the umbilicus, which makes the umbilical depression relatively deeper and maintains the depth.
4. The procedure does not create any new scars on other parts of the body.
5. The flap is created using the midline scar on the abdomen because it reproduces the quality of the normal umbilical skin, which is also composed of scar tissue due to retraction of the umbilical cord.

The concept of increasing the subcutaneous volume by moving the subcutaneous pedicle has never been reported, making this procedure unique. The procedure is an ideal umbilical reconstruction method for use in infants, who usually have very little subcutaneous fat.

26.2 Technique

The first step in our procedure is to design a reverse V-shaped incision line using the midline abdominal scar as the base of the V shape (which corresponds to the position of the planned umbilicus) (Fig. 26.1). The design thus revises the abdominal scar. A rabbit-head-shaped skin flap is then designed in a reverse V shape. The part of the flap that corresponds with the rabbit-head's ears (E) is used to create the two lateral walls of the umbilicus, the forehead (H) is used to create the superior wall, the face (F) is used to create the bottom, and the neck is used to create the inferior wall. A spindle is incorporated into the design to enable resection and plication of the remaining scar on the cranial side of the flap (Fig. 26.2).

The next step is to elevate the flap. Subcutaneous pedicles are created that will be used to attach the parts of the flap from the bilateral rabbit ears to the forehead on each side of the flap. They run diagonally outward from the cranial to the caudal side. Some perforating arteries from the bilateral inferior epigastric arteries are located around the umbilicus, especially below it. The abdominal perforator arteries usually supply blood to the subcutaneous pedicles. The rabbit-head-shaped flap also includes the abdominal scar tissue, whose blood supply is generally unreliable. The pedicle thus stabilizes the blood circulation of the narrow ear parts and the entire upper half of the flap.

The created flap is now moved caudally and is used to reconstruct the umbilical depression. The part of the flap that corresponds to the rabbit's neck is turned under so it can be tucked under the skin on the caudal side of the reconstructed umbilicus, thereby creating the inferior wall of the umbilical depression. The upper wall is created using the part of the flap that corresponds to the rabbit's forehead. The ear parts are folded back caudally on both sides to create the two sides of the umbilical depression. Then the flap's subcutaneous pedicles are moved caudally, thereby loosening the pedicles to create subcutaneous tissue with sufficient height around the

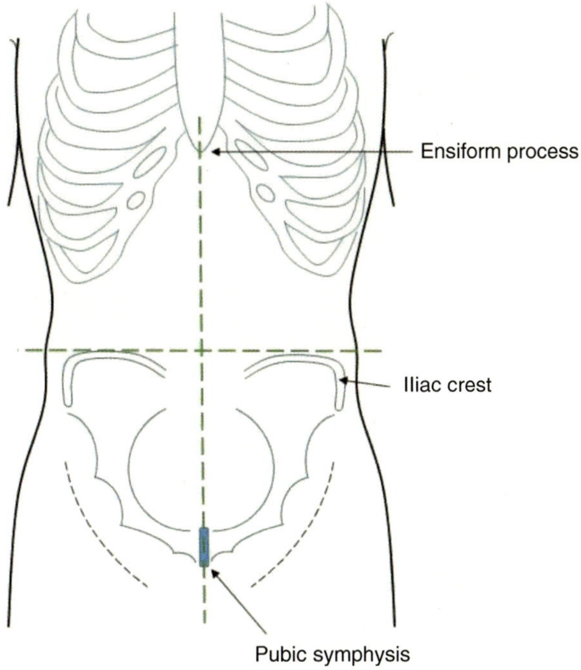

Fig. 26.1 Location for umbilical reconstruction. The appropriate site for umbilical reconstruction is where the midline between the ensiform process and the center of the pubic symphysis transects the line drawn from the highest level of the crest of one ilium to the same point on the other side

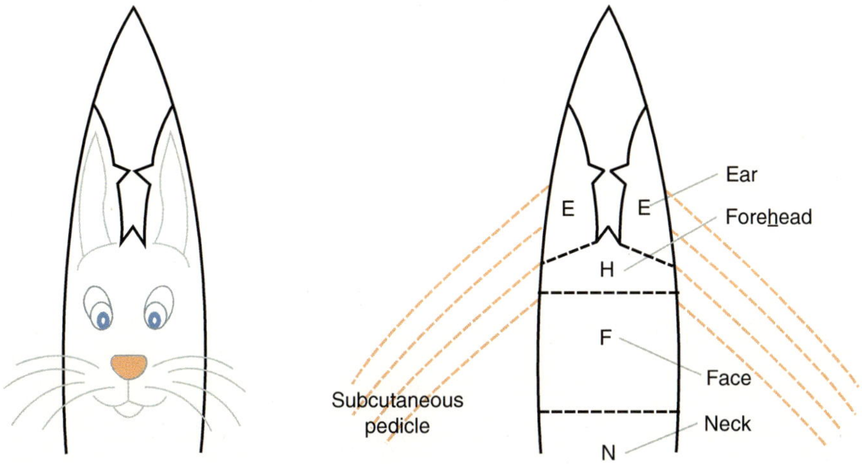

Fig. 26.2 (*Left*) Design of the rabbit-head-shaped flap. (*Right*) The flap is located at the planned reconstruction site on the scar on the cranial side, with the two long ears being used as pedicles caudally. The flap consists of five parts of the rabbit's head: bilateral ears (*E*), forehead (*H*), face (*F*), and neck (*N*). The midline scar cranial to the flap is removed and plicated. The bilateral subcutaneous pedicles attached to the ear (*E*) and forehead (*H*) parts run diagonally and then lateral caudally

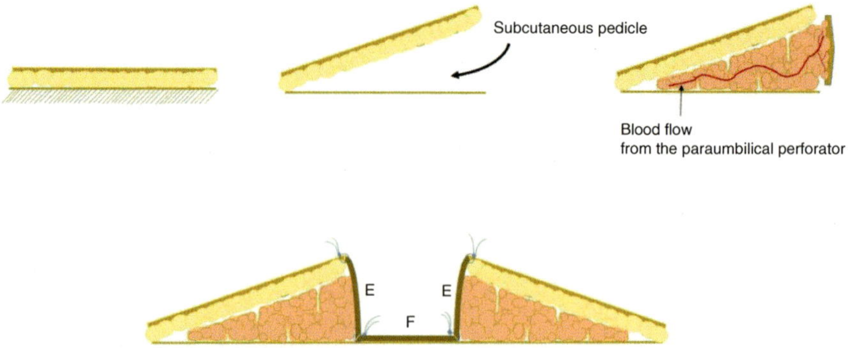

Fig. 26.3 Change in subcutaneous tissue volume. (*Top left*) Soft tissue condition around the umbilicus before subcutaneous pedicle grafting. (*Top middle*) Skin with subcutaneous fat is peeled away to make a space for subcutaneous pedicle insertion. (*Top right*) Change in the subcutaneous tissue volume after subcutaneous pedicle grafting. (*Bottom*) After the umbilicus is reconstructed

umbilicus (Fig. 26.3). The dog ear parts, formed by folding back the rabbit's ears, are used to deepen the upper wall of the umbilical depression and create wrinkles (Fig. 26.4). The rabbit ear parts of the flap are then trimmed to ensure that the shape of the umbilical wall is even on the two sides. The three small triangular flaps are then inserted at three locations around the umbilicus to prevent postoperative shrinkage caused by scar contraction. After suturing each of the flaps, a bolster suture is added to the lower wall of the umbilical depression to prevent it from becoming shallow (Fig. 26.4).

The case of a 22-year-old woman who required umbilical reconstruction is outlined in Fig. 26.5.

26.3 Discussion

Problems complicating reconstruction of an umbilicus in cases of a postoperative umbilical defect include the presence of a postoperative scar on the abdominal midline and, in the case of infants, a limited amount of abdominal skin and an extremely thin subcutaneous fat layer on the abdominal wall caused by tight closure of the abdominal wall. Consequently, reconstructing an umbilicus that appears natural with sufficient depth is often difficult. To achieve a natural-appearing umbilicus, one can imagine the umbilical depression as a box and then reconstruct its base and four walls. This concept is the standard for umbilical reconstruction, with some operative methods already having been reported [6, 7, 10]. The authors' method is also based on this simple box concept. Reconstructing the umbilicus with a sufficiently large flap alone, however, offers two-dimensional solution for a three-dimensional umbilical depression that is difficult to reconstruct and preserve. To reconstruct a deep, natural-appearing umbilicus, we added subcutaneous pedicles to the flap to be used for areas from the side walls to the upper walls of the umbilical depression (i.e., with the rabbit-head-shaped flap, it would be the area from the parts corresponding to the rabbit's ears to the forehead).

A subcutaneous pedicle is different from a skin pedicle because the length and width of the subcutaneous pedicle change during loosening or extension. That is, when it is shortened, its width and thickness expand. Vice versa, when the pedicle is

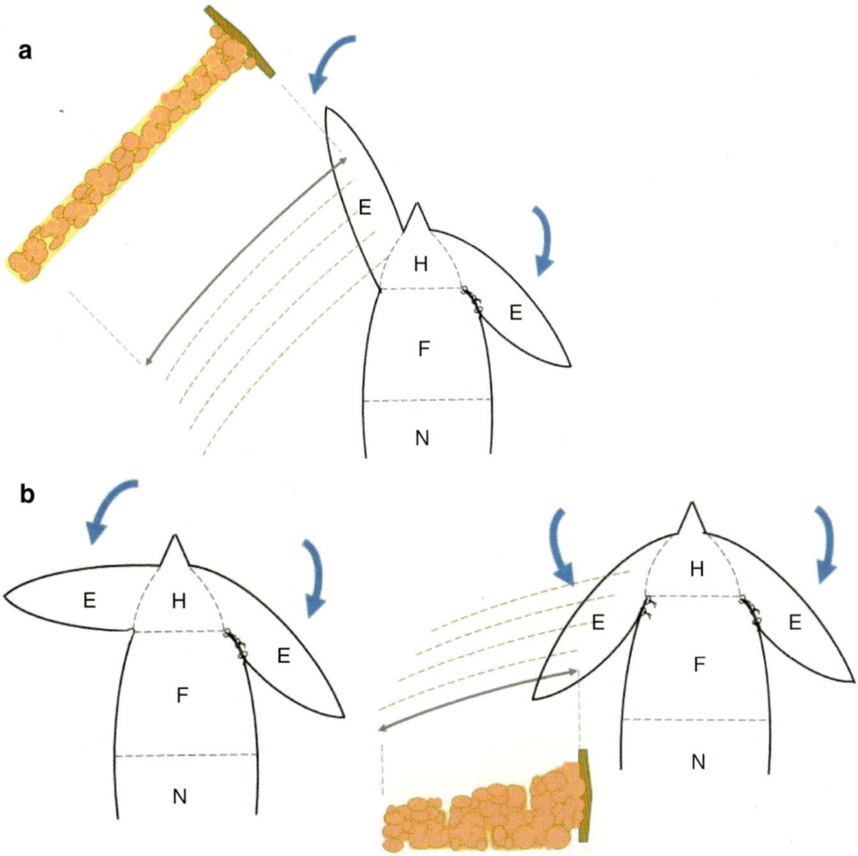

Fig. 26.4 Operative procedure. (**a**) Bilateral ear parts are turned down and sutured to the facial part (*F*). Distortion between the ear (*E*) and forehead (*H*) parts sharpens the folding angle between the forehead (*H*) and face (*F*) parts and the forehead (*H*) and ear (*E*) parts. Bilateral ear (*E*) parts become the lateral wall of the umbilicus (imagined as a box), and the forehead part (*H*) becomes the upper wall. The facial (*F*) and neck (*N*) parts become the bottom and lower walls of the umbilicus, respectively. The section of the subcutaneous pedicle and ear part of the flap are shown on the left. (**b**) The ear parts (*E*) are folded back caudally on both sides to create the two lateral walls of the umbilical depression. At this time, a dog ear deformity occurs at the suture end of the *F* and *E* parts, deepening the depression on the cranial side. The section of the subcutaneous pedicle after moving to the caudal side is shown. (**c**) (*Left, right*) Reconstructed umbilicus with sufficient depth

Fig. 26.4 (continued)

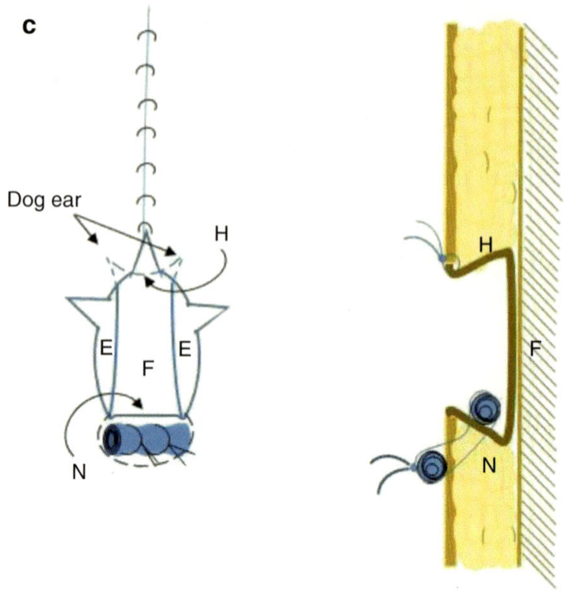

elongated, it becomes narrow and thin. These characteristics are used to increase the subcutaneous fat volume around the umbilicus. The subcutaneous pedicle is moved diagonally from cranial to caudal direction. The length of the pedicle then shrinks and thickens, thereby increasing the volume of the subcutaneous fat tissue. Using this procedure, the authors were able to reconstruct a three-dimensional umbilical depression of sufficient depth. Increasing the volume of subcutaneous tissue surrounding the umbilicus, thereby increasing the thickness, is a major difference between this procedure and previous methods [2–9]. Adding bilateral subcutaneous pedicles is also useful for stabilizing blood flow to dermal flaps that contain a scar, particularly to the long parts of the flap corresponding to the rabbit's ears in the model.

When reconstructing the umbilicus, another important point (other than its morphology) is skin texture. After the umbilical cord retracts, the umbilicus is composed of scar tissue alone. There are multiple uneven wrinkles in the umbilical depression, with the skin texture therefore different from that of the surrounding abdominal skin. To solve this problem, abdominal scar tissue was used to recreate skin texture. Although a method using normal skin (not scarred skin) has been reported, the authors could not recreate the texture of umbilical skin [7, 8]. The advantage of method compared with the other is that we do not create any new scars on normal skin.

Another problem is that the circular scar surrounding a reconstructed umbilicus tends to contract, making the umbilicus smaller. To avoid this problem, three small triangular flaps were created and inserted into the skin surrounding the umbilicus. No narrowing caused by scar contraction was observed in the patients.

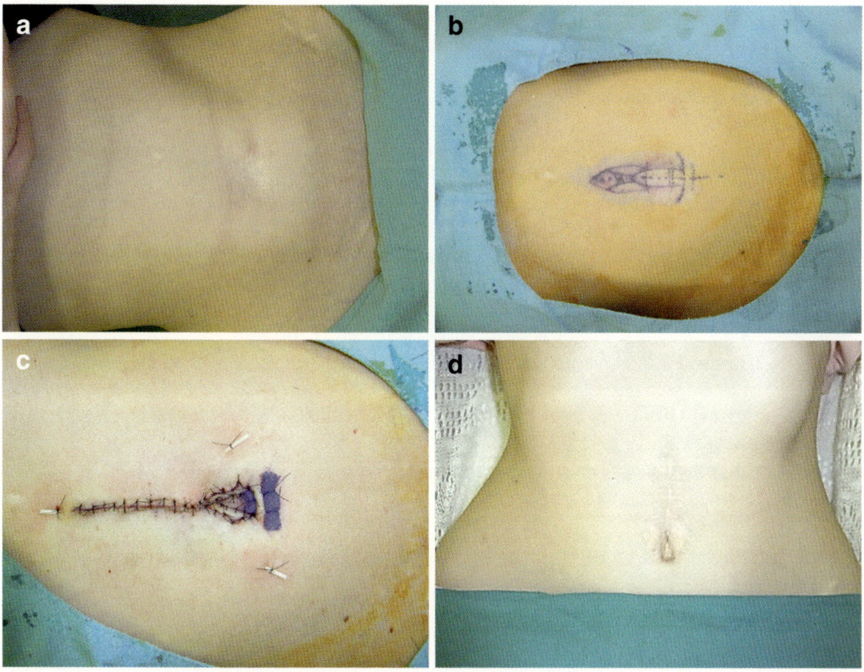

Fig. 26.5 This 22-year-old woman had a stoma that was created at the center of the abdomen for treating ulcerative colitis. An umbilical defect appeared after stomal closure. Umbilicoplasty was performed using the described procedure. (**a**) Preoperative abdominal wall. (**b**) Design of the flap. (**c**) After surgery. (**d**) Eight months postoperative. We obtained the permission of reuse of these images from Katsuseido shuppan [11]

26.4 Conclusions

An operative procedure is presented for repairing postoperative umbilical defects. This method has been used in more than 10 patients. The scar flap adapted completely in all cases, with no complications. It was also possible to reconstruct a permanent umbilical depression with satisfactory shape and sufficient depth. Thus, using a rabbit-head-shaped scar flap with bilateral subcutaneous pedicles is a safe, useful procedure for reconstructing a natural-appearing umbilical depression of sufficient depth.

References

1. Watanabe K, Kiyokawa K, Yamauchi T, Rikimaru H, Nishi Y, Koga N, Migita H. New umbilicoplasty procedure for postoperative umbilical defect using a rabbit head–shaped scar flap with bilateral subcutaneous pedicles. Plast Reconstr Surg. 2009;123(6):1724–8.

2. Borges AF. Reconstruction of the umbilicus. Br J Plast Surg. 1975;28(1):75–6.
3. Kirianoff TG. Making a new umbilicus when none exists. Plast Reconstr Surg. 1978;61(4):603–4.
4. Itoh Y, Arai K. Umbilical reconstruction using a cone-shaped flap. Ann Plast Surg. 1992;28(4):335–8.
5. Sugawara Y, Hirabayashi S, Asato H, Yoshimura K. Reconstruction of the umbilicus using a single triangular flap. Ann Plast Surg. 1995;34(1):78–80.
6. Ohnishi K, Yang YL, Maruyama Y. A new lunch box-type method in umbilical reconstruction. Ann Plast Surg. 1995;35(6):654–6.
7. Yotsuyanagi T, Nihei Y, Sawada Y. A simple technique for reconstruction of the umbilicus, using two twisted flaps. Plast Reconstr Surg. 1998;102(7):2444–6.
8. Park S, Hata Y, Ito O, Tokioka K, Kagawa K. Umbilical reconstruction after repair of omphalocele and gastroschisis. Plast Reconstr Surg. 1999;104(1):204–7.
9. Iida N, Ohsumi N. Reconstruction of umbilical hypogenesis accompanied by a longitudinal scar. Plast Reconstr Surg. 2003;111(1):322–5.
10. Southwell-Keely JP, Berry MG. Umbilical reconstruction: a review of techniques. J Plast Reconstr Aesthet Surg. 2011;64(6):803–8.
11. Koga K, Kiyokawa K. The umbilicoplasty for the umbilical defect (Saikesson ni taisuru Saikeiseijutsu) Keiseigeka. 2013;56(1):53–8.

Chapter 27
Neo-umbilicoplasty as an Option in Umbilical Reconstruction in Anchor-Line Abdominal Dermolipectomy in Postoperative Gastroplasty

Ernando Luiz Ferraz Cavalcanti

27.1 Introduction

Plastic surgery after major weight loss following bariatric surgery is increasingly being performed within our specialized field, and, from among the numerous surgical techniques available, the modified vertical abdominoplasty [1], such as the anchor-line abdominoplasty, is recommended for selected cases with abdominal skin excess in both horizontal and vertical directions [2].

Very often, even in conventional surgery, umbilicoplasty procedures represent a weak point in the results of abdominoplasty. Thus, over a number of decades, some studies have been published seeking to obtain better aesthetic results [3–5], with both transposition and isolation techniques [6], such as neo-umbilicoplasty or umbilical reconstruction techniques [7–9], whether associated or not, to the presence of a midline scar [10, 11].

In the case of ex-obese patients, almost all isolated umbilical scars during abdominoplasty have very long pedicles, with difficult accommodation and attachment to the aponeurosis, generating borderline vascularization and difficulties in defining shape. Furthermore, in many situations, hygiene is impaired. Skin pain, dehiscence, prolonged healing, depigmentation, stenosis, and scar hypertrophy are some of the passive complications that may occur [12], clearly generating a more labor-intensive postoperative period.

It is expected that in the search for improved results, the development of existing techniques and the creation of new ideas or technical details related to abdominoplasty and umbilical reconstruction in these patients may enhance the existing

E.L.F. Cavalcanti, M.D.
Instituto de Medicina Integrada Professor Fernando Figueira,
Rua Ferreira Lopes, 249, Apart 702, Casa Amarela, Recife, Pernambuco, Brazil, CEP 52060-200
e-mail: ernandolfc@hotmail.com

M.A. Shiffman (ed.), *Adult Umbilical Reconstruction*,
DOI 10.1007/978-3-319-43887-0_27

surgical armaments, thus bringing about greater satisfaction for patients and surgeons alike.

Anchor-line abdominoplasty, well reported in the literature, is an excellent dermolipectomy option in patients with major weight loss and who present with an associated midline scar, such as that of gastroplasty. The neo-umbilicoplasty technique described in this study is an umbilical reconstruction method, which is easy to perform and that provides improved aesthetic and natural results, with a lower incidence of complications over the transposition umbilicoplasty, and greater satisfaction for the author and patients [13].

27.2 Technique

The patient is marked in a standing position in order to define the midline vertical detachment, followed by the arcuate marking of the pubic area with the patient lying down. In most cases, the confluence point of the two marks is below the level of the umbilicus (Fig. 27.1).

After general anesthesia or blockade, with the patient in a supine position without lifting the back, a midline incision is made from the xiphoid to the lowest mark of the pubis, with transection and navel detachment of the umbilical stump. The

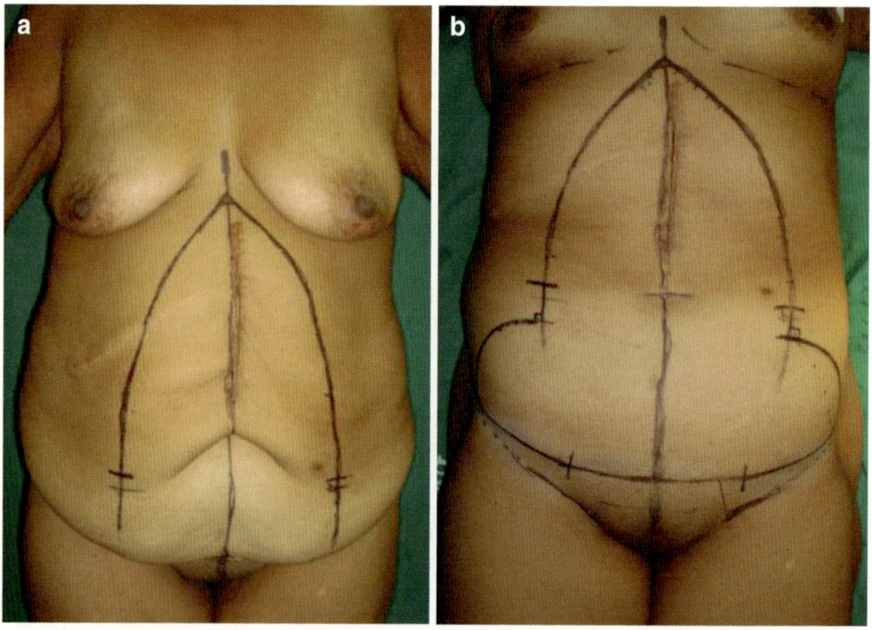

Fig. 27.1 (**a**) Marking of the flaps in the standing position. (**b**) Marking of the flaps in the supine position

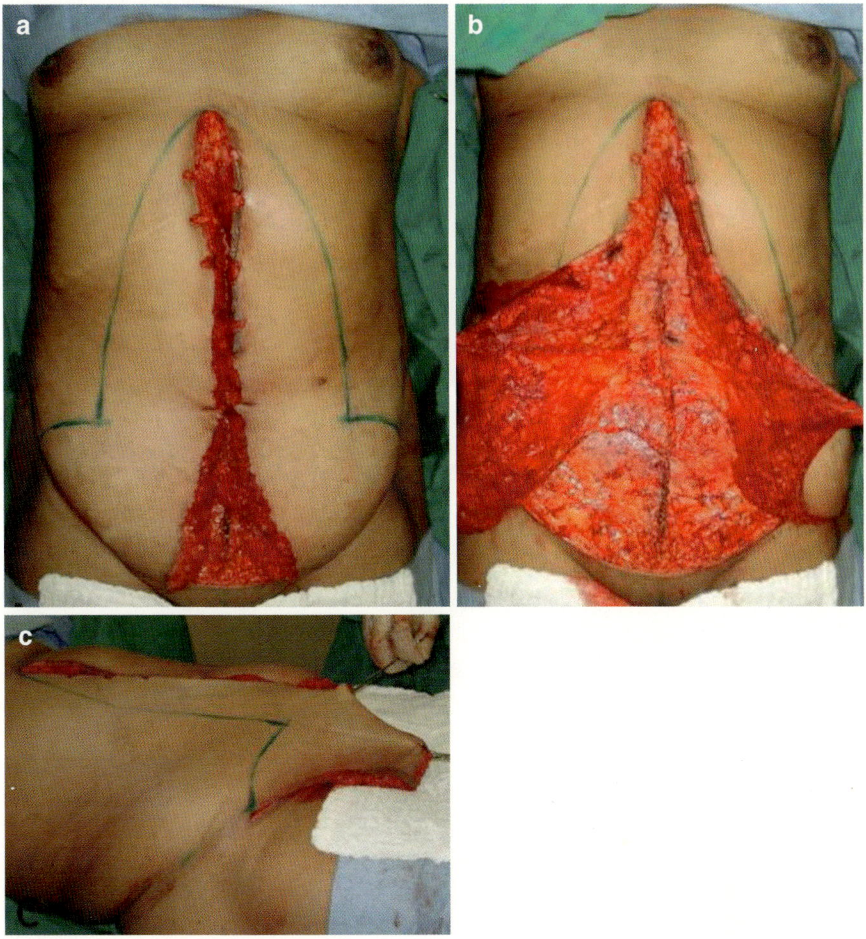

Fig. 27.2 (**a**) Detachment of the dermal fat flaps. (**b**) Finished medial plication. (**c**) Medial and downward traction of the flaps with the definitive marking of the intersection points of the incisions

dermal fat flap is drawn sideways in a supra-aponeurotic plane up to the marking, isolating any umbilical and/or incisional hernias. The skin is then incised along the arcuate pubic markings and the upper flap detached back to the marks where the vertical and horizontal lines intersected (Fig. 27.2).

Xipho-pubic spindle plication of the aponeurosis is performed with solid and stranded double polydioxanone suture (PDS) II 1, and at this moment, any hernias are repaired. The width of the spindle coincides with the limits of the lateral detachment of the flaps (Fig. 27.2). The abdominal flaps are then drawn medial and downward toward the middle of the lower incision, and the intersection point of the vertical and horizontal incisions was marked (Fig. 27.2).

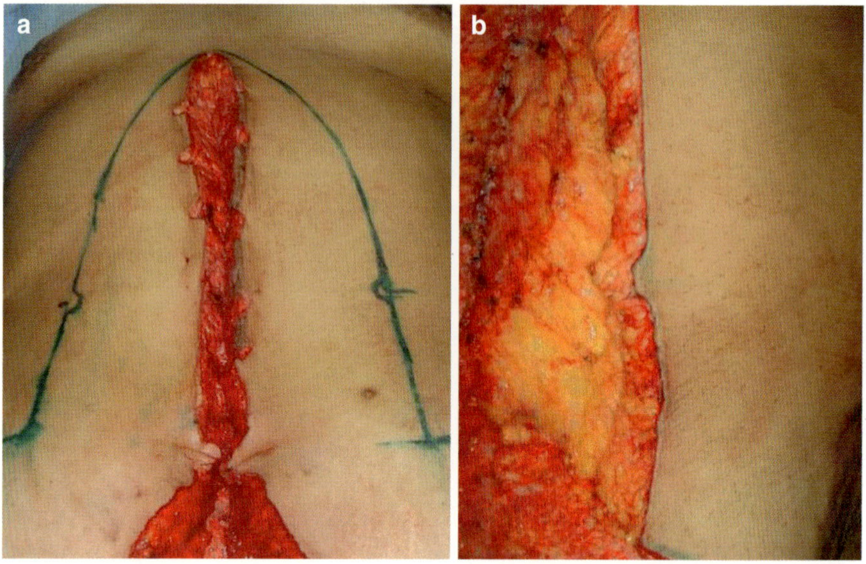

Fig. 27.3 (**a**) Marking the neo-umbilical flaps. (**b**) After resection of the surplus abdominal flaps

At around 10 cm above this point, coinciding with the level of the iliac crests or with the previous positioning of the amputated umbilical stump, two small hexagonal side flaps are marked on the vertical incision line (Fig. 27.3). All the demarcated skin is incised again, and finally the surplus tissue was removed.

These flaps are exclusively dermal, since they are defatted at the base (Fig. 27.4). The subcutaneous layer below the flap is not resectioned, but is folded laterally to allow for some lateral filling of the neo-navel, thus providing it with better depth. Five sutures with mononylon 3–0 are required so as to fix the dermal flaps to the aponeurosis, 3 midline and 2 around 0.5–1 cm to the side of the central point, like the Southern Cross. Figures 27.5, 27.6, 27.7, 27.8, 27.9, and 27.10 show details of the procedure.

Suturing the midline fatty tissue is undertaken with polyglactin (Vicryl®) 0 or 1, fixing the Scarpa's fascia to the aponeurosis in order to reduce supraumbilical subcutaneous dead space. The surgical wound is closed at deep and superficial dermal levels with mononylon 3–0 or 4–0 and poliglecaprone (Monocryl®) 4–0 (Fig. 27.11). A closed suction drain can be placed subcutaneously along the infraumbilical region, but more recently the use of adhesion sutures with Vicryl® 3–0 made this item not necessary.

Figures 27.12, 27.13, and 27.14 present some of the results obtained with the anchor-line abdominoplasty with the described neo-umbilicoplasty.

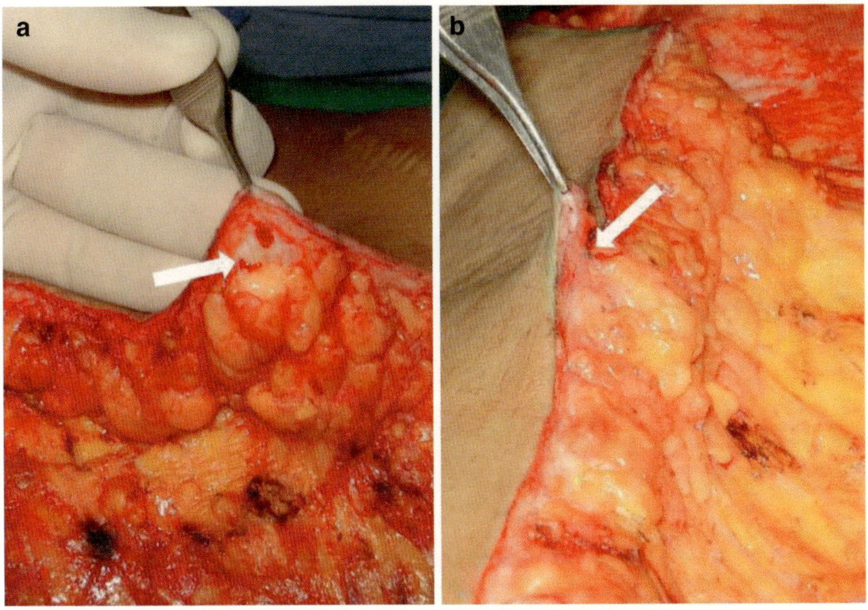

Fig. 27.4 (**a**, **b**) Neo-umbilical flap. The arrows indicate detachment from the base, thus leaving an exclusively dermal flap

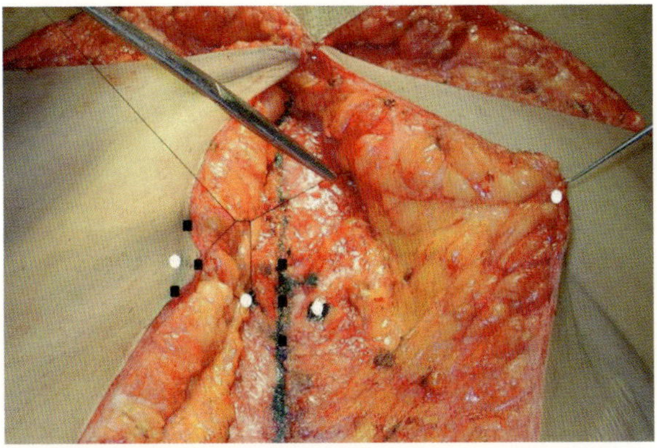

Fig. 27.5 Fixation sutures of the neo-umbilical flaps to the aponeurosis. White circles indicate sutures on the base of the flaps, about 1 cm laterally midline, each side; the black squares indicate the midline sutures

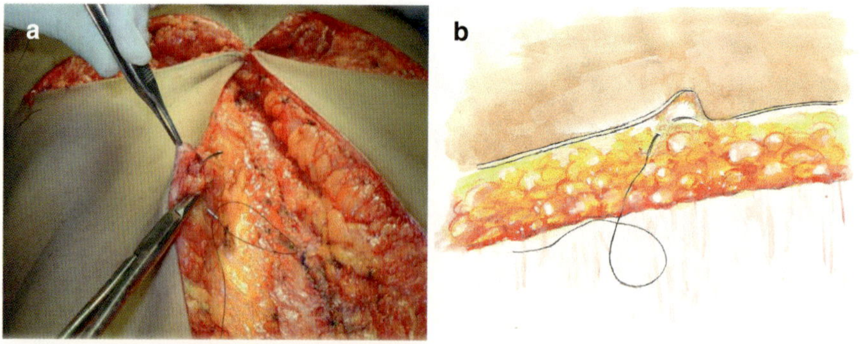

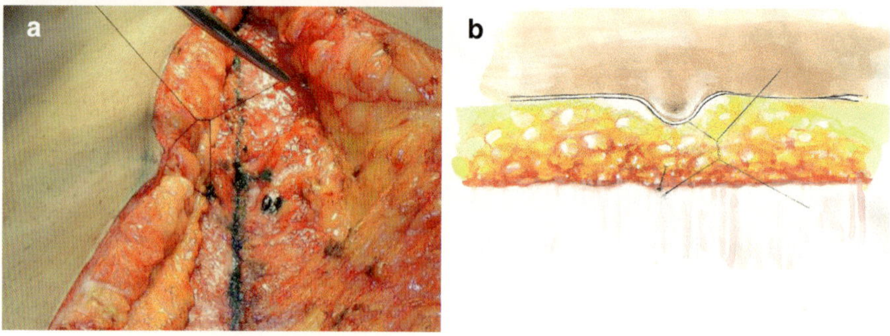

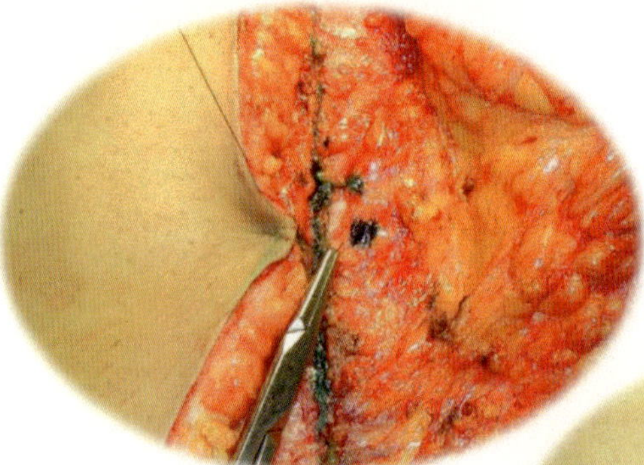

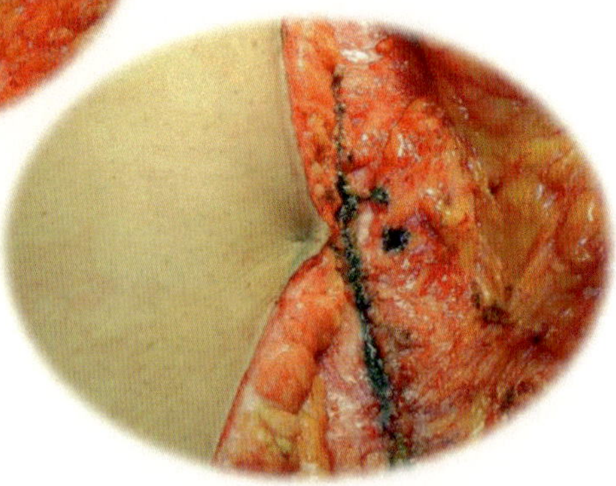

Figs. 27.6, 27.7, 27.8, 27.9 Fig. 27.6 (**a**, **b**) Subcuticular closure. Fig. 27.7 (**a**, **b**) Adipose tissue closure. Figs. 27.8–27.9 Skin closure of abdominal wound with formation of closure at site of neoumbilicus

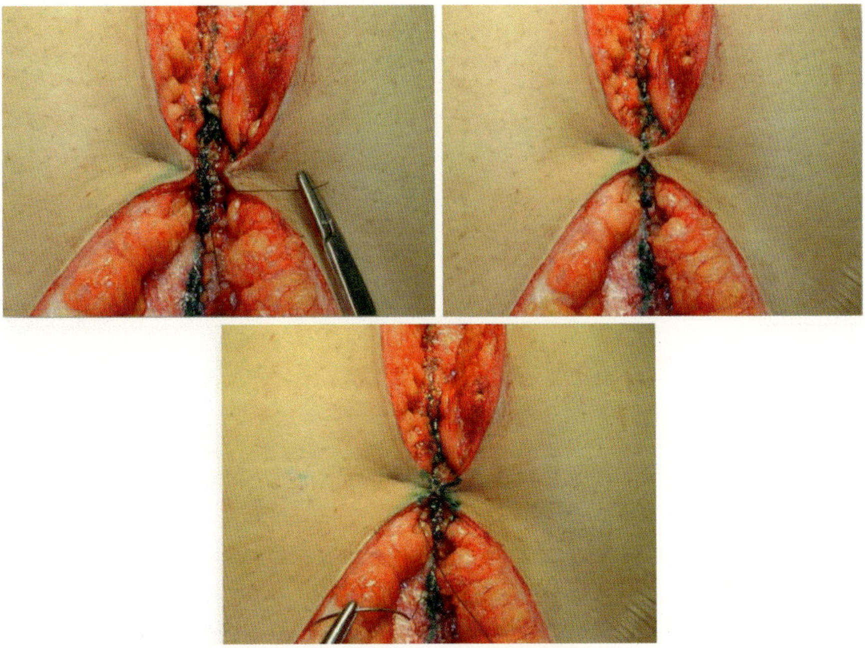

Figs. 27.6, 27.7, 27.8, 27.9 (continued)

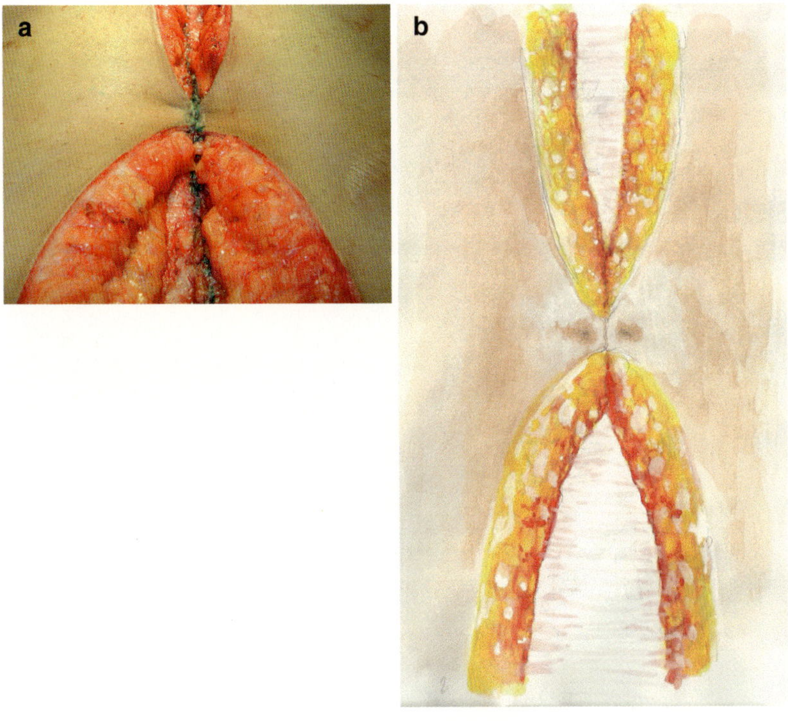

Fig. 27.10 (**a**, **b**) Before fixation of neo-umbilicus to fascia

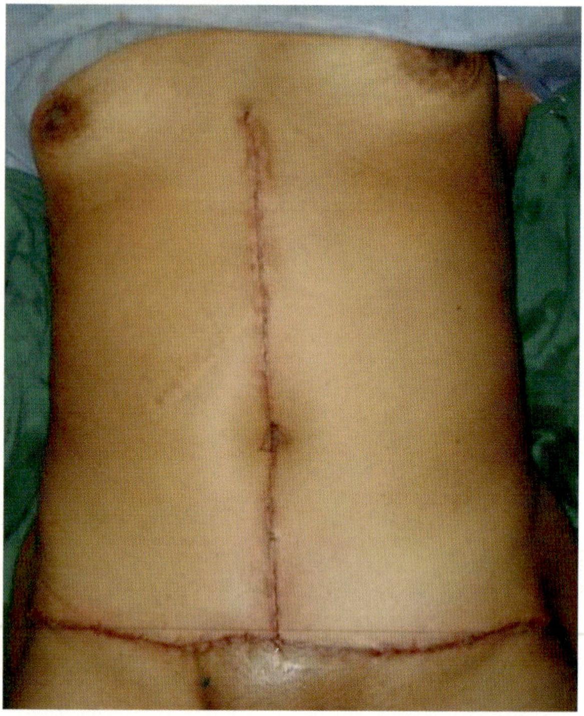

Fig. 27.11 Final closure

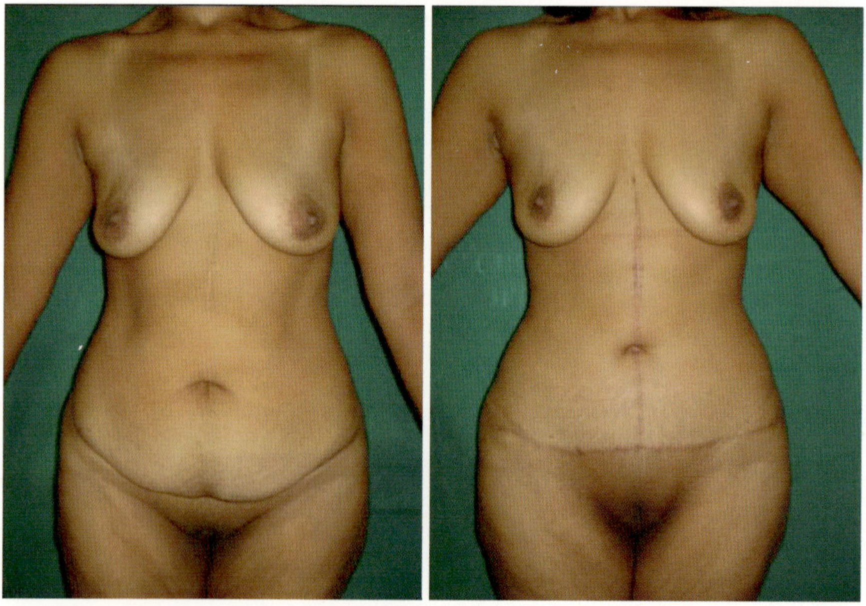

Fig. 27.12 (*Left*) Preoperative. (*Right*) Six months postoperative following anchor-line abdominoplasty plus neo-umbilicoplasty

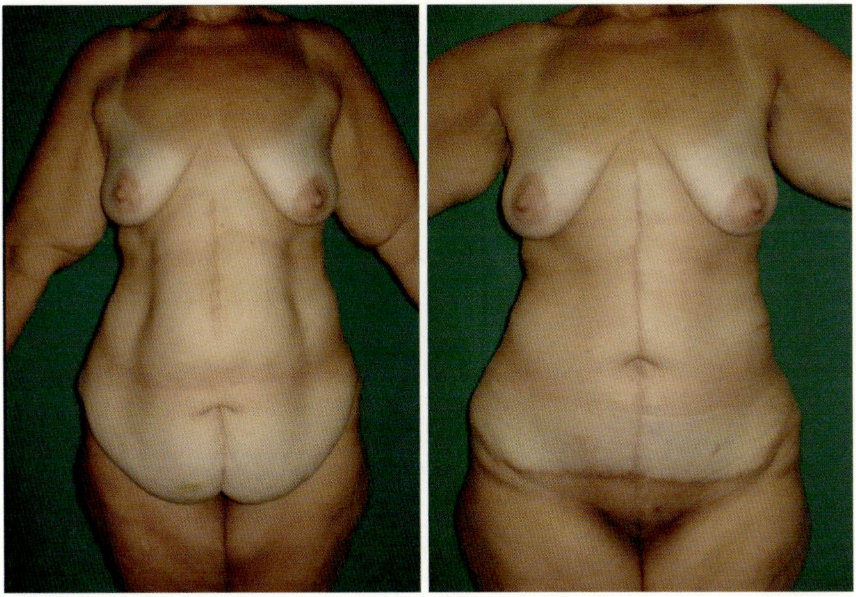

Fig. 27.13 (*Left*) Preoperative. (*Right*) Nine months postoperative after anchor-line abdominoplasty plus neo-umbilicoplasty

27.3 Discussion

Bariatric surgery has increasingly moved closer into the field of plastic surgeons, and quantitative and qualitative psychological analyses have demonstrated a significant improvement in the life quality of their patients [14].

The anchor-line dermolipectomy is a highly favored technique in large post-bariatric surgery centers and has provided good results, with a short surgical time and low complication rates, especially when the patient is able to attain a BMI as close as possible to the ideal [12]. Borud et al. [15] compared the procedures of various authors together with their complications and observed a tendency for major complications in more extensive surgery of total body contouring.

The umbilicus, on the other hand, is very often the site that generates dissatisfaction in abdominal dermolipectomies, regardless of the technique employed. Any type of umbilical reconstruction that aims at good aesthetic results should strive for a number of important features, such as appropriate size, shape, location, and depth. Meanwhile, with the presence of a scar, it would be more desirable not to encounter any complications, such as stenosis, unsightly scars, hypertrophy, or widening. There is a trend toward greater acceptance when periumbilical scars are narrower and less visible [16].

With regard to the question of size and shape, Craig et al. [17] assessed the umbilici of 147 women and found that the highest marks from an aesthetic viewpoint were from those with a medium to small, more vertical format, with or without the presence of an upper "curtain" of skin.

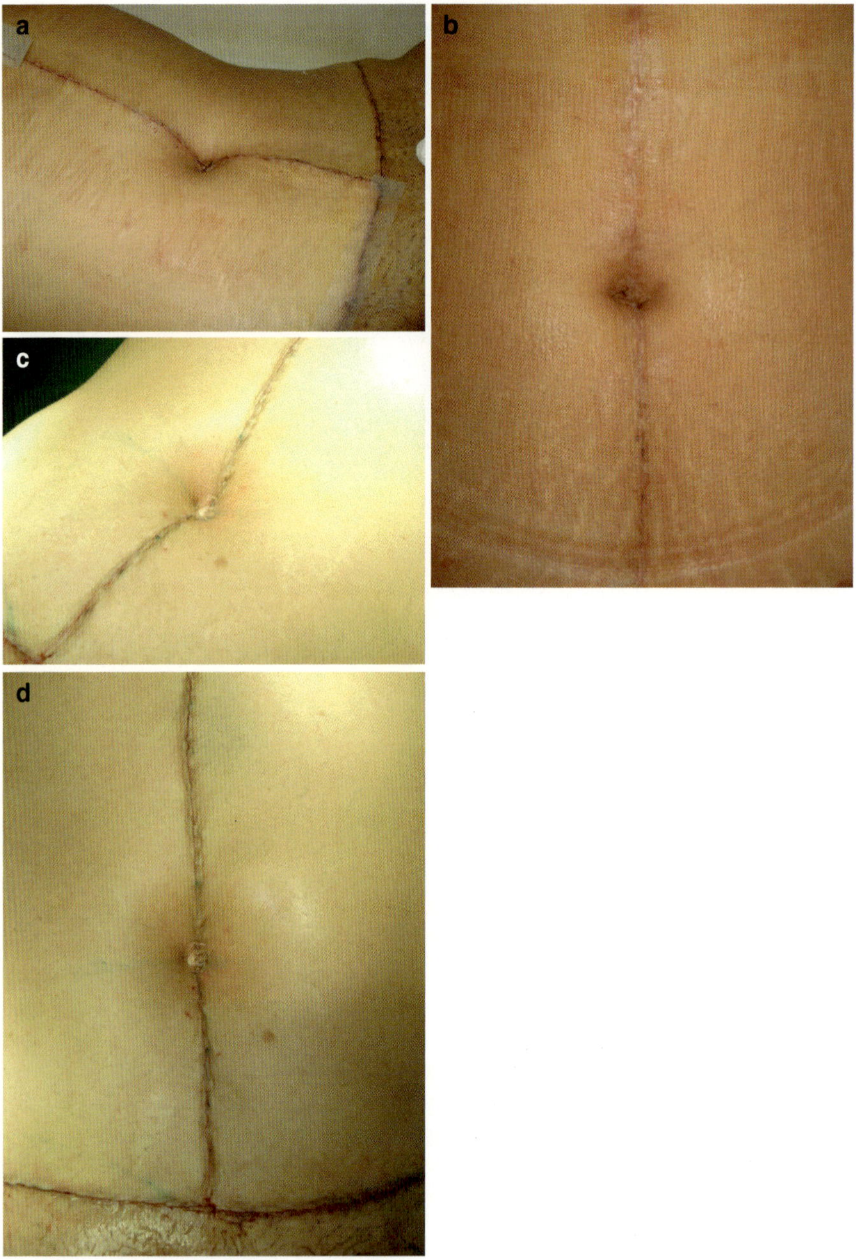

Fig. 27.14 (**a–d**) Final surgical aspect of neo-umbilicoplasties

An Indian study assessed 75 young women with a mean BMI of 29.9 kg/m2 and concluded that the umbilicus was positioned at an average height ratio of 1.6: 1 between the xiphoid and the pubic symphysis. The average depth was found to be 1.16 cm [18]. An association between the reference points of the iliac crests and the area of the amputated umbilical stump are sufficient and appropriate in determining the proper umbilical positioning encountered in the performed neo-umbilicoplasties. With regard to depth, we believe that the good fixation of the neo-navel flaps with nonabsorbable suture was able to maintain the depth of the umbilicus.

Several techniques have been described that attempt to achieve more discreet scarring, associated with more natural umbilicus [16]. Malic et al. [19] compared 2 transposition umbilicoplasty techniques and obtained between 15 and 58 % scar revisions, despite obtaining good results. With ex-obese patients, the pedicle of these umbilical stumps is long, difficult to handle, and is borderline vascularization, which from the viewpoint of both patients and surgeons represents the worst results. The incidence of specific complications with the umbilicus has not been fully described in the literature and has therefore remained underreported. Cortes et al. [12] observed that out of 39 operated patients, 8 % were discovered to be suffering from complications.

Currently, two new techniques of neo-umbilicoplasty like this have been described in literature with good and similar results [20, 21].

27.4 Conclusions

The neo-umbilicoplasty technique described here is an easy procedure for umbilical reconstruction, reproductive, with good aesthetic results and low rate of complications, and providing great satisfaction for the patients. Complaints mostly related to rhomboid umbilicoplasty, like visible scars, widened scars, "umbilicus ball," darkened umbilicus, "strange umbilicus," are not reported in patients undergoing neo-umbilicoplasty.

The anchor technique employed presents limitation in resections of the lateral surplus, although the abdomen resection presents satisfactory results.

References

1. Costa LF, Landecker A, Manta AM. Optimizing body contour in massive weight loss patients: the modified vertical abdominoplasty. Plast Reconstr Surg. 2004;114(7):1917–23.
2. Persichetti P, Simone P, Scuderi N. Anchor-line abdominoplasty: a comprehensive approach to abdominal wall reconstruction and body contouring. Plast Reconstr Surg. 2005;116(1):289–94.
3. Delerm A. Refinements in abdominoplasty with emphasis on reimplantation of the umbilicus. Plast Reconstr Surg. 1982;70(5):632–7.

4. Craig SB, Faller MS, Puckett CL. In search of the ideal female umbilicus. Plast Reconstr Surg. 2000;105(1):389–92.
5. Akbas H, Guneren E, Eroglu L. Natural looking umbilicus as an important part of abdominoplasty. Aesthetic Plast Surg. 2003;27:139–42.
6. Lee MJ, Mustoe T. Simplified technique for creating a youthful umbilicus in abdominoplasty. Plast Reconstr Surg. 2002;109(6):2136–40.
7. Baack BR, Anson G, Nachbar JM, White DJ. Umbilicoplasty: the construction of a new umbilicus and correction of umbilical stenosis without external scars. Plast Reconstr Surg. 1996;97(1):227–32.
8. Yotsuyanagi T, Nihei Y, Sawada Y. A simple technique for reconstruction of the umbilicus, using two twisted flaps. Plast Reconstr Surg. 1998;102(7):2444–6.
9. Sevin A, Sevin K, Senen D, Erdogan B. A new method for umbilicus reconstruction: preliminary report. Aesthetic Plast Surg. 2006;30(5):589–91.
10. Masuda R, Takeda A, Sugimoto T, Ishiguro M, Uchinuma E. Reconstruction of the umbilicus using a reverse fan-shaped flap. Aesthetic Plast Surg. 2003;27(5):349–53.
11. Franco D, Medeiros J, Farias C, Franco T. Umbilical reconstruction for patients with a midline scar. Aesthetic Plast Surg. 2006;30:595–8.
12. Cortes JES, Oliveira DP, Sperly A. Abdominoplastias em âncora em pacientes ex-obesos. Rev Bras Cir Plást. 2009;24(1):57–63.
13. Cavalcanti ELF. Neoumbilicoplastia como opção de reconstrução umbilical nas dermolipectomias abdominais em âncora pós-gastroplastia. Rev Bras Cir Plást. 2010;25(3):509–18.
14. Junior WC, Modolin M, Gobbi CIC, Gemperli R, Ferreira MC. Abdominoplastia circunferencial em pacientes após cirurgia bariátrica: avaliação da qualidade de vida pelo critério adaptativo. Rev Bras Cir Plást. 2009;24(1):52–6.
15. Borud LJ, Colwell AS. Optimization of patient safety in postbariatric body contouring: a current review. Aesthetic Surg J. 2008;28(4):437–42.
16. Rosique MJF, Rosique RG, Lee FDI, Kawakami H, Glattstein N, Mélega JM. Estudo comparativo entre técnicas de onfaloplastia. Rev Bras Cir Plást. 2009;24(1):47–51.
17. Craig SB, Faller MS, Puckett CL. In search of the ideal female umbilicus. Plast Reconstr Surg. 2000;105(1):389–92.
18. Abhyankar SV, Rajguru AG, Patil PA. Anatomical localization of the umbilicus: an Indian study. Plast Reconstr Surg. 2006;117(4):1153–7.
19. Malic CC, Spyrou GE, Hough M, Fourie L. Patient satisfaction with two different methods of umbilicoplasty. Plast Reconstr Surg. 2007;119(1):357–61.
20. Silva FN, Oliveira EA. Neo-onfaloplastia na abdominoplastia vertical. Rev Bras Cir Plást. 2010;25(2):330–6.
21. Donnabella A. Reconstrução anatômica da cicatriz umbilical. Rev Bras Cir Plást. 2013;28(1):119–23.

Chapter 28
New Technique for Neo-umbilicoplasty

Michel E. Pfulg and João Bastos Martins

28.1 The Aesthetic Importance of the Umbilicus

The central location in the abdomen makes the umbilicus an aesthetically important structure in both males and females. It is acknowledged as the most visible and recognized landmark of the abdominal wall. Its size, shape, contour, and position have been subject of study, and multiple techniques have been published searching for the ideal umbilicus. Different opinions exist on this subject. Most authors favor an almond or slight T-shaped with the longest axis in the vertical direction [1]. Some consensus exists on small being preferable to large, a vertical ellipse being preferable to a circle and an "inny" being preferable to an "outie." In the majority of cases, a horizontal skin fold is seen in the upper part of the aesthetically pleasant umbilicus, creating a small superior hood.

In a conventional abdominoplasty with umbilicus transposition, there are also different approaches to the umbilicus. In order to achieve the desirable result described above, we prefer to use a "V" shape incision that allows us to create an umbilicus that meets the aesthetic demands (Fig. 28.1).

M.E. Pfulg, M.D. (✉)
Laclinic Montreux, Avenue de Collonge 43, 1820, Montreux-Territet, Switzerland
e-mail: m.pfulg@laclinic.ch

J.B. Martins
Plastic and Reconstructive Surgery Department, Hospital São José (Central Lisbon Hospital Center), Lisbon, Portugal

M.A. Shiffman (ed.), *Adult Umbilical Reconstruction*,
DOI 10.1007/978-3-319-43887-0_28

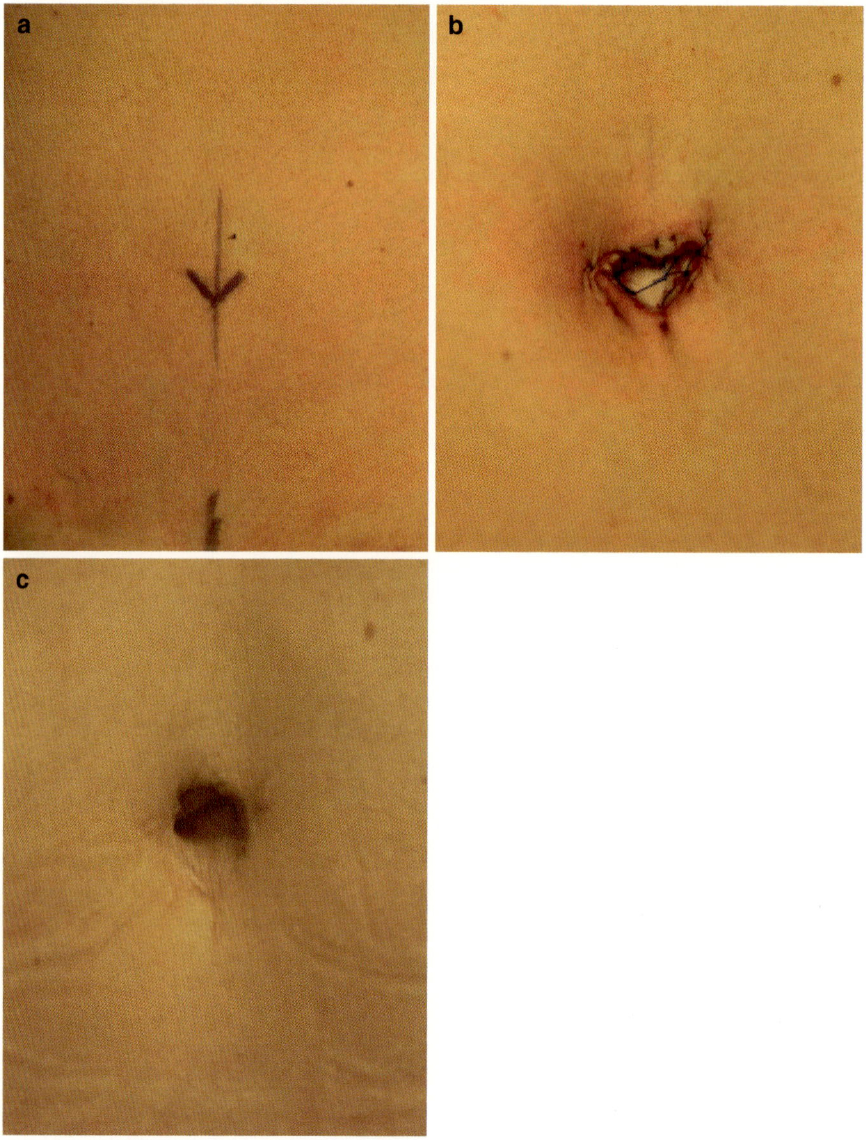

Fig. 28.1 (**a**) The authors' planned V-shape incision. (**b**) Final appearance intraoperatively. (**c**) Follow-up showing a deep, circular umbilicus with a superior hood

28.2 Reconstruction of the Totally Absent Umbilicus

Reconstruction of a destroyed umbilicus after umbilical herniorrhaphy was first reported by McMillan in 1955 [2]. An absent or destroyed umbilicus may result from congenital absence, inflammatory destruction, surgical procedures, or excision from skin cancer (Table 28.1).

Table 28.1 Causes for an absent/destroyed umbilicus [16]

Congenital absence	Bladder exstrophy
	Gastroschisis
	Omphalocele
	Cloacal exstrophy
Inflammatory destruction	Periumbilical necrotizing fasciitis
	Umbilical sepsis
Surgical procedures	Umbilical herniorrhaphy
	Abdominoplasty
	Laparotomy
Skin cancer	Direct excision

The techniques used for reconstruction can follow two main principles: (1) the use of skin or pedicle flaps that remain attached to the abdominal fascia to create the basis of the umbilicus for a small tubular structure [3–7] or (2) the use of the neighboring skin from the abdominal wall to create the depressed tubular structure of the umbilicus [8–15]. In addition to the former group of techniques, sometimes a cartilage graft can be used to improve shape [16]. The authors have the opinion that the unpredictable flap vascularization from the deeper abdominal wall should favor the latter group.

Independently from the technique used, the neo-umbilicus should have a natural morphology, a sufficient and prominent depression, and must be created without causing too many additional scars. Almost all reconstructed umbilici come along with a horizontal or a vertical scar on the skin of the abdominal wall. This is necessary to decrease the amount of skin around the exterior circumference of the umbilicus in order to obtain sufficient depth of the umbilicus. Marconi [5] and later Bartsich [17] have described purse-string methods. Although this is a very simple technique, the long-term results have not been described. The question is, as with the circumareolar mastopexia, if the circular scar will not stretch and the umbilicus flatten.

28.3 Patient Selection

As in any other field of plastic surgery, the correct indication for a procedure is a fundamental key in achieving a successful result. Surgical techniques should be selected as the best solutions to ensure a desirable and predictable result while minimizing morbidity and postoperative disability. This umbilicoplasty technique needs to be combined with either a vertical or horizontal scar over the umbilical position to be able to guarantee sufficient size of the umbilicus. The suitable patient should present a destroyed or absent umbilicus, with no signs of acute inflammation on the periumbilical area and have already a vertical midline scar or accept to have one. To avoid tension on skin closure, there should be enough abdominal tissue to ensure an easy closure in the midline. Usually this is always possible, and it will also improve the patient's waist circumference. The creation of a neo-umbilicus is often required

Table 28.2 Most common indications for neo-umbilicoplasty

Previously completely liberated umbilicus
After total resection of the umbilicus
Following purse-string suture techniques
Central abdominal striae
Midline dehiscence
Umbilical hernia

after a previous abdominoplasty. In some techniques of suprapubic skin resection, the umbilicus is not resected but completely detached from the underlying fascia. If a secondary abdominoplasty needs to be performed with further and wider resection of excess of skin, often the umbilicus needs to be resected. In other techniques with circum-umbilical skin resection and purse-string tightening, the remaining umbilicus is extremely deformed and can no longer be used. Often patients consult after a total resection of the umbilicus following hernia surgery or complicated laparotomies. Common indications for neo-umbilicoplasty found in our practice are listed on Table 28.2.

A careful assessment of the abdominal wall is imperative; the surgeon should evaluate the abdomen for existing scars, skin compliance and elasticity, rectus abdominus muscle diastasis, and the existence of periumbilical hernias. If there is the indication for concomitant procedures in the abdominal wall, they can be performed on the same surgical period.

28.4 Personal Technique

The technique demonstrated here was presented at the International Symposium, ASAPS meeting in Vancouver, Canada, and published in 2005 [18]. The aim of this simple technique is to create a harmonious umbilicus of adequate size, orientation, and depth together with a natural shape. The main advantage of this original method is that it is simple, reproducible, and has very few complications. The authors consider this technique as a personal preference in vertical scar abdominoplasties and umbilical reconstructions.

28.4.1 Surgical Technique

Preoperative markings should be done previously with the patient standing. A triangular skin flap is designed within the elliptical skin excision over the umbilicus either in a vertical or horizontal direction. When using a vertical ellipse, care should be taken to avoid extending the vertical excision line cranially between the breasts. Usually the surgeon can use the old umbilicus scar as reference to decide where to locate the neo-umbilicus in the midline. In cases where this is not possible or this reference scar is not

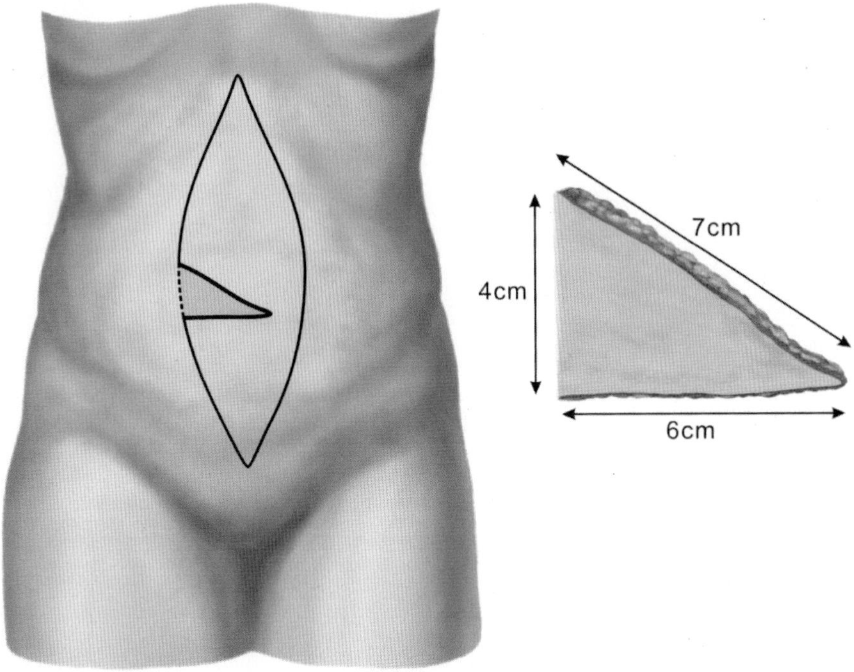

Fig. 28.2 Flap design

available, the body morphology of each patient has an important influence in the location of our flap. The umbilicus depression usually reaches down to the umbilical fascia. It should be placed about 3 cm above the superior iliac spine or at the highest level of the iliac crest [19, 20]. The procedure starts with the incision along the elliptical markings, through the skin and superficial fascia, reaching the rectus abdominus fascia, which should be kept intact. While dissecting the central tissue to be resected, a thin layer of fat and areolar tissue should be preserved just superficial to the rectus fascia. Throughout the course of dissection, meticulous hemostasis must be maintained to ensure minimal intraoperative blood loss. One side of the triangular flap is attached to the remaining skin border. This side of the triangle measures about 4 cm, while the other two borders measure 7 and 6 cm, respectively (Fig. 28.2). If the patient already has a longitudinal scar that will intercept the designed flap, compromising the distal tip of the triangle, the 6 cm distance might be shortened to the point where the longitudinal scar crosses the flap (Fig. 28.3). As a direct consequence, the longer limb of the triangle, marked before as 7 cm, will have to be designed shorter in order to meet the "new" distal flap corner 4/0 nylon simple sutures are used to close the skin in the neo-umbilicius area.

After wide supra-fascial undermining, correction of the rectus diastasis is performed. Outlining the medial borders of the rectus muscles first marks the myofascial plication limits. Usually these markings should design an ellipse from the xiphoid process to the pubic symphysis. The plication is done using a continuous

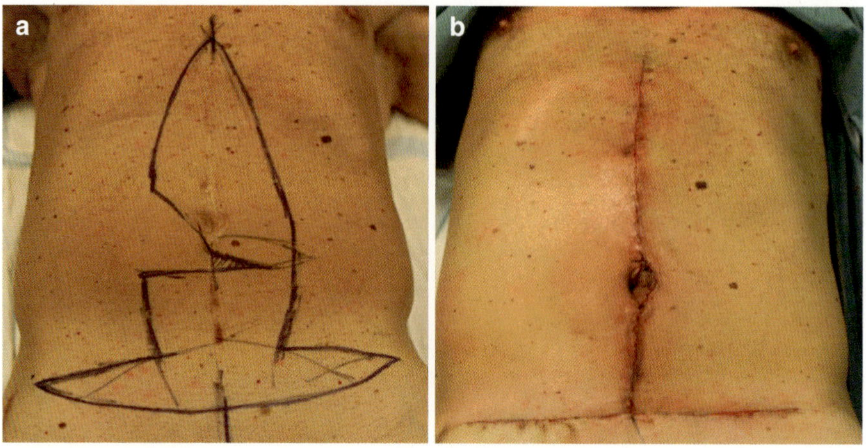

Fig. 28.3 Clinical case with previous deep longitudinal scar. (**a**) Preoperative markings showing shortening of the flap horizontal dimensions to ensure distal flap survival. (**b**) Immediate postoperative result

interlocking non-resorbable suture. For safety reasons, it can be performed in a double line of closure.

The triangular flap is then approached. In the heavier patient, this flap will be too bulky, and it should be thinned making sure to keep the subdermal plexus intact as well as a thin layer of fat, to ensure the distant flap survival. If the surgeon has doubts on the survival of the most distal tip of the triangle, it should be discarded. Over the longest side of the triangle, the flap is folded onto itself (Fig. 28.4) and sutured upon itself, producing the desired cone shape for the umbilicus. The tip of this conical skin structure is then firmly attached in the midline to the fascia of the abdominal wall by a 2/0 resorbable suture. The redundant skin around the neo-umbilicus is resected, and the wound closure is performed using a 2/0 slow resorbable suture for the deep tissues (Scarpa's fascia) and a 3/0 slow resorbable suture for subcutaneous closure, ensuring the minimum tension on the skin. For skin closure, a resorbable intracuticular running suture can be used. In the end of the procedure, some liposuction using a gentle cannula can be performed to diminish the possible bulk on the base of the flap.

28.4.2 Postoperative Care

As the postoperative care is related to the type of abdominoplasty associated with the neo-umbilicoplasty, the operation can be performed as an outpatient or inpatient procedure. As in all abdominoplasty procedures, early ambulation is recommended, and if drains are used they are left in place until discharge in <30 mL in 24 h (usually 3–4 days). Suture material is removed from the vertical and/or horizontal incisions on day 10–12. Umbilical sutures should be removed after week 3. After suture removal, the authors recommend the use of silicone taping for a period of 4–6 months for scar improvement. The use of a compressive band is recommended for 4–8 weeks, depending on the degree of skin undermining and liposuction extension. Some patients will benefit from lymphatic drainage on the postoperative period. It can be started 1 week after the operation and should be performed by an experienced

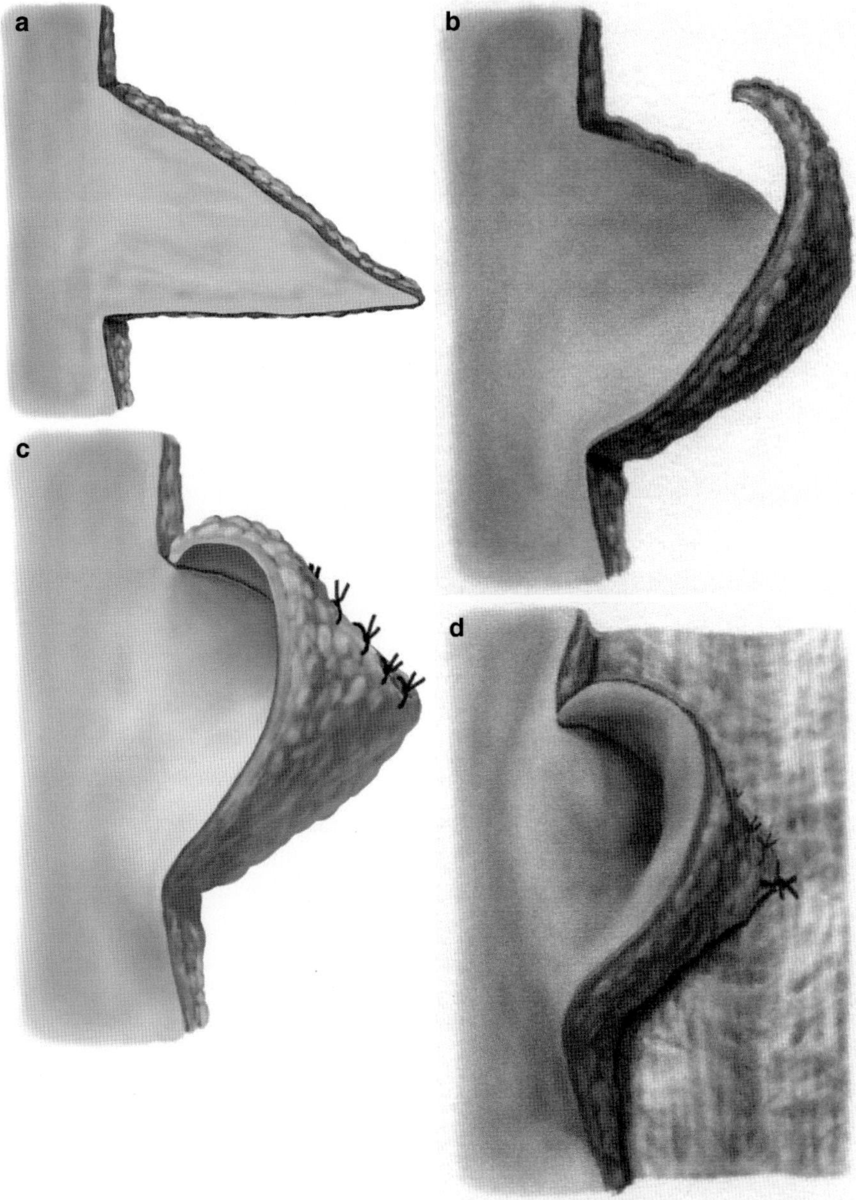

Fig. 28.4 (**a**) The flap after dissection. (**b**) Folding of the flap. (**c**) Suturing of the flap upon itself. (**d**) Suturing the resulting cone to the abdominal wall fascia. (**e**) Abdominal wound closure after skin trimming

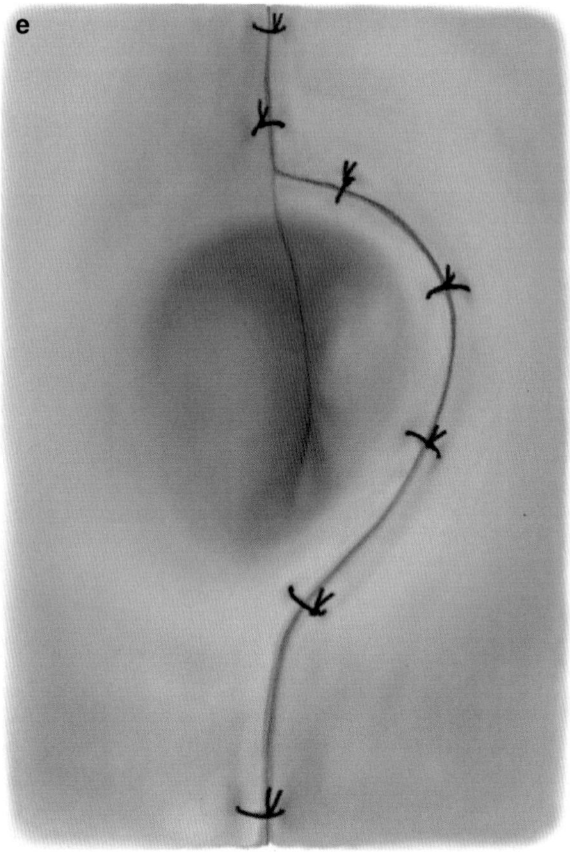

Fig. 28.4 (continued)

professional. If no fascial reconstruction/plication is performed, the patient may return his sporting activities on weeks 4–6 postoperative.

Regarding the neo-umbilicoplasty procedure alone, the only possible complications will be the same as with any other surgical procedure: dehiscence, infection, epitheliolysis, and flap necrosis. The latter two have never occurred in the authors' hands, and the former two are hypothetical, occurring very rarely as in all random flap procedures. Seroma, hematoma, and deep venous thrombosis occurrence will be dependent on the type of abdominoplasty performed and won't be related to the neo-umbilicoplasty.

28.5 Clinical Cases

Four clinical cases are presented with different indications to demonstrate the versatility of the procedure.

28.5.1 Case 1

This is a male patient who had a previous umbilical hernia repair with complete removal of the umbilicus. Patient also presents with a distended abdomen and an important diastasis of the rectus abdominus muscles (Fig. 28.5). With this technique, a flat abdomen with a natural-looking umbilicus was achieved (Fig. 28.5).

28.5.2 Case 2

This is a female patient who was submitted to a failed surgical correction of post-partum striae with a purse-string technique (Fig. 28.6). A very good aesthetic result was achieved.

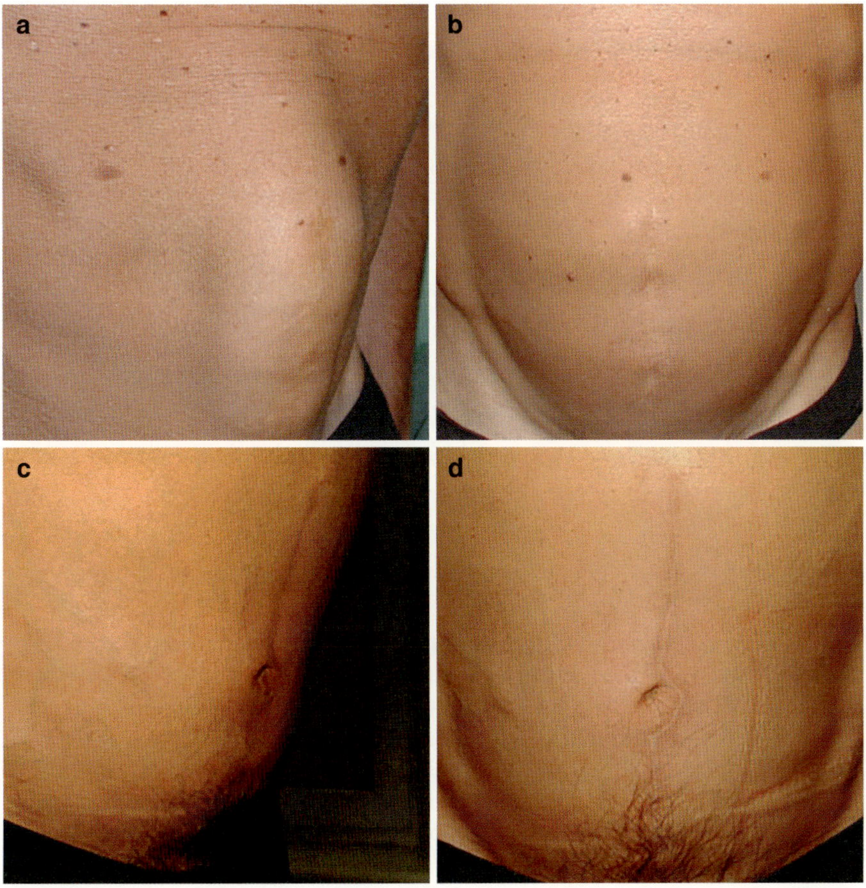

Fig. 28.5 (**a**, **b**) Rectus abdominus diastasis, distended abdomen, and completely absent umbilicus. (**c**, **d**) Three months after diastasis correction with a flat abdomen and a natural-looking umbilicus

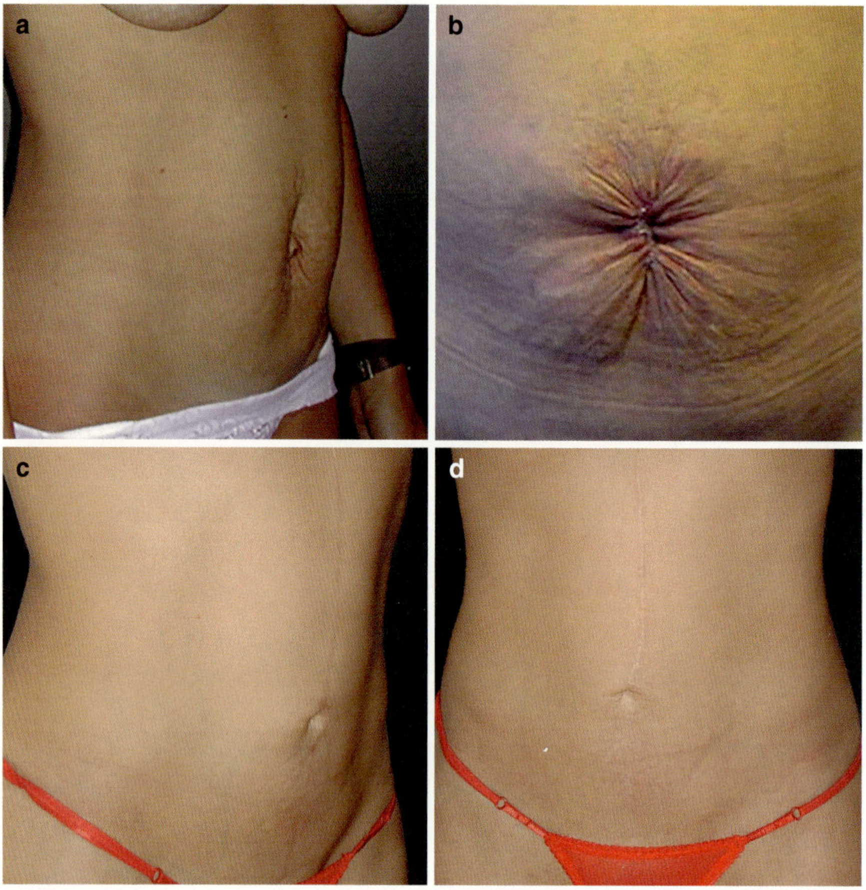

Fig. 28.6 (**a**, **b**) Failed surgical correction of postpartum striae with a purse-string technique. Poor aesthetic result and partial necrosis. (**c**, **d**) Six months after neo-umbilicoplasty using the presented technique

28.5.3 Case 3

This is a female patient with postpartum periumbilical striae, rectus abdominus muscle diastasis, and umbilical hernia (Fig. 28.7). Her main concern was to remove the striae, specially the upper ones. Our technique allowed us to remove the striae and correct both the diastasis and umbilical hernia while achieving an aesthetically pleasant umbilicus. Her main concern was to remove the striae, specially the upper ones. Our technique allowed us to remove the striae and correct both the diastasis and umbilical hernia while achieving an aesthetically pleasant umbilicus.

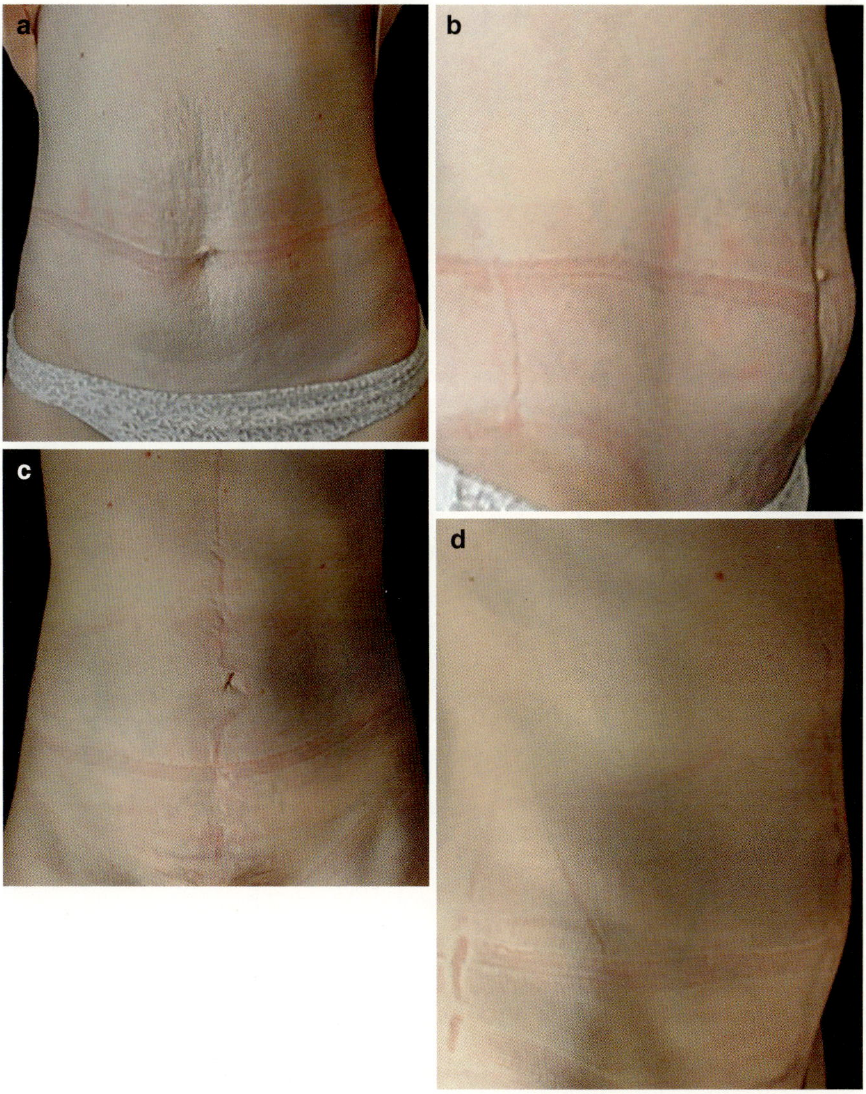

Fig. 28.7 (**a**, **b**) Postpartum periumbilical striae, rectus abdominus muscle diastasis, and umbilical hernia. (**c**, **d**) Four months postoperatively

28.5.4 Case 4

This is a case of a male patient who was submitted to a colon cancer removal through a laparotomy approach, 3 years previously. The postoperative period was complicated by a soft-tissue infection. He now presents with severe scar adherence to the

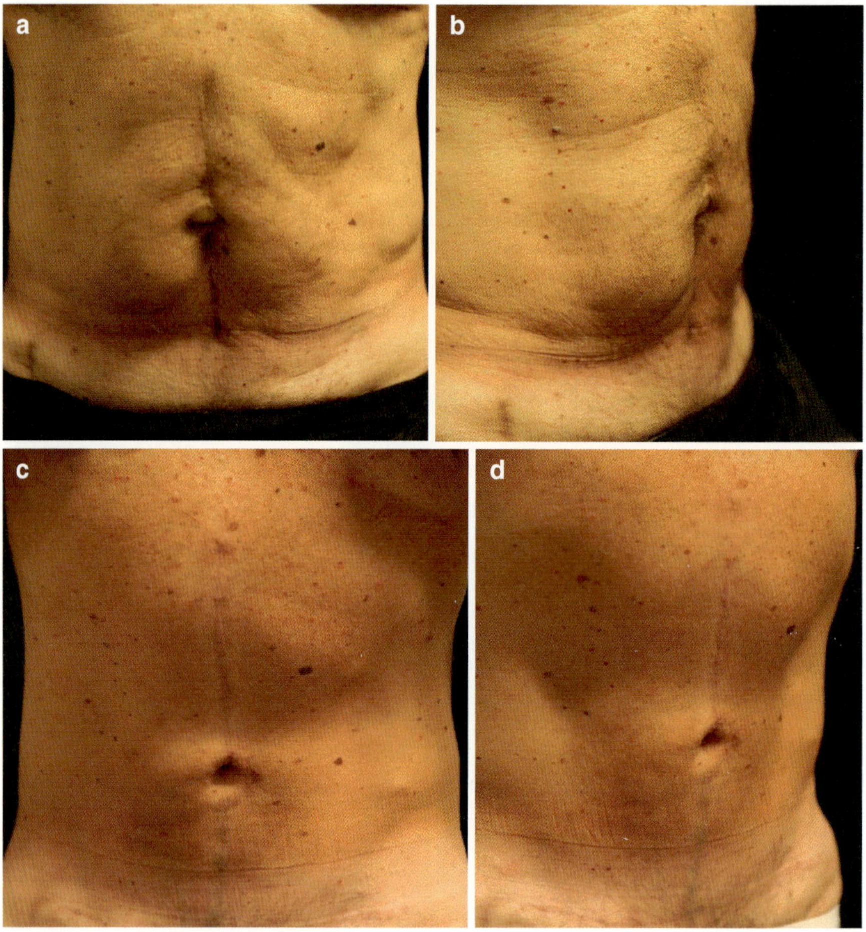

Fig. 28.8 (**a**, **b**) Scar adherence, umbilicus deformation, and muscle diastasis after laparotomy complicated by soft-tissue infection 3 years previously. (**c**, **d**) Long-term results

abdominal fascia, umbilicus deformation, and a rectus abdominus muscle diastasis (Fig. 28.8). The authors' technique allowed the repair of the muscles, corrected the scar, and recreated a normal umbilicus.

28.6 Conclusions

Although this neo-umbilicoplasty technique needs to be combined with a vertical (or horizontal) scar, the final aesthetic result is extremely positive. Most patients accept these scars in order to get an aesthetically pleasant umbilicus, and other patients already present this scars from previous procedures. In addition to creating an umbilicus that is centered, vertically oriented, presents a superior hood, and has some degree of periumbilical depression, it allows the correction of different abdominal deformities.

It is an easy technique with a short learning curve and a very generous versatility. Together with patients' satisfaction, this is the reason why we treasure this technique as a "lifeboat" every surgeon should possess as it can successfully reconstruct a completely absent umbilicus and at the same time correct demanding sequel from previous surgeries.

References

1. Craig SB, Faller MS, Puckett CL. In search of the ideal female umbilicus. Plast Reconstr Surg. 2000;105:389.
2. McMillan WM. Surgery of umbilical hernia with reconstruction of an artificial umbilicus. Q Bull Northwest Univ Med Sch. 1955;29(4):379–82.
3. Iida N, Ohsumi N. Reconstruction of umbilical hypogenesis accompanied by a longitudinal scar. Plast Reconstr Surg. 2003;111:322–5.
4. Itoh Y, Arai K. Umbilical reconstruction using a cone-shaped flap. Ann Plast Surg. 1992;28:335–8.
5. Marconi F. Reconstruction of the umbilicus: a simple technique. Plast Reconstr Surg. 1995;95:1115–7.
6. Shinohara H, Matsuo K, Kikuchi N. Umbilical reconstruction with an inverted C–V flap. Plast Reconstr Surg. 2000;105:703–5.
7. Yotsuyanagi T, Nihei Y, Sawada Y. A simple technique for reconstruction of the umbilicus, using two twisted flaps. Plast Reconstr Surg. 1998;102:2444–6.
8. Lee SL, DuBois JJ, Greenholz SK, Huffman SG. Advancement flap umbilicoplasty after abdominal wall closure: post-operative results compared with normal umbilical anatomy. J Pediatr Surg. 2001;36:1168–70.
9. Borges AF. Reconstruction of the umbilicus. Br J Plast Surg. 1975;28:75–6.
10. Miller MJ, Balch CM. 'Iris' technique for immediate umbilical reconstruction. Plast Reconstr Surg. 1993;92:754–6.
11. Feyaerts A, Mure PY, Jules JA, Morel-Journel N, Mouriquand P. Umbilical reconstruction in patients with exstrophy: the kangaroo pouch technique. J Urol. 2001;165:2026–7.
12. Sugawara Y, Hirabayashi S, Asato H, Yoshimura K. Reconstruction of the umbilicus using a single triangular flap. Ann Plast Surg. 1995;34:78–80.
13. Baack BR, Anson G, Nachbar JM, White DJ. Umbilicoplasty: the construction of a new umbilicus and correction of umbilical stenosis without external scars. Plast Reconstr Surg. 1996;97:227–32.
14. Jamra FA. Reconstruction of the umbilicus by a double V–Y procedure. Plast Reconstr Surg. 1979;64:106–7.
15. Onishi K, Yang YL, Maruyama Y. A new lunch box-type method in umbilical reconstruction. Ann Plast Surg. 1995;35:654–6.
16. Matsuo K, Kondoh S, Hirose T. A simple technique for reconstruction of the umbilicus, using a conchal cartilage composite graft. Plast Reconstr Surg. 1990;86:149–51.
17. Bartsich SA, Schwartz MH. Purse-string method for immediate umbilical reconstruction. Plast Reconstr Surg. 2003;112:1652–5.
18. Pfulg M, Van de Sijpe K, Blondeel P. A simple new technique for neo-umbilicoplasty. Br J Plast Surg. 2005;58:688–91.
19. Koshy CE, Taams KO. Umbilicoplasty. Plast Reconstr Surg. 1999;104:1203–4.
20. Dubou R, Ousterhout DK. Placement of the umbilicus in an abdominoplasty. Plast Reconstr Surg. 1978;61:291–3.

Chapter 29
The Double-Opposing "Y" Technique for Umbilicoplasty in Abdominoplasty and for Umbilical Reconstruction After Omphalectomy

Luca A. Dessy and Marco Mazzocchi

29.1 Introduction

The abdomen plays a leading role in the aesthetic image of the upright human body, and the umbilicus is an important structure for both aesthetic and symbolic standpoints. The umbilicus defines the median abdominal sulcus and contributes to the curved shape of the inferior abdomen. Its absence leads to an unnatural abdominal appearance and an abnormally shaped or misplaced umbilicus may draw undue attention to the central abdomen.

The umbilicus is embryonic in origin and is prone to give rise to poor-quality scars. The umbilicus itself has been described as a depressed scar surrounded by a natural skin fold that measures 1.5–2 cm in diameter and lies anatomically within the midline at the level of the superior iliac crests, 10–12 cm superior to the pubic hairline [1, 2]. Its shape is quite variable, either round or oval, depending on the postnatal scarring of the umbilical cord. It is generally flat and vertically oriented in younger individual, and, later, it develops hooding and deepening of the stalk as fat accumulates along the deep fat pocket around the umbilicus [3, 4]. A transverse orientation generally occurs with aging in combination with weight gain, contributing to a deeper umbilical stalk and an overall widened appearance [5]. Commonly, a wide and deep umbilicus or an exceedingly small umbilicus is considered unattractive. The presence of outward protrusion is also considered unappealing [1].

L.A. Dessy, M.D., Ph.D. (✉)
Department of Plastic and Reconstructive Surgery, Sapienza University of Rome, Via Irpinia 8, Assemini (CA), 09032, Italy
e-mail: lucadessy@hotmail.com

M. Mazzocchi, M.D.
Department of Surgery and Biomedical Science, Section of Plastic Surgery, University of Perugia, Via S. Andrea delle Fratte, Perugia 06100, Italy
e-mail: mazzocc@mclink.it

M.A. Shiffman (ed.), *Adult Umbilical Reconstruction*,
DOI 10.1007/978-3-319-43887-0_29

Appealing characteristics include a moderately small umbilical size with an overall vertical orientation.

Since the development of abdominoplasty to treat redundant skin and fatty tissues of the abdomen, there has been a continuing evolution in the performance of umbilical reposition or reconstruction. The goal of umbilical repositioning is to create natural-looking morphology and minimal residual scars, achieving an aesthetically pleasing result [6]. No single type of umbilicoplasty has had completely satisfied these aesthetic targets.

Many surgical procedures have been described to reposition the umbilicus during abdominal dermolipectomy. Some authors have proposed the use of different types of cutaneous incisions to improve the reconstructed umbilical shape and to disguise the periumbilical scar. Others have advised the use of skin graft, local flaps, or conchal cartilage composite graft to recreate the anatomical shape of the umbilicus [7–26].

The majority of the existing procedures propose a circular incision of the umbilical cone to release it from its original position. This procedure inevitably leads to the retraction of the circular incision and to the stenosis of the neo-umbilical depressed scar; moreover, the scars may be quite evident with these techniques [7]. The use of a cutaneous incision with a "Y" or a "double-Y" shape has improved the aesthetic result and has demonstrated less scarring in the umbilical region [25, 26].

In this chapter, we describe a modified versatile technique for umbilicoplasty using a double-opposing "Y" cutaneous incision on the abdominal skin to reproduce the shape of the umbilicus in all patients candidates for abdominoplasty requiring umbilical repositioning or reconstruction [27–29].

29.2 Surgical Technique

In case of umbilical repositioning, the first step is to isolate the umbilicus. The skin is sharply incised in a vertical elliptical shape, taking care to keep a small skin island around the umbilical scar. Once the cutaneous incision is made, the skin is detached at the lowest level, releasing the umbilicus. Minimal fat is included in the umbilical pedicle to preserve the adventitial blood supply. After the abdominal musculofascial plication, if diastasis of rectus muscles required it, the umbilical dermis is attached to the abdominal rectus fascia superiorly, inferiorly, and on both the lateral sides with absorbable sutures (poliglecaprone 25 4/0). These sutures ensure replacement of the umbilicus in the abdominal midline, pull the scar deeply within the umbilicus, and create depth and vertical orientation. The suture bite between the dermis of the umbilicus and the rectus fascia depends on the adipose panniculus thickness, and it is easily varied. In patients with a thin habitus, it is important to plicate the periumbilical fascia sufficiently to create an inverted umbilicus. The umbilical stalk is embedded during the plication of the abdominal fascia. The elliptical umbilical island is tightened against the tensed abdominal fascia without distortion. The site of umbilicus repositioning in the abdominal flap is

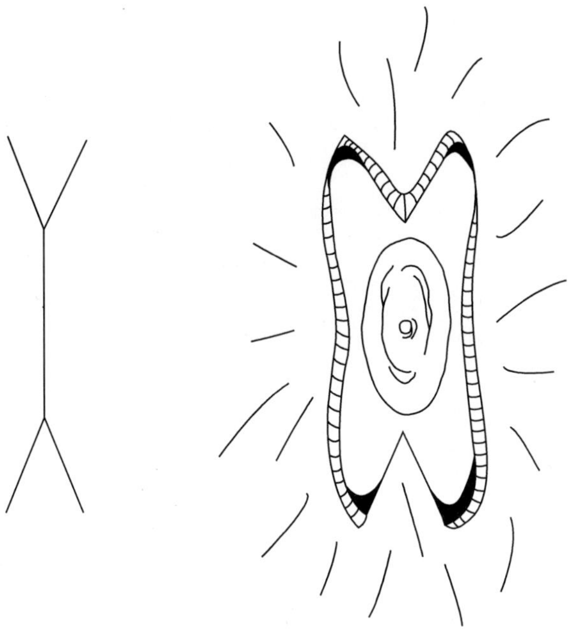

Fig. 29.1 Double-Y cutaneous mark on the abdominal wall: the vertical size must be approximately the same of the original umbilicus; the angle and the size of the four lateral incisions can be modified according to the width we want to obtain

determined by the projection of the original umbilicus. A xipho-pubic line is marked. With one hand beneath the abdominal flap on the tightened umbilicus and the other hand on the abdominal flap, the correct position of the new umbilicus on the abdominal flap is determined. A small double-opposing "Y" cutaneous incision is made in this point (Fig. 29.1).

A patient may have its umbilicus removed during abdominal surgical procedures, such as the repair of ventral incisional hernias. When umbilical reconstruction is required, after the elevation of the adipocutaneous superior abdominal flap and after the repair of eventual ventral incisional hernias requiring omphalectomy (if umbilical reconstruction is performed at the same time), the site of the new umbilicus reconstruction is determined by obtaining on the tensed abdominal flap the crossing point between two lines, the vertical xipho-pubic line and the horizontal line traced above the anterosuperior iliac spines. A small double-opposing "Y" cutaneous incision is made in this point (Figs. 29.1 and 29.2).

The vertical size of the united limbs of the opposing "Y" must be approximately the same of the original umbilicus; the angle and the size of the four lateral incisions can be modified according to the width we want to obtain. Defatting is performed through the vertical incision, which allows easy visualization of the umbilicus. It is important to defat an area 2–3 cm surrounding the umbilicus (Fig. 29.2). This can be done through the double-opposing "Y" incision.

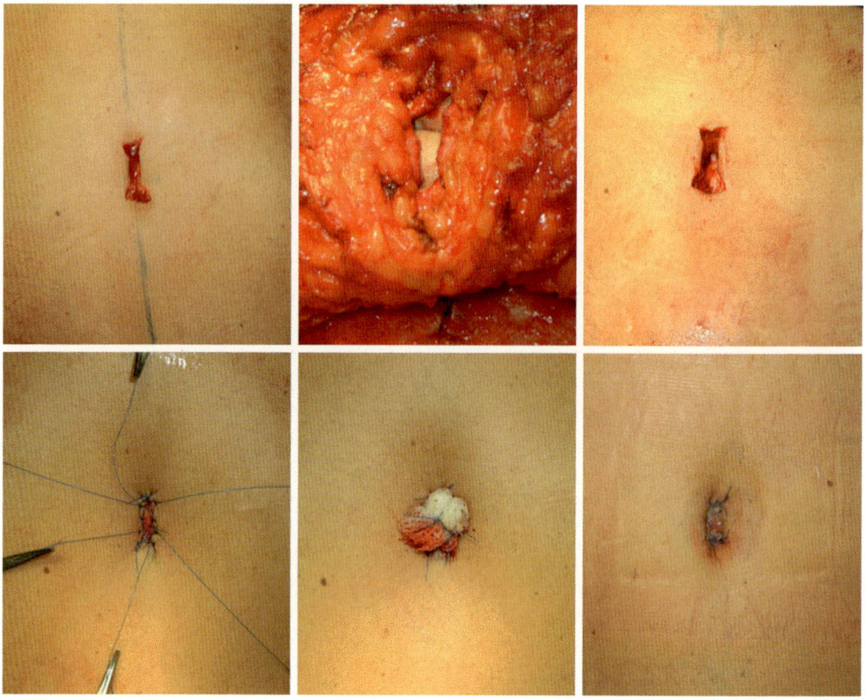

Fig. 29.2 Umbilical reconstruction. (*Top left*) Double-Y cutaneous incision on the abdominal wall. (*Top center*) Defatting. (*Top right*) Double-Y cutaneous incision after defatting. (*Bottom left*) Margins of the double-opposing "Y" incision are sutured to the abdominal fascia with no absorbable sutures leaving a small elliptical and vertically oriented area of uncovered fascia corresponding to the umbilical hollow (nylon 4/0). (*Bottom center*) Dressing with paraffin gauze. (*Bottom right*) Neo-umbilicus 1 week after surgery

Two drains are placed under the tailored abdominal flap, and the lower abdominal wound is sutured in a tension-free position.

In case of umbilical repositioning, the umbilical skin is sutured to the surrounding abdominal skin with no absorbable sutures of nylon 4/0 (Fig. 29.3). In case of umbilical reconstruction, the margins of the double-opposing "Y" incision are sutured to the abdominal fascia with no absorbable sutures of nylon 4/0 leaving a small elliptical and vertically oriented area of uncovered fascia corresponding to the umbilical hollow (Figs. 29.2 and 36.4). Four of these sutures are left longer and tied over a paraffin gauze patch to ensure deep umbilicus positioning (Fig. 29.4).

29.3 Discussion

The umbilicus is the most important aesthetic component of the abdominal wall; it requires optimal reconstruction during abdominoplasty because the umbilical scar is the only visible mark that can disclose a performed abdominoplasty. The

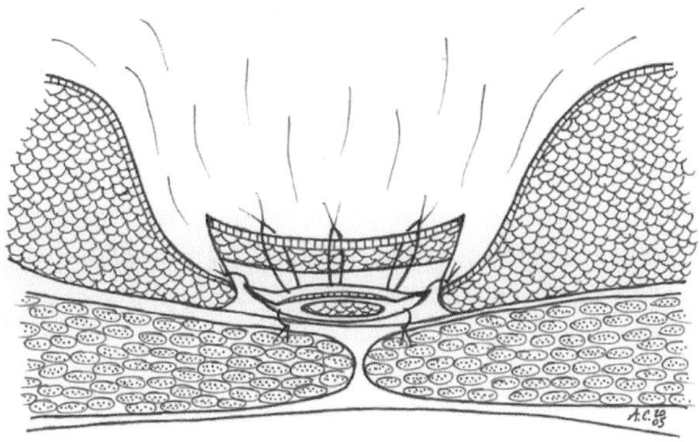

Fig. 29.3 Section of a repositioned umbilicus: the umbilical dermis is attached to the abdominal rectus fascia superiorly, inferiorly, and on both the lateral sides with absorbable sutures (poliglecaprone 25 4/0)

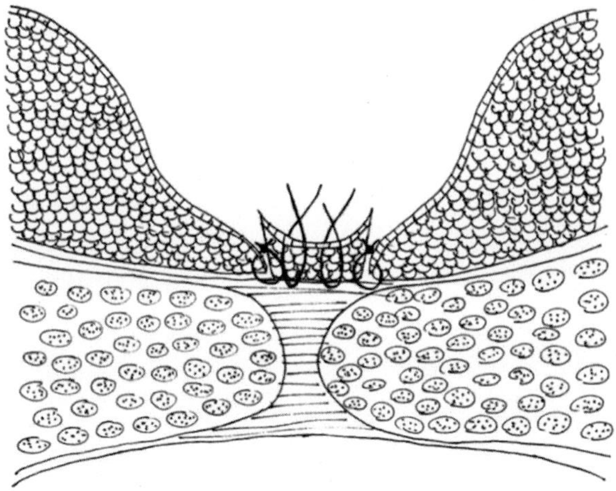

Fig. 29.4 Section of a neo-umbilicus: the margins of the double-opposing "Y" skin flaps are directly sutured to the abdominal rectus fascia superiorly, inferiorly, and on both the lateral sides with no absorbable sutures (nylon 4/0)

umbilicus represents the only natural scar on the body; its absence or grotesque shape may be distressing [1]. Until the late 1950s, the umbilicus was routinely discarded during abdominoplasty [30]. This leads to unattractive results and could cause problems such as omphalitis related to material accumulation [6]. Initially, reconstruction techniques resulted in circular scars which tend to contract, causing umbilical stenosis [14]. Various methods have been advocated to prevent a circular periumbilical scar [8, 10, 13, 31–34].

The aesthetic considerations for umbilical repositioning during abdominoplasty are position, depth, shape, and scar location. An anatomic umbilicus should have a normal slant superiorly, a superior hood, a natural shape (cylindrical with a wide attachment to the abdominal wall fascia and a central mamelon), and it should not have any external scars, especially concentric scars around the umbilical ring, which could result in stenosis [30]. Recent evaluation of the ideal umbilicus has shown that youthful and thin individuals have a small and vertically oriented umbilicus, whereas the older or more obese ones have a rounder, transversely oriented and hooded umbilicus [3, 20].

The main idea of creating an aesthetically pleasing umbilicus is to imitate a more natural-looking one in relation to the patient's body type. The evidence of the anatomical variation of umbilical shape supports this. The most common umbilical shape is the T-shaped one, followed by the oval, vertical, and horizontal shapes, respectively [18]. The majority of the women show a superior hood and a small umbilicus without protrusion. Heavier women tend to have a larger and more transversely oriented umbilicus, whereas in thinner women, the umbilicus has a more oval and vertical orientation. Interestingly, the size of a subject's abdomen does not seem to influence umbilical shape [18].

Our modified technique combines different well-known principles: an elliptical vertical excision of the old umbilicus, a firm suture of the umbilicus to the abdominal fascia, and a double-opposing "Y" cutaneous incision of the abdominal flap. This procedure creates umbilical depth, ensures optimal position, pulls the scar deep in the umbilicus, and allows achieving different shapes according to the skin incision (Figs. 29.5 and 29.6). In fact, increasing the dimension of the residual cutaneous surface of the umbilicus and varying the size of the vertical incision, we can extend or shorten the size of the umbilicus; instead, varying the size and the angle of the four lateral incisions, we can widen or narrow the umbilicus. Any umbilical

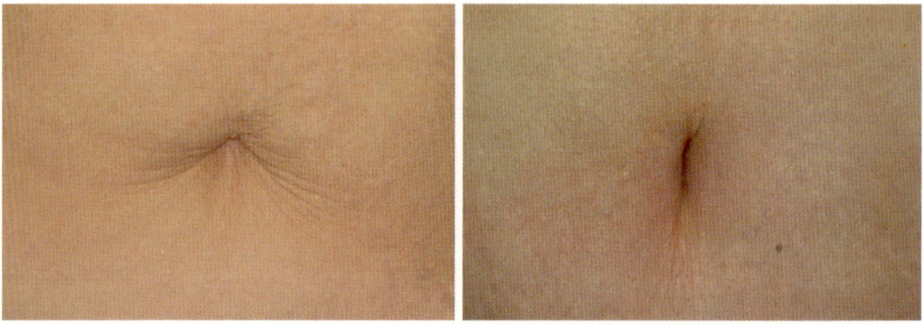

Fig. 29.5 (*Left*) Preoperative umbilicus. (*Right*) Twelve months postoperative after umbilicus repositioning

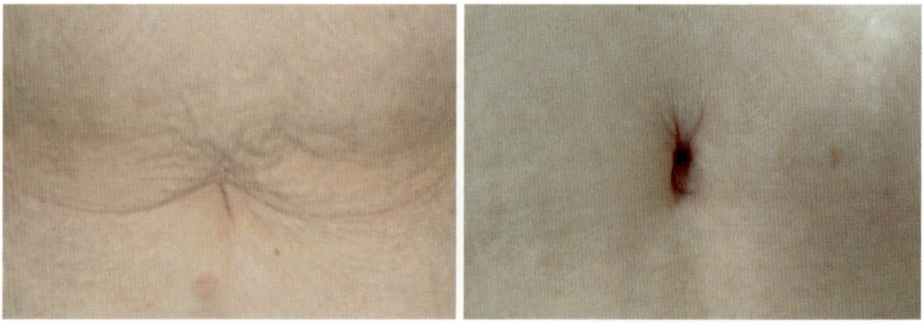

Fig. 29.6 (*Left*) Preoperative umbilicus. (*Right*) Eighteen months postoperative after umbilical reconstruction after laparocele correction

size can be created with this method, and the versatility of this procedure allows to obtain a depressed umbilical scar without any visible scarring on the abdominal skin. This technique can be performed either in obese or thin patients, and different umbilical depths can be created as desired.

Although other methods have been performed to decrease scar visibility, the majority of these methods eventually create a larger round-shaped umbilicus [7, 25]. Others have described suturing of the umbilicus to the superficial muscle fascia; however, they used a sequence of triangular incisions in the abdominal flap that creates a rounder and larger umbilicus [25]. Some techniques are performed without incisions in the abdominal flap [7]; this prevents scars but needs the use of a purse-string suture to recreate the umbilical pattern [7]. The double-opposing "Y" incision in the abdominal flap, compared to circular, half-circular, or triangular incisions, reinforces the vertical orientation of the umbilicus. Defatting the abdominal flap from outside allows easy visualization of the umbilicus, which eliminates the time-consuming and frustrating experience of trying to find the umbilicus after the abdominal flap is positioned and sutured inferiorly.

A variety of techniques have been developed to create hooding of the umbilicus [20]. This hooding may create a natural-looking umbilicus but may leave more superficial and highly visible incisions. The unpredictable nature of the effect of the skin, weight changes, and gravity may modify the position of this artificially created superior fold. Although it is considered natural, hooding is more associated with increased abdominal girth and increased age [33, 34]. It may impair the goal of creating a thinner and more youthful appearance of the abdomen.

29.4 Conclusions

The authors' technique effectively hides scars and produces an appealing umbilicus. The repositioning of the umbilicus is accurate and predictable. The technique is easy to learn and simple to perform and requires no complex skin flaps, cartilage grafts, or difficult suture placement. Additionally, the technique is versatile in abdominoplasty and can be used effectively in different clinical situations, as well as in primary reconstruction of the umbilicus. This technique can be applied to any patient of any build or size. This approach balances the aesthetic issues of shape, depth, scar location, and quality of the umbilicus obtaining a stable result and a youthful and thin appearance of the abdomen.

References

1. Baroudi R. Umbilicoplasty. Clin Plast Surg. 1975;2(3):431–48.
2. Dubou R, Ousterhout DK. Placement of the umbilicus in an abdominoplasty. Plast Reconstr Surg. 1978;61(2):291–3.

3. Psillakis JM, Appiani E, de la Plaza R. Color atlas of aesthetic surgery of the abdomen. New York: Thieme Medical Publishers; 1991. p. 6–7.
4. Markman B, Barton Jr FE. Anatomy of the subcutaneous tissue of the trunk and the lower extremity. Plast Reconstr Surg. 1987;80(2):248–54.
5. Teimourian B, Marefat S. Body contouring with suction-assisted lipectomy. In: Cohen M, editor. Mastery of plastic and reconstructive surgery, vol. 3. Boston: Little Brown; 1994. p. 2186–200.
6. Akbas H, Güneren E, Eroglu L, Uysal OA. Natural-looking umbilicus as an important part of abdominoplasty. Aesthet Plast Surg. 2003;27(2):139–42.
7. Schoeller T, Wechselberger G, Otto A, Rainer C, Schwabegger A, Lille S, Ninković M. New technique for scar less umbilical reinsertion in abdominoplasty procedures. Plast Reconstr Surg. 1998;102(5):1721–3.
8. Delerm A. Refinements in abdominoplasty with emphasis on reimplantation of the umbilicus. Plast Reconstr Surg. 1982;70(5):632–7.
9. Hoffman S. A simple technique for locating the umbilicus in abdominoplasty. Plast Reconstr Surg. 1989;83(3):537–8.
10. Juri J, Juri C, Raiden G. Reconstruction of the umbilicus in abdominoplasty. Plast Reconstr Surg. 1979;63(4):580–2.
11. Kurul S, Uzunismail A. A simple technique to determine the future location of the umbilicus in abdominoplasty. Plast Reconstr Surg. 1997;100(3):753–4.
12. Sugawara Y, Hirabayashi S, Asato H, Yoshimura K. Reconstruction of the umbilicus using a single Triangular flap. Ann Plast Surg. 1995;34(1):78–80.
13. Vernon S. Umbilical transplantation upward and abdominal contouring in lipectomy. Am J Surg. 1957;94(3):490–2.
14. De Lacerda DJ, Martins DM, Marques A, Brenda E, de Moura Andrews J. Umbilicoplasty for the abdomen with a thin adipose layer. Br J Plast Surg. 1994;47(5):386–7.
15. Otto A, Wechselberger G, Schoeller T, Lille S. A method of reconstructing a natural-looking umbilicus in abdominoplasty. Ann Plast Surg. 1997;39:435.
16. Lim TC, Tan WT. Managing the umbilicus during abdominoplasty. Plast Reconstr Surg. 1996;98:1113.
17. Miller MJ, Balch CM. "Iris" technique for immediate umbilical reconstruction. Plast Reconstr Surg. 1993;92:754.
18. Craig SB, Faller MS, Puckett CL. In search of the ideal female umbilicus. Plast Reconstr Surg. 2000;105:389.
19. Masud R, Takeda A, Sugimoto T, et al. Reconstruction of the umbilicus using a reverse fan-shaped flap. Aesthet Plast Surg. 2003;27:349.
20. Lee MJ, Mustoe TA. Simplified technique for creating a youthful umbilicus in abdominoplasty. Plast Reconstr Surg. 2002;109:2136.
21. Iida N, Ohsumi N. Reconstruction of umbilical hypogenesis accompanied by a longitudinal scar. Plast Reconstr Surg. 2003;111:322.
22. Niranjan NS, Staiano JJ. An anatomical method for re-sitting the umbilicus. Plast Reconstr Surg. 2004;113:2194.
23. Ramirez OM. Abdominoplasty and abdominal wall rehabilitation: a comprehensive approach. Plast Reconstr Surg. 2000;105:425.
24. Santanelli F, Mazzocchi M, Renzi L, Cigna E. Reconstruction of a natural-looking umbilicus. Scand J Plast Reconstr Surg Hand Surg. 2002;36(3):183.
25. Masshida H, Montegut W, Phillips R. A method of reconstructing a natural-looking umbilicus in Abdominoplasty. Ann Plast Surg. 1997;38:228.
26. Cannistrà C, Pecorelli E. Umbilical restoration in Abdominal dermolipectomy: a simple double-Y, double-M technique. Aesthetic Plast Surg. 1999;23:364.
27. Mazzocchi M, Dessy LA, Figus A. A versatile technique for repositioning of the umbilicus in abdominoplasty. Plast Reconstr Surg. 2008;121(5):357e–8.

28. Mazzocchi M, Trignano E, Armenti AF, Figus A, Dessy LA. Long-term results of a versatile technique for umbilicoplasty in abdominoplasty. Aesthet Plast Surg. 2011;5(4):456–62.
29. Dessy LA, Fallico N, Trignano E, Tarallo M, Mazzocchi M. The double opposing "Y" technique for umbilical reconstruction after omphalectomy. Ann Ital Chir. 2011;82(6):505–10.
30. Baack BR, Anson G, Nachbar JM, White DJ. Umbilicoplasty: the construction of a new umbilicus and correction of umbilical stenosis without external scars. Plast Reconstr Surg. 1996;97:227.
31. Avelar JM. Abdominoplasty: technical refinement and analysis of 130 cases in 8 years' follow-up. Aesthet Plast Surg. 1983;7:205.
32. Matsuo K, Kondoh S, Hirose T. A simple technique for reconstruction of the umbilicus, using a conchal cartilage composite graft. Plast Reconstr Surg. 1990;86:149.
33. Ribeiro L, Muzy S, Accorsi A. Omphaloplasty. Ann Plast Surg. 1991;27:457.
34. Pitanguy I. Abdominal lipectomy: an approach to it through an analysis of 300 consecutive cases. Plast Reconstr Surg. 1967;40:384.

Chapter 30
Umbilical Reconstruction for Patients with Midline Scars

Diogo Franco, João Medeiros, and Talita Franco

30.1 Introduction

Numerous techniques have been described for umbilical reconstruction using grafts or local flaps [1–16], some with interesting results [5, 14, 16, 17]. There are different opinions on what a normal umbilicus should look like [2, 4, 7, 10, 12, 18]. Restoring the original appearance and minimizing the stigma resulting from previous procedures are the main goals. The ideal would be to achieve them with a minimum of scarring.

The indication for a neo-umbilicoplasty can vary from total [5, 11, 13, 18, 19] to previous surgery sequelae or bariatric surgery [1–4, 6–10, 12, 15–17, 19–21].

Through to the late 1980s, vertical scars on the abdominal wall were relatively common, due mainly to cholecystectomies. The introduction of laparoscopic surgery, which was quickly accepted worldwide, significantly reduced the number of such scars. However, during the 1990s, the development of bariatric surgery for fast weight loss purposes resulted in the appearance of patients with extreme levels of flaccidity not found in those losing weight more slowly. These patients began to accept and even demand more extensive cutaneous resections, showing little concern for large scars, provided that the flaccidity was corrected. For abdominoplasties, the low horizontal scars that were the usual aesthetic standard ceased to be satisfactory because they did not resolve vertical flaccidity. The rule thus became a vertical midline cut associated with a horizontal suprapubic incision. The dermal-adipose resections needed to correct massive amounts of excess skin after bariatric surgery resuscitated the anchor-shaped incisions that had largely dropped out of use and now were returning to a greater extent.

D. Franco, M.D., M.A., Ph.D. (✉) • J. Medeiros, M.D., M.A., Ph.D.
T. Franco, M.D., M.A., Ph.D.
Plastic Surgery Department, Federal University of Rio de Janeiro (UFRJ),
Rua Ramon Franco, 98 – Urca, Rio de Janeiro Cep 22290-290, Brazil
e-mail: contato@diogofranco.com; clinicajoaomedeiros@gmail.com; talita@openlink.com.br

M.A. Shiffman (ed.), *Adult Umbilical Reconstruction*,
DOI 10.1007/978-3-319-43887-0_30

Once again produced quite frequently, vertical abdominal scars may broaden or become hypertrophic, with the umbilicus exteriorized through them not contributing to an improved appearance.

Paradoxically, the existence of a vertical scar justifies a vertical elliptical resection, paving the way for shaping an umbilicus with an excellent appearance that is even better than those resulting from traditional omphaloplasties, as it avoids the usual surrounding scar.

In navel reconstructions on patients with a previous midline scar, we use the technique described by Franco [22].

30.2 Operating Technique

The existence of large longitudinal midline scars, such as those left after intra-cavity abdominal operations, or areas with poor vascularization at the new umbilicus site recommends the resection of these areas or scars and the use of lateral-pediculated rectangular flaps for neo-omphaloplasties. This allows the surgeon to work with better-vascularized tissues, eliminating or reducing previous scars by bringing them to the midline and adjusting the depth of the new umbilicus through the size of the flaps. This is a simple procedure with an easy learning curve.

The incision consists of an elliptical cut surrounding the existing scars but preserving two small rectangular skin flaps pediculated on the edges of the incision, one on each side at the ideal height for positioning the umbilicus. It is recommended that the flaps consist of scar-free skin. These flaps are sutured to each other, forming a small tube whose extremity, after inversion, will be fixed to the aponeurotic plane through three or four mononylon 4-0 sutures (Figs. 30.1 and 30.2).

The extent of the previous vertical scar resection will depend on the presence of hernias or requests for improvement in its appearance (Fig. 30.3).

The rest of the vertical abdominal incision is sutured in three planes, as usual in an abdominoplasty. It is convenient to leave a small gauze plug in the neo-formed umbilical cavity that will assist with the adaptation of the tubular flap to the deeper planes, also avoiding adherence between the sutured edges. This plug will be changed every day until the sutures are removed, with no areas of the wound left open.

The resection of the previous scar and the preparation of the umbilicus with lateral pedicle flaps obtained from fibrosis-free areas endow the abdominal tissues with greater flexibility while lessening the possibility of vascular difficulties. This technique also offers other advantages:

1. Provides an umbilical cavity with a good depth. The dimensions of the flap and consequently the depth of the umbilicus will be adapted to the thickness of the adipose panicle, being longer in overweight patients and shorter in thin patients.
2. Results in a neo-umbilicus without a surrounding scar, reducing the possibilities of postoperative shrinkage and stenosis.

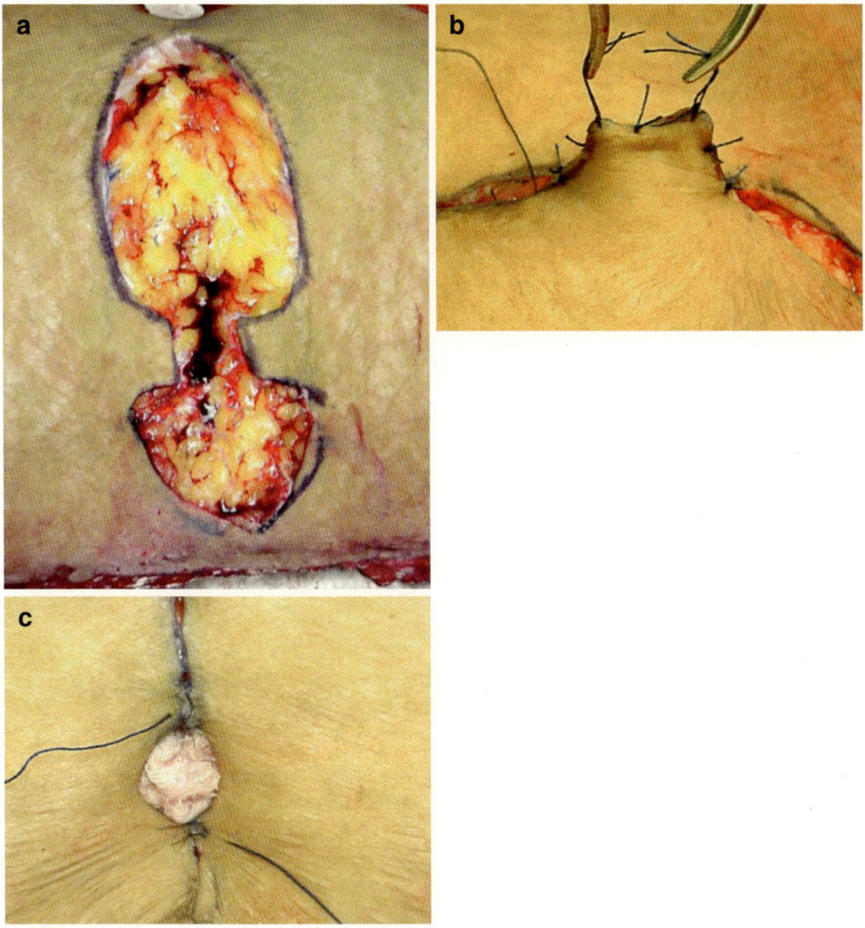

Fig. 30.1 (**a**) Maintenance of lateral cutaneous flaps after excision of previous scar. (**b**) Traction of sutured flaps shows the depth of the new navel. These flaps will be inverted and fixed to the aponeurosis. (**c**) Packing of the reconstructed cavity is recommended until suture removal

3. Interrupts tension along the vertical scar, which is less likely to become hypertrophic, with a better appearance.

This technique is not restricted to neo-omphaloplasties. It can and must be used even for viable umbilicus, provided that the pedicle is shortened and its circumference reduced enough to allow acceptance of the two cross flaps sutured together (Fig. 30.4).

Patients with paramedian scars from previous operations should not undergo abdominoplasties only through low transverse incision, due to the risk of tissue necrosis between the scar and the midline, where vascularization is poor, in addition to the tension imposed after flap resection. Such operations must begin with a vertical resection that brings the scar to the midline (aesthetically better position),

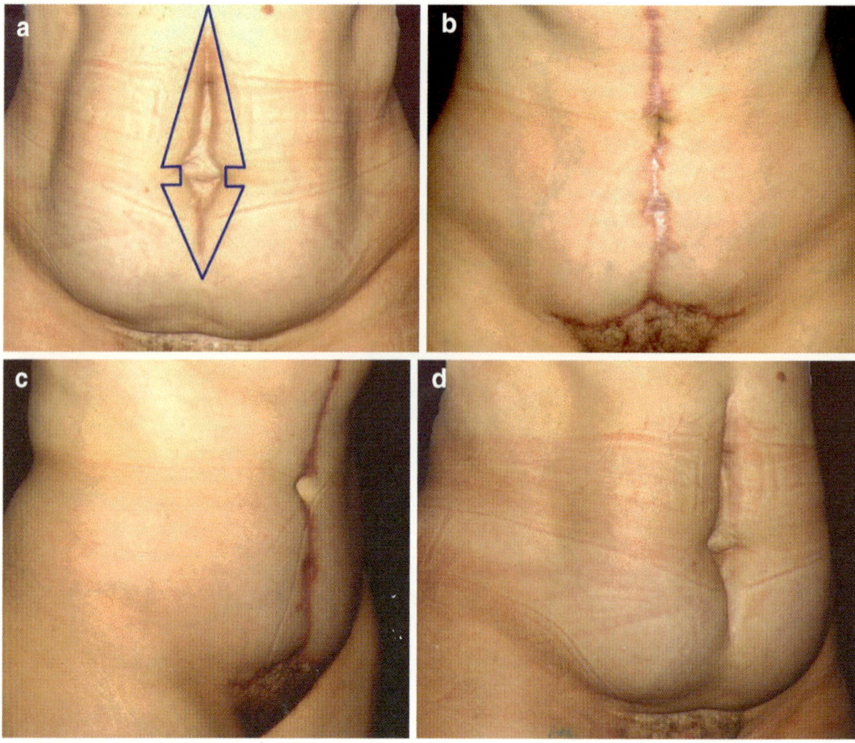

Fig. 30.2 (**a**) Preoperative abdominal scar surgical review. Note the marking of cutaneous flaps for umbilical reconstruction. (**b**) 6-month postoperative. In spite of the salient poor quality scar the reconstructed umbilicus has a good appearance. (**c**) Preoperative oblique view. (**d**) Postoperative

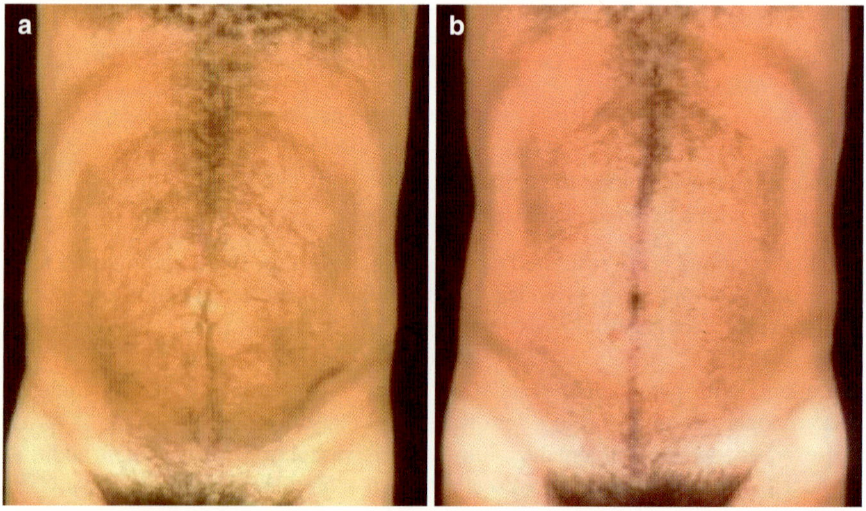

Fig. 30.3 (**a**) Preoperative umbilical hernia correction and abdominal scar revision. (**b**) One year postoperative

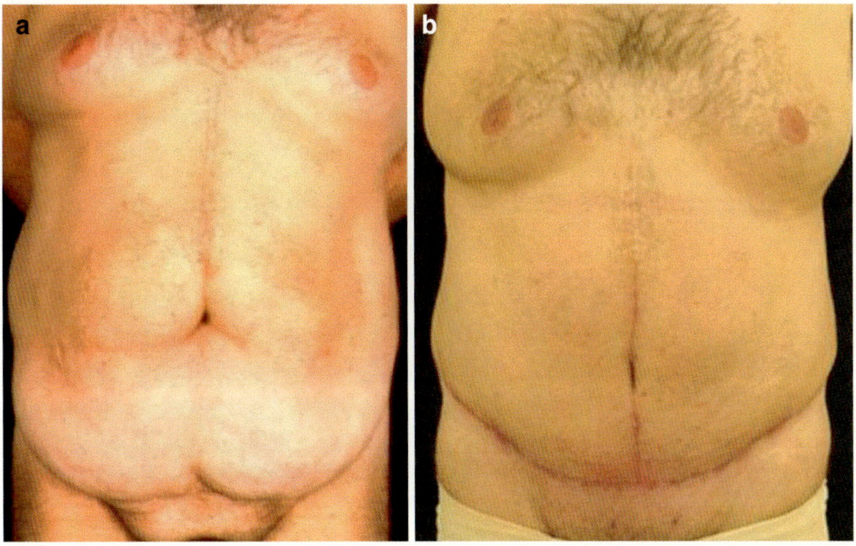

Fig. 30.4 (**a**) Preoperative after bariatric surgery. (**b**) Four months after abdominoplasty and umbilical hernia correction

allowing a neo-umbilicus to be created with the two cross flaps and reducing the length of the suprapubic transverse segment, which is only required if horizontal cutaneous excesses still remains (Fig. 30.5).

30.3 Discussion

Few body areas have prompted as much interest among plastic surgeons as the abdominal wall. Even before medical specialties were established, surgeons aware of the importance of appearance and body comfort tried to correct abdominal deformities, stimulated perhaps because more discreet clothing at that time kept scars better hidden, allowing them to "experiment" with different types of incisions. When umbilical hernias were present, they did not hesitate to resect the umbilicus, together with excess tissue.

More demanding patients wearing more revealing clothes began to safeguard the umbilicus, with resection accepted only in very special cases. Countless techniques appeared for omphaloplasties during abdominoplasties, as well as for neo-omphaloplasties in case of the loss or absence of the umbilicus. The authors of this chapter alone have several publications on the umbilicus, with countless others found in the literature, indicating that there is no unanimity of choice [22–26].

As mentioned in the introduction, two new procedures influenced umbilical techniques and abdominoplasties: video laparotomy, which lessened the need for large incisions, and bariatric surgery, which reintroduced large scars (and not only on the abdomen) in order to correct extreme levels of flaccidity.

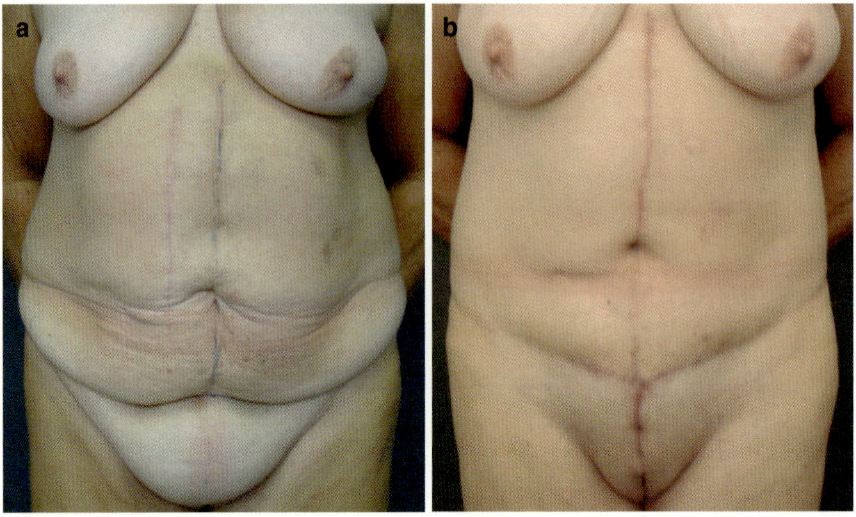

Fig. 30.5 (**a**) Preoperative after bariatric surgery. Note the paramedian scar. (**b**) Eight months after abdominoplasty

Technological development filtered surgical techniques and tactics, leading to the return of some types of conduct that had apparently fallen into disuse. This was what happened with vertical incisions in the abdominal wall, retrieved through post-bariatric abdominoplasties. As a basic principle, plastic surgeons always try to hide their scars, although they are willing to minimize this principle in exchange for significantly improved body shape.

The resection of a vertical dermal-adipose spindle is intended to remove surplus tissues that the traditional low transverse incision abdominoplasty is unable to handle effectively, in addition to helping define the waist more sharply. As an auxiliary advantage, it allows an umbilicus to be created with a good depth without a surrounding scar. The two cross flaps that will form the umbilicus also improve the quality of the long vertical scar, which is interrupted, lessening tension on fibrous tissue.

Although uncommon, paramedian abdominal scars may still be found today. If abdominoplasty is indicated for aesthetic or reconstructive reasons, the vertical elliptical resection encompassing the preexisting scar is to be recommended. The narrow strip of tissue between the scar and the midline is an area with poor vascularization that might be unable to withstand the wide undermining of the abdominal flap, together with the suture tension after excess skin resection. Furthermore, repositioning the scar along the midline is an aesthetic advantage, with the vertical skin resection contributing to better waist definition and allowing the construction of a neo-umbilicus through the technique described above.

References

1. Abenavoli FM, Cusano V, Cucchiara V, D'Amico C, Corvelli L. An idea for umbilicus reconstruction. Ann Plast Surg. 2001;46:194.
2. Baack B, Anson G, Nachbar J, White D. Umbilicoplasty: the construction of a new umbilicus and correction of umbilical stenosis without external scars. Plast Reconstr Surg. 1996;97:227–32.
3. Breuninger H. Navel reconstruction after umbilical melanoma excision. Eur J Plast Surg. 1997;20:325–7.
4. El-Dessouki NI, Shehata SM, Torki AM, Hashish AA. Double half-cone flap umbilicoplasty: a new technique for the proboscoid umbilical hernia in children. Hernia. 2004;8:182–5.
5. Feyaerts A, Mure PV, Jules JA, Morel-Journel N, Mouriquand P. Umbilical reconstruction in patients with exstrophy: the kangaroo pouch technique. J Urol. 2001;165:2026–7.
6. Iida N, Ohsumi N. Reconstruction of umbilical hypogenesis accompanied by a longitudinal scar. Plast Reconstr Surg. 2003;111:322–5.
7. Kajikawa A, Ueda K, Suzuki Y, Ohkouchi M. A new umbilicoplasty for children: creating a longitudinal deep umbilical depression. Br J Plast Surg. 2004;57:741–8.
8. Korachi A, Oudit D, Ellabban M. A simplified technique for umbilical reconstruction. Plast Reconstr Surg. 2004;114:619–21.
9. Masuda R, Takeda A, Sugimoto T, Ishiguro M, Uchinuma E. Reconstruction of the umbilicus using a reverse fan-shaped flap. Aesthetic Plast Surg. 2003;27:349–53.
10. Ozbek S, Ozcan M. Umbilicus reconstruction with modified "unfolded cylinder" technique. Br J Plast Surg. 2005;58:500–3.
11. Park S, Hata Y, Ito O, Tokioka K, Kagawa K. Umbilical reconstruction after repair of omphalocele and gastroschisis. Plast Reconstr Surg. 1999;104:204–7.
12. Pfulg M, Van de Sijpe K, Blondeel P. A simple technique for neo-umbilicoplasty. Br J Plast Surg. 2005;58:688–91.
13. Pinto PA, Stock JÁ, Hanna MK. Results of umbilicoplasty for bladder exstrophy. J Urol. 2000;164:2055–7.
14. Sankale AA, Ngom G, Fall I, Coulibaly NF, Ndove M. Umbilical reconstruction in children. Prospective report of 77 cases. Ann Chir Plast Esthet. 2004;49:17–23.
15. Sawada Y. A method of umbilical reconstruction. Eur J Plast Surg. 1986;9:75–6.
16. Sawada Y. An umbilical reconstruction using subcutaneous pedicle flap. Eur J Plast Surg. 1995;18:185–7.
17. Tamir G, Kurzbart E. Umbilical reconstruction after repair of a large umbilical hernia: the lazy-M and omega flaps. J Pediatr Surg. 2004;39:226–8.
18. Shinohara H, Matsuo K, Kikuchi N. Umbilical reconstruction with an inverted C-V flap. Plast Reconstr Surg. 2000;105:703–5.
19. Bartsich S, Schwartz M. Purse-string method for immediate umbilical reconstruction. Plast Reconstr Surg. 2003;112:1652–5.
20. Schoeller T, Rainer C, Wechselberger G, Piza-Katzer H. Immediate navel reconstruction after total excision: a simple three-suture technique. Surgery. 2002;131:105–7.
21. Yotsuyanagi T, Nikei Y, Sawada Y. A simple technique for reconstruction of the umbilicus, using two twisted flaps. Plast Reconstr Surg. 1998;102:2444–6.
22. Franco D, Medeiros J, Farias C, Franco T. Umbilical reconstruction for patients with a midline scar. Aesthetic Plast Surg. 2006;30:595–8.
23. Franco T, Franco D. Neoomphaloplasty: an old and new technique. Aesthetic Plast Surg. 1999;23:151–4.
24. Franco T, Ferreira da Silva R. Onfaloplastias e neo-onfaloplastias. Folha Med. 1973;67:1047–73.
25. Franco T, Boghossian LC, Silva ALB. Neo-onfaloplastia. Rev Bras Cir. 1985;75:257–60.
26. Tavares Filho JM, Franco D, Franco T. Umbilico e Neoumbilicoplastias Tratado de Cirurgia Plástica após grandes perdas ponderais. São Paulo: Atheneu; 2010. p. 175–87.

Chapter 31
Reconstruction of the Umbilicus Using Rectangular-Shaped Skin Island Flaps

Ken Yamashita, Takatoshi Yotsuyanagi, and Koshiro Arai

31.1 Introduction

The umbilicus can be lost due to surgery for congenital diseases, excision of tumors, and sometimes trauma. Although the umbilicus has no function, it is an important landmark of the abdominal wall, and the absence of the umbilicus has strange impression. Therefore, there have been many reports about reconstruction of the umbilicus. However, reports on reconstruction after tumor removal including the umbilicus are rare. Most reported methods use adjacent skin and are therefore not suitable for a large defect.

The authors describe their reconstructive technique for a large defect including umbilicus and surrounding skin.

31.2 Technique (Figs. 31.1 and 31.2)

After the tumor has been excised, a spindle shape with the same width as that of the defect is made. The longer axis of the spindle should be located on the midline of the trunk even if the defect is shifted in any way from the midline. Then two rectangular-shaped subcutaneous pedicle flaps are made at the cranial and caudal sides of the adjacent skin of the defect. These flaps should be made inside the

K. Yamashita, M.D., Ph.D. (✉) • T. Yotsuyanagi, M.D. Ph.D.
Department of Plastic and Reconstructive Surgery, Sapporo Medical University School of Medicine, 291 S1W16 Chuo-ku, Sapporo, Hokkaido 0608543, Japan
e-mail: yama-ken@sapmed.ac.jp; yamaken@ck9.so-net.ne.jp

K. Arai, M.D.
Department of Plastic and Reconstructive Surgery, Otaru General Hospital, 1-1-1 Wakamatsu 0478550, Otaru, Hokkaido, Japan

M.A. Shiffman (ed.), *Adult Umbilical Reconstruction*,
DOI 10.1007/978-3-319-43887-0_31

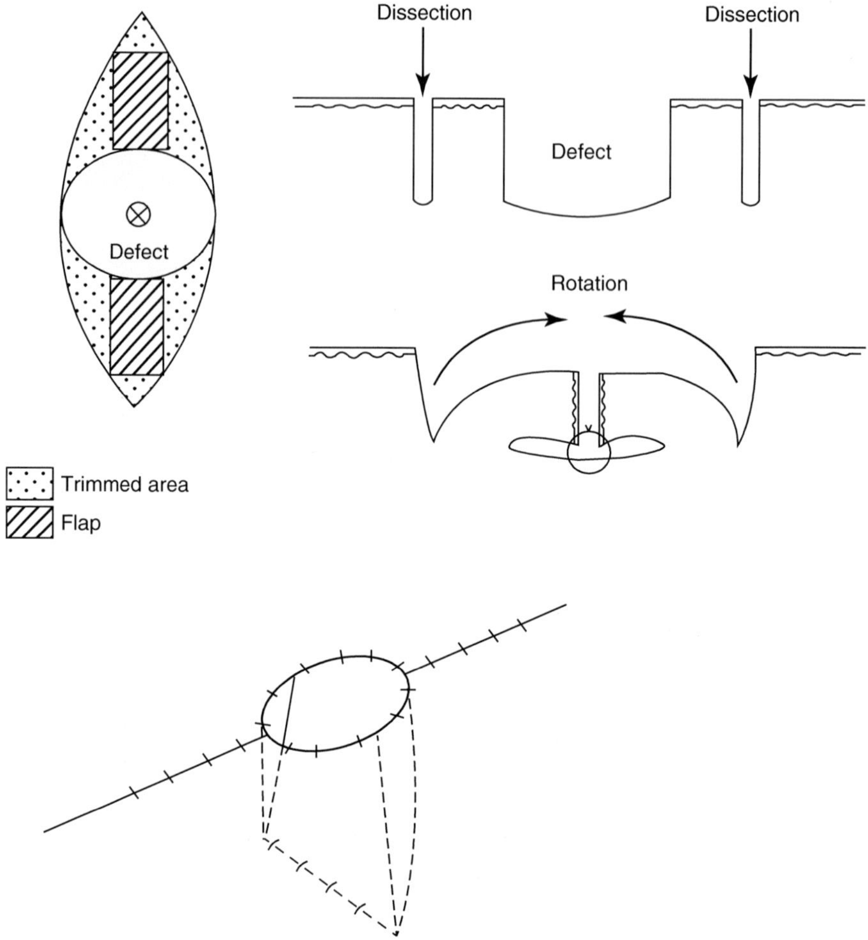

Fig. 31.1 Schematic diagrams of our technique. (*Top left*) Design of the flaps. Flaps should be made inside the dog-ear. (*Top right*) Both flaps are rotated down ventrally, and skin edges are tucked down to the bottom. (*Bottom*) Immediate postoperative

spindle area, which should be removed as a dog-ear, with almost the same sizes. Then the flaps are elevated with care taken not to injure the pedicle. The pedicle should include as much volume of subcutaneous tissue as possible with a perpendicular incision along the flaps, so that the blood supply of the flaps is enough with the penetrating vessels from abdominal fascia. The flaps are rotated down ventrally, and both edges of the flaps are sutured to each other. A skin tube is formed to be used as the lateral wall of the umbilicus. The edges are also tucked down to the rectus fascia tightly at the designed umbilical position. It is better to create a slightly smaller and deeper size as a normal umbilicus. Finally, the skin defect is closed primarily in the midline. The newly formed umbilicus has a sufficient depth with a natural appearance.

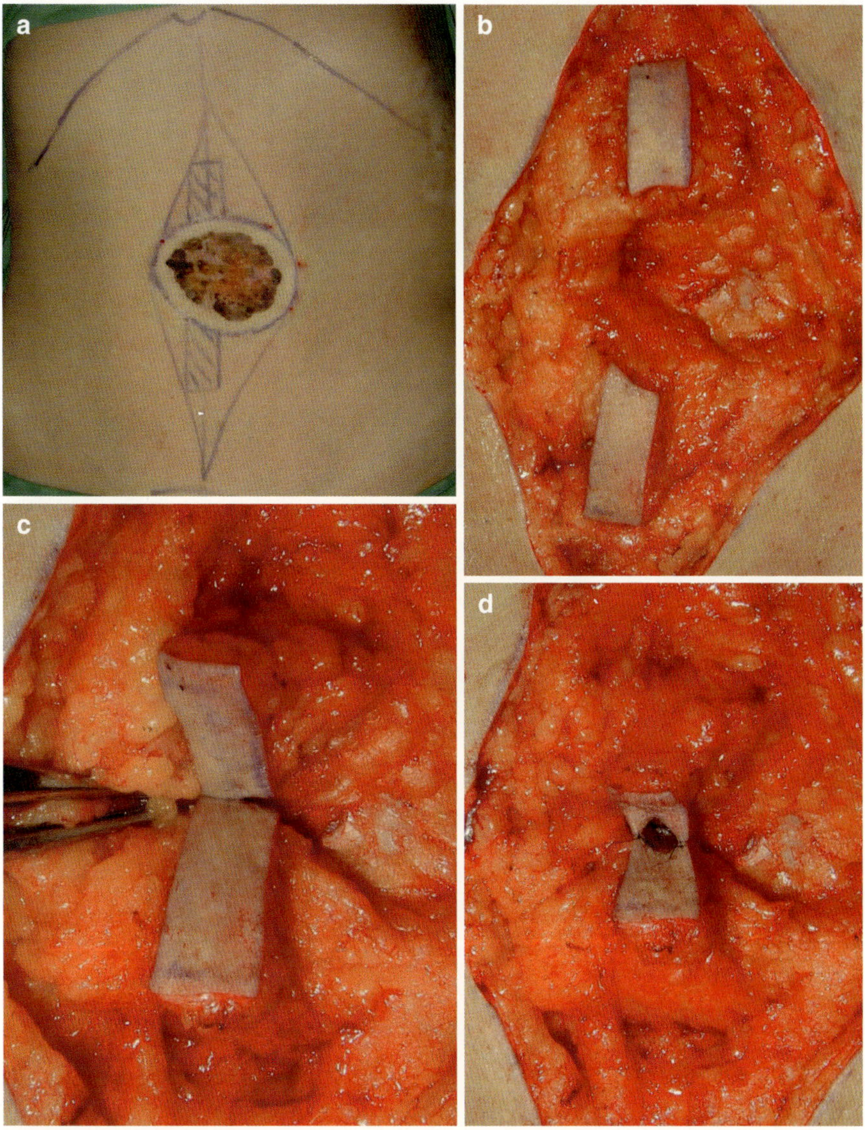

Fig. 31.2 A 78-year-old man with Bowen's disease of the umbilicus. (**a**) Tumor excision line and the flaps. (**b**) After tumor removal, flaps are elevated. (**c**) The flaps are rotated down. (**d**) The flaps are sutured to each other. (**e**) Skin tube. The flaps have thick subcutaneous pedicle. (**f**) Postoperative. (**g**) One year after the operation. (**h**) The umbilicus keeps sufficient depression with a natural appearance

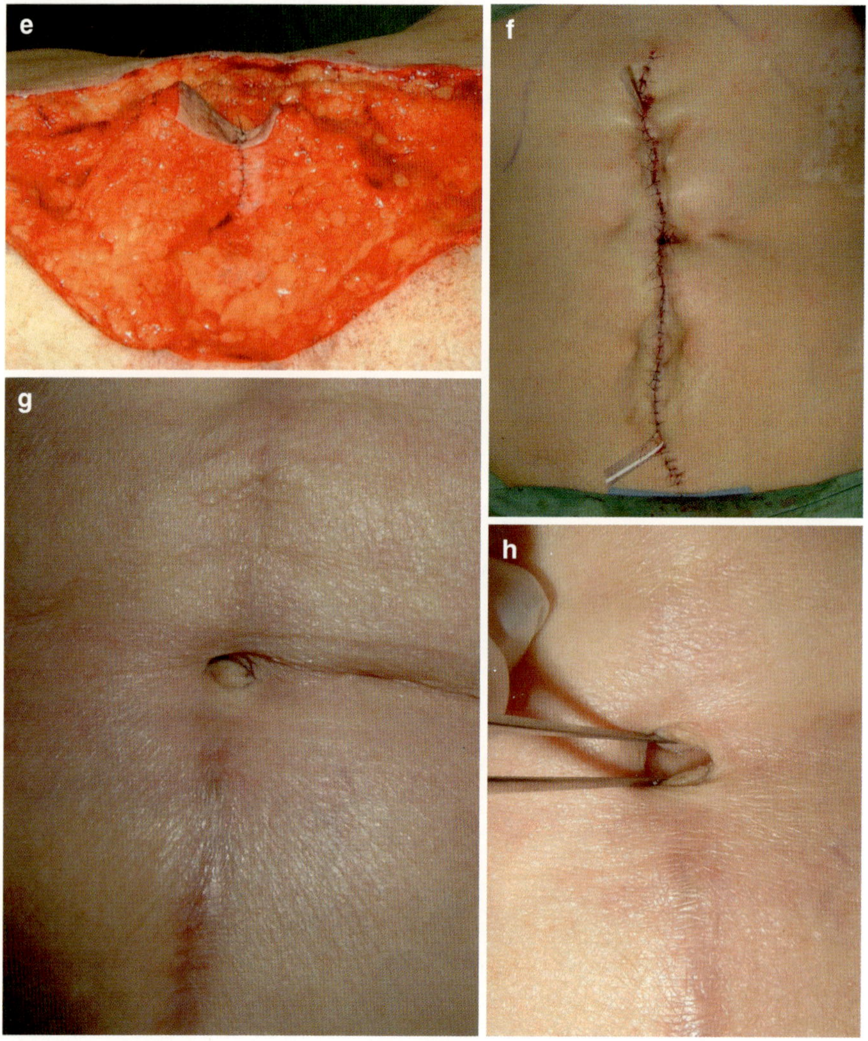

Fig. 31.2 (continued)

31.3 Discussion

The umbilicus can be lost for several reasons such as various abnormalities, trauma, and excision of tumors [1]. Many techniques have been reported for reconstruction of the umbilicus, including skin grafting, the use of local flaps [1–6], and the use of the combination of a local flap and skin grafting [7]. Local flaps are appropriate for making a deep umbilicus and prevent contracture. It is favorable to have skin flaps with sufficient length and width and a thick pedicle to create a deep and natural umbilicus [6]. The use of small flaps will result in insufficient umbilical depth. If the abdominal wall is thin and a thick pedicle cannot be maintained, the opening part of the umbilicus should be shifted cranially from the bottom to have sufficient depth [4, 5]. Because of the sufficient amount of surrounding skin, a deep and natural umbilicus can be created for congenital diseases such as umbilical cord hernias and omphalocele [1–3]. However, it is difficult to reconstruct a large defect including the umbilicus due to tumor removal, and there are few reports about such reconstruction.

The method is more suitable for cases with thick subcutaneous tissue, and a sufficient depth of the umbilicus can be obtained. Even if the amount of subcutaneous tissue is not sufficient, the depth is adjustable by changing the position of the bottom part of the umbilicus. Skin flaps are made within the dog-ear skin that is excised during skin closure, so that no scar is newly created. There is sufficient blood supply from penetrating vessels, and an umbilicus of any size can be made with an easy and safe technique in a short time [6].

Therefore, when the umbilicus is lost with tumor removal, leaving a large defect, the authors' technique is a useful method for primary reconstruction of the umbilicus.

31.4 Conclusions

An effective method for umbilical reconstruction using two rectangular-shaped flaps was described. The flaps can be created within dog-ears, which will be excised, without new scarring. A deep and natural umbilicus can be made by using this procedure.

References

1. Park S, Hata Y, Ito O, Tokioka K, Kagawa K. Repair of mild umbilical hernia. Ann Plast Surg. 1999;42(6):634–7.
2. Hamajima A, Hosaka I. Umbilicoplasty. Jpn J Pediatr Surg. 2002;34(6):676–80.
3. Sawada Y. An umbilical reconstruction using subcutaneous pedicle flap. Eur J Plast Surg. 1995;18:185–7.
4. Yotsuyanagi T, Nihei Y, Sawada Y. A simple technique for reconstruction of the umbilicus, using two twisted flaps. Plast Reconstr Surg. 1998;102(7):2444–6.
5. Yotsuyanagi T, Urushidate S, Sawada Y. Reconstruction of umbilicus using a skin flap. In: Harahap M, editor. Innovative techniques in skin surgery. New York: Marcel Dekker, Inc; 2002. p. 301–7.
6. Arai K, Yamashita K, Suda T, Ikeda K, Yamauchi M, Yotsuyanagi T. Primary reconstruction of the umbilicus, using two rectangular subcutaneous pedicle flaps. J Plast Reconstr Aesthet Surg. 2012;65(1):132–4.
7. Hatoko M, Harashina T. Reconstruction of the umbilicus using a full-thickness skin grafting. Jpn J Plast Reconstr Surg. 1989;32(12):1279–82.

Chapter 32
Umbilical Reconstruction with Double Half-Cone Flap

Alfredo Donnabella and Fernanda Parentoni Santos

32.1 Introduction

Despite depressed and adhered to the profound plans, the umbilicus is the only scar in the human body that anyone wants to possess. Its absence causes significant change in the appearance of the abdomen, thus making it an essential part of its anatomy. The aesthetics of the abdomen is directly related to an agreeable aspect of the umbilicus. Therefore, the umbilicus should have a good shape, an appropriate position, and a natural aspect, and it should not present a stigmatic scar, stenosis, or enlargement. The same applies to its reconstruction.

The umbilicus is described as a depressed scar surrounded by a natural fold of skin approximately 1.5–2.5 cm diameter [1, 2]. Its natural position is described as being the height point on the line that joins the two anterior superior lines of the iliac crests. This point is located between the third and fourth lumbar discs [3–5]. It is known that the position at the horizontal plane can vary superiorly or inferiorly and when the umbilicus is located in a more cranial position gives the abdomen a more gracious aspect [3]. Mauro Deós, a Brazilian plastic surgeon, drew attention to the position of the umbilicus in the horizontal level. The umbilicus located in a more cranial position creates the feeling of a longer abdomen and a narrower hip, normally found in thin patients. When the umbilicus is located more inferiorly, the feeling associated with it is quite the opposite, a short abdomen and a broad hip, which can be found in patients above ideal weight (Fig. 32.1).

A. Donnabella (✉)
Brazilian Society of Plastic Surgery, Private Practice,
Rua Timbiras 3642/504, Belo Horizonte, MG 30140-062, Brazil
e-mail: adonnabella@uol.com.br

F.P. Santos M.D.
Barbacena Medical School, Rua dos Inconfidentes 344/1801, Belo Horizonte,
Barbacena, MG, 30140-120 Brazil
e-mail: nandaparentonists@hotmail.com

M.A. Shiffman (ed.), *Adult Umbilical Reconstruction*,
DOI 10.1007/978-3-319-43887-0_32

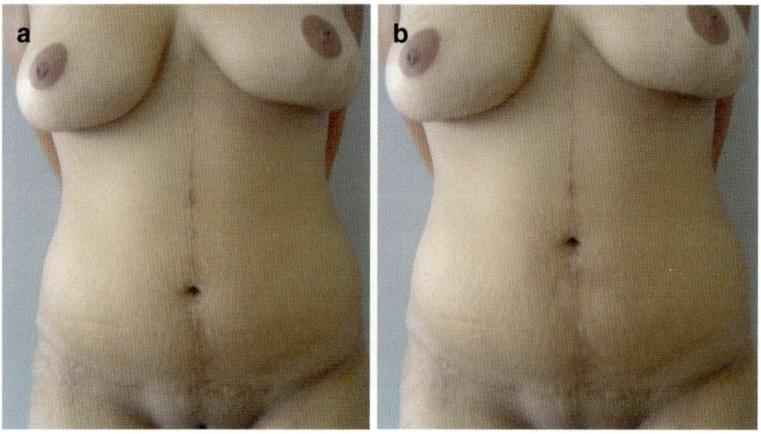

Fig. 32.1 (**a**, **b**) The position of the umbilicus in the horizontal level

Rohrich et al. [4] stated that the clinical and medicolegal implications show that regarding the sagittal plane, the umbilicus exhibits a laterality, to the right or to the left, in 98.3 % of the individuals, which means that only 1.7 % of the umbilicus is truly located at the midline as it is described in a number of works. That position can reach up to 8 % of the width of the abdomen.

Craig et al. make an analysis regarding the most graceful form of the umbilicus: it should be small, with a T silhouette in depth, and be rounded or oval with a discrete fold of skin in its upper portion. A large umbilicus is extremely unaesthetic [1, 5].

The umbilicus is formed by a base (a dome), its corrugated part, and a groove or ring that surrounds it. Its upper portion, which surrounds the depressed portion, is called the impeller.

It is estimated that about 20–30 % of bariatric surgery by laparotomy will develop an incisional hernia, and, in some cases, this hernia encompasses the umbilicus. In these cases, the risk of suffering or necrosis of the umbilicus is elevated, and therefore the primary neo-omphaloplasty is a great option. Its aesthetic results are very good, and a lot of surgeons are choosing this procedure [6, 7].

In order to have a reconstruction that will be as close to the ideal as possible, it is mandatory that every anatomical unit of the element be suitably reconstructed. The key point for the umbilical reconstruction is creating a base where the neo-umbilicus will emerge with the elevation of its edges. This base should be rounded and fixed to the aponeurosis of the rectus abdominis. The umbilicus must have good depth so as to achieve a quite natural look in the reconstruction. Ng [8] has developed a technique for the primary neo-omphaloplasty in the classic abdominoplasty that gives the umbilicus a good shape and manage to have some depth to it. This technique's great trump is the non-removal of the fat in the site of the neo-omphaloplasty. Keeping the fat, the edges of the neo-umbilicus are elevated, getting some depth therein. The removal of the fat around the neo-umbilicus is a huge mistake and should be avoided. With the removal of the fat, the structure that would give sustentation to the lateral wall of the neo-umbilicus is lost.

32.2 Technique

The authors use a modification of the technique proposed by Franco and Medeiros [9] in which the anatomical units such as dome, umbilical groove, and impeller are reconstructed step by step.

In order to reconstruct the umbilicus, be it for total lack of it (in the cases of hernias, destruction by the previous scar, bad formations, tumors, or infections) or for aesthetic reasons, it used two rectangular and parallel flaps that are sutured together and fixed to the aponeurosis of the rectus abdominis. These flaps should measure 1.5 cm height by 2.0 cm wide; however, they can be a little bigger. The flaps should transition with the skin in a curvilinear path and not in a rectum angle. Also, the curvilinear form should be observed in its distal portion (Fig. 32.2). In the case of abdominoplasties, the umbilicus can be eliminated with the surgical piece.

The flap fixation is made with two parallel sutures that bring together the dermis of the flap from one side and the dermis of the flap of the opposite side, reaching also the aponeurosis in the median line. This way, the union of both flaps can be attached by lightly compressing their distal border (Figs. 32.3, 32.4, and 32.5).

With the fixation of both flaps, by compressing their distal border, we can achieve to form the dome or the base of the neo-umbilicus in the aponeurosis. Due to the fact that the dermis from the flap is included at the suture, there is a folding in the flaps, which creates the aspect of the navel groove (Fig. 32.5).

Then, the fat tissue around the umbilicus is approximated with new sutures using Vicryl® 1 (polyglactin) and a 4 cm needle. We should use this big needle so as to include as much fat tissue as possible (Fig. 32.6).

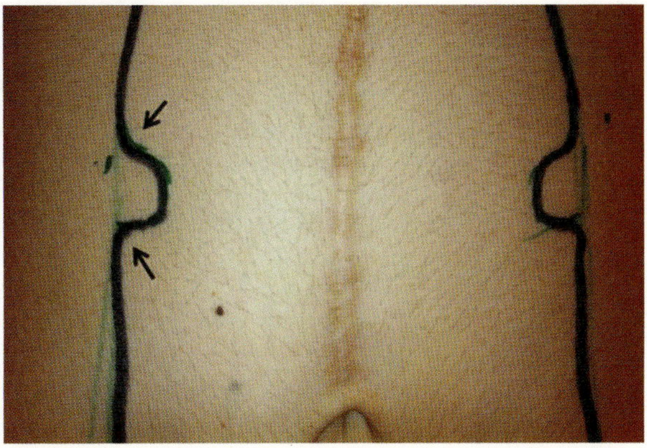

Fig. 32.2 The flaps transition with the skin in a curvilinear path and not in an angle

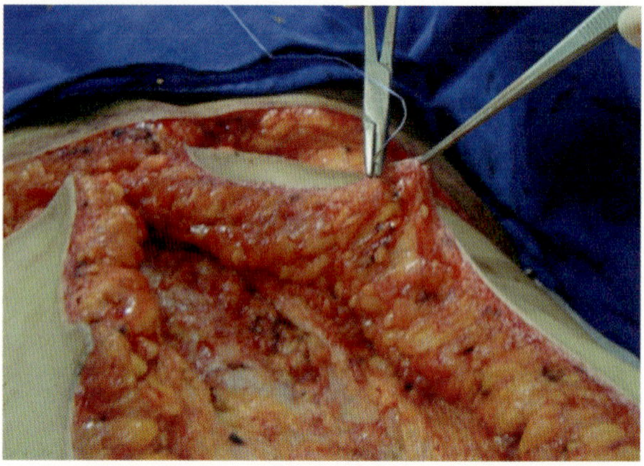

Fig. 32.3 Fixing the neo-umbilicus using the Vicryl® 2.0 (polyglactin)

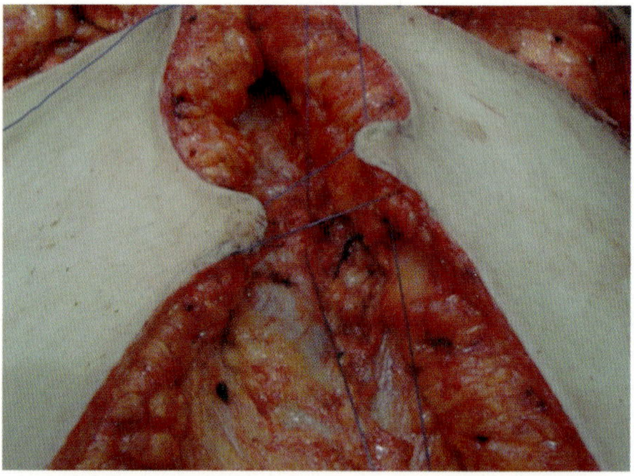

Fig. 32.4 Fixing the neo-umbilicus to the aponeurosis of the rectus abdominis

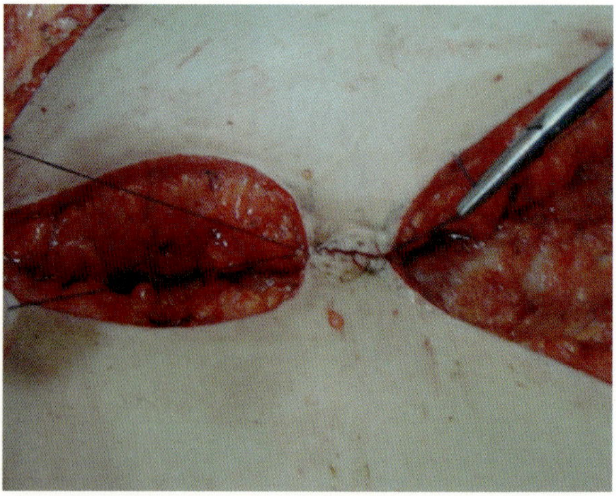

Fig. 32.5 Forming the base of the neo-umbilicus

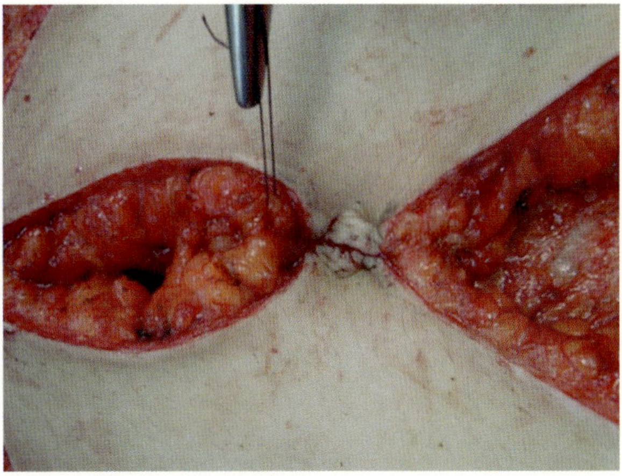

Fig. 32.6 Approximation of the adjacent fat tissue

It is necessary to take care of not putting too much pressure in those stitches, to avoid liponecrosis and the risk of losing this resource. The procedure is concluded with the skin suture (Fig. 32.7). Since the flaps are short, a curvature around the skin in the neo-umbilicus is formed, creating the impeller.

32.3 Discussion

The formation of all anatomical units is achieved: the dome, the groove, and the impeller, besides an adequate depth of the neo-umbilicus. We call attention to the fact that the formation of the base of the neo-umbilicus (dome) is of fundamental importance to a satisfactory reconstruction of the neo-umbilicus. There were no cases of umbilical stenosis, due to the fact that there was not a round scar around the neo-umbilicus. In this way, the stigma of an operated umbilicus is also avoided. Usually, no hypertrophic or keloid scars were observed, although pathological scarring may occur in the vertical scar above or below the umbilicus. In time, it is expected that a ptosis will occur in the cranial portion of the neo-umbilicus, creating a discrete fold, which gives a more natural aspect to the final reconstruction. By keeping the flaps between 1.0 and 2.0 cm, the result is a small and harmonic umbilicus.

With the approximation of the adjacent fat tissue to the neo-umbilicus, an elevation of the boards is achieved which gives the neo-umbilicus the necessary profundity. This approximation of the surrounding fat tissue is essential to define the profundity of the neo-umbilicus. Since it is impossible to make the dome deeper than the aponeurosis, the solution is to elevate the tissues around the neo-umbilicus in order to have the appropriate depth. The tissue available for that maneuver is the adipose tissue. It should be handled with delicacy, because of the real risk of tissue lesion.

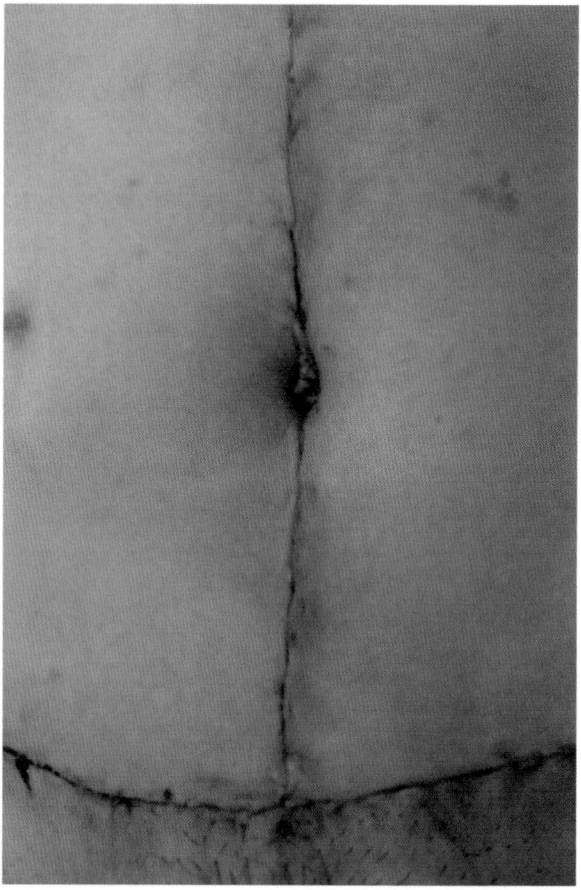

Fig. 32.7 Final aspect of the neo-umbilicus

When we use this technique in the anchor-line abdominoplasty, the technique presented by Silva and Abramo [10] may be used in order to determine the position of the umbilicus in the abdomen, in which a skin big flap is left, and later we define the 1.5–2.0 cm flap. The great difficulty in reconstructing the umbilicus is to achieve the desirable depth in it, especially when the patient does not have enough adipose tissue. The technique presented here which uses the surrounding fat tissue can solve this matter. Keeping a curvature at the base of the flap, instead of the rectum angle, we avoid the approximation of the boarders, and therefore a more rounded umbilicus is created, avoiding a scar that is elongated and closed. These characteristics can be observed in Figs. 32.8, 32.9, and 32.10.

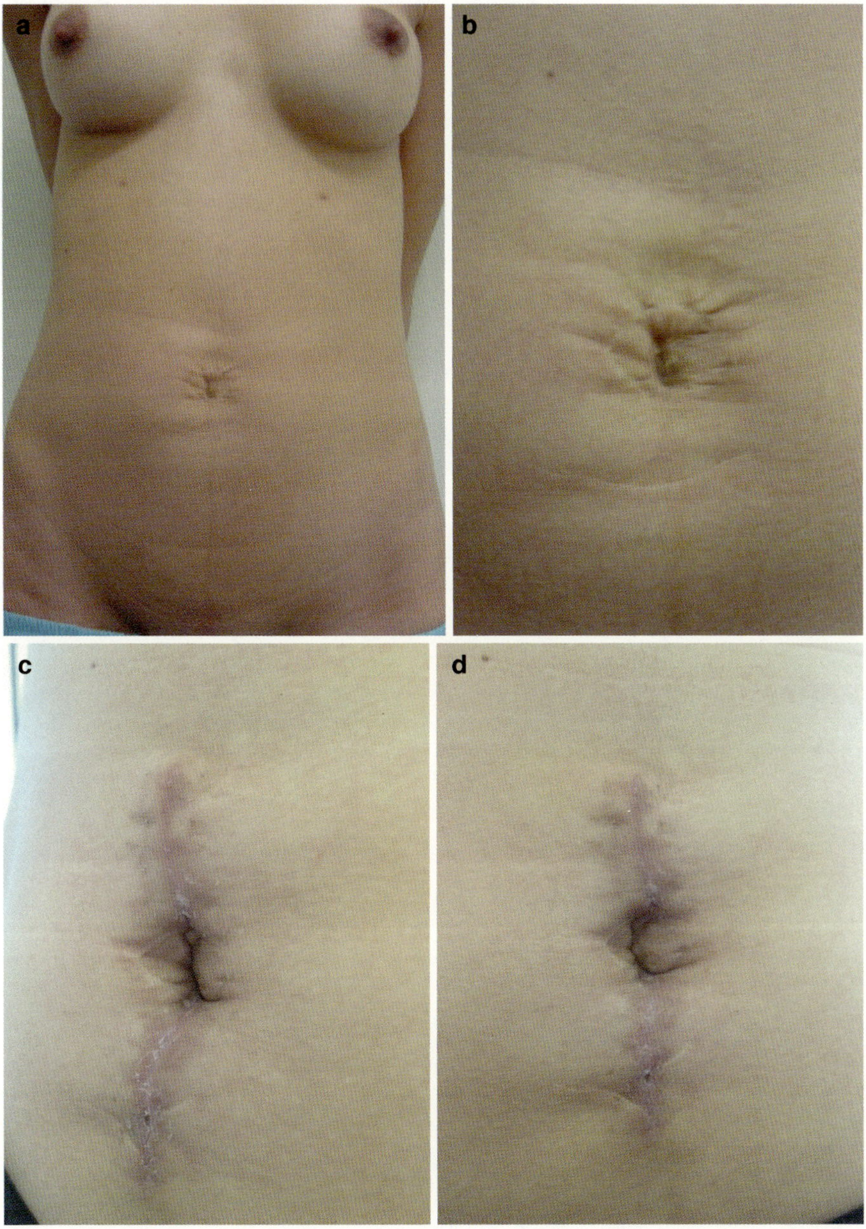

Fig. 32.8 (**a**, **b**) This patient operated on three times and does not have a good aspect of the umbilicus

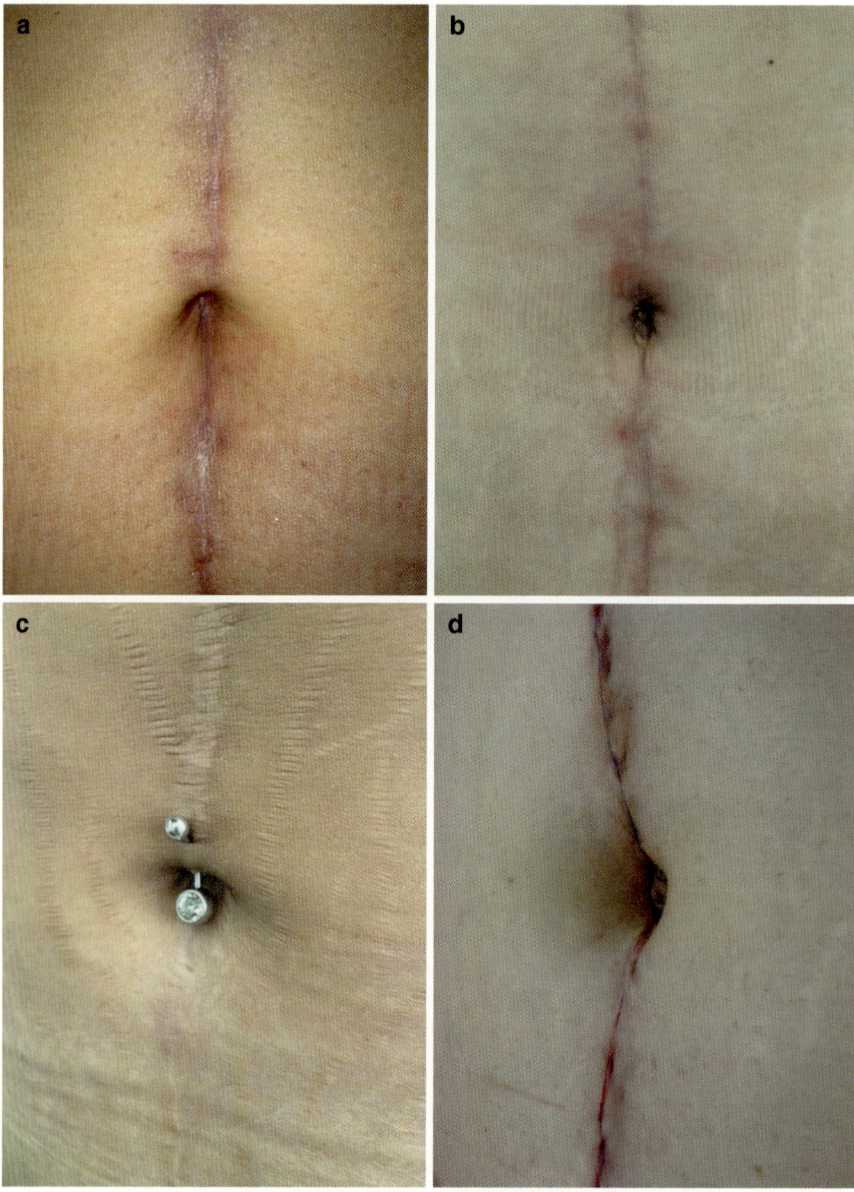

Fig. 32.9 (**a–d**) Postoperative aspect when used in abdominoplasty

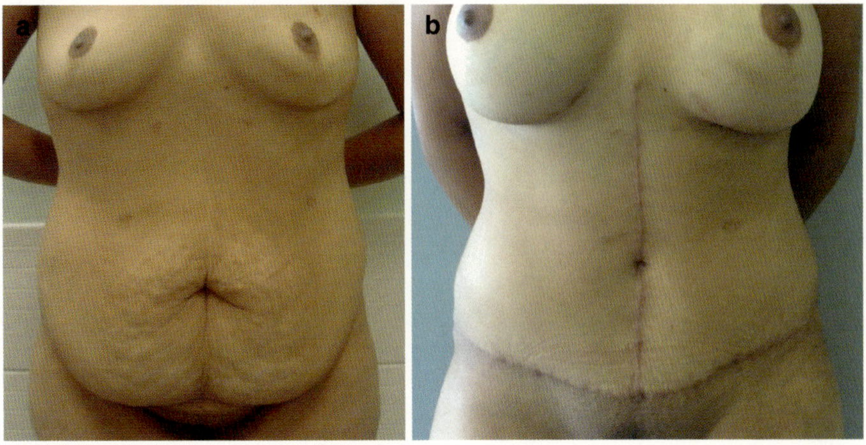

Fig. 32.10 (**a**) Preoperative. (**b**) Anchor-line abdominoplasty using the technique of neo-umbilicus

32.4 Conclusions

The technique for the reconstruction of the umbilicus presented here accounting for the anatomical units provides a very natural look, and in time an excess of skin on the upper part occurs, giving a more graceful appearance to it. The resultant umbilicus exhibits appropriate features of depth and size. The technique avoids the appearance of operated umbilical scar and secondary stenosis because it does not show circular scar and the incision position is in the midline of the neo-umbilicus.

References

1. Craig SB, Faller MS, Puckett CL. In search of the ideal female umbilicus. Plast Reconstr Surg. 2000;105:389–92.
2. Marconi F. Reconstruction of the umbilicus: a simple technique. Plast Reconstr Surg. 1995;95:1115–7.
3. Coetzee T. Clinical anatomy of the umbilicus. S Afr Med J. 1980;57:463–6.
4. Rohrich RJ, Sorokin ES, Brown SA, Gibby DL. Is the umbilicus truly midline? Clinical and medicolegal implications. Plast Reconstr Surg. 2003;112:259–63.
5. Southwell-Keely JP, Berry MG. Umbilical reconstruction: a review of techniques. J Past Reconstr Aesthet Surg. 2011;64:803–8.
6. Cavalcante ELF. Neoumbilicoplastia como opção de reconstrução umbilical nas dermolipectomias abdominais em âncora pós-gastroplastia. Rev Bras Cir Plast. 2010;25(3):509–18.
7. Donnabella A. Reconstrução anatômica da cicatriz umbilical. Rev Bras Cir Plast. 2013;28(1):119–23.
8. Abreu NA. Abdominoplastias: neo-onfaloplastias sem cicatriz e sem excisão de gordura. Rev Bras Cir Plast. 2010;25(3):499–03.
9. Franco D, Medeiros J, Farias C, Franco T. Umbilical reconstruction for patients with a midline scar. Aesthetic Plast Surg. 2006;30:595–8.
10. Silva FN, Abramo E. Neo-onfaloplastia na abdominoplastia vertical. Rev Bras Cir Plast. 2010;25(2):330–6.

Chapter 33
The "Celtic-Cross" Technique for Immediate Umbilical Reconstruction

Emmanuel A. De La Cruz

33.1 Introduction

Loss of the umbilicus after surgical ablative procedures for congenital abdominal wall defects, urachal cyst, and various benign or malignant tumors of the umbilical area can be an embarrassing deformity. There have been several umbiliconeoplasty techniques described in the literature to reconstruct the umbilicus with mixed results. However, there have been very few techniques published in the literature describing the reconstruction of the umbilicus immediately after surgical ablation [1–3]. We present a simple approach to reconstruct the umbilicus immediately after surgical ablation of the umbilicus, which we called the "Celtic-cross" technique [4]. This was the first technique described for immediate umbilical reconstruction, utilizing the midline incision as part of the reconstructive procedure. In our experience, this technique resulted in an aesthetically acceptable newly formed umbilicus.

Although the umbilicus has minimal functional importance and just a mere remnant cicatrix, it is a key aesthetic landmark of the abdomen. Any distortion of the umbilicus, such as a poorly done umbilicoplasty, or even its intentional loss from various surgical procedures can be a frequent cause of concern or complaint from a patient. The optimal umbilical reconstruction technique should be reproducible and aesthetically acceptable with minimal morbidity. The umbiliconeoplasty techniques range from single to three or four pedicled abdominal flaps, the use of grafts, or healing by secondary intention. Miller reported the first immediate umbilical reconstruction in the literature involving a flap resembling an "iris" of a camera lens after wide local excision of a melanoma of the umbilicus [1]. Currently, there are

E.A. De La Cruz, MD, PLLC
Loma Linda University, 2219 Sawdust Road, Unit 1203, The Woodlands, TX 77380, USA
e-mail: info@delacruzplasticsurgery.com

M.A. Shiffman (ed.), *Adult Umbilical Reconstruction*,
DOI 10.1007/978-3-319-43887-0_33

approximately over 30 techniques described for delayed umbilical reconstruction, and there have been very few techniques published in the literature describing the reconstruction of the umbilicus immediately after surgical ablation [1–3].

A simple approach is presented to reconstruct the umbilicus immediately after a midline abdominal incision and surgical ablation of the umbilicus, which we called the "Celtic-cross" technique [5]. This is one of a few methods for immediate umbilical reconstruction, utilizing the midline incision as part of the reconstructive procedure. In our experience, this technique resulted in an aesthetically acceptable newly formed umbilicus.

33.2 Surgical Technique

A Celtic-cross design (Fig. 33.1a) is made over the area to be reconstructed. After flap design is drawn on the abdomen (Fig. 33.1b), a circular incision is then made down to the subcutaneous fat around the umbilicus, creating an island of skin with the previous umbilicus measuring approximately 3 cm in diameter. This is followed by a 2 cm midline incision superiorly and inferiorly. A 2 cm lateral incision is then performed on each side of the circle, creating a "Celtic-cross" configuration (Fig. 33.2) [5]. A 2 cm midline and lateral incisions are optimal to have minimal scarring after this umbiliconeoplasty procedure. Ablation of the umbilicus results in a circular, full-thickness abdominal wall defect. Four local flaps of skin and subcutaneous fat are then made. An upper and lower anchoring sutures of 3-0 PDS are placed in the rectus fascia at the new vertical limits of the umbilicus. The underside or

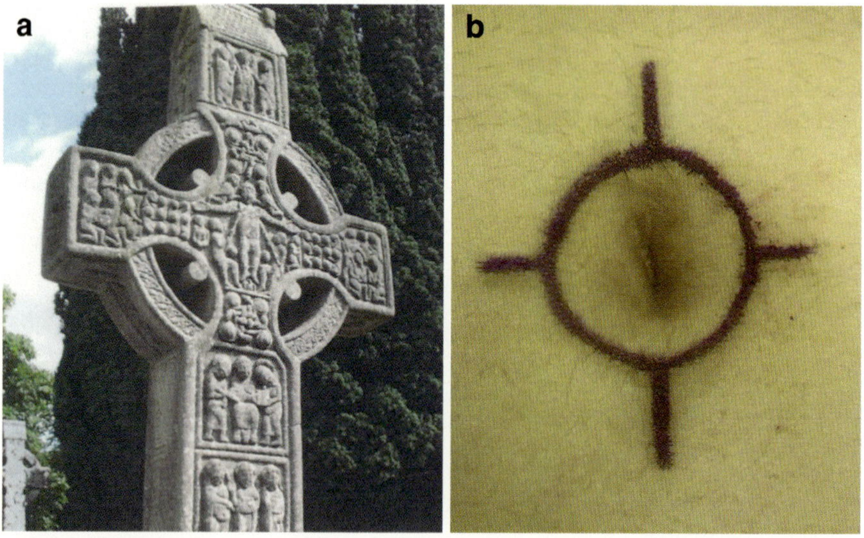

Fig. 33.1 (**a**) Celtic-cross in Dublin, Ireland. (**b**) Celtic-cross design and marking for umbilical reconstruction

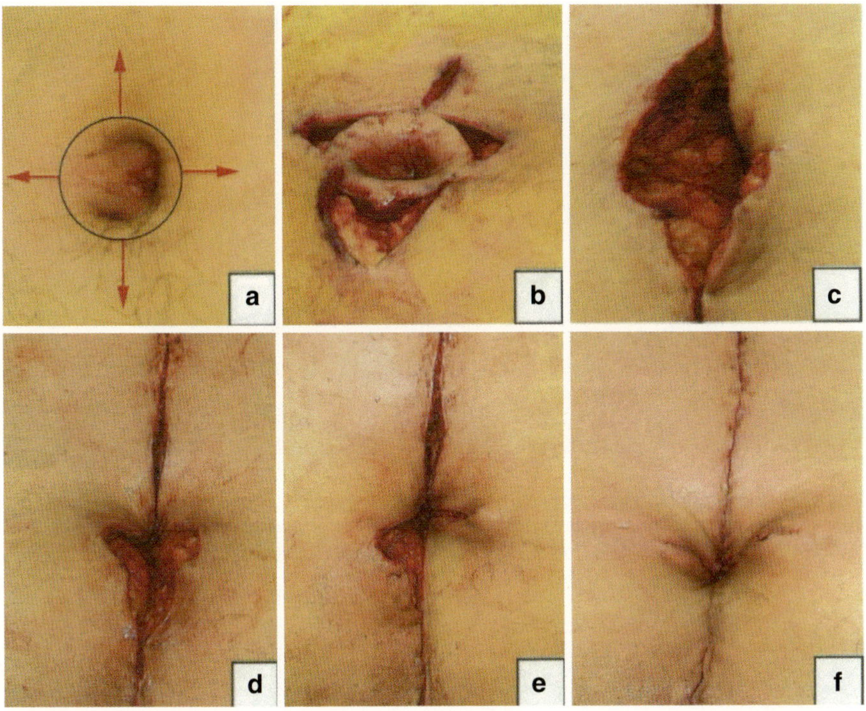

Fig. 33.2 The "Celtic Cross" technique. (**a**) Umbilicus with external urachal sinus. (**b**) A circular incision was performed followed by a 2-cm incision at the three o'clock, six o'clock, nine o'clock, and twelve o'clock positions. (**c–d**) After surgical ablation of the umbilicus, the superior flaps were then anchored onto the rectus sheath. (**e**) The inferior flaps were subsequently anchored onto the rectus sheath. (**f**) After the superior and inferior flaps are anchored and sutured toward the center, the skin is then closed with subcuticular sutures and with derma bond

dermis of each flap is then sutured toward the center to the underlying muscular fascia, causing the depression of the flap (Fig. 33.2) [5]. The superior flaps are first anchored down to the level of the linea alba and rectus sheath. The inferior flaps are similarly anchored onto the rectus muscle fascia. The skin is then reapproximated with 4-0 Monocryl subcuticular sutures and then with Dermabond. Xeroform gauze and a dry ball of gauze are then placed over the neoumbilicus to exert slight pressure over the umbilical area. This keeps the flaps in their adequate position. The gauze is then removed the following day to evaluate the umbilical reconstruction and then repacked with a similar gauze packing and kept for 4–5 days.

This technique can be used for a patient with a previous history of abdominoplasty or umbilicoplasty. The technique is modified by not performing the mid-incision of the "Celtic-cross" design inferiorly. An inverted triangular area superior to the center of the umbilicus is deepithelialized, and the superior flaps are sutured onto the margin of the deepithelialized umbilicus (Fig. 33.3). The inferior portion of the flap is reapproximated as in any umbilicoplasty technique.

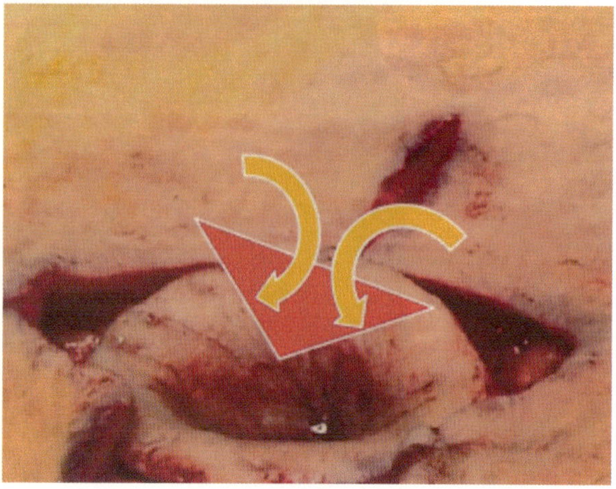

Fig. 33.3 A triangular area over the umbilicus is de-epithelialized. The edges of the superior flaps are then sutured toward the margins of the de-epithelialized area

33.3 Case Reports

33.3.1 Case 1 [5] (Fig. 33.4a)

A 30-year-old male presented with a 4-day history of abdominal pain, fever, and purulent drainage from his umbilicus. Examination revealed an initial temperature of 38.8 °C, 1.5 mm umbilical sinus with purulent drainage, but no periumbilical erythema. No leukocytosis was found on laboratory findings. Antibiotics and intravenous fluids were initiated. Abdominal tomography revealed an inflammatory midline mass posterior to the rectus sheath with no extension to the bladder. The patient was taken to the operating room where an external urachal sinus with inflammation involving the umbilicus was found which required excision of the sinus tract and umbilical cyst with complete surgical ablation of the umbilicus. Immediate umbilical reconstruction was then performed using the "Celtic-cross" technique. Pathology revealed a urachal remnant with no evidence of malignant cells. Postoperatively the patient was discharged with no complications and given a 7-day course of oral antibiotics.

33.3.2 Case 2 [5] (Fig. 33.4b)

A 27-year-old male presented with a 3-week history of abdominal pain and purulent drainage from his umbilicus. On examination the patient was found to be afebrile with an umbilical sinus with purulent drainage but no cellulites. He was found to have mild leukocytosis with a WBC of 12.6. Computed tomography of the

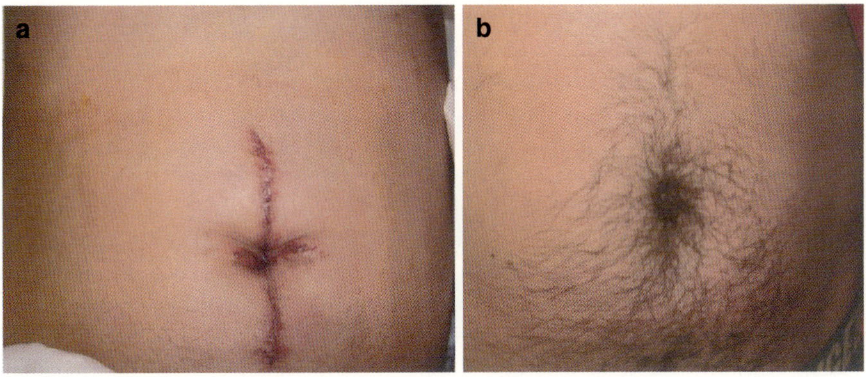

Fig. 33.4 (**a**) Case 1. The appearance of the reconstructed one week after the umbiliconeoplasty. (**b**) Case 2. The neoumbilicus 15 months postoperatively

abdomen/pelvis revealed an 11 cm cystic structure at the umbilicus suspicious for a cyst versus an abscess. The patient was started on piperacillin/tazobactam and subsequently was taken to the operating room. He was found to have a purulent preperitoneal cystic mass requiring a limited laparotomy and complete excision of the umbilical cyst. The cyst was completely removed without any rupture or contamination of the surrounding surgical field. Pathological examination was consistent with a urachal cyst. The patient was discharged with oral augmentin for 7 days. The postoperative course was unremarkable with no evidence of wound infection [5].

33.4 Discussion

There have been numerous umbiliconeoplasty techniques that have been described and reported for acquired or congenital absence of an umbilicus [6–11]. A single-stage immediate umbilical reconstruction is ideal, except in the presence of an infection where a delayed reconstruction is advisable. These delayed reconstruction techniques are designed on an intact abdominal surface which utilizes various local flaps ranging from a double V–Y pattern [10], a twisted vertical rectangular flap [7], a rotated paramedian flap [9] to a triangular skin flap [4]. Often, flaps designed for umbilical reconstruction is combined with a skin or a cartilaginous composite graft [11]. The use of local tissue for umbiliconeoplasty is ideal which accords with Sir Harold Gilles' fundamental principle of plastic and reconstructive surgery to "replace like with like." The best method of umbilical reconstruction should be determined by the plastic surgeon based on the patient's tissue characteristics with a goal of reconstructing a well-proportioned umbilicus and some degree of umbilical depression with a well-concealed scar. The ideal umbilicus should create a permanent, rounded umbilical depression in the mid-abdomen, and the umbilical depression should reach down the umbilical fascia.

Very few techniques described immediate reconstruction after surgical removal of the umbilicus. These techniques ranged from a simple purse-string suture technique [2, 3] to a more innovative progressive rotation of flaps similar to an "iris" of a camera lens [1]. If the abdominal wall bears scars from previous surgery, such as an abdominoplasty, local flaps may be raised to mitigate donor site morbidity. The Celtic-cross technique is a very useful technique since it can utilize the midline incision as part of the procedure. This umbiliconeoplasty technique is ideal in thin- and/or moderate-sized patients with a shallow-depth umbilicus. This technique is applicable to surgical procedures after a midline laparotomy incision that requires surgical ablation of the umbilicus for benign or malignant conditions. It can also be used to reconstruct a neoumbilicus on a previously surgically ablated umbilicus in a patient who will undergo a laparotomy requiring a midline incision. This technique can be modified and used for surgical revision of an umbilicus on a patient with a previous history of umbilicoplasty and/or abdominoplasty.

33.5 Conclusions

The Celtic-cross technique for immediate umbilical reconstruction following surgical ablation of the umbilicus is a very reliable and reproducible umbiliconeoplasty technique that produces a neoumbilicus with a permanent, rounded umbilical depression with a well-concealed scar.

References

1. Miller MJ, Balch CM. "Iris" technique for immediate umbilical reconstruction. Plast Reconstr Surg. 1993;92:754–6.
2. Bartsich SA, Schwartz MH. Purse-string method for immediate umbilical reconstruction. Plast Reconstr Surg. 2003;112:1652–5.
3. Jang HC. A case of immediate umbilical reconstruction after surgical excision of keloid. Korean J Dermatol. 2006;44:187–9.
4. Pfulg M, Van de Sijpe K, Blondeel P. A simple new technique for neo-umbilicoplasty. Br J Plast Surg. 2005;58:688–91.
5. De La Cruz EA, Jaber RK, Tabuenca AD, Joe VC. The Celtic-Cross technique for immediate umbilical reconstruction post-laparotomy and surgical ablation of the umbilicus. J Plast Reconstr Aesth Surg. 2009;62:258–61.
6. Marconi F. Reconstruction of the umbilicus: a simple technique. Plast Reconstr Surg. 1995;95:1115–7.
7. Yotsuyanagi T, Nihei Y, Sawada Y. A simple technique for reconstruction of the umbilicus, using two twisted flaps. Plast Reconstr Surg. 1998;102:2444–6.
8. Abenavoli F, Cusano V, Cucchiara V, D'Amico C, Corvelli L. An idea for umbilicus reconstruction. Ann Plast Surg. 2001;46:194.
9. Borges AF. Reconstruction of the umbilicus. Br J Plast Surg. 1975;28:75–6.
10. Jamra F. Reconstruction of the umbilicus by a double V-Y procedure. Plast Reconstr Surg. 1979;64:106–7.
11. Matsuo K, Kondoh S, Hirose T. A simple technique for reconstruction of the umbilicus, using a conchal cartilage composite graft. Plast Reconstr Surg. 1990;86:149–51.

Chapter 34
Four Flaps Technique for Neoumbilicoplasty

SuRak Eo

34.1 Introduction

As a major aesthetic component of the abdominal wall, the umbilicus is the only scar tissue in the human body which normally remains after birth. An aesthetically pleasing umbilicus has sufficient dimpling and natural superior hooding with an almond shape. Umbilicoplasty is required not only in conditions such as congenital absence due to bladder exstrophy, gastroschisis, omphalocele, and cloacal exstrophy but also in cases of a protruding umbilicus, traumatic umbilical malformation, and after abdominoplasty, breast reconstruction using abdominal tissues, umbilical herniorrhaphy, and laparotomy. Various methods have been employed in order to reconstruct the umbilicus, including the purse-string method [1], the use of several local flaps [2–6], and the use of an ear conchal cartilage graft [7]. Every method has advantages and disadvantages; however, none of the above methods can guarantee optimal results. Here, the author reports his experience with umbilical reconstruction using a technique termed the "four flaps technique" (Fig. 34.1), which may be an easy, simple, safe, and reliable technique, especially in cases where no remaining umbilical tissue is present.

S. Eo, M.D., Ph.D.
Department of Plastic and Reconstructive Surgery, Dongguk University Medical Center, Dongguk University College of Medicine,
27 Dongguk-ro, Ilsandong-gu, Goyang 410-773, South Korea
e-mail: surakeo@yahoo.com

M.A. Shiffman (ed.), *Adult Umbilical Reconstruction*,
DOI 10.1007/978-3-319-43887-0_34

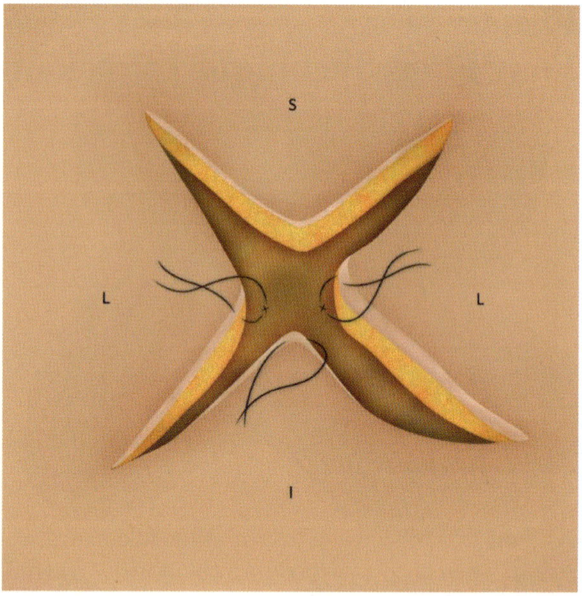

Fig. 34.1 Surgical method employed in the four flaps technique. Three points (the 3, 6, and 9 o'clock abdominal flaps) were anchored to the deep dermis of the umbilicus and linea alba with a 4-0 absorbable suture (*S* superior flap, *L* lateral flap, *I* inferior flap, *X* anchoring point at the appropriate linea alba)

34.2 Technique

In the new umbilicoplasty technique, only neighboring abdominal soft tissue is utilized instead of using remaining umbilical tissue, which is the most distinctive and creative feature of the author's technique. Three of the four newly created flaps (those in the 3, 6, and 9 o'clock directions) are elevated and firmly anchored to the anterior rectus fascial layer. This particular surgical procedure has not previously been reported. The technique was designed for individuals who congenitally lack umbilical tissues (Fig. 34.2) or for use after the excision of a severely hypertrophic and disfigured umbilicus (Fig. 34.3). In both cases, no umbilical tissue was available for use, leaving only the adjacent abdominal soft tissue.

To determine the proper position of the neoumbilicus, two axes were marked on the abdomen as preliminary markings. The transverse axis was marked by connecting both anterior superior iliac spines of the iliac crests, and the vertical axis was marked along the midline of the abdomen in a supine position. An X-shaped incision line was designed (Fig. 34.4). Each of the four triangular flaps had an angle of 90° and the radius of each fan-shaped sector stretched 1 cm over the desired location of the neoumbilicus. The original umbilicus of the patient in Fig. 34.3 consisted entirely of hypertrophic scar tissue, and the scarred umbilicus was completely resected before the reconstruction. After the en bloc excision, a defect was present with a diameter of 3 cm, which led the author to design an X-shaped incision line with limbs of 1.5 cm in length (Fig. 34.3). Under local anesthesia, a skin incision was made, resulting in four flaps in superior, inferior, and lateral positions. The four fan-shaped flaps were then completely detached from the underlying Scarpa's fascia, followed by a defatting procedure, although some subcutaneous fat was

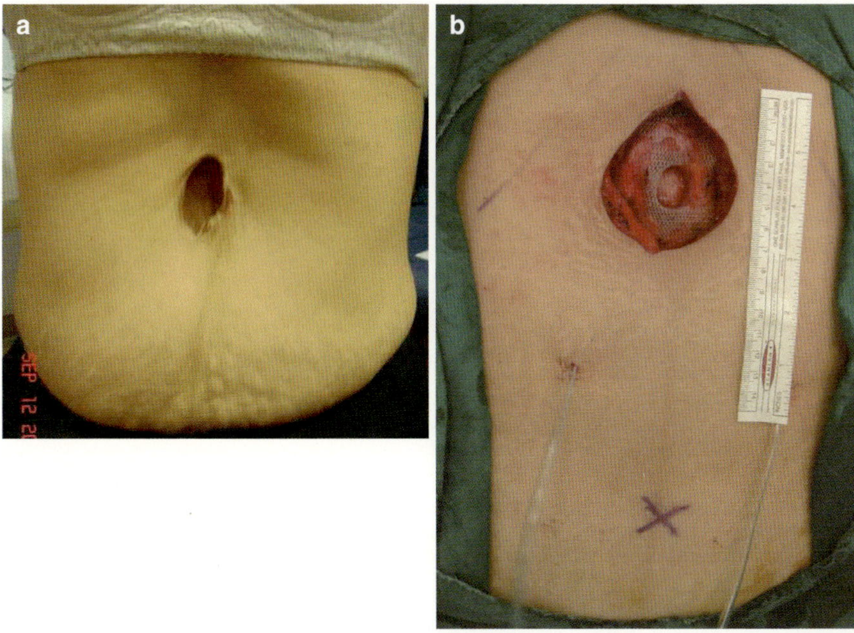

Fig. 34.2 A patient with congenital absence of the umbilicus. (**a**) The 40-year-old female patient showed a congenital absence of umbilical tissue and a soft tissue defect in the epigastric region. (**b**) Beside the removal of epigastric skin and soft tissues, four flaps were designed on the site of preferable location of the neoumbilicus

preserved at the base of the flap. The amount of fat preserved was dependent on the amount of abdominal fat present (Fig. 34.4). After meticulous hemostasis, the dermis of the three non-superior flaps was firmly anchored to the appropriate linea alba in the 3, 6, and 9 o'clock positions with 4-0 absorbable sutures (Vicryl, Ethicon, Somerville, NJ, USA) to produce aesthetically acceptable folding (Fig. 34.5). In the case that a more longitudinal umbilical depression is needed, the inferior flap could be anchored as caudally as possible. The remaining superior flap was not directly fixed to the underlying fascia. Instead, it was used to form the superior hooding. A defatting procedure was performed on the superior flap to a lesser extent than on other flaps, resulting in superior hooding (Fig. 34.4). The skin of each flap was then sutured with 5-0 nonabsorbable nylon sutures (Ethilon, Ethicon, Somerville, NJ, USA). The procedure was completed by packing a small amount of petrolatum gauze in order to ensure that the neoumbilicus remained satisfactorily hollow. Finally, the newly formed umbilicus was immobilized with a tie-over dressing to prevent movement postoperatively, which was maintained for 1 week. After 2 weeks, all of the stitches were removed, and silicone gel (ScarEase Gel, Pillar Surgical, La Jolla, CA, USA) was applied for scar management if necessary. There were no complications such as wound disruption, flap necrosis, hematoma, or infection. In each case, the neoumbilicus retained a sufficient depth during the follow-up period, and both patients were satisfied with their postoperative results (Fig. 34.6).

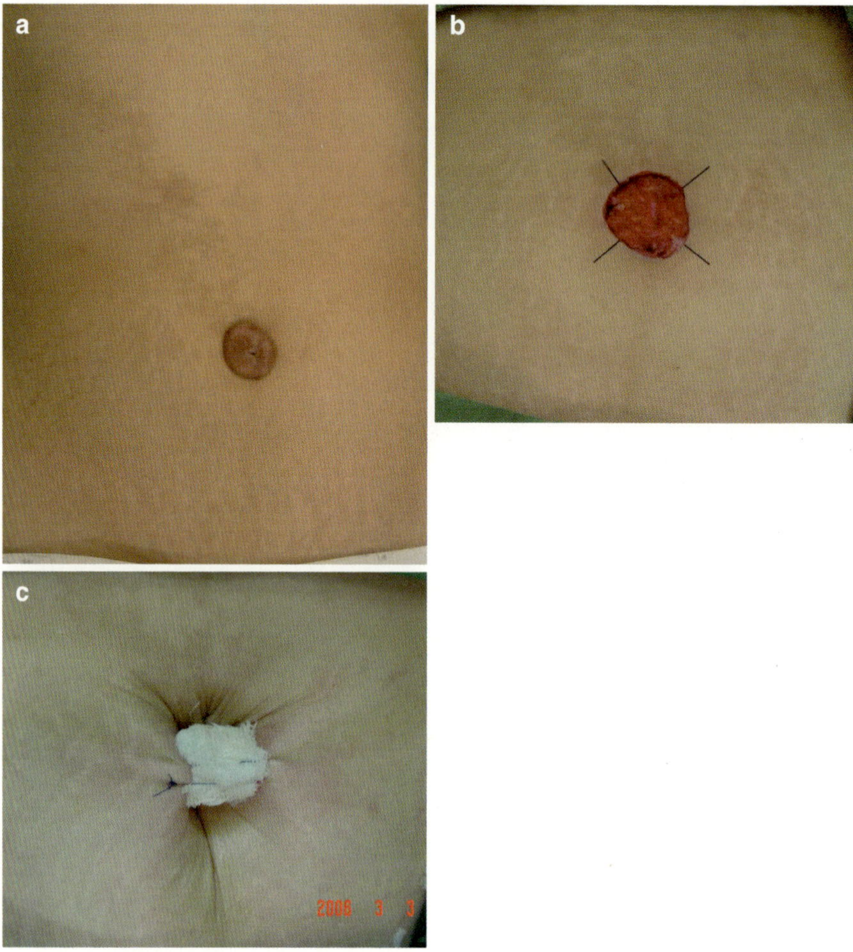

Fig. 34.3 A case of hypertrophic umbilicus. (**a**) Preoperative 40-year-old female with hypertrophic umbilicus. (**b**) After en bloc excision of the hypertrophic scarred umbilicus, an X-shaped incision was designed, starting from the excised skin margin and consisting of four limbs, each 1.5 cm long. (**c**) Tie-over dressing was applied for 1–2 weeks

34.3 Discussion

The umbilicus is located at the midpoint of the lower abdomen and is the major aesthetic unit of the abdominal wall. It is composed almost entirely of dermal and fibrotic tissue, along with a very small amount of subcutaneous fatty tissue, and is usually located approximately 9–12 cm above the superior margin of the mons pubis, slightly above a line connecting the anterior superior iliac spines [8]. The ideal umbilicus should have a natural contour, prominent depth, minimal additional scars, and proper superior hooding. Shinohara et al. [9] emphasized that an

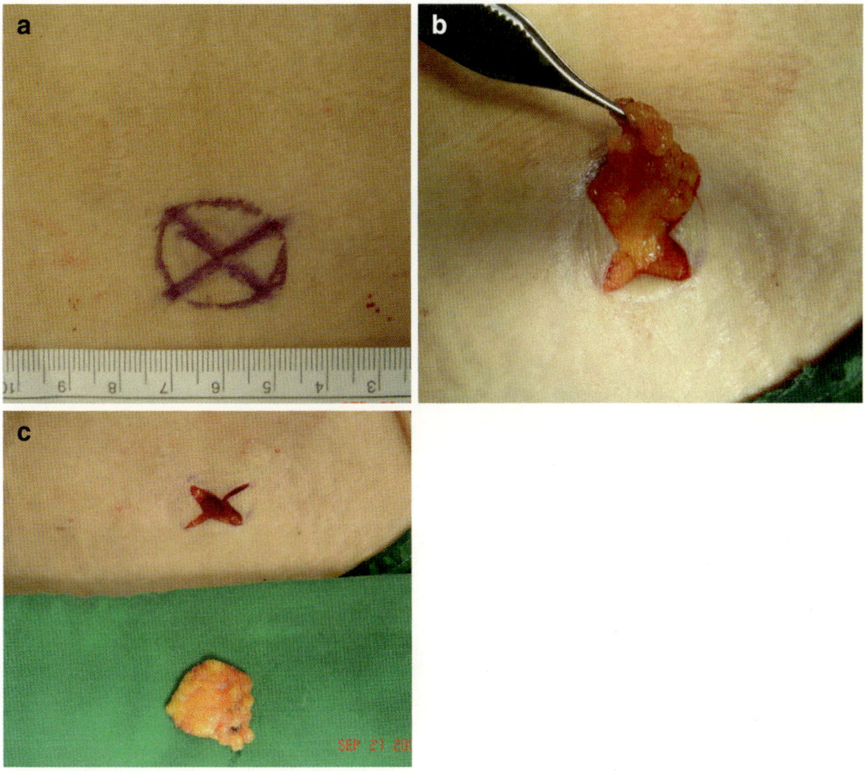

Fig. 34.4 Operative procedures for congenital absence of the umbilicus. (**a**) The design of an X-shaped pattern consisting of four limbs with a length of 1 cm. (**b**, **c**) The four flaps of the neoumbilicus were elevated and abdominal fat was removed

umbilicus with a natural appearance consists of a ring, a tubular wall, a sulcus, and a bottom, without any excess skin that would interfere with the aesthetic aspect of the umbilicus. In addition, Lee et al. [10] suggested that an aesthetically optimal umbilicus must possess the following properties: a vertical ratio of 46:54 (with respect to the xiphoid process and the lower limit of the vulvar cleft), a midline horizontal position, and an oval shape with no hooding or superior hooding.

The absence of the umbilicus is an aesthetically and psychologically frustrating condition for patients and sometimes poses challenges to surgeons [11]. It has recently become common for many people to want an aesthetically pleasing umbilicus because their umbilicus is visible in public when they wear clothes such as crop tops or bikinis. Since many patients have undergone abdominal reconstructive surgery, including procedures involving an inferior epigastric artery perforator flap, developing expertise in umbilical reconstruction has become obligatory for surgeons. However, few reports have addressed reconstructive neoumbilicoplasty after the en bloc excision of the umbilicus, as occurs in surgery treating a disfigured or

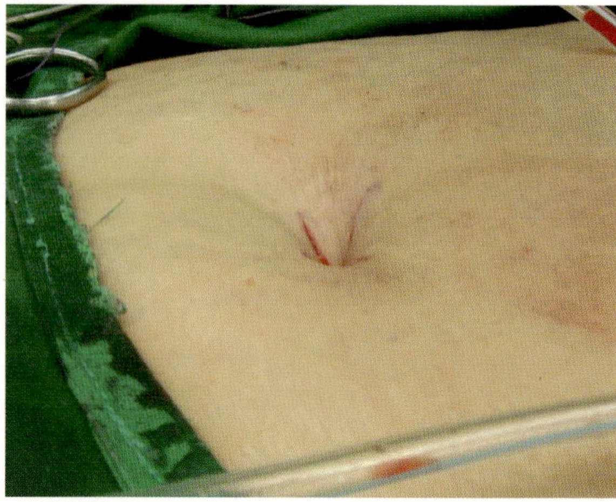

Fig. 34.5 Immediate postoperative after umbilicoplasty. The neoumbilicus shows sufficient depth and natural superior hooding before application of the tie-over dressing

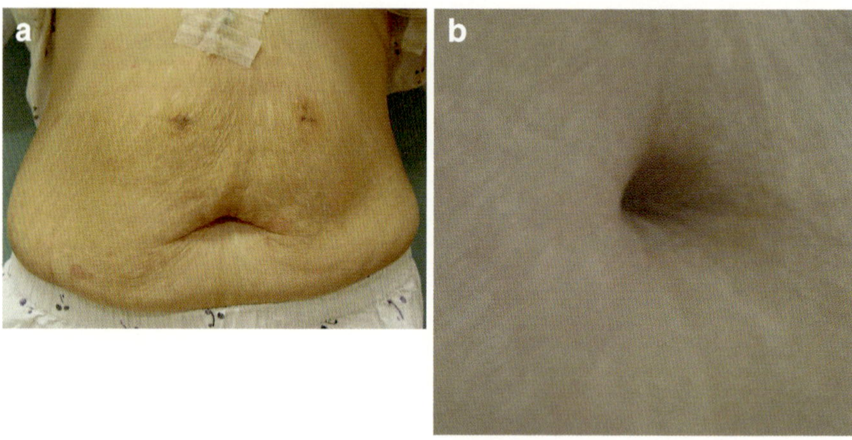

Fig. 34.6 Postoperative patient with a congenitally absent umbilicus. (**a**) Three weeks postoperative. (**b**) Eight years postoperatively, demonstrating the natural appearance of the neoumbilicus with sufficient depth, superior hooding, and minimal additional scarring

hypertrophic umbilicus, umbilical hernia [5], neonatal omphalocele [12], or urachal cancer [13].

Several studies have suggested various surgical techniques for umbilical reconstruction, such as using diversely shaped local flaps, a suture method, and even cartilage grafts [1–7, 9, 11, 14]. The local flap techniques, including an inverted C-V flap [3], yield good short-term results, but these techniques have not yet been used in the absence of remaining umbilical tissue. Miller and Balch [4] introduced the Iris technique for immediate umbilical reconstruction. This technique creates four flaps by making four curvilinear incisions followed by rotating the flaps after a wide resection of the umbilical tissue. However, this procedure leaves a conspicuous dog ear scar around the umbilicus. Bartsich and Schwartz [1] reported a purse-string method for umbilical reconstruction after repairs of recurrent incisional hernia or abdominal surgical procedures such as urachal cyst repair. However, this technique requires thorough wound care for an extended period, as it leaves an open wound after the procedure. Pfulg et al. [2] introduced the use of a triangular flap for umbilical reconstruction after elliptical skin excision over the umbilicus in either a vertical or horizontal direction. It was simple and reproducible with few complications. However, it inevitably results in a long vertical or horizontal scar over the umbilicus to ensure that the neoumbilicus is adequately sized. The major disadvantage of the above techniques is that they use abdominal ground tissue from the abdominal wall. In practice, this is a challenging task for lighter patients and pediatric patients, especially in thin patients, because it is difficult to produce sufficient depth due to lower skin laxity. A neoumbilicus created using those methods may therefore develop a flat appearance over time.

34.4 Conclusions

The techniques described above are either unsatisfactory or too complex [2, 4, 11]. In contrast to those methods, the author left only minimal scars embedded within the dimple. The technique can also be performed on a flat abdominal wall without any remaining umbilical tissue or if there is a partial absence of abdominal skin after the removal of the umbilical tissue. It can also be applied as both delayed and immediate reconstructive procedures with many advantages, including (1) being simple and easy, (2) being appropriate for junior surgeons,(3) involving the manipulation of well-vascularized flaps, (4) yielding satisfactory superior hooding, and (5) resulting in a minimal external scar. Considering these advantages and the fact that it leads to aesthetically satisfactory results, this technique can be widely employed as a useful neoumbilicoplasty technique in patients suffering from an absent or disfigured umbilicus.

References

1. Bartsich SA, Schwartz MH. Purse-string method for immediate umbilical reconstruction. Plast Reconstr Surg. 2003;112(6):1652–5.
2. Pfulg M, Van de Sijpe K, Blondeel P. A simple new technique for neoumbilicoplasty. Br J Plast Surg. 2005;58(5):688–91.
3. Hong YG, Cho JJ. Reconstruction of scarred umbilicus using an inverted c-v flap: a case report. J Korean Soc Plast Reconstr Surg. 2007;34(5):653–5.
4. Miller MJ, Balch CM. "Iris" technique for immediate umbilical reconstruction. Plast Reconstr Surg. 1993;92(4):754–6.
5. El-Dessouki NI, Shehata SM, Torki AM, Hashish AA. Double half-cone flap umbilicoplasty: a new technique for the proboscoid umbilical hernia in children. Hernia. 2004;8(3):182–5.

6. Ricketts RR, Luck SR. Simultaneous umbilicoplasty and closure of small omphaloceles. Surg Gynecol Obstet. 1983;157(6):572–3.
7. Matsuo K, Kondoh S, Hirose T. A simple technique for reconstruction of the umbilicus, using a conchal cartilage composite graft. Plast Reconstr Surg. 1990;86(1):149–51.
8. Friedland JA, Maffi TR. MOC-PS(SM) CME article: abdominoplasty. Plast Reconstr Surg. 2008;121(4 Suppl):1–11.
9. Shinohara H, Matsuo K, Kikuchi N. Umbilical reconstruction with an inverted C-V flap. Plast Reconstr Surg. 2000;105(2):703–5.
10. Lee SL, DuBois JJ, Greenholz SK, Huffman SG. Advancement flap umbilicoplasty after abdominal wall closure: postoperative results compared with normal umbilical anatomy. J Pediatr Surg. 2001;36(8):1168–70.
11. Kirianoff TG. Making a new umbilicus when none exists. Case report. Plast Reconstr Surg. 1978;61(4):603–4.
12. Frigo E, Rettinger-Schimmerl S, Rokitansky AM. Umbilicoplasty in neonates with primary omphalocele closure. Pediatr Surg Int. 1999;15(7):523–4.
13. Park ES, Kim MS, Kim YB. Immediate umbilical reconstruction for urachal cancer. J Korean Soc Aesthetic Plast Surg. 2003;9(2):59–62.
14. Marconi F. Reconstruction of the umbilicus: a simple technique. Plast Reconstr Surg. 1995;95(6):1115–7.

Chapter 35
Enriched Adipose Micrografts (EAM) with Autologous Plasma in the Periumbilical Area

Guillermo Blugerman, Diego Schavelzon, Gabriel Wexler, and Marcelo Lotocky

35.1 Introduction

The use of autologous fat as a filler has been around for over 100 years. In 1893, fat grafts were use to achieve tissue remodeling and improve asymmetries with good results [1]. In 1910 Erich Lexer [2] used autologous fat to improve a depression caused by zygomatic fractures with acceptable results and stable for years, and later, Peer [3] reaffirmed the use and survival of these grafts. The biggest problem remained the need for extirpation of adipose tissue through acceptable skin incisions.

The introduction of liposuction in the 1980s opened new possibilities of obtaining fat and subsequent grafting, without scarring sequelae in the donor area. Our first results were presented at the Brazilian Congress Belo Horizonte in 1986 [4]. Since then we continue to improve our technique, looking for the best protocol to cover all aspects of this procedure that, even being easily reproducible, has a high failure rate if the basic principles of tissue grafting are not respected

This chapter summarizes our current technique of enriched adipose micrografts (EAM), based on the results of the last five consecutive years of its application.

G. Blugerman • D. Schavelzon
B & S Center of Excellence in Plastic Surgery, Buenos Aires, Argentina
e-mail: blugerman@centrosbys.com; drschavelzon@gmail.com

G. Wexler (✉) • M. Lotocky
B & S Center of Excellence in Plastic Surgery, Private Practice, Laprida 1579, Buenos Aires, Argentina
e-mail: gabrielew555@hotmail.com; aliasmarce@hotmail.com

M.A. Shiffman (ed.), *Adult Umbilical Reconstruction*,
DOI 10.1007/978-3-319-43887-0_35

35.2 Healing and Growth Factors

Healing is a process that takes time and compliance with a series of steps that begin with the activation of multiple growth factors. The increased availability of these factors during this process shortens time and improves results, reducing inflammatory reaction and scarring sequelae. The availability of growth factors (GF) at the tissue level may be increased using autologous platelet concentrate obtained from the patient's own blood. GF are polypeptides of amino acids that form a globular protein and belong to the group of cytokines. They are produced in greater quantities by macrophages and platelets.

These cytokines have the ability to join cell membrane receptors that activate or inhibit cellular functions by target cells on which they act. The most studied growth factors are the epithelial growth factor, fibroblast growth factor, and platelet-derived growth factor. The use of growth factors was initiated in the field of maxillofacial surgery and dentistry as a biological material to stimulate bone remodeling, and then its use was expanded to other areas of medical science.

35.3 EAM Indications in the Umbilicus

1. Extreme thinning of the supraumbilical skin triangle, in order to recover subcutaneous tissue thickness. These cases are frequently found in twin pregnancy.
2. Post-liposuction patients with over resection in the periumbilical area. The loss of the periumbilical subcutaneous thickness results in flat umbilicus.

35.4 Surgical Technique

35.4.1 Documentation and Markings

After diagnosis, tissue deficit must be located around the umbilicus: superior, inferior, lateral, combination, or complete periumbilical tissue deficit. A generous donor area must be identified in accordance with the patient. Patient selection and the realistic expectations of possible outcomes are important points to arrive to a good percentage of satisfied patients. Photographs and marks are made in standing position. In some surface defects, a tangential light on the skin is useful for a better documentation and marking of the defects. It is important to use natural-colored long-term markers to avoid erasing landmarks during the procedure. When choosing the donor site, it is important to evaluate the patients' rich in fat tissue areas and the surgeons' preference. There is no heavy evidence on the choice of the donor site in the efficacy of fat grafting, but some studies suggest that there are areas with a higher number of stem cells than others.

35.4.2 Obtaining Inactive Plasma

Before starting the procedure, we draw blood from the patient and the blood is processed to obtain the TP or PRP. Timing is important since after the surgical procedure starts, the platelet count in the patient's blood is lowered. Following our protocol, blood is extracted with a 20 mL sterile syringe for small volume filling and a 40 mL syringe for large volume filling.

The blood is collected in tubes of 8.5 mL containing calcium citrate (BD Vacutainer ACD Solution A) to avoid clotting. The anticoagulated blood is transferred to a separation gel tube (BD Vacutainer SST) that allows mechanical separation of red cells and plasma during centrifugation. The separation process is performed at 3000 rpm for 10 min (this step needs to be adapted to each centrifuging machine). Then the total plasma is in BD Vacutainer SST as seen in Fig. 35.1.

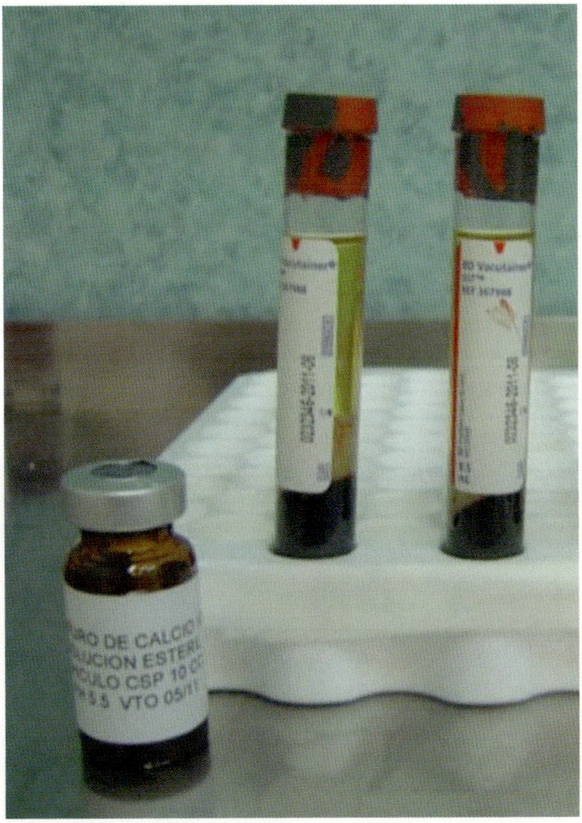

Fig. 35.1 Total plasma after centrifugation in BD Vacutainer SST. On the *right*, calcium citrate for activation

35.4.3 Anesthesia of Donor Area

The use of epinephrine or lidocaine in the donor site has been accused to affect the viability of the graft, but there is no consistent evidence. Following the previous markings, anesthetic infiltration of the donor site is performed using tumescent anesthesia with a solution composed of 0.06 % lidocaine with epinephrine 1:1,000,000 and 12.5 meq of sodium bicarbonate for each liter of saline (0.9 % Na solution). The infiltration is performed using Klein's cannulas connected to the B & S (Blugerman & Schavelzon) peristaltic pump.

35.4.4 Anesthesia of Recipient Site

The receptor area is infiltrated through microcannulas or selected needles according to the area, following presurgical landmarks. The same concentrations of tumescent anesthesia are used, without infiltrating large quantities of liquid. In this way, the receptor area is not distorted, and the anesthetic effect is achieved. For facial treatments, nerve blocks are done as described by Amar and Fox [5].

35.4.5 Preparing Micrografts of Adipose Tissue

The main points to consider when obtaining fat grafts are the degree of tissue invasiveness (patient safety) and tissue viability (efficiency). With this in mind, mechanical damage is minimized in this step.

In the protocol, the procedure requires the use of specific instruments (Fig. 35.2), which we called Micro Graft Fat Cutter (MGFC) or Blugerman Graft Cutter (BGC). In the study by Blugerman et al. [6], University of Frankfurt, it was found that the

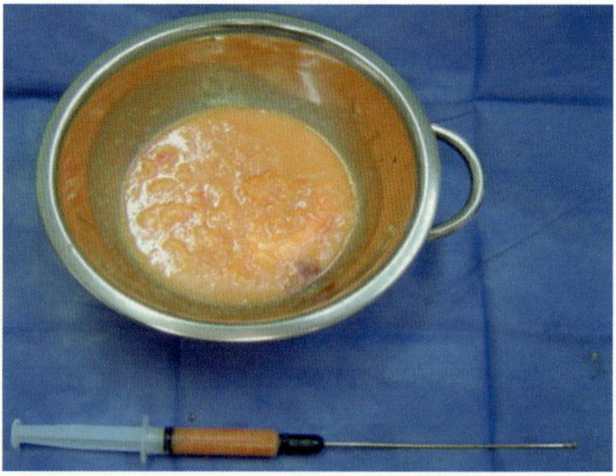

Fig. 35.2 (*Left*) Blugerman Graft Cutter. (*Right*) Micro Graft Fat Cutter

micrografts obtained with both instruments had the same characteristics and survival rate than grafts cut with a scalpel, surpassing those obtained with liposuction cannulas. These instruments are tubular multi-scalpel cannulas that work without suction or vacuum. The cutting edge produces micrografts aided by external compression of the fingers pushing the adipose tissue into the holes to facilitate the splitting of the fat block. Micrografts produced by the actions of MGFC remain suspended in the tumescent solution in the donor area ready for collection.

35.4.6 Collection of Micrografts

To collect the micrografts, a 3–4 mm large hole atraumatic blunt cannula is used. This step is performed with 10 mL syringes at low vacuum pressure, when the volume required is small, or with a B & S peristaltic pump when volume is larger. The B & S peristaltic pump allows to work in a closed circuit for the recovery of grafts. Working in a close circuit reduces the risk of contamination, preventing the entry of large volumes of contaminated air and avoiding the "cyclone" effect inside the bottle. Preventing air contact also avoids fat dehydration reducing the apoptosis rate, thus ensuring vitality of micrografts.

35.4.7 Settling or Centrifugation of the Material

When working with small volumes, the material obtained is centrifuged at 3000 rpm for 3 min, separating the micrografts from the tumescent fluid and the oil, resulting from the rupture of adipocytes. When using volumes exceeding 100 mL, it is preferred to decant the material, without any filtering or transfer.

The special feature of the B & S collecting system is that tissue is pumped through the bottom of the collector, producing washing effect of grafts in the previously sucked fluid. This makes the process of separation by gravity faster and more efficient than using a top-hole bottle. With this system, external washing of the grafts is avoided, reducing the risk of contamination [7–9].

Finally, by reversing the direction of rotation of the peristaltic B & S pump, the tumescent fluid is removed, leaving only the concentrated micrografts ready to use.

35.4.8 Plasma Activation

The platelet concentrate (600,000–1,500,000 × mm) obtained from blood centrifugation has three well-defined layers, the first layer corresponding to the platelet-poor plasma (PPP) and the second corresponding to the platelet-rich plasma (PRP), which is the portion closest to the red blood cells (RBCs) in the third layer.

When using small volume EAM, in which milliliter precision is important, only the PRP is used to prevent dilution of micrografts. When working in body contouring, TP is used, adding the PRP properties to the PPP, which is the residual plasma and contains clotting factors, mainly fibrinogen, thrombin, and calcium molecules that stabilize the blood clot and contribute to a rapid and effective healing of the soft tissues.

In our experience, the use of total plasma (PPP+PRP) in the process has submitted satisfactory and comparable results to the use of PRP, allowing to simplify the procedure and reduce material handling and contamination.

To activate the PRP or TP, 10% CaCl (0.05 cm^3 of CaCl per 3 mL) is added, activating the coagulation cascade.

35.4.9 Preparation of the Recipient Site

Antisepsis of the recipient area is done, and surgical wraps are placed. If the local anesthesia of the recipient region has not been previously done, this is the moment to do it. Depending on the region to be treated, micro-incisions are carried out taking into account the location of the defect and the aesthetic result on the skin.

35.4.10 Injection Technique of EAM

To optimize the viability of enriched adipose micrografts, the mechanical damage of the implanted tissue has to be minimized. Prior to the implantation of micrografts, the technique of pre-tunneling of the subcutaneous tissue (SCT) is done with the spatulated cannula. The spatulated cannula creates paths or tunnels on several levels where the micrografts will be deposited for better distribution. This pre-tunneling should be done with the bevel of the spatulated cannula perpendicularly in respect to the surface of the skin in an attempt to preserve the subdermal plexus, which is highly needed to ensure rapid revascularization and consistent implementation of micrografts. The preservation of the vascular elements also reduces the risk of hematoma, which if present leads to necrosis due to the loss of oxygenation and nutrition of micrografts in their stages.

From the mixture of micrografts and PRP or TP, a gel is obtained (EAM) and is transferred to 1 mL syringes when use for small volume treatment and in 5, 10, or 20 mL when used for large treatment (Fig. 35.3).

Material injection in the periumbilical area is performed using microcannulas of 1 mm and 1.4 mm.

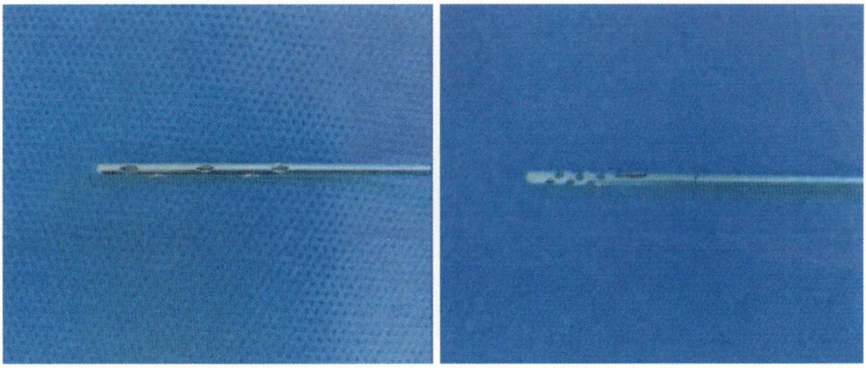

Fig. 35.3 Gel of plasma and fat grafts (EAM)

35.4.11 Re-tunnelization

After the micrografts are injected, the spatula is reintroduced, and new re-tunneling maneuvers are done using the same instrument that will continue to work perpendicularly to the skin. This maneuver will redistribute the grafted tissue more evenly and will reduce the compression exerted from the surrounding tissues to the micrografts.

35.4.12 Postoperation Bandages

At the end of the procedure, a bandage of the micro-incisions with sterile Micropore® tape is done in the recipient's area, exposing the treated area and leaving it free of compression. In the supraumbilical area, Reston® may be applied to keep the implanted areas free from external pressure. The donor site incisions are left opened to promote drainage of the tumescent solution, sterile dressings are placed, and compressive bandaging is applied.

35.5 Risks and Complications Associated with Periumbilical Fat Graft

There were no reported cases of complications related to anesthesia and fat grafting. These complications are rare considering that most cases are performed under local anesthesia with or without sedation, which minimizes the risk of surgery. Blood loss is similar to tumescent liposuction. There are reports of hematoma associated with this procedure, but none were severe or unresolved.

Poor results that do not cover expected are rare. In general the results of this procedure are reported as excellent or good. Most cases reported as unsatisfactory are caused by volume loss of the grafted tissue due to necrosis or reabsorption.

Cases of graft hypertrophy or overgrowth have been documented on rare occasions.

Infections can occur, and cultures should be done with needle aspiration and treated according to cultures.

Persistent erythema is a frequent complication which is hard to differentiate from infection and is caused by the inflammatory process that involves revascularization of grafts and resorption of nonviable graft tissue. Cultures are always negative.

Liponecrosis can occur when the graft is not receiving enough oxygen. This can be the result of a large graft or a poor receptor area. Clinical aspect is similar to infection, and usually a yellowish-brown material drains spontaneously or through puncture.

Other complications include the formation of calcified and noncalcified masses.

35.6 Results

This EAM protocol has been used over the past 8 years. During this period, a total of 25 EAM procedures have been performed around the umbilicus area. The patient and surgeon satisfaction was high in most procedures. If sterile and atraumatic principles are respected, the complication rates are low.

It is important to inform patients about the possibility of reimplantation of new micrografts in the treated area, based on the concept of a progressive increase in volume, so that the patient is prepared for this eventuality. In our case, the need for further sessions of EAM depended on the degree of the defect and the results achieved, with a maximum of three sessions in complex cases (Figs. 35.4 and 35.5). Most second procedures corresponded to minor corrections or minimum volume of tissue irregularities.

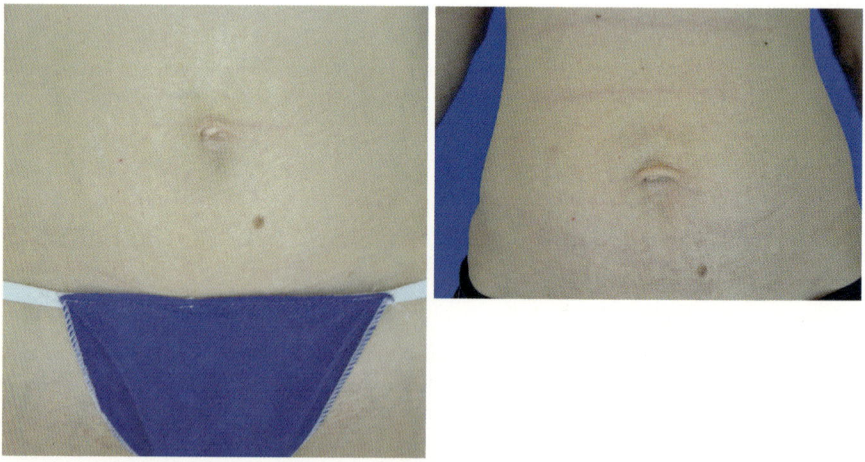

Fig. 35.4 Patient with periumbilical depressions after transumbilical hernioplasty. After 1 month second sessions of EAM (15 and 20 mL)

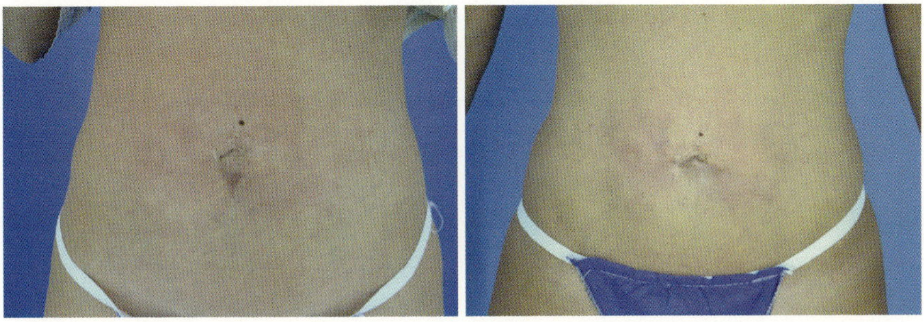

Fig. 35.5 Post-liposuction retraction of the supraumbilical skin. After 2 months of the first session of EAM 13 mL

35.7 Conclusions

The combination of adipose tissue micrografts with concentrate PRP or PT allows us to accelerate the restoration of periumbilical tissues, with a low risk of complications when using autologous material.

We noticed that the resulting gel is easier to inject through the cannula, creating less friction and requiring less pressure for the passage of the micrografts through the syringe to the prefabricated tunnel. Prefabrication of these tunnels reduces the resistance of the tissues to the entrance of the micrografts, facilitating transplantation and uniform distribution. In our experience, the use of EAM has increased fat graft survival in all body areas, further improving the quality of the skin in patients with radiation dermatitis or skin atrophy and achieving greater satisfaction for our patients.

References

1. Neuber GA. Fettransplantation. Chir Kongr Verhandl Deutsch Gesellsch Chir. 1893;22:66.
2. Lexer E. Zwanzig jahr transplantationsforschung in der chirurgie. Arch Min Chir. 1925;138:294.
3. Peer LA. Transplantation of fat. In: Transplantation of tissue. Baltimore: Williams & Wilkins; 1969. p. 165–244.
4. Blugerman G. Metodología actual para Lipoinjerto Autólogo. Actas del XXIII Congreso Brasileiro de Cirugía Plástica. Brasil: Belho Horizonte; 1986.
5. Amar RE, Fox DM. The facial autologous muscular injection (FAMI) procedure: an anatomically targeted deep multiplane autologous fat-grafting technique using principles of facial fat injection. Aesthetic Plast Surg. 2011;35(4):502–10.
6. Blugerman G, Schavelzon D, Podda M, Bonesana G, Pontón A, Chomyzyn A, Martínez L, Izurrategui N. Movilización adiposa interna (liposhifting) con espátula y cortador de microinjertos de grasa. Dermatologia CMQ. 2007;5(2):105–11.
7. Karacalar A, Orak I, Kaplan S, Yildirim S. No-touch technique for autologous fat harvesting. Aesthetic Plast Surg. 2004;28(3):158–64.

8. Shiffman MA, Mirrafati S. Fat transfer techniques: The effect of harvest and transfer methods on adipocyte viability and review of the literature. Dermatol Surg. 2001;27(9):819–26.
9. Smith P, Adams Jr WP, Lipschitz A, Chau B, Sorokin E, Rohrich RJ, Brown SA. Autologous human fat grafting: effect of harvesting and preparation techniques on adipocyte graft survival. Plast Reconstr Surg. 2006;117(6):1836–44.

Chapter 36
Excision and Umbilicoplasty for Umbilical Pilonidal Disease

Nezih Akkapulu and Mehmet Bulent Tirnaksiz

36.1 Introduction

Pilonidal disease is an acquired condition that is commonly found in young male adults. It is believed to be caused by granulomatous inflammation resulting from the irritation of trapped hair shaft between the epidermis and dermis leading to foreign body reaction and multifactorial infection [1–3]. The pilonidal disease was first described in the nineteenth century, and the term pilonidal is derived from the Latin words for hair (pilas) and nest (nidus) [4].

Although, pilonidal disease most commonly occurs in sacrococcygeal region, it has been described in other parts of the body, such as axillary region [5], scalp [6], anal canal [7], interdigital sulcus and hand [8], sternum [9], ear [10], nose [11], and umbilicus [12].

Umbilical pilonidal disease (UPD) is seen less frequently than sacrococcygeal pilonidal disease (SCPD). To date, published studies on this pathology are usually case reports and case series, and no comparative studies have been reported in English literature; thus controversy still surrounds the etiology, pathogenesis, and proper management of the umbilical pilonidal disease (UPD) [13–17].

N. Akkapulu, M.D., FACS (✉)
Department of General Surgery, Ordu Teaching and Research Hospital, Bahcelievler Mahallesi, Yunus Emre Caddesi No: 8/3, 52200 Ordu, Turkey
e-mail: akkapulu@gmail.com

M.B. Tirnaksiz, M.D.
Department of General Surgery, Hacettepe University School of Medicine, Ankara 06230, Turkey
e-mail: mbtirnaksiz@gmail.com

M.A. Shiffman (ed.), *Adult Umbilical Reconstruction*,
DOI 10.1007/978-3-319-43887-0_36

36.1.1 Clinical Features of Umbilical Pilonidal Disease

Umbilical pilonidal disease is commonly found in young male adults. The prevalence of UPD is not accurately known, but has been reported to be in the range of 0.1–0.6 % [17, 18].

A hairy body, lack of personal hygiene, deep umbilical recess, hyperhidrosis, overweight, wearing of tight clothes, belt usage, and history of sacrococcygeal pilonidal disease (SCPD) have been commonly suggested as predisposing factors (Table 36.1). In a study of 31 patients with UPD, various risk factors were compared to 100 volunteers. The report shows hirsute status, wearing tight clothes, and obesity, and familial history of PD was significantly higher in the UPD group [17].

It is believed that UPD and SCPD share the similar pathogenic mechanisms. Hair follicle plays a central role. Repeated microtrauma and tugging action of the urachus result in the development of pits in which hair strands induce local inflammation and foreign body reaction leading to the formation of subcutaneous cavity [13]. On the other side, UPD has lower recurrence rate and smaller amount of fistula tract than SCPD [19].

The two most common symptoms are mild pain and bloody or purulent discharge from the umbilicus [13, 14, 20]. In the presence of acute abscess, patients typically present with a tender, fluctuant mass in the umbilicus, sometimes accompanied by periumbilical cellulitis, fever, and leukocytosis. An acute abscess is the presenting finding in approximately 25 % of patients with UPD [13]. Chronic cases may present with a small and reddish umbilical mass with or without discharge.

Since UPD is a rare occurrence and in its chronic form, the presentation is variable, it may easily be misdiagnosed as any other lesion of the umbilicus. Differential diagnosis for UPD includes embryologic anomalies (omphalomesenteric and urachal

Table 36.1 Predisposing factors for UPD

	Eryilmaz et al. [13]	Kareem [14]	Sarmast et al. [15]	Fazeli et al. [16]	Coskun et al. [17]
Gender (male/female)	24/2	121/13	29/14	39/6	31/4
Age (mean)	22	24	25	22	24.83
BMI (mean)	N/A	24.07	N/A	N/A	23.8*
Obesity (%)	15	1.49	N/A	N/A	N/A
Hirsute status (%)	88	98.5	N/A	93.3	48*
Insufficient personal hygiene (%)	73	30.6	N/A	N/A	61.3**
Deep navel (%)	81	100	N/A	N/A	N/A
Hyperhidrosis (%)	23	N/A	N/A	N/A	N/A
History of SCPD (%)	N/A	32.83	N/A	13.74	19**
Tight clothes (%)	N/A	N/A	N/A	N/A	74*
Belt usage (%)	N/A	N/A	N/A	N/A	80**

BMI body mass index, *SCPD* sacrococcygeal pilonidal disease, *N/A* not available
*$p<0.05$; **$p>0.05$

cysts) or acquired pathologies such as Sister Mary Joseph's nodule, skin tumors, pyogenic granuloma, umbilical hernia, and endometriosis [13, 21]. When diagnosis of UPD is not easy, complementary investigations should be considered [22, 23].

36.2 Treatment

An optimal treatment protocol for UPD includes the following goals: simple intervention, low morbidity and recurrence rate, and fast return to normal activity. Despite these goals, there is no consensus about the ideal treatment of UPD. It should be kept in mind that no single mode of treatment meets all these goals. Analysis of the literature is difficult because of the following reasons: all published studies are case reports and small case series and, therefore, difficult to compare; many treatment modalities have been proposed for the definitive treatment of UPD; results are enormously heterogeneous; and follow-up periods are short or absent.

Treatment options range from non-operative (conservative) modalities to radical surgical procedures such as umbilectomy. Conservative treatment modalities include shaving around the umbilicus, simple incision, and curettage of the sinus with hair extraction [13, 14]. Eryilmaz et al. [13] reported a retrospective case series of 26 patients treated with conservative methods. They found that conservative treatment was successful in 88 % of patients. Healing and recurrence rates were not reported in this study. In a recent retrospective review on conservative treatment, Kareem reports 134 patients treated over 6.5 years. A follow-up period was available in 34 % of patients. Conservative treatment was successful in 76 % of patients without recurrence. Twenty-four percent of patients required more than one therapeutic session [14].

Although conservative techniques are simple to perform and cost-effective, they have not been well evaluated. Surgical excision, which is more effective, remains the therapeutic standard for UPD. Surgical treatment options include umbilectomy with immediate closure, umbilectomy with secondary intention healing, and excision of sinus with umbilicoplasty. Umbilectomy is the most radical procedure with probably the lowest recurrence rate. However, this technique is not cosmetically satisfactory and, therefore, should be considered as a last resort. Compared to umbilectomy, sinus excision and umbilicoplasty appear to achieve similar recurrence rates with better cosmetic results [16, 24].

36.3 Operative Technique for Sinus Excision and Umbilicoplasty

The patient is placed in a comfortable supine position. Spinal or inhalation anesthesia can be used. At our institution, patients receive a first generation cephalosporin for antibiotic prophylaxis. A curvilinear incision (reverse bucket-handle) is made at the inferior rim of the umbilicus from the 3 o'clock position to the 9 o'clock position. The umbilicus proper should be retained in the skin flap. Dissection is carried down to the level of the linea alba and anterior sheaths of the rectus muscle. Umbilicus is everted completely. Sinus pit or pits can now be visualized (Fig. 36.1). A probe can be introduced into the pit or pits or methylene blue can be instilled into the sinus opening to better outline all involved parts (Fig. 36.2). Pit(s) and sinus are then dissected off circumferentially and excised completely (Fig. 36.3). After careful hemostasis is obtained, the apex of the subcutaneous tissue beneath the umbilicus is sutured down to the linea alba with 2/0 absorbable sutures. This produces the desirable ingoing belly button. Further absorbable sutures are used to obliterate the subcutaneous dead space. The incision is closed with a running subcuticular

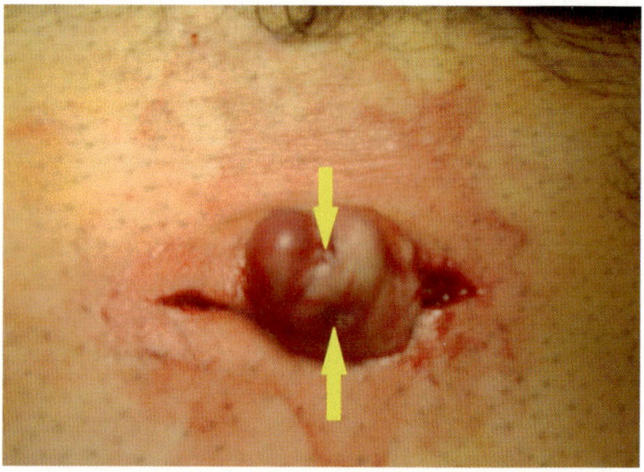

Fig. 36.1 The everted umbilicus. Sinus pits are shown by *arrows* [12]

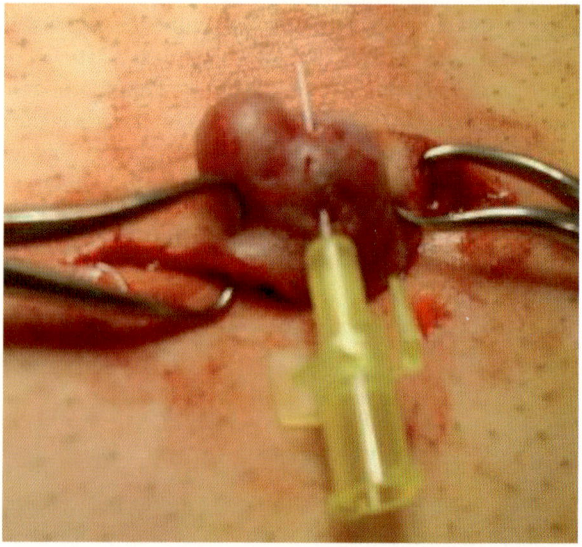

Fig. 36.2 The connecting tract between pits is revealed by a probe

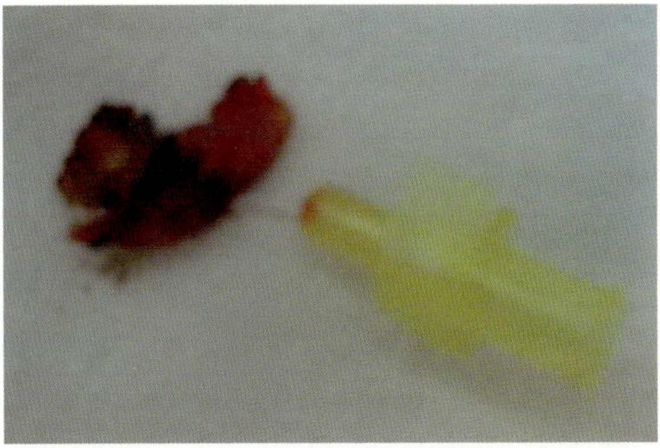

Fig. 36.3 The tissue around the probe is removed

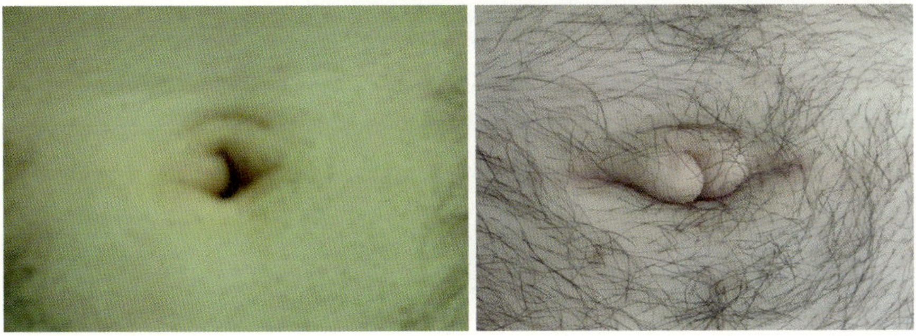

Fig. 36.4 (*Left*) Umbilicus preoperative. (*Right*) After the excision of the pits and sinus [12]

absorbable 4/0 suture and dressed with tissue adhesive. To help prevent a wound seroma, a ball of cotton or gauze should be placed in the umbilicus and held in place with an abdominal binder (Fig. 36.4).

36.4 Conclusions

Umbilical pilonidal disease (UPD) is seen less frequently than sacrococcygeal pilonidal disease (SCPD). This rare occurrence is predominant in young adult males. Treatment options range from non-operative (conservative) modalities to radical surgical procedures. There is no consensus about the ideal treatment of UPD. Conservative measures have not been well evaluated. Surgical excision, which is more effective, remains the therapeutic standard for UPD. Many surgical treatment options have been described in the literature. Umbilectomy is the most radical procedure with probably the lowest recurrence rate. However, this technique is not cosmetically satisfactory and, therefore, should be considered as a last resort. Compared to umbilectomy, sinus excision and umbilicoplasty appear to achieve similar recurrence rates with better cosmesis.

References

1. Hull TL, Wu J. Pilonidal disease. Surg Clin North Am. 2002;82(6):1169–85.
2. Humphries AE, Duncan JE. Evaluation and management of pilonidal disease. Surg Clin North Am. 2010;90(1):113–24.
3. Velasco AL, Dunlap WW. Pilonidal disease and hidradenitis. Surg Clin North Am. 2009;89(3):689–701.
4. Rm H. Pilonidal sinus. Boston Med Surg J. 1880;103:485–6.
5. Sengul I, Sengul D, Mocan G. Axillary pilonidal sinus: a case report. N Am J Med Sci. 2009;1(6):316–8.
6. Pehlivanli F, Karaca G, Pekcici MR, Yildirim K, Karaca B. Pilonidal sinus disease of the scalp. Am Surg. 2012;78(4):E242–3.
7. Aggarwal K, Jain BK, Sharma N, Goel S. Pilonidal sinus of anal canal: a possible unique diagnosis. ANZ J Surg. 2015;85(9):693–4.
8. Ito A, Yoshida Y, Yamamoto O. Case of interdigital pilonidal sinus in a dog groomer. J Dermatol. 2013;40(12):1051–2.
9. Ahmed I, Chan FC, McLaughlin P. Pilonidal abscess of the sternum. Irish J Med Sci. 2002;171(4):237.
10. Woodward WW. A pilonidal sinus of the ear. ANZ J Surg. 1965;35(1):72–3.
11. Paulose KO, Al Khalifa S, Raj SS, Saeed T. Pilonidal sinus of the nose. J Laryngol Otol. 1989;103(12):1210–3.
12. Akkapulu N, Tanrikulu Y. Umbilical pilonidal sinus: a case report. J Med Case. 2011;2(6):272–4. doi:10.4021/jmc348w
13. Eryilmaz R, Sahin M, Okan I, Alimoglu O, Somay A. Umbilical pilonidal sinus disease: predisposing factors and treatment. World J Surg. 2005;29(9):1158–60.
14. Kareem T. Outcomes of conservative treatment of 134 cases of umbilical pilonidal sinus. World J Surg. 2013;37(2):313–7.
15. Sarmast MH, Javaherizadeh H, Shahvari MR. Non-surgical treatment of umbilical pilonidal sinus in adolescent and adult cases. Polski Przeglad Chirurg. 2011;83(12):652–3.
16. Fazeli MS, Lebaschi AH, Adel MG, Kazemeini AR. Evaluation of the outcome of complete sinus excision with reconstruction of the umbilicus in patients with umbilical pilonidal sinus. World J Surg. 2008;32(10):2305–8.
17. Coskun A, Bulus H, Faruk Akinci O, Ozgonul A. Etiological factors in umbilical pilonidal sinus. Indian J Surg. 2011;73(1):54–7.
18. Goodall P. The aetiology and treatment of pilonidal sinus. A review of 163 patients. Br J Surg. 1961;49:212–8.
19. Naraynsingh V, Hariharan S, Dan D. Umbilical pilonidal sinus: a new treatment technique of sinus excision with umbilical preservation. Dermatol Surg. 2009;35(7):1155–6.
20. El-Bakry AA. Discharging umbilicus. Saudi Med J. 2002;23(9):1099–100.
21. Molderez CM, Wouters KB, Bergmans GB, Michiels GK. Umbilical discharge: a review of 22 cases. Acta Chirurg Belg. 1995;95(3):166–9.
22. McClenathan JH. Umbilical pilonidal sinus. Can J Surg. 2000;43(3):225.
23. Abdulwahab BA, Harste K. Umbilical pilonidal sinus. Ugeskr Laeger. 2010;172(41):2848–9.
24. Haj M, Cohen I. Umbilical pilonidal sinus ambulatory surgical technique. J Ambulatory Surg. 2004;11(1–2):37–9.

Part V
History of Tumors of the Umbilicus

Chapter 37
History of Tumors of the Umbilicus

Melvin A. Shiffman

37.1 Introduction

Cullen (1916) [1] (Appendix A) published his cases of benign tumors and primary and metastatic cancers involving the umbilicus and included an extensive review of cases previously published. He stated that Nicaise and Boursier, in 1881 [2], wrote an exhaustive treatise on umbilical diseases. Villar, in 1886 [3], wrote a thesis on umbilical tumors, going into the subject very carefully and making a satisfactory classification of the various umbilical tumors. Hanay (1843) [4] reported a scirrhous carcinoma of the umbilicus.

Nicaise and Boursier (1881) [2] discussed benign tumors such as:

1. Hypertrophic umbilicus
2. Angiomata
3. Lymphocele
4. Benign connective-tissue growths
5. Myxomata
6. Fibromata
7. Papillomata
8. Lipomata
9. Dermoid cysts
10. Sweat gland tumors
11. Adenomyomata

They also described malignancies of the umbilicus including:

1. Primary squamous-cell carcinoma
2. Primary adenocarcinoma

M.A. Shiffman, M.D., J.D.
Private Practice, 17501 Chatham Drive, Tustin, CA 92780-2302, USA
e-mail: shiffmanmdjd@gmail.com

M.A. Shiffman (ed.), *Adult Umbilical Reconstruction*,
DOI 10.1007/978-3-319-43887-0_37

3. Metastatic carcinoma from the stomach, gallbladder, intestine, ovary, and uterus and from other abdominal organs
4. Telangiectatic myxosarcoma
5. Spindle-cell sarcoma
6. Round-cell sarcoma
7. Melanotic sarcoma

Pernice (1892) [5] found 21 cases in the literature that he considered primary carcinoma of the umbilicus.

37.2 Primary Adenocarcinoma

Cullen (1916) [6] thought that primary adenocarcinoma of the umbilicus was possibly from remnants of the omphalomesenteric duct. Glazer (1973) [7] found a primary adenocarcinoma arising in a vitellointestinal duct remnant at the umbilicus.

Ross and Hill (1975) [8] described a case of primary adenocarcinoma of the umbilicus and reviewed the literature. They discussed possible origins of glandular tissue within this area. Multiple connections are present within the umbilicus (vascular, lymphatic, and embryologic) that may give this area access to metastatic lesions. The primary tumors may originate within the usual umbilical tissue (skin and soft tissue). Glands that are not normally present in the region of the umbilicus rarely develop malignant neoplasms. They postulated that glandular tissue may arise either as metaplasia from squamous epithelium or from glandular embryologic rests including omphalomesenteric duct remnants and urachal remnants.

Hernandez et al. (1993) [9] studied the histological and ultrastructural features, as well as the immunoreactivity of one case of uncommon primary papillary and psammomatous adenocarcinoma of the umbilicus. Observations were undertaken in a 9-year follow-up and included the primitive tumor, two local recidives, and inguinal lymphatic metastasis on two occasions. Papillary structures, numerous psammoma bodies, as well as weak and focal positive reactions to CEA and cytokeratin were present in all the tumors. Since these features and their ultrastructural characteristics were identical to primary papillary serous neoplasias of the peritoneum and ovarium, the hypothesis of an origin in coelomic remnants was considered.

Alver et al. (2007) [10] described a case of a primary umbilical adenocarcinoma with short-time survival related to local recurrence and multiple hepatic metastases 6 months after her surgical treatment. Alnaqbi et al. (2007) [11] described a 60-year-old patient with adenocarcinoma arising from the coelomic mesothelium of a hernia sac. The tumor was a serous papillary adenocarcinoma. No primary tumor was found.

Atri et al. (2009) [12] described a 28-year-old male who presented with complaints of discharge from the umbilicus for 1 year duration. Discharge was thick and purulent in nature, associated with off-on pain in the abdomen which was mild to moderate in intensity and non-referred type. On local examination there was a reddish brown swelling of 2.5 × 3.0 cm in size present in the umbilical region which was subcutaneous, round, tender, mobile, and hard in consistency. Operative findings revealed a nodule of 5×5 cm on the umbilicus. Swelling was not seen extending to the peritoneum, and adjacent structures were not infiltrated. Histopathology of the excised nodule was suggestive of adenocarcinoma of umbilicus.

A 51-year-old man with an umbilical mass was reported by Liu (2011) [13]. Surgical biopsy showed infiltrating neoplasm with glandular and focal papillary architecture. FDG PET/CT demonstrated a focus of abnormal uptake located in the umbilicus, without evidence of a primary tumor elsewhere. Further investigations with EGD, colonoscopy, and cystoscopy were all negative for a neoplasm. The whole-body FDG PET/CT is an ideal imaging modality for evaluation of an umbilical lesion, especially identification or exclusion of a primary neoplasm elsewhere.

37.3 Angiomyxoma

Angiomyxoma of the umbilicus was reported by Fortune and Ostor (1980) [14] and Goksever et al. (2010) [15].

37.4 Benign Tumors of the Umbilicus

37.4.1 Teratoma

Teratomas consist of a combination of the tissues from all three blastodermic layers (ecto-, meso-, and endoderm). One distinguishes mature teratomas (cysts), immature teratomas (solid tissue), and malignantly degenerated teratomas.

Brooks (1919) [16] reported the first teratoma of the umbilicus. Chavali et al. (2014) [17] had a patient with immature teratoma at the umbilicus region presenting as exomphalos.

Kreczy et al. (1994) [18] described a case of 10×7×5-cm mass located just at the end of an omphalocele in the umbilical cord of a full-term baby. The tissues of all three germinal layers could be found, but there were no skeletal structures. Five cases were found in the literature from 1887 to 1993, the latest reported in 1985.

Teratomas of the umbilical cord are very rare lesions. They discussed the relationship between the teratoma of the umbilical cord and the holoacardius amorphus.

37.4.2 Hemangioma

There was a case report of umbilical hemangioma by Sathiyathasan et al. (2011) [19].

37.4.3 Heterotopic Liver

Heterotopic liver was noted in the umbilicus by Lee et al. (2011) [20].

37.4.4 Polyp

Kuitin et al. (1979) [21] stated that anomalies of the omphalomesenteric duct (OMD) present a variety of surgical problems. The most readily apparent of these lesions is the umbilical polyp. One-third of patients explored at their hospital and 56 % of patients reviewed had an additional OMD anomaly when explored for an umbilical polyp. The preferred treatment for this lesion should be a minilaparotomy after the presence of intestinal mucosa at the umbilicus is confirmed.

37.4.5 Colonic Mucous Membrane

Rejmanowski et al. (1989) [22] noted heterotopy of colonic mucous membrane in the navel skin of a 1.5-year-old child.

37.4.6 Endometriosis

Endometriosis involving the umbilicus is attributed to Villar (1886) [23] by Cullen (1916) [24] who describes von Noorden's case (1901) [25] and then refers to Mintz (1899) [26] and finally Villar's (1886) case. The citation was "As will be noted from the history, the patient was a woman 39 years of age. There was no evidence of inflammation. Histologic examination in some places showed groups of glands lying in a stroma differing from the ordinary surrounding stroma. These groups of glands were lined with one layer of cylindric epithelium, and the cavities of some of the dilated spaces contained cells that had taken up blood-pigment.

[Von Noorden draws attention to the fact that his case bore a marked resemblance in many ways to Mintz's case. There remains little doubt in my mind that the glands resemble those found in the body of the uterus, and the thickened, dense stroma around them bears a marked resemblance, even with the very low power, to the stroma of the uterine mucosa. The picture, at any rate, is much more suggestive of a glandular growth of uterine origin than of one coming from the sweat-glands. I endeavored, through Professor Doderlein, of Munich, to locate Dr. von Noorden, and, if possible, secure a section of this growth, but have not been successful."—T. S. C.]

> After Glands in a Small Umbilical Tumor. von Noorden [25]… The glands in the lower half of the picture bear quite a resemblance to uterine glands. Those in the center of the field remind one of the pictures seen in the depths of uterine glands, where there is some reduplication of the folds. The gland in the left part of the field is markedly dilated and contains much detritus. It is rather difficult to classify this tumor reported by Villar, but as it presents a few clinical and histologic points suggestive of the group under consideration, I mention it here, although it is not considered in the digest.

Steck and Helwig (1965) [27] stated that the differential diagnosis of a lesion of the umbilicus including hernia, embryological rest masses, and various granulomas, all these must be excluded before diagnosis of cutaneous endometriosis of the umbilicus is confirmed.

According to Wellberry (1999) [28], although retrograde menstruation seems almost certain to be involved in the pathogenesis of endometriosis, that theory does not explain the full spectrum of the disease. For example, endometrial implants are occasionally found in such remote sites as the lung or even the nose. Moreover, endometriosis also occurs, rarely, in men taking large doses of estrogen. The theories of coelomic metaplasia and Müllerian remnant differentiation are better suited than the theory of retrograde menstruation to explain some of these exceptional circumstances.

Endometriosis typically appears as superficial "powder burn" or "gunshot" lesions on the ovaries, serosal surfaces, and peritoneum—black, dark-brown, or bluish puckered lesions, nodules, or small cysts containing old hemorrhage surrounded by a variable extent of fibrosis. Atypical or "subtle" lesions are also common, including red implants (petechial, vesicular, polypoid, hemorrhagic, red flame-like) and serous or clear vesicles [29].

Anaf et al. (2000) [30] reported that microscopically the glandular epithelium is one layer thick with cuboidal or tall cells and eosinophilic cytoplasm. The degree of cyclic changes of the glandular component depends on the amount of fibrous tissue, the amount of stroma around the glands, and the degree of vascularity. Endometriosis in places with native smooth muscle component may induce marked hypertrophy identical to that observed in cases of adenomyosis that leads to the creation of adenomyomata or adenomyomatous nodules.

Douglas and Rotimi (2004) [31] reviewed the clinicopathological characteristics of 34 cases of extragenital endometriosis. Eleven cases were in the intestinal tract and two in the urinary tract, and 21 were in other sites, including the Pfannenstiel scar, inguinal canal, umbilicus, and perineum.

Mechsner et al. (2009) [32] performed immunohistochemical analysis (Ki 67, estrogen/progesterone, CD 10, smooth muscle actin, desmin, caldesmon, von Willebrand factor, cyclooxygenase-2, and VEGF) of umbilical endometriosis and found that these will help establish the diagnosis. Fukuda and Mukai (2010) [33] showed the usefulness of CD10 in identifying the interstitium of ectopic endometriosis.

There are numerous reports of endometriosis of the umbilicus [31, 34–82].

Neoplastic changes can occur in endometriosis [83–87].

References

1. Cullen TS, editor. Embryology, anatomy, and diseases of the umbillicus: together with diseases of the urachus. Philadelphia: WB Saunders Co; 1916. p. 350–458.
2. Nicaise E, Boursier A. Ombilic. Dictionnaire Encyclopedique des Sc. Med Paris. 1881;2 s, xv:140–262, deuxieme ser.
3. Villar F. Tumeurs de l'ombilic. These de Paris; 1886. No. 19.
4. Hannay 1843 scirrhous cancer of the umbilicus. Edin Med Surg J. 1843;lx:313.
5. Pernice L. Die Nabelgeschwülste, Edité par Halle, M. Niemeyer. 1892.
6. Cullen TS. Sarcoma of the umbilicus. In: Cullen TS, editor. Embryology, anatomy, and diseases of the umbilicus: together with diseases of the urachus. Philadelphia: WB Saunders Co; 1916. p. 449–58.
7. Glazer G. Primary adenocarcinoma arising in a vitello-intestinal duct remnant at the umbilicus. Br J Surg. 1973;60(3):247–9.
8. Ross JE, Hill Jr RB. Primary umbilical adenocarcinoma. A case report and review of literature. Arch Pathol. 1975;99(6):327–9.
9. Hernández N, Medina V, Alvarez-Arguelles H, Gutiérrez R, Pérez-Palma J, Díaz-Flores L. Primary papillary psammomatous adenocarcinoma of the umbilicus. Histol Histopathol. 1993;8(4):593–8.
10. Alver O, Ersoy YE, Dogusoy G, Erguney S. Primary umbilical adenocarcinoma: case report and review of the literature. Am Surg. 2007;73(9):923–5. Department of General Surgery, Istanbul University, Cerrahpasa Medical Faculty, Istanbul, Turkey.
11. Alnaqbi KA, Joshi S, Ghazal-Aswad S, Abu Zidan FM. Primary umbilical adenocarcinoma. Singapore Med J. 2007;48(12):e308–10.
12. Atri R, Dhull A, Ksur P, Singh G, Chauhan A. Primary umbilical adenocarcinoma – a case report. Int J Third World Med 2009;9(1). https://ispb.com/IJTWM/9/3696. Accessed 6 July 2015.
13. Liu Y. Primary umbilical neoplasm demonstrated on FDG PET/CT. Clin Nucl Med. 2011;36(7):e67–8.
14. Fortune DW, Ostör AG. Angiomyxomas of the umbilical cord. Obstet Gynecol. 1980;55(3):375–8.
15. Göksever H, Celiloğlu M, Küpelioğlu A. Angiomyxoma: a rare tumor of the umbilical cord. J Turk Ger Gynecol Assoc. 2010;11(1):58–60. http://www.ncbi.nlm.nih.gov/pmc/articles/PMC3939307/. Published online 2010. Accessed 7/12/15.
16. Brooks B. Umbilical teratoma: a report of a case containing pancreas and intestine. Ann Surg. 1919;69(6):603–5.
17. Chavali LV, Bhaskar RV, Reddy JB. Immature teratoma at umbilicus region presenting as exomphalos: a case report with review of literature. Indian J Med Paediatr Oncol. 2014;35(3):231–3.
18. Kreczy A, Alge A, Menardi G, Gassner I, Gschwendtner A, Mikuz G. Teratoma of the umbilical cord. Case report with review of the literature. Arch Pathol Lab Med. 1994;118(9):934–7.
19. Sathiyathasan S, Jeyanthan K, Hamid R. Umbilical hemangioma: a case report. Arch Gynecol Obstet. 2011;283:15.
20. Lee SY, Chang, Nam W, Suh JH. Heterotopic liver in the umbilicus: a case report. Basic Applied Pathol. 2011;4(1):30–2. http://onlinelibrary.wiley.com/doi/10.1111/j.1755-9294.2010.01084.x/full. Accessed 10 July 2015.
21. Kutin ND, Allen JE, Jewett TC. The umbilical polyp. J Pediatr Surg. 1979;14:741–4.
22. Rejmanowski T, Madej M, Brzostek A, Zwoliński K. Heterotopy of colonic mucous membrane in the navel skin of a 1.5 year old child. Pediatr Pol. 1989;64(3):187–8.
23. Villar F. Tumours de l'ombilie. These de Paris; 1886, obs. 68.
24. Cullen TS. Embryology, anatomy, and diseases of the umbilicus: together with diseases of the urachus. Philadelphia: WB Saunders Co; 1916. p. 350–458.

25. von Noorden W. Ein Schweissdrusenadenom mit Sitz im Nabel und ein Beitrag zu den Nabelgeschwtilsten. Deutsche Zeitschr f Chir. 1901;lix:215.
26. Mintz W. Das wahre Adenom des Xabels. Deutsche Zeitschr f Chir. 1899;li:545.
27. Steck WD, Helwig EB. Tumors of the umbilicus. Cancer. 1965;18:907–15.
28. Wellbery C. Diagnosis and treatment of endometriosis. Am Fam Physician. 1999;60:1753–68.
29. Kennedy S, Bergqvist A, Chapron C, D'Hooghe T, Dunselman G, Greb R, et al. ESHRE guideline for the diagnosis and treatment of endometriosis. Hum Reprod. 2005;20:2698–704.
30. Anaf V, Simon P, Fayt I, Noel J. Smooth muscles are frequent components of endometriotic lesions. Hum Reprod. 2000;15:767–71.
31. Douglas C, Rotimi O. Extragenital endometriosis – a clinicopathological review of a Glasgow hospital experience with case illustrations. J Obstet Gynaecol. 2004;24(7):804–8.
32. Mechsner S, Bartley J, Infanger M, Loddenkemper C, Herbel J, Ebert AD. Clinical management and Immunohistochemical analysis of umbilical endometriosis. Arch Gynecol Obstet. 2009;280(2):235–42.
33. Fukuda H, Mukai H. Cutaneous endometriosis in the umbilical region: the usefulness of CD10 in identifying the interstitium of ectopic endometriosis. J Dermatol. 2010;37(6):545–9.
34. Weller CV. Endometriosis of the umbilicus.Am J Pathol 1935;11 (2): 281–6. Boggs R. Endometriosis of the umbilicus: vicarious menstruation following hysterectomy. Arch Surg. 1938;37(4):642–50.
35. Latcher JW, Oneonta NY. Endometriosis of the umbilicus. Am J Obstet Gynecol. 1953;66:161–8.
36. Beirne MF, Berkheiser SW. Umbilical endometriosis a case report. Am J Obstet Gynecol. 1955;69:895–7.
37. Scott RB, Nowak RJ, Tindale RM. Umbilical endometriosis and the Cullen sign. Obstet Gynecol. 1958;11:556–69.
38. Williams HE, Barsky S, Storino W. Umbilical endometria (silent type). Arch Dermatol. 1976;112:1435–6.
39. Harvey E. Umbilical endometriosis. Acta Obstet Gynecol Scand. 1976;112:1435–6.
40. Michowitz M, Baratz M, Stavorosky M. Endometriosis of the umbilicus. Dermatologica. 1983;167:326–30.
41. Igawa HH, Ohura T, Sugihara T, Hosokawa M, Kawamura K, Kaneko Y. Umbilical endometriosis. Ann Plast Surg. 1992;29:266–8.
42. Berqvist A. Different types of extragenital endometriosis: a review. Gynecol Endocrinol. 1993;7(3):207–21.
43. Yu C, Perez-Reyes M. MR appearance of umbilical endometriosis. J Comput Assist Tomogr. 1994;18(2):269–71.
44. Hill AD, Banwell PE, Sangwan Y, Darzi A, Manzies-Gown N. Endometriosis and umbilical swelling. Clin Exp Obstet Gynecol. 1994;21:28–9.
45. Huang PH, Tsai RY, Chen MJ, Chan HL. Cutaneous endometriosis of the umbilicus – report of a case and review of the literature. Dermatol Sin. 1995;13:103–9.
46. Chen TH. Umbilical endometriosis. Eur J Plast Surg. 1998;21(1):51–2.
47. Munoz H, Waxtein L, Vega ME, Cortes R, Hojyo MT, Dominguez-Soto L. An ulcerated umbilical nodule. Arch Dermatol. 1999;135(9):1113–8.
48. Loverro G, Mei L, Vicino M, Cormio G, Selvaggi L. Umbilical endometriosis. J Gynecol Surg. 2001;17(2):65–8.
49. Zollner U, Girshcick G, Steck T, Dietl J. Umbilical endometriosis without previous pelvic surgery: a case report. Arch Gynecol Obstet. 2003;267:258–60.
50. Lorenzo E, Fernández-Corona A, Garcia-Merayo M, Sals S, Hernández-Rodriguez JL. Endometriosis umbilical. Clin Invest Ginecol Obstet. 2004;31(9):335–7.
51. Razzi S, Rubegni P, Sartini A, De Simone S, Fava A, Cobellis L, Fimiani M, Petraglia F. Umbilical endometriosis in pregnancy: a case report. Gynecol Endocrinol. 2004;18(2):114–6.

52. Kerr OA, Mowbray M, Tidman MJ. An umbilical nodule due to endometriosis. Acta Derm Venereol. 2005;86(3):277–8.
53. Hartigan CM, Holloway BJ. MR imaging features of endometriosis at the umbilicus. Br J Radiol. 2005;78(932):755–7.
54. Onesti MG, Cigna E, Buccheri EM, Alfano C. Endometriosi ombelicale pnmaria. Dermatol Clin. 2005;2:75–8.
55. Sutton C, Adamson GD, Jones KD. Modern management of endometriosis. Oxon: Taylor & Francis; 2006.
56. Lovino F, Ruggiero R, Irlandese E, Gili E, Loschiavo F. Management of a rare occurrence. Chir Ital. 2007;59(6):895–9.
57. Victory R, Diamond D, Johns A. Villar's nodule: a case report and systematic literature review of endometriosis externa of the umbilicus. J Minim Invasive Gynecol. 2007;14:23–32.
58. Rai R, Sathyamoorthy A, D'Souza C. Umbilical endometriosis. J Clinic Diagn Res. 2008;2(6):1203–6.
59. Lee A, Tran HT, Walters RF, Yee H, Rosenman K, Sanchez MR. Cutaneous umbilical endometriosis. Dermatol Online J. 2008;14(10):23.
60. Dessy LA, Buccheri EM, Chiummariello S, Gagliardi DN, Onesti MG. Umbilical endometriosis, our experience. In Vivo. 2008;22:811–5.
61. Elm MK, Twede JV, Turiansky GW. Primary cutaneous endometriosis of the umbilicus: a case report. Cutis. 2008;81(2):124–6.
62. Wiegratz I, Kissler S, Engels K, Strey C, Kaufmann M. Umbilical endometriosis in pregnancy without a previous surgery. Fertil Steril. 2008;90(1):199.e17–20.
63. Bagade PV, Guirguis MM. Menstruating from the umbilicus as a rare case of primary umbilical endometriosis: a case report. J Med Case Rep. 2009;3:9326.
64. Pavalli VB, Mamdouh MG. Menstruating from the umbilicus as a rare case of primarily umbilical endometriosis: a case report. J Med Case Rep. 2009;3:9326.
65. Chatzikokkinou P, Thorfin J, Angelidis IK, Papa G, Trevisan G. Spontaneous endometriosis in an umbilical skin lesion. Acta Dermatovenerol Alp Panonica Adriat. 2009;18(3):126–30.
66. Bagade PV, Guirguis MM. Menstruating from the umbilicus as a rare case of primary umbilical endometriosis: a case report. J Med Case Reports. 2009;3:9326.
67. Panicker R, Pillai N, Nagarserkar U. Villar's nodule: a rare presentation of external endometriosis. Med J Armed Forces India. 2010;66(1):70–1.
68. Dadhwal V, Gupta B, Dasgupta C, Shende U, Deka D. Primary umbilical endometriosis: a rare entity. Arch Gynecol Obstet. 2010;283 Suppl 1:119–20.
69. Skidmore RA, Woosley JT, Katz VL. Decidualized umbilical endometriosis. Int J Gynecol Obstet. 1996:52(3):269–73. Int J Surg 2010;8(2):109–11.
70. Fedele L, Frontino G, Bianchi S, Borruto F, Ciappina N. Umbilical endometriosis: a radical excision with laparoscopic assistance. Int J Surg. 2010;8(2):109–11.
71. Kyamidis K, Lora V, Kanitakis J. Spontaneous cutaneous umbilical endometriosis: report of a new case with immunohistochemical study and literature review. Dermatol Online J. 2011;17(7):5.
72. Fernandas H, Maria NJ, Pailoor K, Kini R. Primary umbilical endometriosis – diagnosis by fine needle aspiration. J Cytol. 2011;28(4):214–6.
73. Weng CS, Yang YC. Villar's nodule — umbilical endometriosis. N Engl J Med. 2011;364:e45.
74. Singh A. Umbilical endometriosis mimicking as papilloma to general surgeons: a case report. Australas Med J. 2012;5(5):272–4.
75. Kesici U, Yenisolak A, Kesici S, Siviloglu C. Primary cutaneous umbilical endometriosis. Med Arh. 2012;66(5):353–4.
76. Efremidou EI, Kouklakis G, Mitrakas A, Liratzopoulos N, Polychronidis AC. Primary umbilical endometrioma: a I rare case of spontaneous abdominal wall endometriosis. Int J Gen Med. 2012;5:999–1002.
77. Ashraf F, Yasmin N, Islam JA, Choiidhury FR, Guha K. Umbilical endometriosis in a 39 years old parous woman: a case report. J Shaheed Suhrawardy Med Coll. 2012;4(2):65–7.

78. Fancellu A, Pinna A, Manca A, Capobianco G, Porcu A. Primary umbilical endometriosis. Case report and discussion on management options. Int J Surg Case Rep. 2013;4(12):1145–8.
79. Joycerani D, Mondal S, Paul S, Pramanik SR. Primary umbilical endometriosis: a rarity. J Hum Reprod Sci. 2014;7(4):269–71.
80. Pariza G, Mavrodin CI. Primary umbilical endometriosis (Villar's nodule) – case study, literature revision. Chirurgia (Bucur). 2014;109(4):546–9.
81. Daniel Paramythiotis D, Stavrou G, Panidis S, Panagiotou D, Chatzopoulos K, Papadopoulos VN, Michalopoulos A. Concurrent appendiceal and umbilical endometriosis: a case report and review of the literature. J Med Case Reports. 2014;8:258.
82. Omori M, Oqawa T, Nara M, Hashi A, Hirata S. Umbilical endometriosis with giant degenerated uterine leiomyomas: a case report. Gynecol Oncol Case Rep. 2014;9:18–20.
83. Heaps JM, Nieberg RK, Berek JS. Malignant neoplasms arising in endometriosis. Obstet Gynecol. 1990;75(6):1023.
84. Yantiss RK, Clement PB, Young RH. Neoplastic and preneoplastic changes in gastrointestinal endometriosis: a study of 17 cases. Am J Surg Pathol. 2000;24:513–24.
85. Slavin RE, Krum R, Dinh TV. Endometriosis-associated intestinal tumors: a clinical and pathological study of 6 cases with a review of the literature. Hum Pathol. 2000;31:456–63.
86. Chen KTK. Endometrioid adenocarcinoma arising from colonic endometriosis mimicking primary colonic carcinoma. Int J Gynecol Pathol. 2002;21:285–8.
87. Jones KD, Owen E, Berresford A, Sutton C. Endometrial adenocarcinoma arising from endometriosis of the rectosigmoid colon. Gynecol Oncol. 2002;86:220–2.

Part VI
Malignant Tumors of Umbilicus

Chapter 38
Umbilical Metastasis: Current Viewpoint

Raimondo Gabriele and Marco Conte

38.1 Introduction

Umbilical nodules are rare and can be classified as benign or malignant. Benign tumors include cutaneous endometriosis, foreign body granuloma, melanocytic nevi, papilloma, fibroma, epithelial inclusion cysts, epidermoid cysts, seborrheic keratosis, abscess, omphalitis, pilonidal sinus, keloid, hernia, and myxoma. Primary umbilical malignancies are less common than metastatic by a ratio of nearly 1:8 [1–7]. These include adenocarcinoma, sarcomas, malignant melanomas, basal cell carcinomas, and squamous cell carcinomas. Clinically they cannot be differentiated from secondary tumors. More frequently (80 % of cases) umbilical malignant lesions are represented by intra-abdominal neoplasm metastases [8–15]. In the last instance, these lesions also are named "Sister Mary Joseph nodule" (SMJN). In 1949 Sir Hamilton Bailey first used this eponym in his book *Physical Signs in Clinical Surgery* to describe umbilical metastases, in honor of Sister Mary Joseph, superintendent nurse and surgical assistant of Dr. William Mayo at St. Mary's Hospital in Rochester (at present Mayo Clinic, Minnesota). Sister Mary Joseph was the first to note the link between umbilical nodules and intra-abdominal malignancy [16–26].

R. Gabriele, M.D. (✉) • M. Conte, M.D.
Department of Surgery "Pietro Valdoni", "Sapienza" Università di Roma,
Via G.n. Lancisi 2, 00161 Rome, Italy
e-mail: raimondo.gabriele@uniroma1.it; m_conte@hotmail.it

M.A. Shiffman (ed.), *Adult Umbilical Reconstruction*,
DOI 10.1007/978-3-319-43887-0_38

38.2 Epidemiology

We have analyzed the scientific literature of the last decade (2005–2015), and using the keywords "Sister Mary Joseph's nodule" and "umbilical metastases," we found a total of 125 scientific papers on the subject. Results are useful for the purposes of our study with 108 manuscripts for a total of 253 cases of umbilical metastases observed.

The umbilicus is the favorite venue of intra-abdominal metastasis of tumors. The umbilical nodule may represent the early symptom of malignancy to diagnose or the recurrence of a cancer already known [3, 11, 27–43]. In 80 % of cases, the umbilical lesion is the first sign of malignancy, whereas 20 % appear after the diagnosis and/or treatment of the primary tumor (Table 38.1). The SMJN shows with a higher incidence in females with a ratio of 1.7:1 (Table 38.2). The fifth and sixth decades are the age groups most represented (Table 38.3).

The gastrointestinal tract is the most common location (40 %) of the primary tumors followed by the genitourinary tract (37 %) and other locations (12 %). In the 11 %, primitive neoplasms are unknown (Tables 38.4 and 38.5).

Ovarian carcinoma is the most frequent site of primaries (71 %) followed by the pancreas (33 %), stomach (31 %), and colon-rectum (15 %) (Tables 38.6 and 38.7). Histological findings show that most cases involved metastasis of adenocarcinoma [3, 5–11, 13, 20–32, 35–65].

Table 38.1 Clinical presentation of SMJN

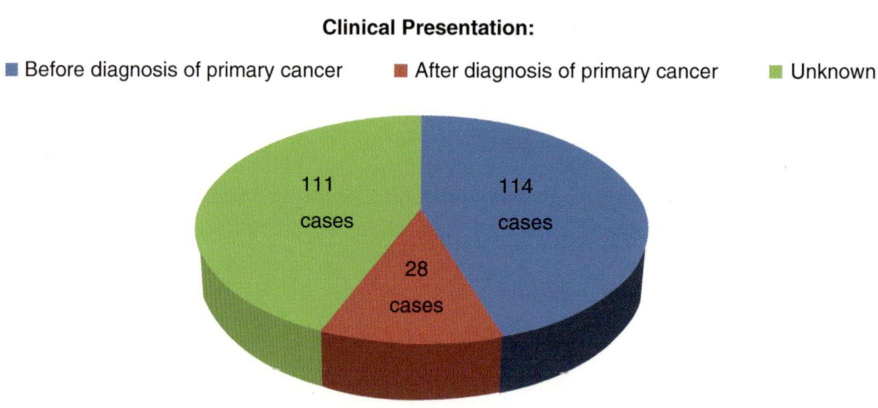

Table 38.2 Distribution of patients according to sex

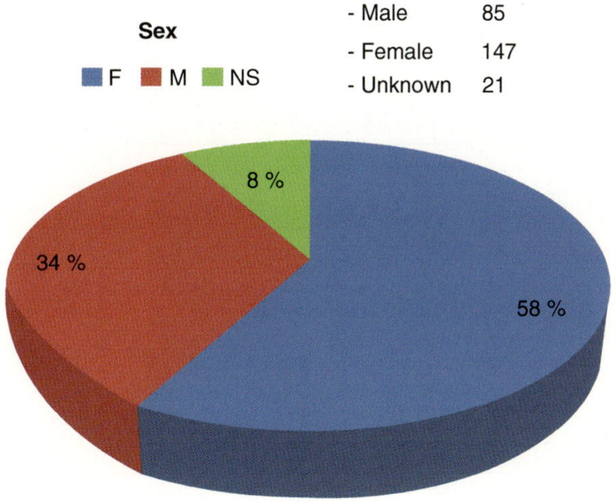

Table 38.3 Distribution of patients according to age group

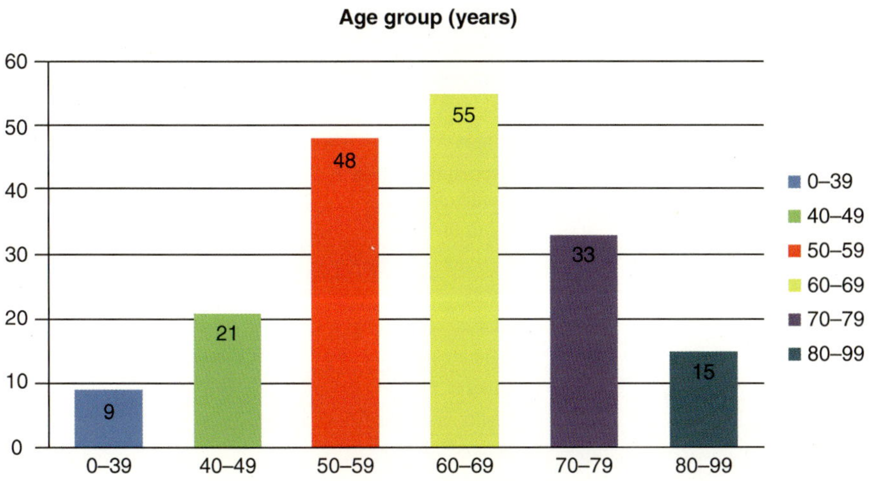

Table 38.4 Distribution of patients according to organ systems

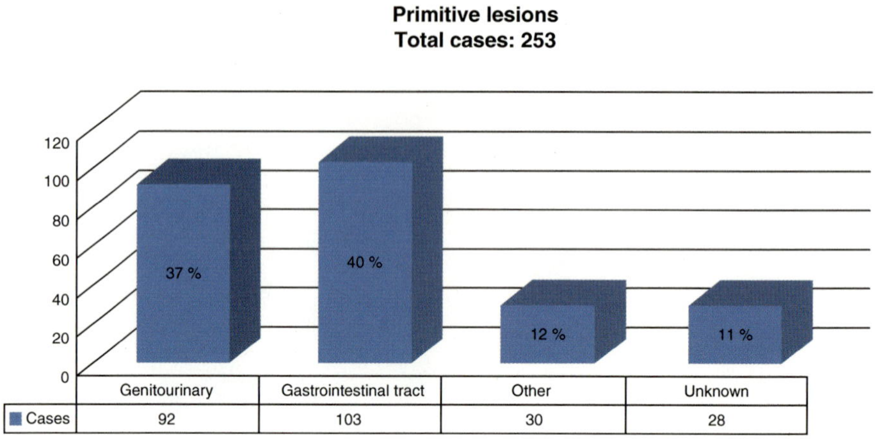

Table 38.5 Distribution of patients according to primary site of malignancy

Organ system	*n*
Gastrointestinal tract	*103*
Colon	16
Stomach	31
Gallbladder	13
Pancreas	34
Others	9
(Appendix 3, anus 1, esophagus 2, ileum 2, duodenum 1)	
Genitourinary	*92*
Prostate	6
Ovary	65
Uterus	11
Bladder	3
Others	7
(Fallopian tubes 3, kidney 2, urachus 1, penis 1)	
Others	*30*
Pulmonary	5
Lymphoma	6
Neuroendocrine	2
Peritoneal mesothelioma	9
Breast	1
Liver	2
Melanoma	2
DSRCT	3
(Desmoplastic small round cell tumor)	

Table 38.6 Gastrointestinal tract: distribution of patients according to primary tumor site

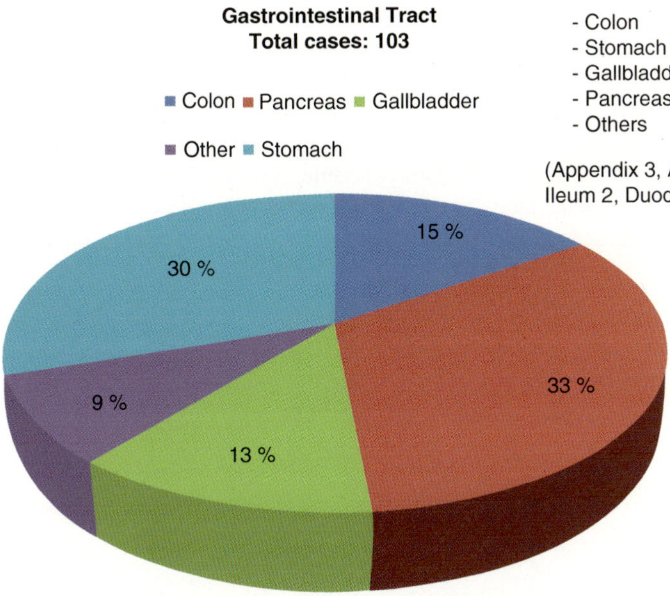

- Colon 16
- Stomach 31
- Gallbladder 13
- Pancreas 34
- Others 9

(Appendix 3, Anus1, Esophagus 2, Ileum 2, Duodenum 1)

Table 38.7 Genitourinary tract: distribution of patients according to primary tumor site

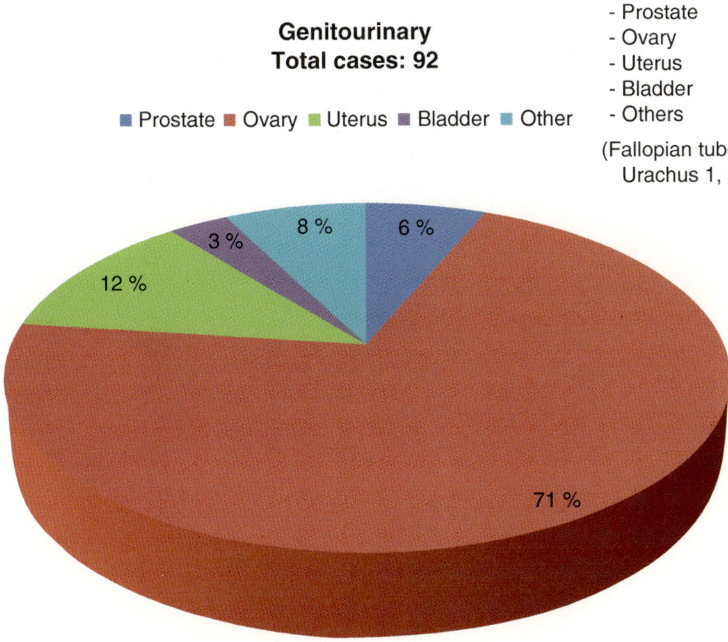

- Prostate 6
- Ovary 65
- Uterus 11
- Bladder 3
- Others 7

(Fallopian tubes 3, Kidney 2, Urachus 1, Penis 1)

38.3 Clinical Findings

Umbilical metastasis nodule presents as an occasionally painful lump of hard-fibrous consistency, irregular edges, attached to the anterior abdominal wall. The surface may be ulcerated and necrotic, with hematic, serous, purulent, or mucous discharge. The size is usually between 0.5 and 2 cm, although lesion up to 10 cm has been reported (Fig. 38.1). Instead of a distinct nodule, it may also present as a diffuse induration of the subcutaneous tissue. The primary symptoms of an internal cancer may be a painless umbilical mass that is misdiagnosed as an umbilical hernia.

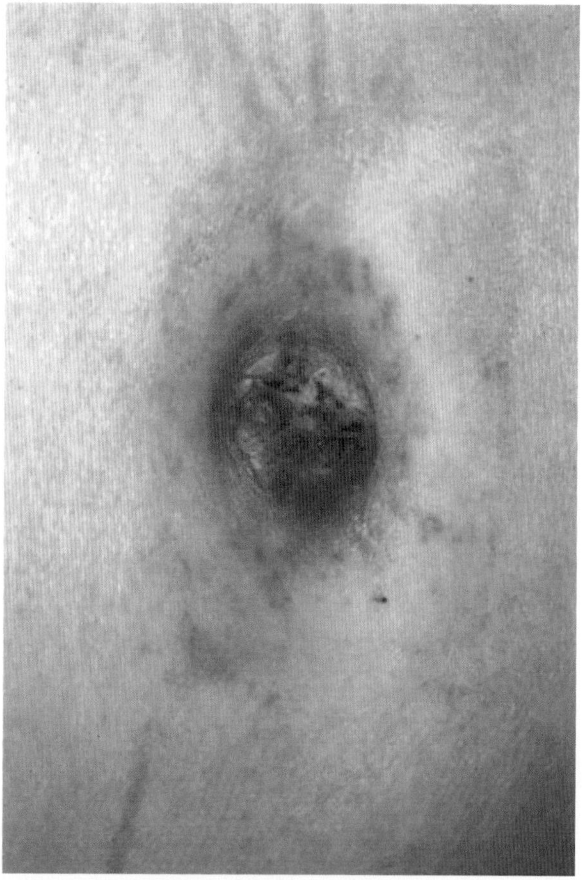

Fig. 38.1 Umbilical lump covered by the erythematous skin

38.4 Pathophysiology

A full understanding of the mechanisms whereby the tumor spreads to the umbilicus remains unclear. However, following anatomical criteria, several hypotheses have been proposed.

The umbilical ring is a scar invaginated on the abdominal wall between the transversalis fascia and peritoneum. After birth, the fetal cord structures develop into ligaments or peritoneal folds: (1) the median umbilical ligament secondary to the obliterating urachus, (2) medial umbilical ligaments (which are obliterated umbilical arteries), and (3) the ligamentum teres (obliterated left umbilical vein) that continues into (4) the falciform ligament. On the lateral umbilical folds, the inferior epigastric vessels and, sometimes, a vestigial vitelline duct connecting the umbilicus to the ileum can be recognized. The umbilical region shows a rich arterial supply that includes the inferior epigastric and deep circumflex iliac branches of the external iliac artery and the superior epigastric branch of the internal mammary artery.

The venous drainage includes several anastomotic branches, coming from cranially the axillary vein, through the internal mammary vein, and, caudally, the femoral vein through the superficial epigastric vein. In addition, the umbilicus may be connected with the portal system, through small umbilical veins.

The lymphatic system connects the umbilical region to the axillary, inguinal, and para-aortic lymph nodes. The deep lymphatic system passes along the falciform ligament, pierces the diaphragm, and enters the anterior mediastinum or courses to the nodes around the iliac arteries [66–73].

All these systems (arterial, venous, and lymphatic) as described represent possible routes by which metastatic tumor cells could implant into the umbilical region.

It is reasonable to suggest that direct extension of tumor through the peritoneum is the preferred route for gastrointestinal tumors. Furthermore, the common association between hepatic and umbilical metastases might suggest that the tumor spreads from the primary site to the liver through the portal system and then, through the lymphatic and/or venous channels, to the umbilicus. It is still unclear if the umbilical tumor spread precedes the hepatic spread or vice versa.

Renal cell carcinoma typically spreads via extrarenal extension, lymphatic dissemination, or venous invasion by the tumor. Intraperitoneal spread may occur as a result of disruption of the renal capsule [3, 11, 34–38, 74–87]. The dissemination of neoplastic cell through the urachus is assumed to be the mechanism for the bladder cancers.

Hematogenous, lymphatic, and venous spread all represent valid mechanisms of tumor spread from gynecological cancers [3, 6–9, 11, 25–38, 63–77].

38.5 Discussion

Metastatic cancer of the umbilicus, known as Sister Mary Joseph nodule, is typically associated with visceral malignancy. It is an uncommon and rare manifestation of an abdominopelvic neoplasm (1–3 %). Usually it indicates disseminated disease and poor prognosis surgically not amenable in the majority of cases [71, 88–103].

Statistical data analysis of last 10 years, over 253 cases of umbilical metastases published in 108 scientific papers, showed interesting details, sometimes different from those previously reported. SMJN predominates in female (147 cases, 58 %) than male (85 cases, 34 %) with a ratio of 1.7:1. The remaining 8 % is not specified by some authors in their work. The reasons for this gender difference remain unclear. The higher incidence is found between the fifth and sixth decades (57 %) with highest peak between 60 and 69 years (30 %).

In 88 % of cases (225 out of 253), we are able to diagnose the primary neoplasm, whereas in 11 % of cases, the source of primary site of the tumor remains unknown. SMJN can be the first clinical sign of a not yet identified malignancy or a manifestation of recurrence in a patient with a previous malignancy [52–67, 104–107]. In the majority of cases (80 %), umbilical metastasis represents the first manifestation of intra-abdominal malignancy, whereas in 20 % of cases, it is detected during or after management and treatment of primary tumor.

Noninvasive diagnostic techniques of SMJN include: ultrasonography, dermoscopy, computerized tomography (CT) scan, and positron emission tomography (PET) imaging. The aim of these procedures is to increase the suspicion of an umbilical metastatic tumor. In this last instance, excisional biopsy with histopathological evaluation is mandatory to achieve the diagnosis and to find the possible primary site. Fine-needle aspiration cytology is more indicated in those cases of recurrence umbilical metastasis to support histological behavior of a previously treated malignancy [14–32, 41–47, 108–118].

The gastrointestinal tract is the most frequent location of the primary malignancy among the organ systems (40 %), followed by the genitourinary tract (37 %). In 12 % of cases, other organs are affected (respiratory, lymphopoietic, neuroendocrine, peritoneal, mammary, liver, melanocytic, and desmoplastic small round cell tumors (DSRCT)). In 11 % the origin site is unknown. The ovary is the most common site of primary neoplasm, representing 28.8 % of all primary tumors and 70.6 % of those of the genitourinary tract followed by the uterus (11/92 cases), prostate (6/92), bladder (3/92), fallopian tubes (3 cases), kidney (2 cases), and urachus (1 case), and the penis (1 case) is the remainder.

Pancreatic cancer is the recently most common site of gastrointestinal tract (33 %) and the second of all primary neoplasm (15.1 %). Usually it is localized to the tail and the body, rarely to the head.

Then in decreasing order of frequency, we find the stomach (30 %), the colorectum (15.5 %), and the biliary tree (12.5 %). Others nearly 9 % are evaluated (appendix three cases, esophagus two cases, ileum two cases, duodenum one case, and anus one case).

SMJN is usually considered a sign of advanced primary malignancy and represents widespread metastasis with an associate poor prognosis [9–24, 54–68, 84–90, 119].

Survival rates in these patients range from 2 to 11 months after the discovery of umbilical lesion, even if isolated cases of greater survival are reported in international literature [3–29, 44–77, 88–114].

Current statistical data do not show notable difference in survival when the umbilical malignancy is diagnosed before eventual treatment of primary neoplasm (9.7 months) comparing with those when the umbilical lesion appears after primary tumor treatment (7.6 months).

Normally the finding of SMJN almost certainly establishes the inoperability of the patient, except those cases which necessitate a palliative or emergency surgical treatment.

Aggressive and combined approach (surgery with chemotherapy and/or radiotherapy) may be useful in isolated cases to increase survival. To make this choice, we must take care of the stage of cancer and the patient's clinical condition.

A careful analysis of the data reported in the literature regarding the correlation between the primary tumor and umbilical metastases leads to the belief that these patients are frequently affected by primary tumors that usually have a slow and progressive clinical course, with a low and nonspecific initial symptoms, such as neoplasms of the ovary, pancreatic body-tail, prostate, as well as gastric gland. The diagnosis of these tumors occurs most often in advanced stage with widespread metastases and poor prognosis. That may explain the negative prognostic significance of SMJN, which therefore is always a valuable indicative sign of advanced cancer.

References

1. Ittyachen AM, Krishnamoorthy S, Shanavas A. Sister Mary Joseph's node. Am J Med. 2014;127(5):e7–8.
2. Heymann WR. Sister Mary Joseph nodule: impact on the clinician. Cutis. 2013;91(1):7–8.
3. Ghimire S, Giri S, Pathak R, Martin MG. Sister Mary Joseph's nodule in a patient with metastatic small cell lung cancer. J Community Hosp Intern Med Perspect. 2015;5(3):27388.
4. José RJ, Hawley L. Sister Mary Joseph's nodule. QJM. 2013;106(8):779.
5. Rahman MT, Nakayama K, Rahman M, Nakayama N, Ishikawa M, Katagiri A, Katagiri H, Ishibashi T, Iida K, Miyazaki K. Sister Mary Joseph's nodule associated with rare endometrial squamous cell carcinoma. Arch Gynecol Obstet. 2012;286(3):711–5.
6. Balsarkar DJ, Jakhere S. Sister Mary Joseph nodule. Indian J Gastroenterol. 2012;31(1):36–8.
7. Gaiser MR, Schäkel K, Helmbold P. Lest we forget: Sister Mary Joseph and her nodule. Int J Dermatol. 2013;52(5):587–8.
8. Chalya PL, Mabula JB, Rambau PF, McHembe MD. Sister Mary Joseph's nodule at a University teaching hospital in northwestern Tanzania: a retrospective review of 34 cases. World J Surg Oncol. 2013;11:151.
9. Davar S, Hanna D. Sister Mary Joseph's nodule. J Cutan Med Surg. 2012;16(3):201–4.
10. Dodiuk-Gad R, Ziv M, Loven D, Schafer J, Shani-Adir A, Dyachenko P, Rozenman D. Sister Mary Joseph's nodule as a presenting sign of internal malignancy. Skinmed. 2006;5(5):256–8.

11. Piura B, Meirovitz M, Bayme M, Shaco-Levy R. Sister Mary Joseph's nodule originating from endometrial carcinoma incidentally detected during surgery for an umbilical hernia: a case report. Arch Gynecol Obstet. 2006;274(6):385–8.
12. Masmoudi A, Boudaya S, Charfeddine A, Dammak A, Amouri M, Khabir A, Marrekchi S, Bouassida S, Sallemi T, Krichen MS, Turki H, Zahaf A. Sister Mary Joseph's nodule: report of five cases. Int J Dermatol. 2008;47(2):134–6.
13. Yamashita S, Sakon M, Hiura Y, Nakano K, Higaki N, Murakami M, Hayashida H, Kan K, Ichihara T. A case of metastases of umbilicus (Sister Mary Joseph's nodule). Gan To Kagaku Ryoho. 2008;35(12):2112–4.
14. Akhtar K, Zaheer S, Ahmad S, Sherwani RK. Sister Mary Joseph's nodule: a rare cytologic presentation. Clin Pract. 2011;1(1):e6.
15. Miranda A, Alves M, Lopes F, Fonseca T. Sister Mary Joseph' nodule. Rev Clin Esp (Barc). 2014;214(4):e47.
16. Chirapongsathorn S, Kamath PS. Sister Mary Joseph's nodule. Mayo Clin Proc. 2015;90(2):310.
17. Ahmed S, Rashid S, Kue-A-Pai P, Cheungpasitporn W. Sister mary joseph's nodule: what lies beneath? N Am J Med Sci. 2013;5(3):252.
18. Papalas JA, Selim MA. Metastatic vs primary malignant neoplasms affecting the umbilicus: clinicopathologic features of 77 tumors. Ann Diagn Pathol. 2011;15(4):237–42.
19. Brunelli M, Manfrin E, Miller K, Eccher A, Gobbo S, Reghellin D, Chilosi M, Remo A, Martignoni G, Menestrina F, Bonetti F. Her-2/neu evaluation in Sister Mary Joseph's nodule from breast carcinoma: a case report and review of the literature. J Cutan Pathol. 2009;36(6):702–5.
20. Fairchild A, Janoski M, Dundas G. Sister Mary Joseph's nodule. CMAJ. 2007;176(7):929–30.
21. Zadeh VB, Kadyan R, Al-Abdulrazzaq A, Al-Otaibi S, Sarhan A, Najem N. Sister Mary Joseph's nodule: a case of umbilical cutaneous metastasis with signet ring cell histology. Indian J Dermatol Venereol Leprol. 2009;75(5):503–5.
22. Kar JK, Kar M. Sister Mary Joseph's nodule (SMJN). J Assoc Physicians India. 2012;60:114.
23. Esperto H, Canha C, Meira E. Sister Mary Joseph's nodule. Acta Med Port. 2012;25(4):258.
24. Tso S, Brockley J, Recica H, Ilchyshyn A. Sister Mary Joseph's nodule: an unusual but important physical finding characteristic of widespread internal malignancy. Br J Gen Pract. 2013;63(615):551–2.
25. Wronski M, Klucinski A, Krasnodebski IW. Sister Mary Joseph nodule: a tip of an iceberg. J Ultrasound Med. 2014;33(3):531–4.
26. Abu-Hilal M, Newman JS. Sister Mary Joseph and her nodule: historical and clinical perspective. Am J Med Sci. 2009;337(4):271–3.
27. Handa U, Garg S, Mohan H. Fine-needle aspiration cytology of Sister Mary Joseph's (paraumbilical) nodules. Diagn Cytopathol. 2008;36(5):348–50.
28. Yendluri V, Centeno B, Springett GM. Pancreatic cancer presenting as a Sister Mary Joseph's nodule: case report and update of the literature. Pancreas. 2007;34(1):161–4.
29. Albano EA, Kanter J. Images in clinical medicine. Sister Mary Joseph's nodule. N Engl J Med. 2005;352(18):1913.
30. Fill S, Taran A, Schulz HU, Kahl S, Kalinski T, Smith B, Costa SD. Sister Mary Joseph's nodule as the first sign of pregnancy-associated gastric cancer: a case report. World J Gastroenterol. 2008;14(6):951–3.
31. Ehmann LM, Fiegl M, Wollenberg A. Multiple Sister Mary Joseph's nodules in a patient with gastric cancer. Dtsch Med Wochenschr. 2011;136(25-26):1365–8.
32. Haruki T, Nakamura H, Kubouchi Y, Taniguchi Y, Miwa K, Adachi Y, Fujioka S, Ito H. Sister Mary Joseph's nodule that originated from lung adenocarcinoma. Gen Thorac Cardiovasc Surg. 2011;59(3):212–5.
33. Singh H, Sharma P, Reddy RM, Bal C, Malhotra A, Kumar R. Sister Mary Joseph nodule in endometrial carcinoma: detection with FDG PET/CT. Clin Nucl Med. 2013;38(6):e263–4.
34. Husein-ElAhmed H, Aneiros-Fernandez J, Arias-Santiago S, Naranjo-Sintes R. Sister Mary Joseph's nodule as a metastasis of ovarian adenocarcinoma. Int J Dermatol. 2010;49(9):1045–6.

35. Wijekoon NS, Samarasekera DN. Sister Mary Joseph's nodule as the sole presenting feature of disseminated squamous cell cancer of the esophagus: a rare case. J Gastrointest Cancer. 2007;38(2-4):99–101.
36. Psarras K, Symeonidis N, Baltatzis M, Notopoulos A, Nikolaidou C. Umbilical metastasis as primary manifestation of cancer: a small series and review of the literature. J Clin Diagn Res. 2014;8(10):17–9.
37. Huang YY, Chen YL, Huang SH, Huang CY. Huge uterine leiomyoma combined with umbilical inclusion cyst mimicking a Sister Mary Joseph's nodule. Taiwan J Obstet Gynecol. 2015;54(1):81–3.
38. Hori T, Okada N, Nakauchi M, Hiramoto S, Kikuchi-Mizota A, Kyogoku M, Oike F, Sugimoto H, Tanaka J, Morikami Y, Shigemoto K, Ota T, Kaneko M, Nakatsuji M, Okae S, Tanaka T, Gunji D, Yoshioka A. Hematogenous umbilical metastasis from colon cancer treated by palliative single-incision laparoscopic surgery. World J Gastrointest Surg. 2013;5(10):272–7.
39. Ullery BW, Wachtel H, Raper SE. Sister Mary Joseph's nodule presenting as large bowel obstruction: a case report and brief review of the literature. J Gastrointest Surg. 2013;17(10):1832–5.
40. Bolanaki H, Courcoutsakis N, Kouklakis G, Kakolyris S, Karayiannakis AJ. Sister Mary Joseph's nodule as the first sign of pancreatic carcinoma. J Gastrointest Cancer. 2012;43:254–7.
41. Mashimo Y, Horimatsu T, Miyamoto S. Umbilical metastasis (Sister Mary Joseph's nodule) from esophageal squamous cell carcinoma. Clin Gastroenterol Hepatol. 2011;9(8):A20.
42. Barboza-Quintana O, Alvarado-Bernal YL, Flores-Gutiérrez JP, Ancer-Rodríguez J, Garza-Guajardo R. Diagnosis of carcinosarcoma metastatic to the umbilicus by fine needle aspiration biopsy: a case report. Acta Cytol. 2010;54(5 Suppl):819–22.
43. Al-Wadi K, Bernier M. Sister Mary Joseph's nodule. J Obstet Gynaecol Can. 2010;32(8):721.
44. Kurt S, Camuzcuoglu H, Camuzcuoglu A, Dicle N, Tinar S. Umbilical metastasis of serous component as a first sign of mixed type epithelial ovarian cancer. Eur J Gynaecol Oncol. 2009;30(4):455–7.
45. Lee CK, Chang YW, Jung SH, Jang JY, Dong SH, Kim HJ, Kim BH, Chang R. A case of Sister Mary Joseph's nodule as a presenting sign of gastric cancer. Korean J Gastroenterol. 2008;51(2):132–6.
46. Ohta S, Yamakawa Y, Hasegawa T, Tateno M, Matsui K. Advanced ovarian cancer with Sister Mary Joseph's nodule—a case report. Gan To Kagaku Ryoho. 2007;34(1):117–9.
47. Shih YI, Chen PM, Chen PC, Hsiao LT. Lymphoma presenting as Sister Mary Joseph's nodule sparing intra-abdominal involvement. Int J Hematol. 2006;83(3):194.
48. Kim YW, Srodon M, Bristow RE. Stage IV micropapillary serous ovarian carcinoma: a report of three cases. Int J Gynecol Pathol. 2005;24(3):235–8.
49. Limmathurotsakul D, Rerknimitr P, Korkij W, Noppakun N, Kullavanijaya P, Rerknimitr R. Metastatic mucinous cystic adenocarcinoma of the pancreas presenting as Sister Mary Joseph's nodule. JOP. 2007;8(3):344–9.
50. Kolwijck E, Boss EA, van Altena AM, Beex LV, Massuger LF. Stage IV epithelial ovarian carcinoma in an 18 year old patient presenting with a Sister Mary Joseph's nodule and metastasis in both breasts: a case report and review of the literature. Gynecol Oncol. 2007;107(3):583–5.
51. Al-Mashat F, Sibiany AM. Sister Mary Joseph's nodule of the umbilicus: is it always of gastric origin? A review of eight cases at different sites of origin. Indian J Cancer. 2010;47(1):65–9.
52. Lee HL, Kwon YI, Song SY. Umbilical metastasis: Sister Mary Joseph's nodule. Clin Gastroenterol Hepatol. 2011;9(3):e20.
53. Shimizu H, Maegawa J, Ho T, Yamamoto Y, Mikami T, Nagahama K. Cutaneous metastasis of pancreatic carcinoma as an initial symptom in the lower extremity with obstructive lymphedema treated by physiotherapy and lymphaticovenous shunt: a case report, review, and pathophysiological implications. Lymphology. 2010;43(1):19–24.
54. Wu YY, Xing CG, Jiang JX, Lu XD, Feng YZ, Wu HR. Carcinoma of the right side colon accompanied by Sister Mary Joseph's nodule and inguinal nodal metastases: a case report and literature review. Chin J Cancer. 2010;29(2):239–41.

55. Papalambros A, Sigala F, Vouza EG, Hepp W, Antonakis P. Sister Mary Joseph's nodule as primary localized malignant mesothelioma. Report of a case. Zentralbl Chir. 2011;136(2):172–4.
56. Wang F, Chen H, Zhang X. Sister Mary Joseph's nodule derived from lung cancer. Indian J Dermatol Venereol Leprol. 2011;77(5):609–11.
57. Powell JL. Powell's pearls: eponyms in medical and surgical history. Sister Joseph's Nodule; Sister MaryJoseph (1856–1939). J Surg Educ. 2011;68(5):442–3.
58. Munoz J, Chacra W, Hanbali A, Ali H. Sister Mary Joseph's nodule. BMJ Case Rep. 2011;2011: bcr 0620114349.
59. Ozaki N, Takamori H, Baba H. Sister Mary Joseph's nodule derived from pancreatic cancer. J Hepatobiliary Pancreat Sci. 2011;18(1):119–21.
60. Cetin B, Benekli M, Bulutay P, Akyurek N, Cura E, Coskun U, Buyukberber S. Sister Mary Joseph's nodule as a rare sign of lymphoma. Int J Hematol. 2011;94(2):209–12.
61. Bai XL, Zhang Q, Masood W, Masood N, Tang Y, Cao CH, Fu QH, Zhang Y, Gao SL, Liang TB. Sister Mary Joseph's nodule as a first sign of pancreatic cancer. World J Gastroenterol. 2012;18(45):6686–9.
62. De Kock I, Dekeyzer S, Smet BS, Delrue L. Sister Mary Joseph nodule. JBR-BTR. 2013;96(6):394.
63. Zhang CJ, Sun GP, Liu H, Peng WR, Xiong FX, Pan YY, Da J. Primary clear cell adenocarcinoma of the peritoneum presents as Sister Mary Joseph's nodule: a case report and literature review. Eur J Gynaecol Oncol. 2014;35(6):745–8.
64. Menzies S, Chotirmall SH, Wilson G, O'Riordan D. Sister Mary Joseph nodule. BMJ Case Rep. 2015;2015. pii: bcr 2014206808.
65. Iavazzo C, Madhuri K, Essapen S, Akrivos N, Tailor A, Butler-Manuel S. Sister Mary Joseph's nodule as a first manifestation of primary peritoneal cancer. Case Rep Obstet Gynecol. 2012;2012:467240.
66. Sengupta S, Church E, Chia KV. Sister Mary Joseph's nodule: recurrent endometrial adenocarcinoma presenting as an umbilical metastasis. J Obstet Gynaecol. 2009;29(2):170–1.
67. Scudeler D, Wakely Jr PE. Fine needle aspiration biopsy of gastrointestinal stromal tumor presenting as an umbilical mass (Sister Mary Joseph's Nodule). Ann Diagn Pathol. 2006;10(2):100–3.
68. Giner Galvañ V, Ferrández MG, Martínez J, Esteban MJ, Kuehn S. Sister Mary Joseph's nodule as non-Hodgkins lymphoma clinical presentation. Rev Clin Esp. 2005;205(3):143–4.
69. Renner R, Sticherling M. Sister Mary Joseph's nodule as a metastasis of gallbladder carcinoma. Int J Dermatol. 2007;46(5):505–7.
70. Sina B, Deng A. Umbilical metastasis from prostate carcinoma (Sister Mary Joseph's nodule): a case report and review of literature. J Cutan Pathol. 2007;34(7):581–3.
71. Liu CY, Yong CC, Wu SC, Lin CY, Chen CL, Wang CC. Sister Mary Joseph's nodule associated with hepatocellular carcinoma. Surgery. 2010;147(1):167–8.
72. Cheva A, Stavrakis T, Paraskevas G, Papadimitriou N, Kakoutis E, Makrantonakis A. Sister Mary Joseph's nodule as the sole presenting sign of gastric signet ring cell adenocarcinoma. Gastroenterol Clin Biol. 2010;34(10):565–8.
73. Liu Y. Primary umbilical neoplasm demonstrated on FDG PET/CT. Clin Nucl Med. 2011;36(7):e67–8.
74. Heller DS. Lesions of the umbilicus: what the minimally invasive gynecologic surgeon needs to know about the belly button. J Minim Invasive Gynecol. 2012;19(6):680–3.
75. Tsuruya K, Matsushima M, Nakajima T, Fujisawa M, Shirakura K, Igarashi M, Koike J, Suzuki T, Mine T. Malignant peritoneal mesothelioma presenting umbilical hernia and Sister Mary Joseph's nodule. World J Gastrointest Endosc. 2013;5(8):407–11.
76. Khalfallah M, Chaker Y, Dziri C. Sister Mary Joseph's nodule showing adenocarcinoma of pancreas. Tunis Med. 2011;89(10):790–1.
77. Golovanova EV, Chikunova BZ, Mel'kina ES, Shliakhovskiĭ IA, Efremov LI. Difficulties in vivo diagnosis of mucinous adenocarcinoma of vermiform appendix with metastasis in the navel. Eksp Klin Gastroenterol. 2011;11:91–6.

78. Nakamura M, Tamura J, Takaki R, Ohshiro M, Akamine M, Naha Y, Hirata T, Kinjo F, Fujita J. Sister Mary Joseph's nodule. Intern Med. 2009;48(19):1775.
79. Shen Z, Yang X, Chen L, Hao F, Zhong B. Sister Mary Joseph's nodule as a diagnostic clue to metastatic colon carcinoma. J Clin Oncol. 2009;27(19):e1–2.
80. Gabriele R, Conte M, Egidi F, Borghese M. Umbilical metastases: current viewpoint. World J Surg Oncol. 2005;3(1):13.
81. Shah S, Gupta S, Shet T, Maheshwari A, Wuntkal R, Mohandas KM. Metastatic clear cell variant of hepatocellular carcinoma with an occult hepatic primary. Hepatobiliary Pancreat Dis Int. 2005;4(2):306–7.
82. Colla TG, Lovatto L, Duquia RP. Case for diagnosis: umbilical metastasis of pancreatic carcinoma (Sister Mary Joseph's Nodule). An Bras Dermatol. 2009;84(3):297–8.
83. Pereira WA, Humaire CR, Silva CS, Fernandes LH. Sister Mary Joseph's nodule: a sign of internal malignancy. An Bras Dermatol. 2011;86(4 Suppl 1):S118–20.
84. Jing H, Zhang Y, Li F. Sister Mary Joseph Nodules on 99mTc HYNIC-TOC scintigraphy in patients with neuroendocrine tumors. Clin Nucl Med. 2015;40(2):166–8.
85. Reichert MC, Farmakis G, Bohle RM, Lammert F, Zimmer V. Cholangiocarcinoma presenting as Sister Mary Joseph's nodule: case report and short review of the literature. J Gastrointest Cancer. 2014;45(2):231–3.
86. Jarry J, Nguyen V, Imperato M. A fishy nodule. Gastroenterology. 2012;142(1):e26–7.
87. Pontinen T, Melin A, Varadi G, Khanmoradi K, Chewaproug D, Kung SC, Zaki R, Ortiz J. Cutaneous metastasis of pancreatic adenocarcinoma after kidney transplant: a case report and review of the literature. Exp Clin Transplant. 2010;8(4):273–6.
88. Setty B, Blake MA, Holalkere NS, Blaszkowsky LS, Fischman A. Laparoscopic scar: a mimicker of Sister Mary Joseph's nodule on positron emission tomography/CT. Australas Radiol. 2006;50(5):507–9.
89. Inadomi T. Sister Mary Joseph's nodule: a clue to finding pancreatic cancer in a patient previously affected by gastric cancer. Eur J Dermatol. 2005;15(6):492–4.
90. Rosado Rubio C, Alvarez Alamo V, Ortiz Sierra MC, Domínguez MF. Sister Mary Joseph nodule secondary to rectal adenocarcinoma. Rev Esp Geriatr Gerontol. 2010;45(4):241–2.
91. Li F, Yu J, Yang Z. Sister Mary Joseph's nodule originating from primary duodenal adenocarcinoma. Am J Med Sci. 2012;344(1):40.
92. Zhang Z, Wang J, Huang J, Yu X. Umbilical metastasis derived from early stage rectal cancer: a case report. World J Surg Oncol. 2014;12:82.
93. Aljehani Y. An unusual cause for Sister Mary Joseph's nodule: a case report. Oman Med J. 2014;29(6):458–60.
94. Nikolaou M, Zyli P, Stamenkovic S, Koniari K, Psachoulia C, Kalofonos HP. Sister Mary Joseph's nodule in advanced ovarian cancer. J Obstet Gynaecol. 2013;33(2):214–5.
95. Vaughn JE, Gopal AK. Relapsed mantle cell lymphoma presenting as sister Mary Joseph nodule. Case Rep Med. 2010;2010:708348.
96. Abdulqawi R, Ahmad S, Ashawesh K. A rare cause of Sister Mary Joseph's nodule. Swiss Med Wkly. 2007;137(39–40):559–60.
97. Tsai HW, Yuan CC, Wang PH. Umbilicus as the only site of metastasis in recurrent ovarian cancer. J Chin Med Assoc. 2006;69(5):233–5.
98. Tomaszewska K. Sister Mary Joseph's nodule disclosing an ovarian cancer. Ginekol Pol. 2005;76(9):735–7.
99. Lee WJ, Chou CJ. Sister Mary Joseph's nodule. Emerg Med J. 2006;23(12):956.
100. Xiao J, Li JD, Xu MM, Zhu AN, Feng YL. Umbilicus metastasis in patients with epithelial ovarian cancer : clinical features of 21 patients. Zhonghua Yi Xue Za Zhi. 2013;93(25):1986–8.
101. Zhou HY, Wang XB, Gao F, Bu B, Zhang S, Wang Z. Cutaneous metastasis from pancreatic cancer: A case report and systematic review of the literature. Oncol Lett. 2014;8(6):2654–60.
102. Gupta P, Kumari A, Kriplani A, Bhatla N. Sister Mary Joseph's nodule as the first and only sign of recurrence in a case of stage Ia carcinoma ovary. BMJ Case Rep. 2014;2014. pii: bcr 2013201779.

103. Datta S, Sengupta SG, Bhattacherjee S, Ghosh M. Umbilical nodule, an uncommon presentation of gastric malignancy. J Assoc Physicians India. 2012;60:51–3.
104. Genders RE, Bonsing BA, van der Molen A, Lavrijsen S. Image of the month. Sister Mary Joseph nodule. Arch Surg. 2011;146(3):361–2.
105. Salemis NS. Umbilical metastasis or Sister Mary Joseph's nodule as a very early sign of an occult cecal adenocarcinoma. J Gastrointest Cancer. 2007;38(2-4):13–4.
106. Fukuda H, Saito R. A case of Sister Mary Joseph's nodule from prostatic cancer. J Dermatol. 2006;33(1):46–51.
107. Kruczek K, Nabhan C. Sister Mary Joseph nodule from prostate cancer. J Am Osteopath Assoc. 2012;112(7):462.
108. Higuchi M, Shibata-Kikuchi S, Ito T, Gondo C, Takahara M, Moroi Y, Furue M. Marked melanocyte colonization of pigmented Sister Mary Joseph's nodule from intrahepatic cholangiocarcinoma. Eur J Dermatol. 2014;24(1):125–6.
109. Deb P, Rai RS, Rai R, Gupta E, Chander Y. Sister Mary Joseph nodule as the presenting sign of disseminated prostate carcinoma. J Cancer Res Ther. 2009;5(2):127–9.
110. Kirshtein B, Meirovitz M, Okon E, Piura B. Sister Mary Joseph's nodule as the first presenting sign of primary fallopian tube adenocarcinoma. J Minim Invasive Gynecol. 2006;13(3):234–6.
111. Métivier Jr D, Bonardel G, Rouquie D, Gontier E, Chargari C, Dechaud C, Foehrenbach H, Chapuis O. 18F-FDG PET/CT imaging of Sister Mary Joseph's nodule. Clin Nucl Med. 2012;37(5):486–8.
112. Jacques J, Mesturoux L, Vong C, Legros R, Loustaud-Ratti V. An umbilical nodule. Rev Med Interne. 2014;35(1):73–4.
113. Sharma A, Sharma V. Image diagnosis: Sister Mary Joseph nodule. Perm J. 2014;18(2):132.
114. Agrawal V, Garg PK, Mohanty D, Jaswal V. Umbilical nodule in cholangiocarcinoma. Sister Mary Joseph Nodule. Saudi J Gastroenterol. 2012;18(5):345–6.
115. Larentzakis A, Theodorou D, Fili K, Manataki A, Bizimi V, Tibishrani M, Katsaragakis S. Sister Mary Joseph's nodule: Three case reports. Case J. 2008;1(1):182.
116. Doros L, Kaste SC, Rodriguez-Galindo C. Sister Mary Joseph's nodule as presenting sign of a desmoplastic small round cell tumor. Pediatr Blood Cancer. 2008;50(2):388–90.
117. Mun JH, Kim JM, Ko HC, Kim BS, Kim MB. Dermoscopy of a Sister Mary Joseph nodule. J Am Acad Dermatol. 2013;68(6):e190–2.
118. Salinas F, Martínez L, Egea J, López J. Sister Mary Joseph's nodule. Med Clin (Barc). 2007;129(3):120.
119. Prabhu R, Krishna S, Shenoy R, Natarajan A. Pancreatic cancer presenting as a Sister Mary Joseph's nodule. BMJ Case Rep. 2013;2013. pii: bcr 201320101020.

Chapter 39
Umbilical Tumors

Saleh Abdel-Kader and Fikri M. Abu-Zidan

39.1 Introduction

The umbilicus is an abdominal scar that persists after the fall of the umbilical cord (the only root for food and gas exchange of the fetus). No wonder, the umbilicus is related to various embryological remnants including the vitellointestinal duct, the urachus, the falciform ligament, and the vesicoumbilical ligaments (Fig. 39.1) [1].

A wide variety of tumors occur in the umbilicus, mostly metastatic from the viscera. These metastases are attributed to the generous vascular and fetal connections of the umbilicus. Umbilical tumors account for about 10 % of all tumors affecting the anterior abdominal wall. The majority are benign (80 %) while malignancy is rare (20 %) [2]. Majority of umbilical tumors are secondary to intra-abdominal malignant disease, while primary umbilical tumors are extremely rare [3].

S. Abdel-Kader, PhD, MRCS
Department of Surgery, Faculty of Medicine, Ain Shams University, Cairo, Egypt

Department of General Surgery, Al-Ain Hospital, Al-Ain, UAE
e-mail: sa154cairo@hotmail.com

F.M. Abu-Zidan, M.D., Ph.D. (✉)
Department of Surgery, College of Medicine and Health Sciences, UAE University, 17666, Al-Ain, UAE
e-mail: fabuzidan@uaeu.ac.ae

M.A. Shiffman (ed.), *Adult Umbilical Reconstruction*,
DOI 10.1007/978-3-319-43887-0_39

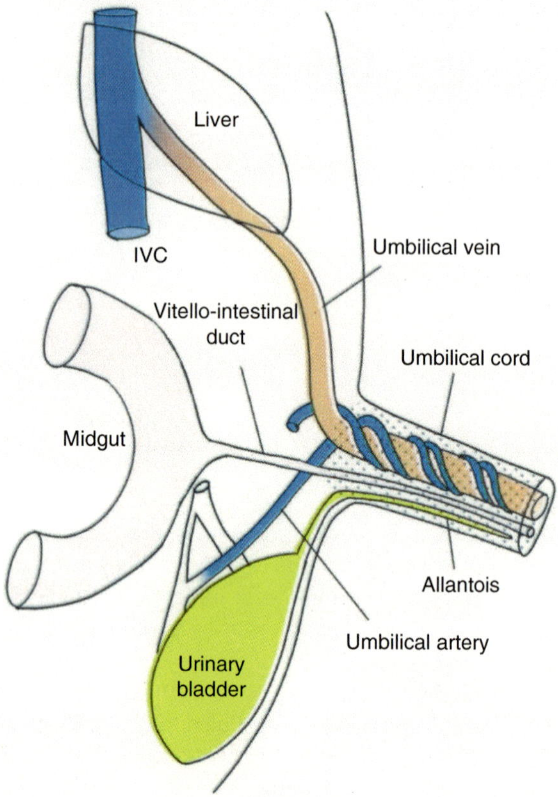

Fig. 39.1 The relationship of the umbilicus to different embryological structures including (1) the vitellointestinal duct, (2) the allantois, (3) the umbilical vein, and (4) the umbilical arteries (Illustrated by Mohammad Abu-Zidan, undergraduate student, UAE University, UAE)

39.2 Umbilical Anatomy

The umbilicus is a wrinkled scar covered by a normal skin at the linea alba, midway between the xiphoid process and symphysis pubis at the previous site of disconnected umbilical cord. The periumbilical tissues form the thinnest part of the abdominal wall. The umbilical fascia, which supports the floor of the umbilicus, is a condensation of the fascia transversalis and is firmly adherent to the deeper peritoneum and to superficial linea alba.

Figure 39.1 shows the relationship between the umbilicus and the different remnants of the embryological structures. They form various peritoneal folds and ligaments. These include: (1) the obliterated residual of the vitellointestinal duct. It once connected the yolk sac to the terminal ileum and may persist in adulthood as Meckel's diverticulum, (2) the urachus (median umbilical ligament) which is the obliterated allantois that connected the umbilicus to the roof of the urinary bladder, (3) the falciform ligament which is the remnant of the umbilical vein that drained to the inferior vena cava carrying oxygenated blood, and (4) the vesicoumbilical ligaments on the sides of the urachus, which were the umbilical arteries originating from the internal iliac arteries and carrying deoxygenated blood to the placenta [4].

39.3 Clinical Manifestations

Patients having umbilical tumors usually present with an umbilical swelling of variable sizes. This can be painful and misdiagnosed as obstructed umbilical hernia. The swelling may ulcerate and bleed resembling infected umbilical pilonidal abscess. The tumor may completely replace the umbilicus [5]. Patients may have nausea, vomiting, weight loss, constipation, pain, melena, or other symptoms depending on the origin of the tumor or extent of its metastasis.

Umbilical metastasis was first reported in 1864 by Storer [6] who called it "Sister Mary Joseph's nodule." It may be the first presenting sign in patients with unknown malignant disease. This nodule may occur as dermal, subcutaneous, or peritoneal deposit. It usually presents as firm, irregular nodule or exfoliative umbilical mass that may ulcerate and become painful. It may occasionally discharge serous fluid and may become infected and bleed. It may have different colors including normal skin, red, blue, purple, brown, or black color. This depends on the depth of tumor penetration into the skin, its vascularity, and the presence of inflammation and hemorrhage.

Patients may also present with periumbilical erythema due to hyperemia. This hyperemia results from obstruction of the cutaneous lymphatic vessels by the tumor [7]. Rarely, patients may develop periumbilical ecchymosis (Cullen's sign), due to intrahepatic tumor hemorrhage or hemorrhagic ascites. In such cases the ecchymosis is likely to be due to blood tracking along the falciform ligament. Periumbilical hemorrhage caused by malignancy is an ominous predictor of high mortality [8].

39.4 Histopathology

Primary umbilical tumors can be adenocarcinoma, melanoma, carcinoid tumor, and serous carcinoma of the peritoneum [9]. The absence of sebaceous or sweat glands in the umbilicus cannot explain the origin of primary adenocarcinomas. Nevertheless, they may stem from metaplasia of the squamous epithelium or the glandular components of the vitellointestinal duct and the urachus [5]. Adenocarcinomas arising from the columnar epithelium covering the embryonic remnant of the umbilical cord are identical to primary papillary serous neoplasia of the peritoneum and ovaries. It may originate from coelomic remnants. Primary umbilical adenocarcinoma could also arise from preexisting endometrioma and from the mesothelium of the hernia sac [10].

Table 39.1 Common organs as the source for Sister Mary Joseph's nodules by their ordered frequency

Ovaries
Stomach
Colorectal and small bowel
Pancreas
Endometrium
Cervix
Breast
Gallbladder
Lung
Prostate

Table 39.2 Primary site of carcinomas in 121 men and 176 women having Sister Mary Joseph's nodule

Site	Men	Women	Combined (%)
Stomach	36 (30 %)	16 (9 %)	52 (17.5 %)
Rectum, colon, and small bowel	30 (25 %)	21 (12 %)	51 (17.2)
Pancreas	22 (18 %)	14 (8 %)	36 (12.1 %)
Lung	4 (3 %)	—	4 (1.3 %)
Ovary	–	60 (34 %)	60 (20.2 %)
Endometrium	–	21 (12 %)	21 (7.1 %)
Cervix	–	9 (5 %)	9 (3 %)
Gallbladder	–	5 (3 %)	5 (1.7 %)
Breast	–	5 (3 %)	5 (1.7 %)
Prostate	2 (2 %)	—	2 (1 %)
Others	6 (5 %)	9 (5 %)	15 (5.1 %)
Unknown	21 (17 %)	16 (9 %)	37 (12.5 %)
Total	121 (100 %)	176 (100 %)	297 (100 %)

Data were retrieved from Dubreuil et al. [1], Data were used with permission [1]

Table 39.1 shows the most common sites of metastasis to the umbilicus by their frequency and their percentages as reported by Dubreuil et al. [1]. Table 39.1 summarizes the findings of Table 39.2, which shows the most frequent sites of umbilical metastasis ordered by their frequency.

There are other rare causes for umbilical malignancy. Uncommonly, adenocarcinoma arising from Meckel's diverticulum may invade the umbilicus [11]. Furthermore, umbilical Paget's disease was described in a patient with prostatic cancer. Both the umbilicus and prostate are derived from a similar embryonic origin, the cloaca [12]. Other rare tumors that spread into the umbilicus include carcinoid tumors, leiomyosarcoma, granulosa cell tumor, myxoid liposarcoma of the stomach, small cell carcinoma of the lung, myeloma, peritoneal mesothelioma, adenoacanthoma of the uterus, hepatoma, transitional cell carcinoma, and mixed Mullerian tumors [13]. Non-Hodgkin's lymphoma and acute myeloid leukemia were reported to metastasize to the umbilicus producing a rapidly growing ulcerative lesion [14, 15].

Table 39.3 Pathological varieties of malignant tumors that spread to the umbilicus

Adenocarcinoma
Squamous cell carcinoma
Melanoma
Carcinoid
Leiomyosarcoma
Granulosa cell tumor
Myxoid liposarcoma of the stomach
Small cell carcinoma of the lung
Peritoneal mesothelioma
Adenoacanthoma of the uterus
Hepatoma
Transitional cell carcinoma of the bladder
Papillary serous carcinoma of peritoneum
Umbilical Paget's disease
Mixed Mullerian tumor
Myeloma
Non-Hodgkin's lymphoma
Acute myeloid leukemia

Table 39.4 Routes of spread of malignancy to the umbilicus

Contiguous extension
Umbilical hernia
Iatrogenic spread
Embryological remnant spread
Lymphatic spread
Arterial spread
Venous spread

Histologically, most metastatic lesions are adenocarcinoma followed by squamous cell carcinoma. The immune profile of the tumor can indicate its origin. Tumors arising from the urachus are predominantly transitional epithelium in origin but occasionally have glandular epithelium. They usually affect the males and present with suprapubic mass and difficult micturition [3]. Table 39.3 shows the different histopathological varieties of malignant tumors that spread to the umbilicus.

39.5 Pathophysiology of Malignant Disease Spread

The umbilicus has numerous embryonic vascular and lymphatic connections which make it vulnerable to neoplastic cell deposition. Table 39.4 shows different routes in which tumors can metastasize to the umbilicus and vise versa. These include the following.

39.5.1 Contiguous Extension

The umbilicus is directly related to the extraperitoneal tissue, making the spread from peritoneal surface to the umbilicus very likely [2]. The most common example is the ovarian cancer contiguous spread to metastasize to the umbilicus. Vascular or lymphatic spread is not the cause of metastasis in this condition [16].

39.5.2 Umbilical Hernia

Sometimes the tumor cells become embedded in an old umbilical hernia and can be misdiagnosed as incarcerated umbilical hernia [3].

39.5.3 Iatrogenic Spread

After laparoscopic surgery, port-site metastasis can occur at the umbilicus. This occurs either via direct invasion through the thin wall at the incision site or due to tracking of tumor cells into the incision at surgery. Rarely, these metastases are associated with hidden intra-abdominal malignancy [17].

39.5.4 Embryological Remnant Spread

Although embryological remnants were thought to play a major role in metastasis to the umbilicus, it seems that it has minor role compared with other routes for spread [18].

39.5.5 Lymphatic Spread

Lymphatic connections exist between periumbilical skin and deep lymphatic network; para-aortic, internal mammary; and external iliac nodes [19]. Other connections are present with the superficial abdominal lymphatic network and axillary and inguinal lymph nodes. Cutaneous lymphoscintigraphy revealed unusual patterns of lymphatic spread [20]. Lymphatic spread is predominantly a retrograde lymphatic permeation [21]. In addition, the umbilicus is the point of intersection of numerous lymphatic networks. This explains the high risk of lymphatic spread to the umbilicus and also the high risk of dissemination from it [22].

39.5.6 Venous Spread

The vertebral venous system is very important for cutaneous spread of the umbilical tumors. The venous drainage of the umbilicus goes into different directions including: (1) the axillary veins through the lateral thoracic veins, (2) the femoral veins through the superficial epigastric veins, (3) the portal vein through small veins in the ligamentum teres, and finally (4) the vertebral veins, which connect the abdominal wall veins with the head and neck veins. This route is important because it bypasses the portal, pulmonary, and caval veins [21, 23].

39.5.7 Arterial Spread

Malignant cells can migrate through bloodstream to be implanted in the umbilicus [24].

39.6 Differential Diagnosis

Table 39.5 shows the differential diagnosis of an umbilical swelling. Many benign diseases are found in the umbilicus, such as inflammation, pilonidal sinus, fistulas, hernias, and endometriosis. Endometriosis usually presents as a brownish red nodule which characteristically increases in size and becomes painful during

Table 39.5 Benign and malignant umbilical lesions

Benign lesions
Cutaneous endometrioma
Pilonidal abscess and fistula
Incarcerated umbilical hernia
Vitellointestinal cyst
Congenital polyps
Skin and subcutaneous tissue lesions (papilloma, nevi, fibroma, lymphangioma, epithelial inclusion cyst)
Malignant lesions
Metastatic tumors
Primary adenocarcinoma
Squamous cell carcinoma
Basal cell carcinoma
Adenocarcinoma of urachal remnants
Malignant melanoma
Myosarcoma

menstruation. It may bleed especially during menses. It represents about 10% of extrauterine endometrial tissue in all women at childbearing age [25]. The differential diagnosis also includes granuloma (pyogenic, foreign body), urachal duct cyst, omphalomesenteric duct abnormalities, keloid, epithelial inclusion cyst, and benign and malignant tumors [26, 27]. Adenocarcinoma is uncommon and is difficult to be distinguished from secondary deposits (Sister Mary Joseph's nodule) [28].

39.7 Diagnostic Workup

Complete clinical examination is of great importance to achieve the correct diagnosis. A detailed examination of the umbilicus and periumbilical area should be performed during the assessment of a known cancer patient. Alternatively, when an umbilical tumor is suspected, a full clinical examination should be performed to try to find the source of metastasis. Table 39.1 shows the organs from which metastasis commonly originates.

Table 39.6 shows the suggested workup when a malignant umbilical tumor is proven by histopathology. Laboratory investigations include a complete blood cell count, liver function test, urea, creatinine, and electrolytes. Tumor markers like CA125, CA19-9, and carcinoembryonic antigen (CEA) are helpful both for the diagnoses and prognosis of the disease.

High-resolution ultrasound scan can detect small nodules located few centimeters beneath the skin. It can also demonstrate the solid nature of the umbilical nodule [11]. Furthermore, it may detect peritoneal masses, lymphadenopathy, liver metastases, or ascites.

Table 39.6 Workup for patients having umbilical tumors

Blood investigations
Complete blood cell count
Liver function tests
Tumor markers: CA125, CA 19-9, CEA
Radiology
Ultrasound
Computed tomography
MRI
PET
Procedures
Fine needle aspiration
Excisional biopsy
Upper gastrointestinal endoscopy
Lower gastrointestinal endoscopy
Laparoscopy
Laparotomy

A computed tomography scan (CT scan) may reveal intra-abdominal mass, hypertrophic lymph nodes, and locally advanced tumors [29]. PET-CT scan is a useful modality to discover primary lesions of hidden malignancy [30].

Umbilical masses should be biopsied to reach a histopathological diagnosis. This includes fine needle aspiration of the nodule. The cytological examination can provide a rapid and reliable diagnosis, especially in patients with documented malignancy [13]. Alternatively umbilical masses should be excised for a definite diagnosis [27]. Immunohistochemistry of the fine needle aspiration (FNA) may guide the diagnosis in particular patients with unknown primary tumors [31]. Upper and lower gastrointestinal endoscopy may be useful in defining the primary origin of the tumor. Exploratory laparotomy may be indicated when the origin of the tumor cannot be identified. Diagnosis of primary umbilical carcinoma is reached only by exclusion [3].

39.8 Treatment

The treatment of primary umbilical adenocarcinoma is surgical followed by adjuvant chemotherapy. Different oncological surgical modalities are implemented. The standard treatment is complete radical excision of the tumor with adequate safety margin. Abdominal exploration is indicated to rule out existence of a primary tumor that had not been discovered before surgery [32]. Sentinel lymph node biopsy must be carried out in patients with primary skin malignant lesions [33]. Unnecessary handling, palpation, and probing should be avoided. Debulking surgery followed by adjuvant chemotherapy is the offered palliative treatment for advanced malignant tumors. Surgical cytoreduction by omentectomy is an option for unresectable malignant umbilical tumors. Metastatic deposits if treated by aggressive surgical excision including resection of primary tumor will show occasional long-term survival [34]. Reconstruction of the umbilicus is seldomly needed after surgical excision of the malignant lesion. Plastic surgeons have many techniques for reconstruction especially after surgery for benign lesions. These techniques include double V-Y procedures, local flaps, bilateral advancement flaps, circumferential rotation flaps, and local flaps combined with conchal cartilage composite graft [35].

39.9 Prognosis

The presence of an umbilical metastatic mass usually carries a poor prognosis indicating a widespread tumor. Untreated patients may survive up to 11 months from the time of diagnosis [11] Few patients (13.5 %) with umbilical metastasis remain alive after 2 years. Prolonged survival in cases of solitary umbilical metastasis has been reported. These cases require aggressive surgery and chemotherapy [1]. Primary malignant umbilical tumors which arise from the skin, such as squamous cell carcinoma, basal cell carcinoma, and malignant melanoma, have a favorable outcome if excised early [33]. However, the prognosis is still not well defined for the primary adenocarcinoma because they are extremely rare [32]. More case reports of primary umbilical tumors will help to elucidate the pathogenesis, diagnosis, therapeutic options, and prognosis of these tumors [5].

39.10 Learning Points

1. Majority of umbilical malignant tumors are metastatic while primary malignancy is rare.
2. Generous vascular and embryologic connections of the umbilicus explain the reason for umbilical metastasis.
3. Thorough examination of the umbilicus should be a routine part of the assessment of a known cancer patient.
4. Primary malignant umbilical tumors are diagnosed by exclusion of metastasis to the umbilicus.
5. Aggressive surgery and chemotherapy may be required for solitary metastasis to the umbilicus or primary malignant umbilical tumors.
6. The presence of umbilical metastasis indicates a poor prognosis.

Acknowledgment The authors thank Professor Suhail Al-Salam, FRCPath, Department of Pathology, College of Medicine and Health Sciences, UAE University, Al-Ain, UAE, for reviewing the final manuscript of this book chapter.

References

1. Dubreuil A, Dompmartin A, Barjot P, Louvet S, Leroy D. Umbilical metastasis or Sister Mary Joseph's nodule. Int J Dermatol. 1998;37(1):7–13.
2. Blumenthal NJ. Umbilical tumours. A case report and review of the literature. S Afr Med J. 1980;58:457–8.
3. Alnaqbi KA, Joshi S, Ghasal-Aswad S, Abu Zidan FM. Primary umbilical adenocarcinoma. Singapore Med J. 2007;8:e308–10.
4. Coll DM, Meyer JM, Mader M, Smith RC. Imaging appearances of Sister Mary Joseph nodule. Pictorial review. Br J Radiol. 1999;72:1230–3.
5. Alver O, Ersoy YE, Dogusoy G, Erguney S. Primary umbilical adenocarcinoma: case report and review of the literature. Am Surg. 2007;73:923–5.
6. Storer HR. Circumscribed tumor of the umbilicus closely simulating umbilical hernia. Boston Med Surg J. 1864;lxx:73.
7. Fajobi O, Jafri Z, Vadgama N, Cannon E, Myint F. Retroperitoneal non-Hodgkin's lymphoma presenting as periumbilical erythema. J Am Acad Dermatol. 2005;53:527–8.
8. Mabin TA, Gelfand M. Cullen's sign, a feature of liver disease. Br Med J. 1974;1:493–4.
9. Ransom DT, Patel SR, Keeney GL, Malkasian GD, Edmonson JH. Papillary serous carcinoma of the peritoneum. A review of 33 cases treated with platin-based chemotherapy. Cancer. 1990;66:1091–4.

10. Glazer G. Primary adenocarcinoma arising in a vitello-intestinal duct remnant at the umbilicus. Br J Surg. 1973;60:247–9.
11. Gabriele R, Conte M, Egidi F, Borghese M. Umbilical metastases: current viewpoint. World J Surg Oncol. 2005;3:13.
12. Remond B, Aractingi S, Blanc F, Verola O, Vignon D, Dubertret L. Umbilical Paget's disease and prostatic carcinoma. Br J Dermatol. 1993;128(4):448–50.
13. Majmudar B, Wiskind AK, Croft BN, Dudley AG. The Sister (Mary) Joseph Nodule; its significance in gynaecology. Gynecol Oncol. 1991;40:152–9.
14. Tam C, Turner H, Hicks RJ, Seymour JF. Diffuse large B-cell non-Hodgkin's lymphoma presenting as Sister Joseph's nodule. Leuk Lymphoma. 2002;43:2055–7.
15. Beynet D, Oro AE. Leukemia cutis presenting as a Sister Mary Joseph nodule. Arch Dermatol. 2004;140:1170–1.
16. Goodheart RS, Cooke CT, Tan E, Matz LR. Sister Mary Joseph's nodule. Med J Aust. 1986;145:477–8.
17. Clair DG, Lautz DB, Brooks DC. Rapid development of umbilical metastases after laparoscopic cholecystectomy for unsuspected gallbladder carcinoma. Surgery. 1993;113:355–8.
18. Scarpa FJ, Dineen JP, Boltax RS. Visceral neoplasia presenting at the umbilicus. J Surg Oncol. 1979;11:351–9.
19. Uren RF, Howman-Giles RB, Thompson JF, Shaw HM, McCarthy WH. Lymphatic drainage from peri-umbilical skin to internal mammary nodes. Clin Nucl Med. 1995;20(3):254–5.
20. Chakraborty AK, Reddy AN, Grosberg SJ, Wapnick S. Pancreatic carcinoma with dissemination to umbilicus and skin. Arch Dermatol. 1977;113(6):838–9.
21. Touraud J, Lentz N, Dutronc Y, Mercier E, Sagot P, Lambert D. Umbilical cutaneous metastasis (or Sister Mary Joseph's nodule) disclosing an ovarian adenocarcinoma}. Gynecol Obstet Fertil. 2000;28(10):719–21.
22. Glover RP, Waugh JM. The retrograde lymphatic spread of carcinoma of the "rectosigmoid region". Its influence on surgical procedures. Surg Gynecol Obstet. 1946;82:434–48.
23. Batson OV. The role of the vertebral veins in metastatic processes. Ann Intern Med. 1942;16:38–45.
24. Brodland DG, Zitelli JA. Mechanism of metastasis. J Am Acad Dermatol. 1992;27:6–8.
25. Albrecht LE, Tron V, Rivers JK. Cutaneous endometriosis. Int J Dermatol. 1995;34:261–2.
26. Banerjee I, Pratap D. Umbilical adenoma. Int Surg. 1977;62:608–10.
27. Ioannidis O, Cheva A, Stavrakis T, Paraskevas G, Papadimitriou N, Kakoutis E, Makrantonakis A. Sister Mary Joseph's nodule as the sole presenting sign of gastric signet ring cell adenocarcinoma. Gastroenterol Clin Biol. 2010;34(10):565–8.
28. Fourati M, El Euch D, Haouet H, Boussen H, Haouet S, Mokni M. Ben Osman Dhahri A. Adenocarcinoma of the umbilicus. Ann Dermatol Venereol. 2004;131(4):379–81.
29. Shetty MR. Metastatic tumour of the umbilicus: a review 1830–1989. J Surg Oncol. 1990;45:212–5.
30. Lee CK, Chang YW, Jung SH, Jang JY, Dong SH, Kim HJ, et al. A case of Sister Mary Joseph's nodule as a presenting sign of gastric cancer. Korean J Gastroenterol. 2008;51:132–6.
31. Hernandez N, Medina V, Alvarez-Arguelles H, Gutierrez R, Perez-Palma J, Diaz-Flores L. Primary papillary psammomatous adenocarcinoma of the umbilicus. Histol Histopathol. 1993;8:593–8.
32. Febrero B, Ruiz de Angulo D, Ortiz MA, Lopez MJ, Parrilla P. Primary adenocarcinoma of the navel: an uncommon entity. Cir Esp. 2014;92(6):436–8.
33. Zaccagna A, Siatis D, Pisacane A, Giacone E, Picciotto F. Surgical treatment of primary melanoma of the umbilicus with sentinel lymph node biopsy and plastic reconstruction: case report and review of literature. EJSO. 2011;37:233–6.
34. Dalrymple JC, Bannatyne P, Russell P, Solomon HJ, Tattersall MH, Atkinson K, Carter J, Duval P, Elliott P, Friedlander M, et al. Extraovarian peritoneal serous papillary carcinoma. A clinicopathological study of 31 cases. Cancer. 1989;64:110–5.
35. Etter L, Cook JL. Basal cell carcinoma of the umbilicus: a case report and literature review. Cutis. 2003;71:123–6.

Chapter 40
Surgical Approaches for Melanocytic Nevi and Malignant Melanoma of the Umbilicus

Christoph R. Loeser, Edgar Dippel, Adrien Daigeler, Soraya Navysany, and Laurenz Schmitt

40.1 Introduction

Malignant melanoma in the navel is a rather rare finding despite the fact that we treat around 300 new cases of melanoma each year in skin cancer centers like the one in Ludwigshafen. On the other hand, patients present with nevi in the umbilicus quite often. Depending on the exact location at the superficial or deeper part of the navel, the individual sensitivity, and the form of the tunnel like structure, clinical observation and dermoscopic evaluation are impaired, if possible at all. Due to these limitations, complete removal of the lesion in an outpatient setting with histological examination might prove a sensitive decision. Useful approaches for these rather frequent but for the uninitiated difficult-to-reach lesions are presented. Once a melanoma is histologically proven, complete removal with an appropriate security margin is mandated, eventually requiring reconstructive procedures.

C.R. Loeser, MD (✉) • E. Dippel, M.D. • S. Navysany, M.D.
Skin Cancer Center, Ludwigshafen Hospital, Bremserstr. 79, 67063 Ludwigshafen, Germany
e-mail: loeserc@klilu.de; dippele@klilu.de; sorayan@gmx.net

A. Daigeler, M.D.
Department of Plastic Surgery, Burn Center, Hand Center, BG-University Hospital Bergmannsheil, Bochum, Germany
e-mail: daigeler@hotmail.com

L. Schmitt, M.D.
Clinical Centre Dermatology and Allergology, Department Dermatosurgery, University Hospital Aachen, Aachen, Germany
e-mail: laurenzschmitt@gmx.de

M.A. Shiffman (ed.), *Adult Umbilical Reconstruction*,
DOI 10.1007/978-3-319-43887-0_40

40.2 Technique

Surgical approaches for the minimal invasive removal of melanocytic lesions and melanoma of the navel.

40.2.1 Melanocytic Nevi

Melanocytic nevi frequently appear in the navel. Quite often, the lesion inside the navel is completely hidden (Fig. 40.1). When revealed by lateral tension, the lesion is only partially exposed. In these cases, clinical and dermoscopic evaluation can be impaired or impossible. Whenever clinical and dermoscopic evaluation is inconclusive, surgical removal for histologic evaluation is advisable. The navel is usually a cone-shaped, inverted structure with a high grade of individual variation in size and depth. For some people, the navel is a highly sensitive region, and manipulation can cause a certain amount of discomfort. Naturally, the deeper the lesion is located, the more difficult it is to reach. While it is not possible to widen the access to deeper planes of the navel without destruction, there is an easy way to bring lower parts of the navel to the surface. This is achieved by lifting the tissue on the base of the umbilicus upwards. One has to be careful handling the tissue of the lesion in question. Any pressure might distort the tissue, thereby impairing the histologic evaluation. A very effective way to lift the base of the navel while preserving the tissue of the lesion is by employing so-called traction sutures [1, 2]. After infiltration with local anesthesia, we place one or more 4–0 Vicryl sutures. The placement and the number of sutures depend on the shape of the navel, the size of the lesion, and the exact location of the lesion inside the navel.

If dealing with a papillomatous lesion, the traction suture can be placed beneath the tissue using a large needle. The lesion is then lifted and excised with a scalpel. This approach is most appropriate, if healing should take place by secondary intention. While excising, the surrounding and underlying tissue moves back to its original place, thereby becoming inaccessible again to further suturing. This method is preferred in rather unsuspicious, exophytic lesions, when surgery is also considered for esthetic reasons. Usually, additional traction sutures will be placed, to stabilize the field of surgery (Fig. 40.1). When a primary closure is intended, they are kept in place until the wound is closed (Fig. 40.2). To avoid removal of sutures, we usually use absorbable material. Contact with water like showering is encouraged from day two after surgery. Longer exposure to water like bathing or swimming should be avoided for approximately 10 days. Due to an atraumatic technique in handling the tissue, we have never experienced complications like wound infections. The removal of lesions in the navel is best performed with assistance for holding the traction sutures while handling the lesion and the closure. Anyway, there are ingenious ways to accomplish the task single-handed. Then we use sort of a ring, here built by wound clamps (consider single use instrument for that purpose). Four traction

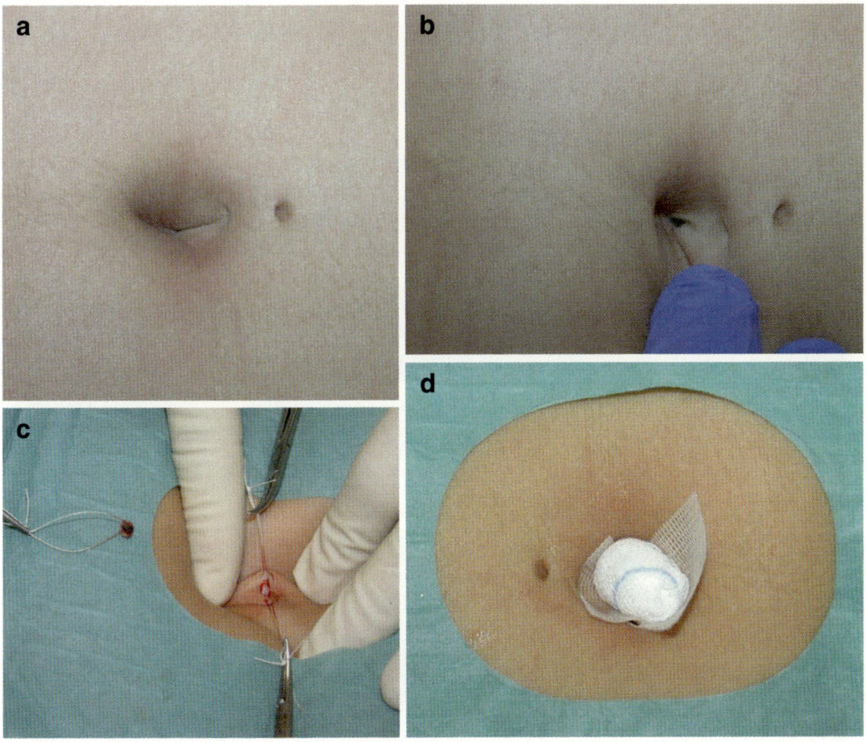

Fig. 40.1 (**a**) Navel of a 25-year-old woman. A melanocytic lesion is completely hidden. Note voluntary porous-like scarring due to piercing. (**b**) Melanocytic lesion on the base of the same navel as in figure 1, now partly exposed. (**c**) Two traction sutures close to the lesion exposed the site of surgery. The atypical nevus was secured by an additional suture. (**d**) Placement of gauze following surgery

sutures were quickly placed after local anesthesia and attached to the clamp construction (Fig. 40.3). Then removal of the lesion was performed under stable conditions. Suturing was done after releasing the two opposite traction sutures on the left and on the right to relief tension, while those up and down remained until after the closure.

40.2.2 Malignant Melanoma

Melanoma of the navel seems to be a rarity. When histologically proven, tumor depth is key to the recommendation for additional margin. While microscopically controlled surgery might be sufficient for in situ melanoma [3], margins of 1 cm (below 2 mm thickness) and 2 (if above) are established [4]. Depending on the site and the individual shape of the navel, a melanoma might grow

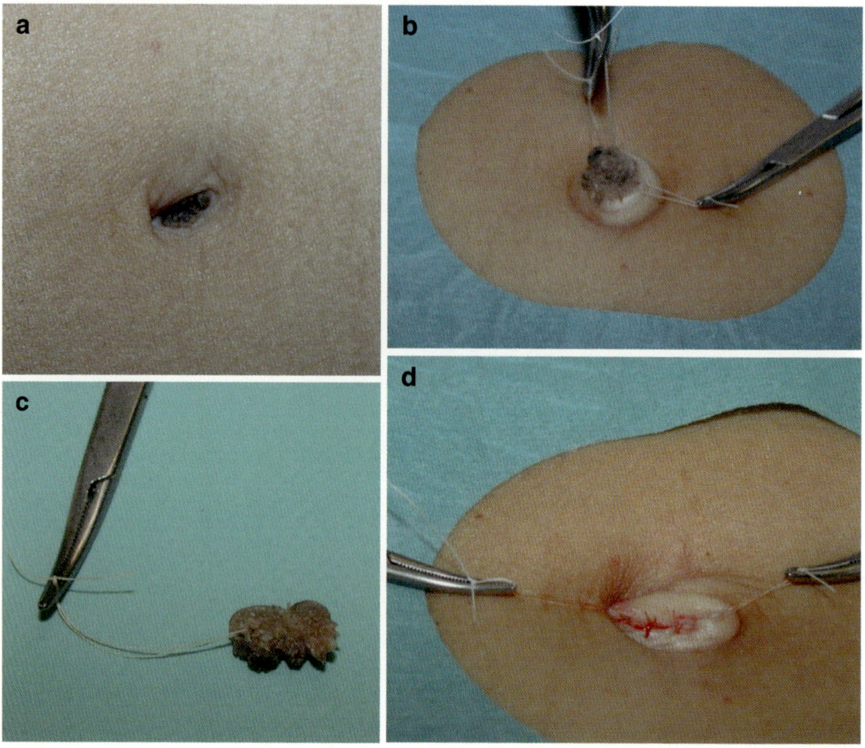

Fig. 40.2 (**a**) Papillomatous lesion at the base of the navel. (**b**) Auxiliary suture placed beneath the nodule lifting the base of the navel with first traction suture in place. (**c**) Exophytic lesion immediately after removal. (**d**) After suturing with resorbable material facilitated by two traction sutures shortly before their removal

undetected for extended periods of times. Therefore, chances for high-risk tumors are increased. This possibly leads to extensive surgery, including sentinel lymph node biopsy, which can be performed in one setting [5]. Depending on the amount of adipose tissue, deep defects are created. While several approaches are known [6, 7], we prefer a one-step procedure [8]. If the tumor thickness is above 2 mm, a security margin of 2 cm to all sides is established (Fig. 40.4). A circular excision is performed with a scalpel, and the tissue is then mobilized with scissors. By lifting the tissue, the abdominal part of the navel is exposed, and a clamp is positioned as deep as possible. A strong ligation seals the abdomen. The wound edges are fixed to the abdominal fascia by absorbable sutures. In our example, an additional circular suture was placed (Fig. 40.4). The central part heals by secondary intention. When exposed, one sees dominant scarring in the middle of the abdomen. For necessary follow-ups, the essential clinical inspection is unimpaired. In a normal standing position, the scar is completely hidden, and, depending on the nutrition state of the patient, the abdomen gives a natural appearance.

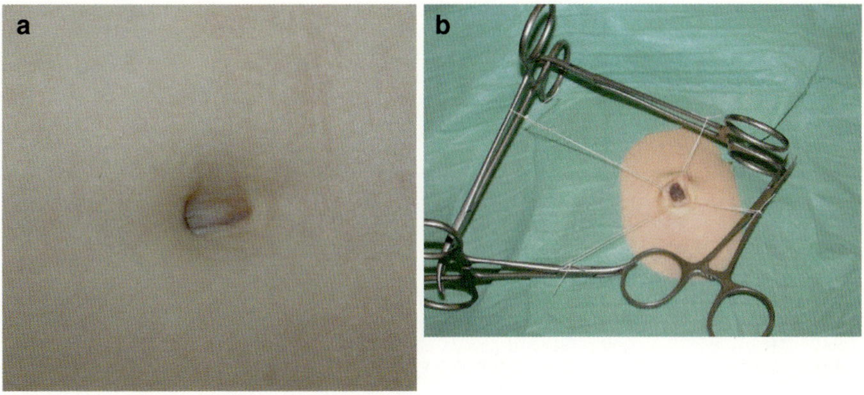

Fig. 40.3 (**a**) Melanocytic lesion completely hidden on the base of the navel. (**b**) Exposure of lesion in navel of figure 9 with four traction sutures placed to four sides on construction of surgical clamps

40.3 Discussion

If a patient presents with a lesion inside the navel for removal, the surgeon is confronted with two problems. In the first place, the lesion is difficult to access and partially or completely hidden from view. Secondly, the surrounding tissue is flexible, and it is difficult to establish a stable plane for cutting. While radiosurgery might be an option, use of lasers should be avoided, since it is crucial to preserve the tissue for histologic examination. It might be possible to facilitate access by other means, like clamps or hooks. In our opinion, the use of traction sutures is the most elegant and least traumatic way to achieve easy access and to make office surgery possible. We therefore recommend the use of tractions sutures as a convenient tool for umbilical surgery.

Since melanoma of the navel is quite rare, it is difficult to find surgeons experienced in treating this condition. A dermatologist might see a melanoma of the navel once or twice in his or her career, if at all. However, when confronted with the problem, a multidisciplinary approach might me sensible. In the case presented above, umbilical surgery was conducted by a plastic surgeon in cooperation with a dermatologic surgeon, followed by bilateral inguinal sentinel lymph node biopsy. After previous abdominal surgery or in case of occult umbilical hernia, the bowels might be closer to the surgical field than expected. Therefore, an occult hernia should be investigated before surgery, and collaboration with a surgeon is advisable. While dermatologic surgery is mostly done in local or tumescent anesthesia, in extensive surgery, patients can profit from general anesthesia as in our case. While several methods for the reconstruction of the navel were pondered before surgery, we finally decided on the most simple approach, by just recreating the scar, which the umbilicus originally consists of, without making additional cuts. In retrospect, the circumferential suture should be omitted, as well as a swab, which

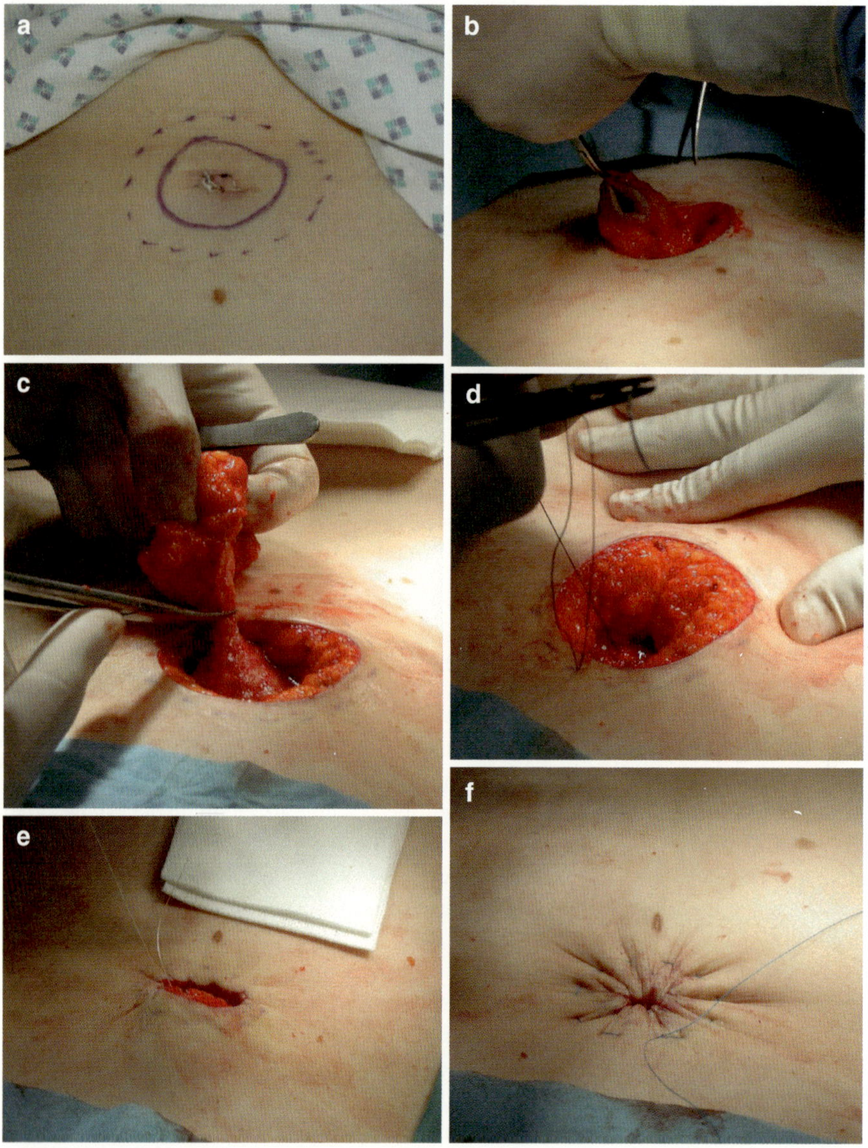

Fig. 40.4 (**a**) A security margin of at least 2 cm is marked on the skin before surgery. (**b**) After deep circular incision, the tissue is freed by preparation with scissors. (**c**) Positioning of a clamp on the base of the outer portion of the navel before ligation. (**d**) Ligation in place before deep attachment of the surrounding wound edges. (**e**) Circular suture before tying. (**f**) Finished closure with additional circular suture in place (which could be omitted in retrospect). (**g**) Ten days after surgery with swab removed. Note scarring of suture for swab on four sides. (**h**) Three months after surgery when navel is revealed by tension. (**i**) Three months after surgery in normal standing position

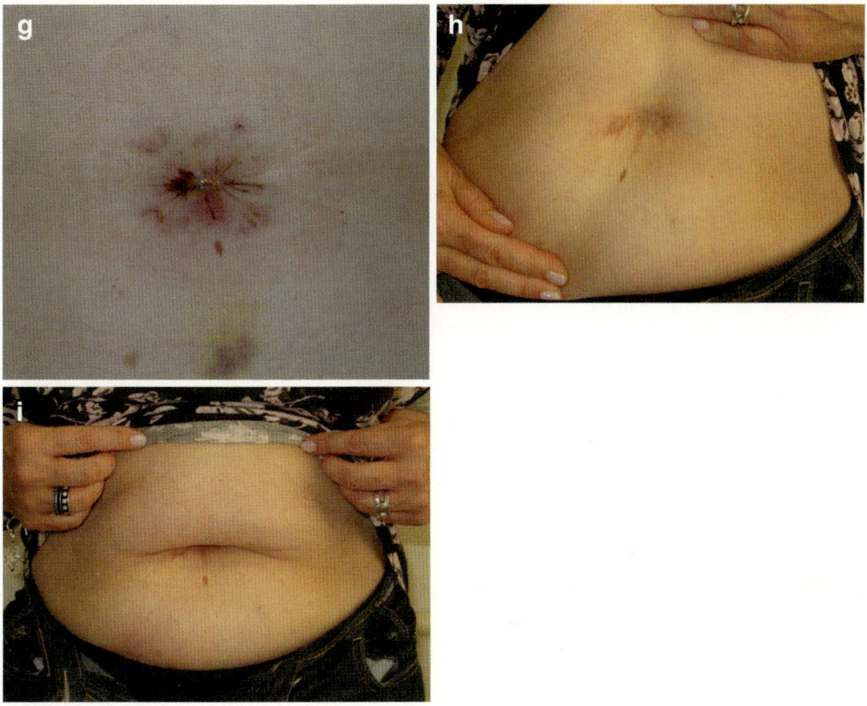

Fig. 40.4 (continued)

was temporarily sutured above the new navel. It might only have caused unnecessary scarring, while the natural shrinkage of the concave area through healing be secondary intention for the central part might have achieved the same outcome. In our example, complete healing occurred in the matter of 6 weeks [9]. The patient was most delighted that she was able to access public areas like spas without noticeable scars. She never felt mutilated, since in an upright position the abdomen looked completely natural.

40.4 Conclusions

Any bothersome melanocytic lesion in the navel should be removed and histologically investigated. Excision can be achieved by using minimally traumatic techniques as described above. When melanoma is detected, complete removal is mandatory. Additional security margins need to be added according to tumor thickness. Healing by secondary intention should always be considered and can be facilitated by approximating sutures. While performing umbilical surgery, one should always keep in mind that the navel itself is just a very special type of scar.

References

1. Goodrich RG, Lane JE, Kent DE. Use of intra-operative traction sutures in dermatologic surgery as an aid in visualization and stabilization in the operative field. Dermatol Surg. 2006;32:1272–3.
2. Loeser C. The traction suture—a universal tool. J Dtsch Dermatol Ges. 2007;5(10):940–2.
3. Loeser C, Rompel R, Breuninger H, Möhrle M, Häfner HM, Kunte C, Hassel J, Hohenleutner U, Podda M, Sebastian G, Hafner J, Konz B, Kaufmann R, German Society for Dermatosurgery. Microscopically controlled surgery (MCS). J Dtsch Dermatol Ges. 2010;8(11):920–5.
4. Pflugfelder A, Kochs C, Blum A, Capellaro M, Czeschik C, Dettenborn T, Dill D, Dippel E, Eigentler T, Feyer P, Follmann M, et al. Malignant melanoma S3-guideline "diagnosis, therapy and follow-up of melanoma". J Dtsch Dermatol Ges. 2013;11 Suppl 6:1–116.
5. Zaccagna A, Siatis D, Pisacane A, Giacone E, Picciotto F. Surgical treatment of primary melanoma of the umbilicus with sentinel lymph node biopsy and plastic reconstruction: case report and review of the literature. Eur J Surg Oncol. 2011;37:233–6.
6. Yoshiyasu I, Katsuyki A. Umbilical reconstruction using a cone-shaped Flap. Ann Plast Surg. 1992;28:335–8.
7. Breuninger H, Zimmermann C. Umbilical reconstruction after excision of melanomas in the area of the umbilicus. Hautarzt. 1996;47:273–5.
8. Miller MJ, Balch CM. "Iris" technique for immediate umbilical reconstruction. Plast Reconstr Surg. 1992;92(4):754–6.
9. Navysany S, Daigeler A, Dippel E, Loeser C. Reconstruction of the umbilicus after malignant melanoma. J Dtsch Dermatol Ges. 2013;11(5):462–4.

Chapter 41
Robotic-Assisted Excision of Urachal Adenocarcinoma with Umbiliconeoplasty

Paul G. Morrison and Chad R. Tracy

41.1 Introduction

The embryologic structure, the allantois, typically involutes before birth to become the urachus, which is anatomically referred to as the umbilical ligament. Various urachal anomalies occur when this developmental process fails. The anomalies are characterized by the pattern of patency: patent urachus (entire tract patent), urachal cyst (patency within the central portion of the remnant), umbilical-urachal sinus (umbilical side patent), and vesicourachal diverticulum (bladder side patent) [1].

The primary malignant histology of the urachus is adenocarcinoma in 90% of cases [2, 3]. It is thought to occur from chronic inflammation, infection, or sloughing of cells within the incompletely involuted urachus. A variety of subtypes exists: mucinous, enteric, mixed, and signet ring [4]. Regardless of subtype, complete surgical resection of the tumor with negative margins is the cornerstone of oncologic management. In localized disease, complete excision is the standard of care and potentially curative [2]. Further multimodal therapy is not typically warranted [2, 5]. Early surgery was performed in the open setting with radical cystectomy, urachal excision, and umbilectomy. However, similar oncologic outcomes were demonstrated in partial cystectomy with urachal excision [6], which obviated prior radical approaches and need for urinary diversion. Minimally invasive laparoscopic and robotic-assisted techniques are now practiced with the goal of ensuring wide local excision for cancer control while minimizing surgical morbidity, postoperative pain, and convalescence time [2].

P.G. Morrison, M.D. • C.R. Tracy, M.D. (✉)
University of Iowa, Departments of Urology,
200 Hawkins Dr, 3RCP, Iowa City, IA 52242-1089, USA
e-mail: paul-morrison@uiowa.edu; chad-tracy@uiowa.edu

M.A. Shiffman (ed.), *Adult Umbilical Reconstruction*,
DOI 10.1007/978-3-319-43887-0_41

41.2 Epidemiology

Urachal adenocarcinoma is a rare entity representing 0.35–0.7 % of all bladder malignancies [7]. However, it represents 22–35 % of all bladder adenocarcinomas [7]. A slight male-to-female predominance of approximately 2:1 has been noted [4, 6, 8], and median age is typically 50 years (range 16–87) [4, 6].

41.3 Evaluation

Patients may present with microscopic or gross hematuria, mucusuria, a palpable midline subumbilical mass, drainage from the umbilicus, or by incidental findings on cross-sectional imaging [7, 9]. Cystoscopy and CT imaging are key diagnostic exams. A mass at the dome of the bladder is the hallmark finding, but often cystoscopy may appear normal [10]. If a mass is visible, cystoscopic biopsy can be performed to confirm the diagnosis. CT imaging should identify a cystic or solid mass in the urachus and provides necessary staging evaluation to rule out metastatic disease and lymph node involvement (Fig. 41.1) [10]. Calcifications within the mass may be present and are suggestive of urachal adenocarcinoma [4]. Signs of local infection (reddened, fluctuant umbilical mass) are not specific as they may be present in benign [10] or malignant disease [9]. In patients with asymptomatic entirely cystic masses that are unable to be biopsied via cystoscopy, it may be difficult to establish a preoperative diagnosis of malignancy. In the setting of equivocal findings, patients should undergo surgical resection for therapeutic and diagnostic purposes.

41.4 Technique

41.4.1 Positioning and Port Placement

The patient is brought to the operative suite and general anesthesia is induced. Securement of the chest with tape or straps is essential for later steep Trendelenburg positioning [10]. The patient is placed in dorsal lithotomy position in order to allow cystoscopic access to the bladder. Abdominal access for pneumoperitoneum is attained superior to the umbilicus via commonly described laparoscopic techniques (Veress needle or Hassan). Anticipating umbilectomy, the 12 mm camera port is placed 3–5 cm supraumbilical in the midline. Diagnostic laparoscopy can be performed to visualize related injuries, tumor characteristics, abdominal adhesions, and bladder anatomy relative to the urachal mass. Remaining port placement is similar in configuration for robotic bladder diverticulectomy or radical cystectomy [10–12]. Two 8 mm robotic ports are placed approximately 6–10 cm inferior to the

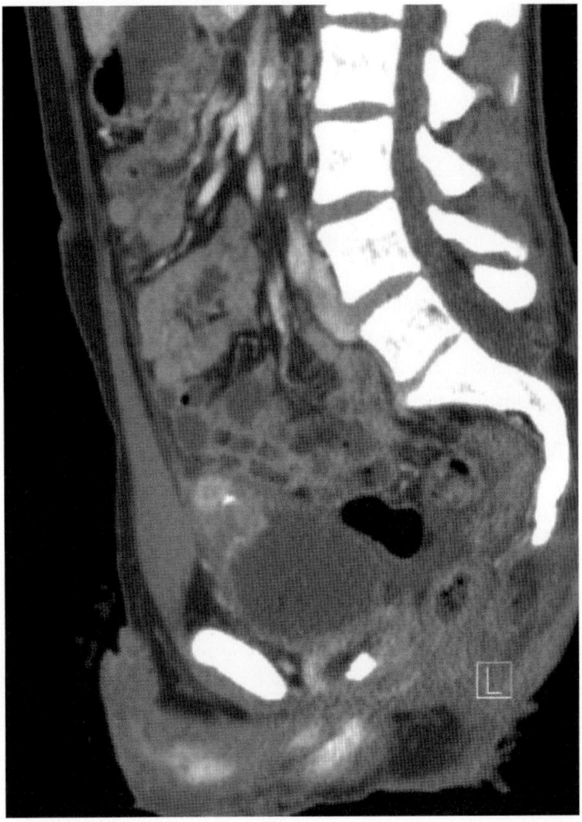

Fig. 41.1 CT image showing an enhancing anterior wall bladder mass and calcification extending into the urachal remnant

camera port along the external boarder of the rectus muscle. Additional ports are placed at surgeon discretion. A 5–12 mm assistant port can be placed in the midaxillary line at the level of the umbilicus [9].

41.4.2 Alternate Access Strategy

A preperitoneal subumbilical approach has been described as an alternative access strategy for urachal excision [13, 14]. A 1–2 cm subumbilical incision is made. Dissection is performed through the subcutaneous tissues to the level of the posterior rectus sheath. A preperitoneal balloon dilator is then passed over the posterior rectus sheath to dissect it off the anterior abdominal wall. After deflation of the balloon dilator, the umbilicus is circumscribed and deposited in the abdominal cavity. The camera port is placed several centimeters supraumbilical or it may be placed through the umbilical defect. The fascia is then closed as applicable to ensure adequate pneumoperitoneum. The remainder of the surgery proceeds in the transperitoneal fashion with the same port configuration as above.

41.4.3 Cystoscopy

Cystoscopy is performed prior to bladder and urachal dissections. It may be employed prior to port placement; however, it can be strategically utilized after port placement to visualize the intended partial cystectomy margin from both intraperitoneal and cystoscopic views (Fig. 41.2) [10, 12]. This can help ensure adequate margins of resection through use of electrocautery to delineate the line of partial cystectomy. Following cystoscopy, a Foley catheter is placed, which can be used to distend or empty the bladder during laparoscopic mobilization.

41.4.4 Urachal Excision

The patient is reclined in steep Trendelenburg to facilitate gravity retraction of the bowels out of the pelvis. Once the robot is docked, dissection begins in an inverted V shape from the level of the umbilicus to the bladder. The dome of the bladder is then fully mobilized by dissection into the space of Retzius, and a plane is developed to dissect the urachus free from its anterior attachment. If not previously completed at the time of cystoscopy, the bladder is inflated with irrigant, and the peritoneum overlying the bladder dome is scored with electrocautery, assuring a 2–3 cm rim of normal bladder beyond any notable tumor [12, 13, 15]. Careful dissection is performed through sequential layers of the bladder until only mucosa is remaining. The bladder should be drained via Foley catheter at this point to prevent potential tumor spillage. Cystotomy is made and circumferential electrocautery is

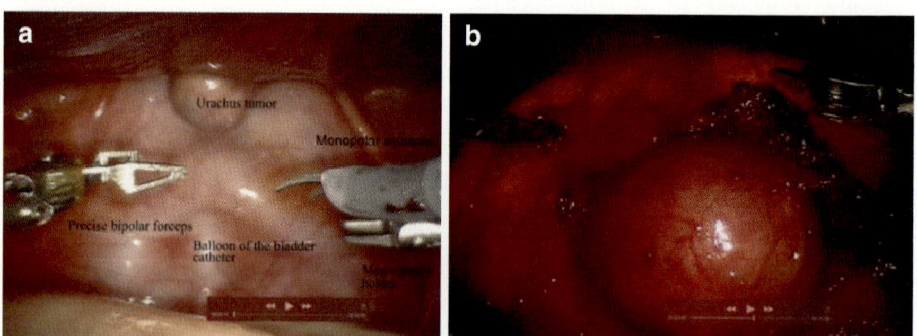

Fig. 41.2 (**a**) Abdomen and pelvis are inspected after the entry into the peritoneal cavity. The urachus tumor is identified as well as pelvic anatomical landmarks. (**b**) Flexible cystoscopy with transillumination to define the endoluminal boundaries of the mass [12] (Used with permission)

utilized to free the bladder dome margin. If the cystotomy is large, internal retention sutures may be placed between the anterior cystotomy and abdominal wall to aide in reconstruction. Cystotomy closure is performed with 2–0 absorbable suture in two layers, with the first layer approximating the mucosa and the second seromuscular imbricating layer providing muscular apposition and strength. Sterile saline is flushed into the bladder via the Foley catheter to ensure watertight closure.

Two options for excision of the urachus are described: intracorporeal division at the level of the umbilicus or extracorporeal en bloc excision [2, 11, 12, 15]. With the intraperitoneal approach, the urachus is divided at the level of the umbilicus and deposited in an Endo Catch™ bag (Covidien, Mansfield, MA) [11, 12, 15]. The umbilicus is then excised extracorporeally after undocking the robot. Alternatively, the specimen can be left intact in the intracorporeal location and removed through the umbilicus en bloc [2]. Frozen section will confirm the presence of malignancy in uncertain cases and ensure adequate surgical margins. Confirmed malignancy necessitates lymph node dissection. With the intracorporeal approach, the surgeon may opt to perform an umbilical-sparing procedure in the event of benign frozen section pathology [10].

41.4.5 Lymph Node Dissection

In cases of confirmed malignancy or highly suspicious lesions, extended bilateral pelvic lymph node dissection may be performed prior to urachal excision and partial cystectomy. As mentioned above, an alternate approach defers lymphadenectomy until confirmation of malignancy by frozen section of the urachal specimen. The template of lymphadenectomy corresponds to the template performed with radical cystectomy for invasive urothelial carcinoma. Dissection of the external iliac node packet is performed along the external iliac artery from the common iliac bifurcation to Cooper's ligament distally. The lateral border is the genitofemoral nerve and the medial border is the external iliac artery. Dissection of the internal iliac and obturator node packets is excised working along the internal iliac artery and obturator canal.

41.4.6 Umbilical Excision and Umbiliconeoplasty

Following completion of the partial cystectomy, the robot is undocked and the ports are removed under direct visualization. A skin incision is made around the umbilicus, and the entire umbilicus is encircled and dissected free with a cone of tissue around the umbilicus to assure negative margins. An Alice or Kocher clamp placed on the umbilicus can be helpful for providing traction during this step in the procedure. If the urachal specimen was not previously excised, the specimen is removed en bloc. If the urachal remnant was excised and deposited in an Endo

Catch™ bag, then only the umbilicus specimen is excised. After removal of all lymphadenectomy, urachal, and umbilical specimens, a surgical drain through one of the robotic port sites may be placed at surgeon discretion. The umbilical fascial defect is closed with synthetic monofilament suture.

Attention is then turned to umbiliconeoplasty. There are numerous techniques described for umbilical reconstruction, but the majority are delayed reconstructions on an intact abdomen [16, 17]. Four main techniques have been described for immediate umbilical reconstruction at the time of the umbilectomy.

The "iris" technique was described in 1993 to reconstruct the umbilicus after wide local excision of a melanoma [18]. Four full-thickness local flaps of skin and subcutaneous fat are marked out in the tissue surrounding the defect. Each flap is equal in size and shape with a 1.5 cm wide base and a length one-fourth the circumference of the defect. The tips of the four flaps are sutured together and then to the abdominal wall with nonabsorbable suture. Working from the center toward the periphery, the adjacent iris flaps are approximated and uneven edges are revised. This technique results in a pattern like the iris or diaphragm of a camera lens with scars radially oriented from the center.

The method was described by Bartsich et al. [19] in 2002 for umbiliconeoplasty after urachal cyst excision. Eight interrupted, absorbable sutures are utilized around the circumference of the defect to tack the dermis to the abdominal wall. These sutures are left untied while a nonabsorbable purse-string suture is placed around the circumference. The interrupted sutures are tied to produce the indentation, and then the purse string is tied to the desired umbilical size and to align the skin edge with the tacking sutures. The small remaining skin defect at the center of the purse string is packed and allowed to heal by secondary intention.

The "Celtic cross" technique was utilized in 2007 to repair the umbilical defects following urachal and umbilical resection (Fig. 41.3) [17]. The Celtic cross pattern is marked out on the intact umbilicus. The circular incision is made in the Celtic cross and then the radial cardinal direction extension incisions are made superiorly, inferiorly, and bilaterally. The circular incision is further dissected and the umbilicus specimen is excised from the pattern. Four local flaps remain around the circular defect. The corners of the flaps are then brought toward the center with anchoring 2–0 Vicryl. The tips of the superior flaps are first anchored to the rectus fascia, and then the inferior flaps are likewise anchored to the rectus fascia. The four incision lines are then approximated with 4–0 monocryl subcuticular sutures and Dermabond® (Ethicon, Somerville, NJ).

A one-stage umbiliconeoplasty procedure described in 2013 is particularly helpful when a midline subumbilical incision has already been made as part of the umbilical and urachal excision procedure [16]. Two triangular subumbilical flaps are created by skin incision and then dissection to the level of the rectus fascia with a base-to-side ratio of 1:2.5. The flap is first thinned appropriately to help recreate the umbilical indentation, and then the flaps are rotated 180° and sutured to each other. This creates one large triangular flap that is pointed superiorly. Three anchor sutures are placed on the fascia 3–4 cm below the umbilicus and sutured to the skin

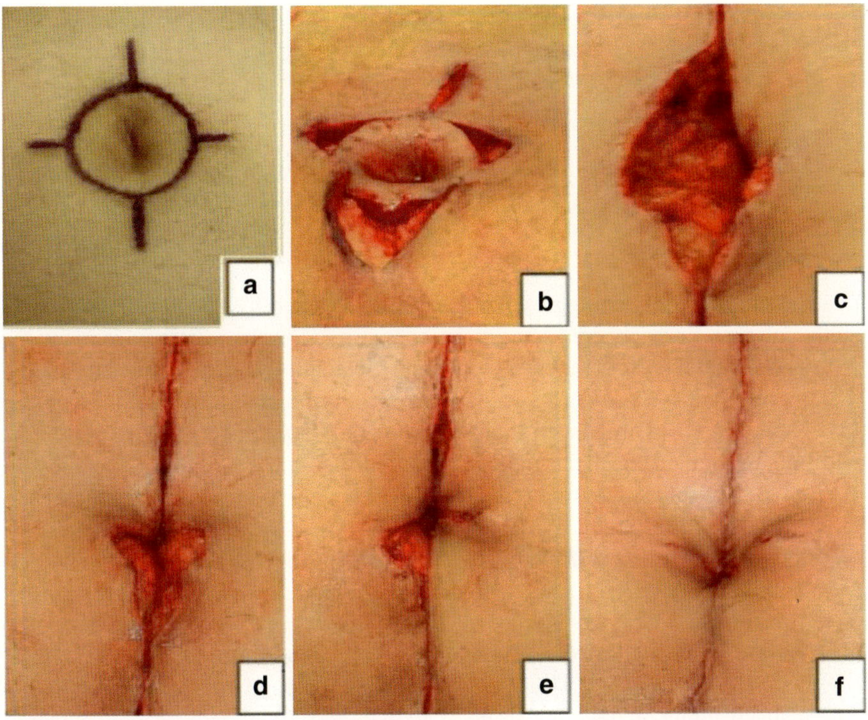

Fig. 41.3 The "Celtic cross" technique. (**a**) Umbilicus with external urachal sinus. (**b**) A circular incision is made followed by a midline incision superiorly and inferiorly and a lateral incision on each side. (**c, d**) After surgical ablation of the umbilicus, the superior flaps are then anchored down at the level of the linea alba and rectus sheath. (**e**) The inferior flaps are then similarly anchored on to the rectus muscle fascia. (**f**) After the superior and inferior flaps are anchored and sutured toward the center, the skin is then reapproximated with 4/0 monocryl subcuticular sutures and Dermabond® [17] (Used with permission)

flap. A free needle is then threaded with both ends of the suture and sewn to the abdominal wall to anchor the skin flap down to the abdominal wall. The flap is sutured with 5–0 Vicryl to the edge of the umbilical defect. The cranial side of the defect is closed in a V-Y fashion, which helps develop the umbilicus into an elliptical, vertically oriented shape. Remaining untied 3–0 nylon sutures are tied to reconstruct the umbilical fossa at the appropriate depth.

41.4.7 Postoperative Care

Patients are admitted for inpatient recovery and may be discharged, if appropriate, on postoperative day one. A surgical drain, if placed, can be assessed prior to discharge for quantity of fluid output and the presence of high fluid creatinine.

The drain is typically removed prior to discharge provided there are no concerns about urine leakage. Following discharge, the Foley catheter is left in place for 7–10 days, at which time a cystogram may be performed to confirm watertight closure prior to catheter removal [2, 10–12].

41.5 Discussion

Urachal carcinoma is an aggressive disease with generally poor prognosis, especially for tumors discovered late in the course [8]. Surgical therapy remains the only proven effective treatment modality [5]. Neoadjuvant and adjuvant chemotherapy reports have been largely anecdotal with typically unsuccessful responses [5]. Ashley et al. [8] reviewed their series of 66 consecutive patients presenting with metastatic and localized disease and identified a 5-year cancer-specific survival of 49 %. The authors found that on univariate analysis, positive surgical margins (*HR* 4.7), high tumor grade (*HR* 3.6), positive lymph nodes (*HR* 5.1), metastases at diagnosis (*HR* 3.3), advanced tumor stage (*HR* 4.8), failure to perform umbilectomy (*HR* 3.0), and primary radiation therapy (*HR* 2.9) were all associated with and increased risk of death at follow-up ($p<0.05$). However, on multivariate analysis, the only predictors of death were tumor grade (*HR* 3.7) and surgical margins (*HR* 3.8). Herr et al. [6] reported improved prognosis with a 5-year survival rate of 70 % in a group of 50 patients with no radiographic evidence of metastases at the time of diagnosis. Metastatic disease was found at surgery in 2 patients (4 %), and 8 patients (16 %) had positive nodal disease on final pathology. These authors similarly found that positive surgical margins, positive lymph nodes, and pathologic stage, but not tumor grade, were significant predictors of death during follow-up.

In many cases it may be difficult to establish the diagnosis of malignancy prior to surgical resection. In this setting, the presence of a solid mass and/or calcification on preoperative imaging is considered supportive of malignancy [4, 8]. In the study by Ashley et al. [8], 50 % of the tumors were solid, 25 % had a cystic component, and 33 % had macroscopic calcification. Utilization of frozen section is not discussed in the published series as these series primarily address preoperatively confirmed cases of malignancy. When malignancy is not definitively confirmed preoperatively, frozen section may prove highly useful to avoid the morbidity of lymphadenectomy as well as umbilectomy.

While there is some controversy regarding the role of umbilectomy, it is generally recommended in the case of malignant disease in order to confirm adequate surgical margins which are an important predictor of overall survival [6, 8]. However, if margins are otherwise negative, umbilectomy itself has not been established as a proven predictor of outcomes. On univariate analysis, failure to perform umbilectomy had a statistically significant hazard ratio of 3.0, but this was not a significant factor in multivariate analysis [8] Furthermore, the method of umbilectomy differs among the reported series. Many authors advocate en bloc resection [2], whereas others assert a segmental approach with urachectomy followed by umbilectomy [11, 12, 15]. Siefker-Radtke [5] commented that urachal tumors can occur anywhere along the urachus and may contain tumor-containing cystic fluid that could contaminate the peritoneal cavity if transecting the urachus at umbilical level. Additionally, the author anecdotally reports patients having rupture of cystic fluid into the abdominal cavity during transection of the urachus at the umbilical level.

The umbilicus has no functional importance; however, it is the key anatomic landmark of the anterior abdominal wall, and the lack of this structure can be a source of patient dissatisfaction [20]. Although many techniques are described, those described here address immediate reconstruction. Urologists are primarily responsible for the surgical care of urachal malignancy and therefore often assume the additional responsibility of umbilical reconstruction. While aesthetics may be demoted compared to cancer control, it is important to preoperatively plan the umbilical reconstruction in concert with the patient's expectations. Utilizing any of the four techniques will allow successful de novo creation of an aesthetic important feature while sparing patients a secondary surgery. It may be prudent to involve a plastic surgeon in the reconstructive process, especially for patients with high expectations and/or notable participation in activities that place high importance on appearance. Regardless of technique, the principles of reconstruction are to recreate a natural, aesthetically appealing structure using a procedure that is reproducible, reliable, and preferably single staged. The "ideal" umbilicus is described as small, oval, and non-protuberant. It has a ring orifice, tubular wall, and superior hooding with vertical or T-shaped orientation (Fig. 41.4) [20].

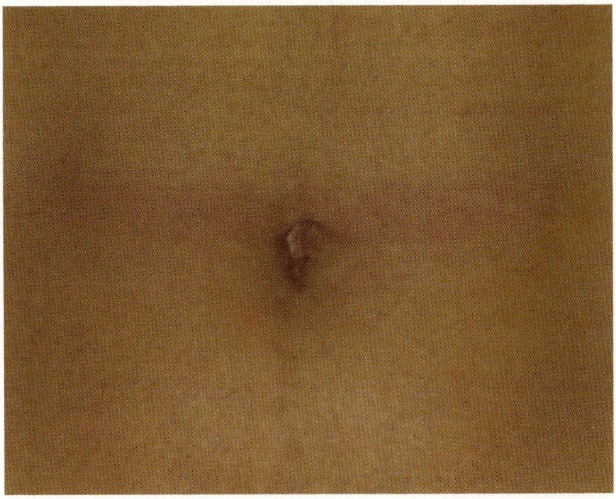

Fig. 41.4 The "ideal" umbilicus [20] (Used with permission)

41.6 Conclusions

Urachal carcinoma has an overall poor prognosis, but wide local excision through partial cystectomy, urachectomy, and umbilectomy is potentially curative for localized disease. Relatively recent evolution in minimally invasive techniques has allowed for robotic-assisted laparoscopic excision of this malignancy, leading to decreased postoperative morbidity compared to open surgery. Due to the rarity of the condition, comparative studies between operative techniques do not exist; however, the knowledge that negative surgical margins is consistently a predictor of survival provides the intuition that robotic techniques should be equivalent if proper margins are attained. Umbilectomy is recommended in all cases of malignancy, though it has not yet been definitively proven necessary by the available studies. Umbilical reconstruction is an essential step in restoring the appearance of the abdominal wall.

References

1. Frimberger DC, Kropp BP. Bladder anomalies in children. In: Wein AJ, Kavoussi LR, Novick AC, Partin AW, Peters CA, editors. Campbell-Walsh urology. 10th ed. Philadelphia: Saunders; 2012. p. 3379–88.
2. Williams CR, Chavda K. En bloc robot-assisted laparoscopic partial cystectomy, urachal resection, and pelvic lymphadenectomy for urachal adenocarcinoma. Rev Urol. 2015;17(1):46–9.
3. Molina JR, Quevedo JF, Furth AF, Richardson RL, Zincke H, Burch PA. Predictors of survival from urachal cancer: a Mayo Clinic study of 49 cases. Cancer. 2007;110:2434–40.
4. Paras Jr FA, Maclennan GT. Urachal adenocarcinoma. J Urol. 2008;180(2):720.
5. Siefker-Radtke A. Urachal carcinoma: surgical and chemotherapeutic options. Expert Rev Anticancer Ther. 2006;6(12):1715–21.
6. Herr HW, Bochner BH, Sharp D, Dalbagni G, Reuter VE. Urachal carcinoma: contemporary surgical outcomes. J Urol. 2007;178(1):74–8.
7. Gopalan A, Sharp DS, Fine SW, Tickoo SK, Herr HW, Reuter VE, Olgac S. Urachal carcinoma: a clinicopathologic analysis of 24 cases with outcome correlation. Am J Surg Pathol. 2009;33(5):659–68.
8. Ashley RA, Inman BA, Sebo TJ, Leibovich BC, Blute ML, Kwon ED, Zincke H. Urachal carcinoma: clinicopathologic features and long-term outcomes of an aggressive malignancy. Cancer. 2006;107(4):712–20.
9. Bockholt NA, Nepple KG, Dahmoush L, Tracy CR. Robotic-assisted laparoscopic excision of urachal sinus found to be mucinous carcinoma: a case for umbilectomy. BJU Int. 2011. http://www.bjuinternational.com/case-studies/robotic-assistedlaparoscopic- excision-of-urachal-sinus-found-to-be-mucinous-carcinomaa-case-for-umbilectomy/
10. Richstone L, Douglas SS. Robotic and laparoscopic bladder surgery. In: Wein AJ, Kavoussi LR, Novick AC, Partin AW, Peters CA, editors. Campbell-Walsh urology. 10th ed. Philadelphia: Saunders; 2012. p. 2386–410.
11. Wadhwa P, Kolla SB, Hemal AK. Laparoscopic en bloc partial cystectomy with bilateral pelvic lymphadenectomy for urachal adenocarcinoma. Urology. 2006;67(4):837–43.
12. Aoun F, Peltier A, van Velthoven R. Bladder sparing robot-assisted laparoscopic en bloc resection of urachus and umbilicus for urachal adenocarcinoma. J Robot Surg. 2015;9(2):167–70.

13. Milhoua PM, Knoll A, Bleustein CB, Ghavamian R. Laparoscopic partial cystectomy for treatment of adenocarcinoma of the urachus. Urology. 2006;67(2):423.e15–17.
14. Wang B, Li X, Ming S, Ma X, Li HZ, Ai Q, Zhang X. Combined extraperitoneal and transperitoneal laparoscopic extended partial cystectomy for the treatment of urachal carcinoma. J Endourol. 2016;30(3):280–285.
15. Hong SH, Kim JC, Hwang TK. Laparoscopic partial cystectomy with en bloc resection of the urachus for urachal adenocarcinoma. Int J Urol. 2007;14(10):963–5.
16. Omori M, Hashikawa K, Sakakibara S, Terashi H, Tahara S, Shibaoka Y, Kimura K, Sano K. One-stage umbilicus reconstruction after resection of urachal cyst. Ann Plast Surg. 2013;71(1):93–5.
17. De La Cruz EA, Jaber RK, Tabuenca AD, Joe VC. The "Celtic cross" technique for immediate umbilical reconstruction post-laparotomy and surgical ablation of the umbilicus. J Plast Reconstr Aesthet Surg. 2009;62(2):258–61.
18. Miller MJ, Balch CM. "Iris" technique for immediate umbilical reconstruction. Plast Reconstr Surg. 1993;92(4):754–6.
19. Bartsich SA, Schwartz MH. Purse-string method for immediate umbilical reconstruction. Plast Reconstr Surg. 2003;112(6):1652–5.
20. Southwell-Keely JP, Berry MG. Umbilical reconstruction: a review of techniques. J Plast Reconstr Aesthet Surg. 2011;64(6):803–8.

Part VII
Benign Tumors of the Umbilicus

Chapter 42
Umbilical Endometriosis

Carla I.J.M. Theunissen and Frank F.A. IJpma

42.1 Introduction

42.1.1 Case

First of all, we will present a case of a painful, livid colored nodule in the umbilicus, which turned out to be umbilical endometriosis. A 47-year-old healthy female presented with a painful and livid colored nodule in the umbilicus, which gradually evolved over the past 6 months. She had no symptoms of dysmenorrhea or cyclical umbilical pain. At physical examination, she had a soft, painful swelling with a diameter of 2 cm in the umbilicus, which was irreducible by gentle digital pressure (Fig. 42.1). Ultrasonography revealed a hypodense nodule of 1.8 cm at the umbilicus (Fig. 42.2). However, a definitive diagnosis could not be established so far. Under the provisional clinical diagnosis, 'irreducible umbilical hernia with probably strangulated fatty tissue in the hernia sac', surgical exploration of the umbilicus was performed. Under general anesthesia, a sub-umbilical incision was made. To our surprise, a subcutaneous, lobulated mass was exposed, which was fixated on the bottom of the umbilicus (Fig. 42.3). The abdominal wall itself was unaffected. The nodule was excised, and histopathological examination revealed connective tissue fragments with irregular tubular formations surrounded by stromal cells. Our patient

C.I.J.M. Theunissen, M.D. (✉)
Department of Plastic Surgery, Isala,
Dokter van Heesweg 2, 8025 AB Zwolle, The Netherlands
e-mail: c.i.j.m.theunissen@isala.nl

F.F.A. IJpma, M.D.
Department of Surgery, University Medical Center Groningen, Postbox 30.001,
9700 RB, Groningen, The Netherlands
e-mail: frankijpma@gmail.com

M.A. Shiffman (ed.), *Adult Umbilical Reconstruction*,
DOI 10.1007/978-3-319-43887-0_42

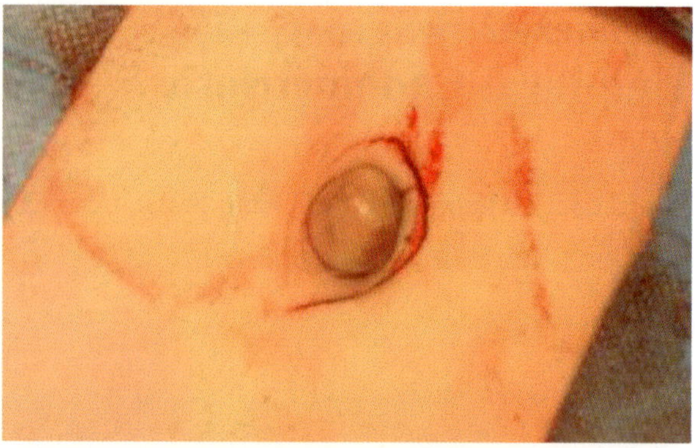

Fig. 42.1 Clinical presentation of a livid, soft, painful swelling in the umbilicus

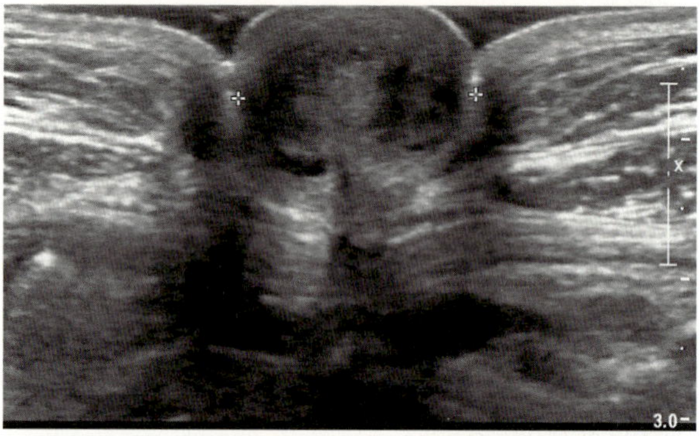

Fig. 42.2 Ultrasonography of the umbilicus demonstrating a hypodense nodule of 1.8 cm at the umbilicus

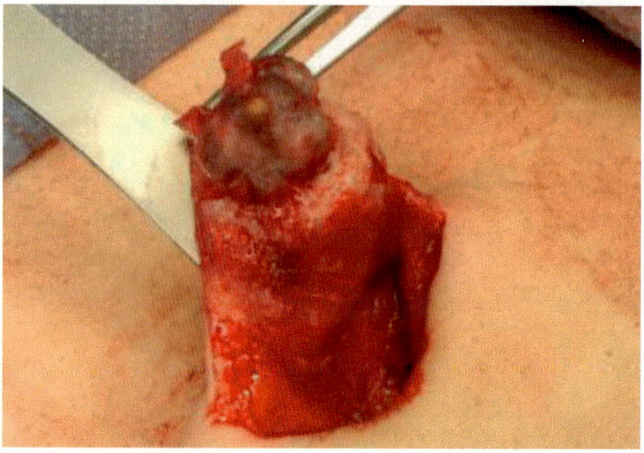

Fig. 42.3 Intraoperative image of a dark discolored, lobulated swelling at the bottom of the umbilicus

was treated by excision of the swelling that turned out to be primary umbilical endometriosis (PUE). Two months after the surgery, she visited the outpatient clinic and reported complete recovery of the painful sensation and swelling in the umbilicus. This case highlights the importance of including PUE in the differential diagnosis of women with a painful umbilical nodule and demonstrates that the diagnosis is often not recognized based on its clinical and radiological appearance [1].

42.1.2 History

Intra-abdominal endometriosis is a common disease, which affects 6–10% of all women in the reproductive age. This disease is defined by the presence of endometrial tissue outside the uterus. Most often the pelvic peritoneum is affected [2, 3]. Common symptoms of endometriosis are dysmenorrhea, noncyclic pelvic pain, infertility, and menorrhagia [2]. The umbilicus is an uncommon site of endometriosis and is affected in 0.5–4% of all women with endometriosis. This condition, also known as Villar's nodule, could have a spontaneous or "primary" nature but can also occur iatrogenic or "secondary" [3]. In English literature, approximately 40 cases of PUE have been described, and in 20–50% of the cases, umbilical endometriosis was misdiagnosed [4]. The pathogenesis of PUE is not fully clarified. Possible explanations for PUE could be the migration of endometrial cells to the umbilicus through the lymphatic system or embryonic remnants in the umbilical fold, such as the urachus and the umbilical vessels. This is proposed as the dissemination theory. Another explanation for PUE could be the retrograde menstruation or implantation theory. Hereby, endometrial tissue refluxes through the fallopian tubes during the menstruation period and from there through the abdominal cavity to organs close by [5–7]. Two more theories have been proposed for the manifestation of endometriosis. The Müllerianosis or embryonic rest theory suggests that Mullerian origin cells produce endometrial foci after a specific stimulus, when these cells are incorporated within other tissue [8]. Finally, the coelomic metaplasia or induction theory suggests that metaplastic transformation of peritoneal mesothelium may result in endometriosis [9]. Secondary umbilical endometriosis (SUE) is often scar related and is caused by iatrogenic dissemination of endometrial cells, for instance, after laparoscopy or laparotomy [2, 3, 6].

42.2 Clinical Manifestation

In most cases, the clinical manifestation of umbilical endometriosis consists of an umbilical nodule with maximal depth of penetration up to the fascial level, such as the abovementioned case [3]. This nodule can be associated with cyclical or continuous umbilical pain, and there can be a bleeding tendency from the nodule in the umbilicus. The color of the nodule can be brown, red, blue, dark, or flesh-colored [5]. Differential diagnoses of umbilical endometriosis are shown in Table 42.1 [5–7].

42.3 Radiological Diagnosis

Literature is scarce about sensitivity and specificity of ultrasonography, CT scan, and MRI in diagnosing umbilical endometriosis. No pathognomonic signs of umbilical endometriosis have been established for one of these imaging techniques. Some

Table 42.1 Differential diagnosis of an umbilical nodule

Benign	Malignant
Cutaneous endometriosis/endosalpingiosis[a]	Sister Mary Joseph node[b]
Hemangioma/vascular malformation	Melanoma
Umbilical hernia/cicatrical hernia	Sarcoma
Sebaceous cyst	Adenocarcinoma
Granuloma Lipoma Abscess Keloid Omphalomesenteric or urachus anomaly and/or infection Desmoid tumor	Lymphoma

[a]Endosalpingiosis: the presence of fallopian tube-like epithelium outside of the fallopian tube
[b]Sister Mary Joseph node: palpable nodule bulging into the umbilicus as a result of metastasis of a malignant tumor in the pelvis or abdomen

information about the size of the nodule and its adherence to surrounding tissues can be observed with ultrasound, CT scan, and MRI [7, 10]. Furthermore, CT scan and MRI are also of little value in diagnosing intra-abdominal endometriosis [11, 12]. Umbilical endometriosis can be diagnosed by histological examination after surgical excision and in many cases the diagnosis will only be established postoperatively with histological examination. With hematoxylin and eosin staining, the presence of endometrial glands and stromal cells in the dermis will eventually lead to the diagnosis [2].

42.4 Treatment

In patients with symptomatic umbilical nodule due to umbilical endometriosis, treatment should be considered. When patients also have clinical symptoms of intra-abdominal endometriosis, referral to a gynecologist is also mandatory besides treatment of umbilical endometriosis. The treatment of endometriosis with hormones can diminish clinical symptoms of umbilical endometriosis temporarily [13]. However, after discontinuation of hormonal therapy, it is likely that symptoms will reoccur. The most frequently used hormones to treat endometriosis are agonist of gonadotropin-releasing hormone (GnRH) and oral contraceptives [2, 5]. In patients with a symptomatic umbilical nodule due to umbilical endometriosis, surgical exploration and excision of the nodule should be considered. Recurrence of umbilical endometriosis after carefully surgical excision is rare [5]. Different methods of surgery are known for umbilical endometriosis under general and local anesthesia. Skin-sparing excision with primary or local flap closure is one of the possibilities [1, 14]. When complete resection of the nodule, fascia, peritoneum, and umbilicus is performed, closure of underlying fascie should be performed with or without closure of the peritoneum [15, 16]. Repair of the fascia requiring a mesh is feasible when a large umbilical hernia or fascia defect is detected [17]. Another treatment possibility is the combination of hormonal therapy and surgery to decrease the size of the nodule before excision is performed [5].

After resection of umbilical endometriosis, reconstruction of the umbilicus is important for the aesthetic appearance of the abdomen. A small, superiorly hooded, and vertically oriented umbilicus with a slight circular depression should be the ideal shape of the umbilicus [18, 19]. In elder patients, a larger, rounder, and more horizontal orientation of the umbilicus is seen [20]. Fixation of the caudal part of the umbilicus to the anterior rectus fascia is necessary when the umbilicus can be preserved to create the circular depression of the umbilicus. In case of omphalectomy a new umbilicus should be created. Different reconstructive options are the use of small flaps of variable sizes, such as a rhombic or triangular flap, that have to be attached to the abdominal fascia to create the basis of the new umbilicus for a conical skin structure [21–23].

42.5 Conclusions

By increasing the awareness of umbilical endometriosis as a potential diagnosis in women with a painful, sometimes discolored, umbilical swelling, we hope this condition will be recognized and treated optimally.

References

1. Theunissen CI, IJpma FF. Primary umbilical endometriosis: a cause of a painful umbilical nodule. J Surg Case Rep. 2015;2015(3):rjv025.
2. Giudice LC, Kao LC. Endometriosis. Lancet. 2004;364:1789–99.
3. Victory R, Diamond MP, Johns DA. Villar's nodule: a case report and systematic literature review of endometriosis externa of the umbilicus. J Minim Invasive Gynecol. 2007;14:23–32.
4. Bektas H, Bilsel Y, Sari YS, Ersöz F, Koç O, Deniz M, Boran B, Huq GE. Abdominal wall endometrioma; a 10-year experience and brief review of the literature. J Surg Res. 2010;164(1):e77–81.
5. Efremidou EI, Kouklakis G, Mitrakas A, Liratzopoulos N, Polychronidis A. Primary umbilical endometrioma: a rare case of spontaneous abdominal wall endometriosis. Int J Gen Med. 2012;5:999–1002.
6. Fancellu A, Pinna A, Manca A, Capobianco G, Porcu A. Primary umbilical endometriosis. Case report and discussion on management options. Int J Surg Case Rep. 2013;4:1145–8.
7. Hensen JH, Van Breda Vriesman AC, Puylaert JB. Abdominal wall endometriosis: clinical presentation and imaging features with emphasis on sonography. AJR Am J Roentgenol. 2006;186:616–20.
8. Batt RE, Yeh J. Mullerianosis: four developmental (embryonic) mullerian diseases. Reprod Sci. 2013;20:1030–7.
9. Matsuura K, Ohtake H, Katabuchi H, Okamura H. Coelomic metaplasia theory of endometriosis: evidence from in vivo studies and an in vitro experimental model. Gynecol Obstet Invest. 1999;47 Suppl 1:18–20.

10. Savelli L, Manuzzi L, Di Donato N, Salfi N, Trivella G, Ceccaroni M, Seracchioli R. Endometriosis of the abdominal wall: ultrasonographic and Doppler characteristics. Ultrasound Obstet Gynecol. 2012;39:336–40.
11. Rousset P, Rousset-Jablonski C, Alifano M, Mansuet-Lupo A, Buy JN, Revel MP. Thoracic endometriosis syndrome: CT and MRI features. Clin Radiol. 2014;69:323–30.
12. Stratton P, Winkel C, Premkumar A, Chow C, Wilson J, Hearns-Stokes R, Heo S, Merino M, Nieman LK. Diagnostic accuracy of laparoscopy, magnetic resonance imaging, and histopathologic examination for the detection of endometriosis. Fertil Steril. 2003;79:1078–85.
13. Saito A, Koga K, Osuga Y, Harada M, Takemura Y, Yoshimura K, Yano T, Kozuma S. Individualized management of umbilical endometriosis: a report of seven cases. J Obstet Gynaecol Res. 2014;40:40–5.
14. Arkoulis N, Chew BK. An unusual case of asymptomatic spontaneous umbilical endometriosis treated with skin-sparing excision. J Surg Case Rep. 2015;2015(3):rjv017.
15. Calagna G, Perino A, Chianetta D, Vinti D, Triolo MM, Rimi C, Cucinella G, Agrusa A. Primary umbilical endometrioma: Analyzing the pathogenesis of endometriosis from an unusual localization. Taiwan J Obstet Gynecol. 2015;54:306–12.
16. Pramanik SR, Mondal S, Paul S, Joycerani D. Primary umbilical endometriosis: A rarity. J Hum Reprod Sci. 2014;7:269–71.
17. Stojanovic M, Radojkovic M, Jeremic L, Zlatic A, Stanojevic G, Janjic D, Mihajlovic S, Dimov I, Kostov M, Zdravkovic M, Stojanovic M. Umbilical endometriosis associated with large umbilical hernia. Case report. Chirurgia (Bucur). 2014;109:267–70.
18. Malic CC, Spyrou GE, Hough M, Fourie L. Patient satisfaction with two different methods of umbilicoplasty. Plast Reconstr Surg. 2007;119:357–61.
19. Visconti G, Salgarello M. The divine proportion "Ace of Spades" umbilicoplasty: A new method of navel positioning and plasty in abdominoplasty. Ann Plast Surg. 2016;76:265–9.
20. Bruekers SE, van der Lei B, Tan TL, Luijendijk RW, Stevens HP. "Scarless" umbilicoplasty: a new umbilicoplasty technique and a review of the English language literature. Ann Plast Surg. 2009;63:15–20.
21. Iida N, Ohsumi N. Reconstruction of umbilical hypogenesis accompanied by a longitudinal scar. Plast Reconstr Surg. 2003;111:322–5.
22. Itoh Y, Arai K. Umbilical reconstruction using a cone-shaped flap. Ann Plast Surg. 1992;28:335–8.
23. Pfulg M, Van de Sijpe K, Blondeel P. A simple new technique for neo-umbilicoplasty. Br J Plast Surg. 2005;58:688–91.

Part VIII
Complications

Chapter 43
Umbilicoplasty Complications

Melvin A. Shiffman

43.1 Introduction

Knowing and understanding the possible complications of umbilicoplasty is extremely important for surgeons performing surgery on the umbilicus. The knowledge will allow the opportunity for the surgeon to avoid the complications and be prepared for treatment of complications that may occur. The possible complications should be discussed with the patient prior to attempting umbilical reconstruction.

43.2 Possible Complications

43.2.1 Adverse Reaction to Anesthesia

Depending on the type of anesthesia utilized, the medications used may have acute allergic reactions. Using general anesthesia when performing abdominal wall surgery with concomitant umbilical reconstruction leaves open all the other possible complications from a general anesthetic that include thromboembolism, heart problems, and pulmonary problems.

When using local anesthesia to perform umbilical reconstruction, there is still the possibility of allergic reaction to the preservative, methylparaben.

M.A. Shiffman, M.D., J.D.
Private Practice, 17501 Chatham Drive, Tustin, CA 92780-2302, USA
e-mail: shiffmanmdjd@gmail.com

M.A. Shiffman (ed.), *Adult Umbilical Reconstruction*,
DOI 10.1007/978-3-319-43887-0_43

43.2.2 Asymmetry

The possibility of asymmetry would include local distortion of the umbilicus such as depression of one side and error in location of the midline for the umbilicus. This may require fat transfer or surgical revision for depression or surgical revision of the location of the umbilicus.

43.2.3 Bleeding

Bruising after umbilical surgery is usually quite light and short-lived. Bleeding usually occurs in small amounts and can be controlled with mild pressure. A small vessel may bleed postoperatively and cause a hematoma. This would require evacuation of the hematoma and control of the vessel with electrocoagulation.

43.2.4 Bulging

Bulging of the flap [1] may occur, but this is rare.

43.2.5 Dehiscence

The wound may break open if the closure is too tight, infection has occurred, or from the patient exerting himself/herself too much, causing tension on the wound. This can be treated by keeping the wound clean and dressed until secondary healing has occurred. Closure of the wound may be attempted but will pull apart at times if the cause was too tight a closure.

43.2.6 Discomfort

There is usually a little discomfort in the umbilical area where the suturing has taken place. This will be relieved after removal of the sutures. Discomfort may be caused by some necessary added procedures around the umbilicus or when flaps are raised to form the neoumbilicus. This will usually subside within a couple of weeks.

43.2.7 Epidermolysis

Epidermolysis is loosening of the epidermis, with extensive blistering of the skin that occurs after injury. Pedreira et al. [1] used a triangular umbilicoplasty with skin flap and noted that there were five cases (2.58 %) of epidermolysis in the umbilical stump. There was complete resolution using moist dressings.

43.2.8 Erythema

Redness or erythema [2] of the flap may occur, but this is transient in nature.

43.2.9 Flattening or Disappearance of Umbilical Depression

Failure to secure the umbilical stalk to the underlying fascia may result in flattening or disappearance of the umbilical depression.

43.2.10 Granulation Tissue

The occurrence of granulations [2] is usually from an open part of the wound. This can occur when sutures pull apart; necrosis or deep sutures do not close the defect at the depths of the neoumbilicus. Granulations will respond well to silver nitrate applicators or swabs. The granulations shrink, and ultimately healing takes place.

43.2.11 Incorrect Positioning

This is usually the failure to pay attention to the new position of the umbilicus and failure to shorten the umbilical stalk. There are many methods to determine the correct position of the umbilicus on the anterior abdominal wall. If the patient has a long umbilical stalk and is obese, the umbilicus can fall to one side or the other. Shortening the umbilical stalk and fastening it to the underlying fascia will prevent displacement.

43.2.12 Infection

Infection occurs in 1–3 % of clean surgeries. Antibiotics may be used postoperatively, but even then infection can occur. When the umbilical reconstruction is performed without other procedures, probably antibiotics can be avoided. Too much use of antibiotics in situations where they may not be needed has resulted in resistant organisms.

Infection in the wound may result in a breakdown of the wound and subsequent granulations. If an abscess occurs, this must be drained and irrigated with sterile saline. Oral antibiotics may be started if none were given postoperatively. If postoperative antibiotics had been used, it is important to try to get a culture and sensitivity and then change the antibiotic.

43.2.13 Loss of Tissue

Tissue may be lost if necrosis occurs. Reconstruction can be performed after complete healing.

43.2.14 Necrosis

Postoperative necrosis can occur from lack of adequate vascularity. If flaps are used for neoumbilicus, the source of the blood supply for the flaps should be identified first and preserved at surgery. The normal umbilicus has two sources of arterial supply, one deep (epigastric vessels) and one superficial (subdermal vessels).

Smoking will cause death of flaps [3, 4] and should be avoided at least 2 weeks before and 2 weeks after surgery. Even one cigarette can cause up to 90 min of lack of blood to a flap [5].

Hematoma can compress the vessels and should be promptly drained. If the flap is pulled too tightly, a portion of the flap may become necrotic.

Treatment of necrosis consists of waiting until the necrotic area sloughs and heals secondarily. If infection is associated with necrosis, then the dead tissues should be debrided, antibiotics started, and the wound cleansed daily until healing occurs. Revision of the umbilicus should be performed after 6 months to allow time for the scar to mature and soften.

43.2.15 Numbness

The umbilicus is supplied by the 10th intercostal nerve superficially, and the superior/anterior epigastric artery supplies the deep part. Local flaps may contain branches of the superficial nerves and supply the neoumbilicus. Numbness of the stalk of the umbilicus is not usually noted.

Division of superficial nerves will result in numbness. This usually improves over a period of 6 months. However, the numbness may be permanent, but over time the patient will stop noticing the numbness.

43.2.16 Pain

Pain in the umbilicus is usually mild and can be easily controlled with pain medications. Most pain occurs from concomitant procedures such as abdominoplasty. One would expect that the pain will subside over time if treated appropriately with medication.

43.2.17 *Pigmentary Changes*

Hyperpigmentation or hypopigmentation can occur but rarely requires treatment.

There are a variety of medications that can be applied to treat hyperpigmentation. Products that contain Kojic acid, ascorbic acid, hydroquinone, or alpha hydroxy acids (AHA) such as glycolic acid are useful. However, exposure to sunlight usually causes the hyperpigmentation to recur.

43.2.18 *Prolonged Healing*

Prolonged healing usually is a result of external substances like smoking or from abnormalities such as diabetes, nutritional state such as low albumin, hypovitaminosis A or C, zinc deficiency, etc.

Smoking must be stopped completely 4 weeks before surgery and 2 weeks after surgery. Metabolic abnormalities should be diagnosed and treated.

43.2.19 *Scar*

Scars are usually hidden within the belly button, but some techniques will have visible scar [6, 7]. Hypertrophic and keloid scars are the result of aberrations of physiologic wound healing. Keloids occur in 15 % of Asians, Hispanics, and Blacks.

Treatment methods include laser, chemical peel, or injections of steroid with 5 FU or bleomycin. Keloids will recur 80 % of the time. Hypertrophic scars occasionally resolve without treatment.

43.2.20 *Seroma*

Seroma is rare but may occur in instances when other procedures are performed in the vicinity. This includes closure of the underlying fascia, resection or revision of a large scar, and local flaps used for reconstruction.

43.2.21 *Swelling*

Swelling will usually resolve within a few weeks. Prolonged swelling may occur. This may require further evaluation, like ultrasound, for diagnosing the cause such as seroma or hematoma.

43.2.22 Umbilical Depression

There may be flattening [6] or disappearance of the umbilicus, but this is usually caused by failure to attach the deepest portion (base) of the umbilical stalk to the underlying fascia or loss of the sutures holding the base to the fascia. This will require surgical correction.

43.3 Unsatisfactory Aesthetic Results

The patient must be informed preoperatively about the limitations of aesthetic appearance in the particular procedure to be performed.

Certainly surgery on an abnormal or absent umbilicus may result in less than normal appearance at the conclusion of surgery. There may be limitations of aesthetics because of scarring from flap reconstruction or removal of a preoperative scar in the center of the abdomen.

Patients, surgeons, and patient families have different ideas about what is the ideal appearance of the umbilicus. An irregular or a "lop-sided" appearance of the belly button may require further surgery to correct. If the patient is totally dissatisfied, further surgery for correction may be necessary.

43.3.1 Unsatisfactory Size

The size of the umbilical opening may be too small (stenosis) or too big. This can be corrected surgically.

43.4 Discussion

Pereira et al. [1] evaluated complications in 194 patients have triangular flap umbilicoplasty.

The five cases of epidermolysis also had hyperchromia. 1.55 % of cases had a slight umbilical narrowing by scar retraction. There was good resolution after using silicone molds for 2 months. The most frequent stigmas associated with umbilicoplasty were not observed in this study, such as necrosis, scar narrowing requiring surgical intervention, enlargement of the umbilical scar circumference, lack of anatomical contours, irregular positioning, or even a streaky appearance caused by marks from external sutures.

References

1. Pereira JFV, Schutz LG, Kostic V, D'Avila CLP, Mateus FN. Umbilicoplastia triangular com retalhodérmico. Rev Bras Cir Plást. 2011;26(3):496–501.
2. Takasu H, Watanabe Y. Umbilicoplasty with 3 triangular skin flaps and excised diamond-shaped skin flap. J Pediatr Surg. 2010;45(10):2041–4.
3. Smoking and its effects on the skin. http://www.dermnetnz.org/reactions/smoking.html. Accessed 1 Jan 2016.
4. Smoking effects on the skin. http://quitday.org/support/skin-health. Accessed 1 Jan 2016.
5. The effect of smoking on the skin. Quit smoking support.com. http://quitsmokingsupport.com/skin.htm. Accessed 1 Jan 2016.
6. Sagna A, Ly A, Fall I. The umbilical cutaneous "Y-to-V" plastic surgery in the care of pedunculated umbilical hernia in the infant and the child. J Pediatr Surg Case Rep. 2014;2(10):480–2.
7. Lee YT, Kwon C, Rhee SC, Cho SH, Eo SR. Four flaps technique for neoumbilicoplasty. Arch Plast Surg. 2015;42(3):351–5.

Chapter 44
Improving Aesthetic Quality of Umbilical Scar in Vertical Abdominal Dermolipectomies: The Opposing Triangular Flaps Technique

André Luís Rosenhaim Monte

44.1 Introduction

The umbilical scar still represents a challenge in abdominoplasties and when unaesthetic by enlargement or stenosis is a factor of patients' dissatisfaction. In patients with vertical umbilical dermolipectomy, this situation is more frequent, since omphaloplasty in these cases is performed in circumferential way, where stenotic or large scars are common. In these surgeries, currently indicated mainly for patients with large weight loss, whose benefit of attained body contouring supplant the aesthetic limitation of vertical scar, we still observe many levels of dissatisfaction toward the unaesthetic umbilical scar.

Thinking about these cases and researching about countless techniques of omphaloplasties and neo-omphaloplasties [1–7], considering the principles of scar healing which corroborate for umbilical scar alteration, we initiated with a mixed technique where the umbilical stump was preserved for the treatment of a patient with stenotic umbilical scar [8]. The result obtained showed satisfactory aesthetic quality and avoided the scar stenosis relapse in a way we could extend its indication for primary use in vertical dermolipectomy.

A.L.R. Monte, M.D.
Private Practice, Porto Alegre, RS, Brazil
e-mail: alrmonte@hotmail.com

M.A. Shiffman (ed.), *Adult Umbilical Reconstruction*,
DOI 10.1007/978-3-319-43887-0_44

44.2 Surgical Technique

Vertical abdominal dermolipectomy marking is something peculiar to each case, depending on the skin flabbiness above and below the umbilicus, ranging from a vertical ellipse only, with small suprapubic compensation, to the classic dermolipectomy in anchor, so that we will not detail this subject.

After marking the vertical ellipse, two lateral and internal rectangular flaps are preserved to this marking, to the approximate height of umbilical stump. This adaption to the original technique we described allows us better posterior precision on umbilical location, as commonly may occur alteration on the position of triangle flaps after the traction of abdominal flaps (Figs. 44.1 and 44.2).

We performed the resection in one block as recommended by Pontes [9], with the preservation of umbilical stump and demarcated rectangular flaps (Fig. 44.3). Then it is made the plication of rectus abdominis muscles, definition of height for umbilical stump pedicle, and correction of hernias, as necessary. Regarding the height of umbilical stump, we usually position it on iliac crest level or slightly above and up to 1 cm of pedicle height. Certain difficulty of umbilical stumps accommodation is observed with excessively long pedicles.

We start the vertical operative wound suture on the surfaces from their extremities, leaving only the umbilical stump area, where this is practically biparted on its laterals, preserving a central segment of approximately 0.5 cm (Figs. 44.4 and 44.5). We marked on the rectangular flaps, precisely on the umbilical stump height, two opposing triangular flaps from 1.5 to 2 cm of base and length, the measure of which varies according to the panniculus adipose height in a way to avoid tension. We resect the skin excess and thus obtain four opposing and similar triangular flaps. We

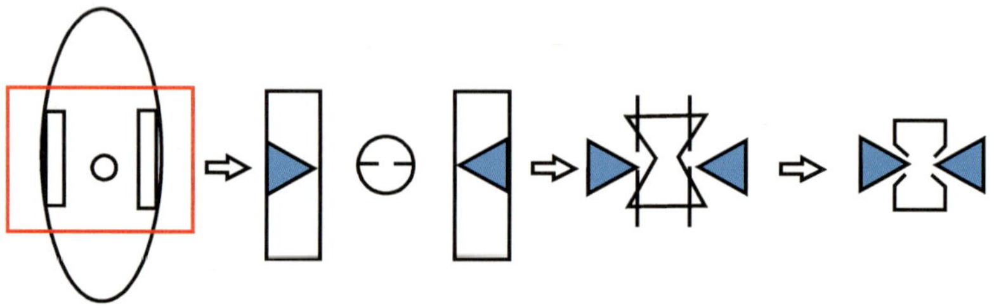

After marking the vertical ellipse, two lateral and internal rectangular flaps are preserve to this marking, to the approximate height of umbilical stump. Close view in red mark.

Perform in-block ressection, preserving the lateral flaps. After the muscle plication and the stump fixation, define the triangualr flaps with 1,5 cm of base and length and them bipart the umbilicus preserving 0,5 to 1,0 cm in the centre.

Resect the skin excess and thus obtain four opposite and similar triangular flaps. Resect the lateral excess of umbilical stump, which facilitates post suture and accommodation.

The apex of the side flaps is anchored with a "U" stitch and interpolates to the umbilical stump flaps. Suture the bottoms of the umbilical flaps and lateral flaps together and the proximal and distal points of the operation wound become closer.

Fig. 44.1 Opposite triangular flaps omphaloplasty technique

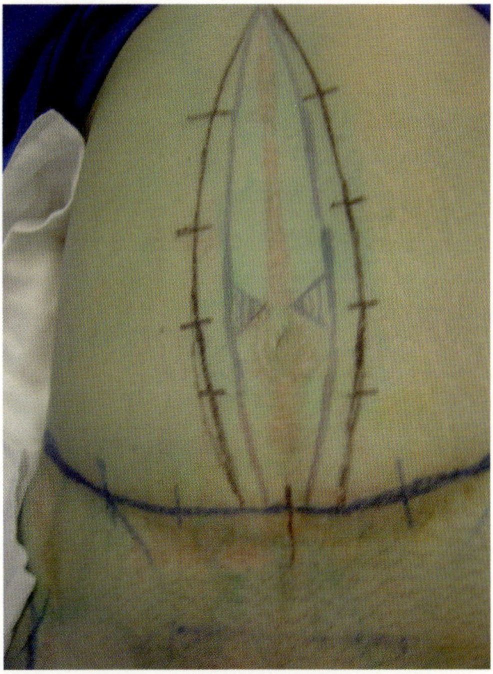

Fig. 44.2 Surgery markings

resect the lateral excess of umbilical stump, which facilitates post suture and accommodation (Fig. 44.6). The apex of lateral flaps is sutured and interpolated to umbilical stump flaps, enabling to be fixed to the aponeurosis.

We perform the routine of subdermal internal sutures with colorless mononylon 4.0 between the flaps and external U sutures (Fig. 44.7). We fixed the sutures to the flaps' base among themselves and conclude the wound edges operative suture approaching the distal and proximal vertices (Figs. 44.8, 44.9, and 44.10). On this stage, it evidences skin redundancy on umbilical stumps' flaps that can be resected again on their laterals or redistributed with compensation sutures, requiring more skills and patience from the surgeon. The bandage/curative is always made with dry gauze turunda (tent), changed daily.

44.3 Discussion

There are highly frequent unsightly and hypertrophic scars in vertical dermolipectomies or abdominoplasties with anchor scar, mainly related to circumferential omphaloplasty usually performed, because of the scar contraction phenomena. The

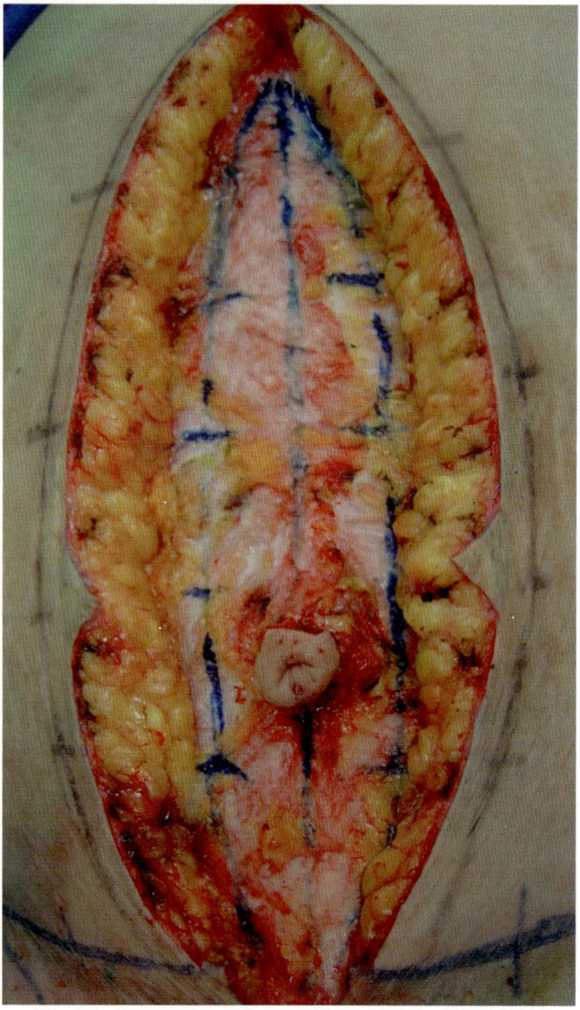

Fig. 44.3 One block resection of the abdominal vertical dermolipectomy. Lateral triangular flaps preserved. Muscle plication markings

reverse situation occurs when we resect too much partial skin ellipses from the vertical operative wound's edges, periumbilical, causing large umbilicus by contrary tensions on itself, usually existent in this type of surgery.

Based on these theories and on the article published by Franco et al. [5], we idealize for treatment of an umbilical stenosis in late postoperative vertical dermolipectomy [8], an additional elliptical resection, where we preserved two lateral triangular flaps to the existing umbilical scar, aiming to enlarge, since, for us, it had insufficient skin. As we needed to break the stenotic ring, it seemed obvious to us bilateral horizontal incisions on this stump, so we could interpolate the triangular flaps (Figs. 44.11, 44.12, and 44.13). We only found difficulties during the final suture,

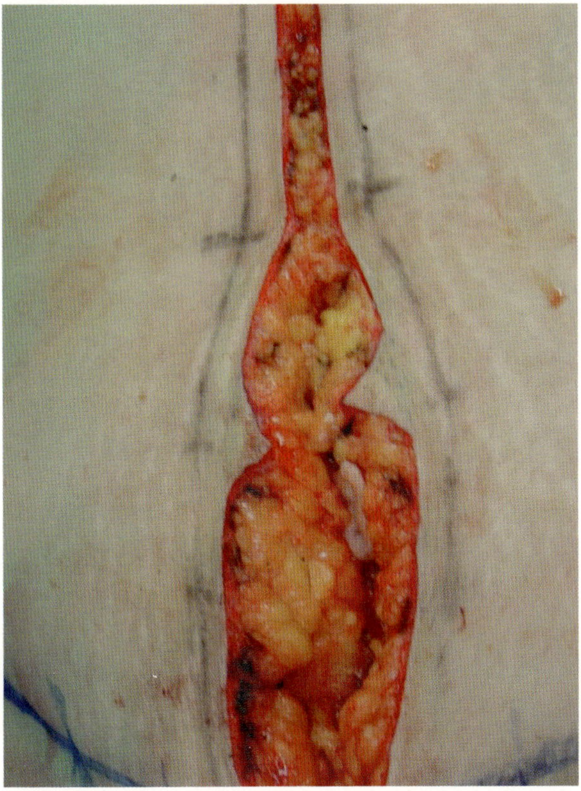

Fig. 44.4 After muscle plication, the operative wound is sutured from their extremities, leaving only the umbilical stump area

where we needed to resect the excess skin of superior and inferior umbilical stump, in a way to facilitate the skin compensation for vertical supra and infraumbilical incision.

The interpolation of these flaps, besides avoiding the umbilical stenosis relapse, also avoided the tension action of enlargement and propitiated a more natural and aesthetic appearance to the belly button due to the absence of lateral scars (Fig. 44.14). This fact motivated us to use it primarily in our cases of vertical abdominoplasties, presenting the same reproducibility of results (Figs. 44.15 and 44.16).

An important technical detail regards the location of triangular flaps concerning existing umbilical scar, so that these may not be made too superiorly, under the risk of obtaining a longer umbilical scar (Figs. 44.17 and 44.18), since the migration of abdominal flap is bigger in its distal portion, besides occurring pubic elevation. So, there is no significant change of position where the lateral flaps are marked, causing few marking errors in some cases. Therefore, due to its unpredictability of positioning, we have performed these marked flaps on a rectangular skin segment preserved bilaterally, designed at the same level as the umbilical stump after traction of the abdominal skin flaps. Triangular flaps may not exceed 2 cm of base; otherwise, we

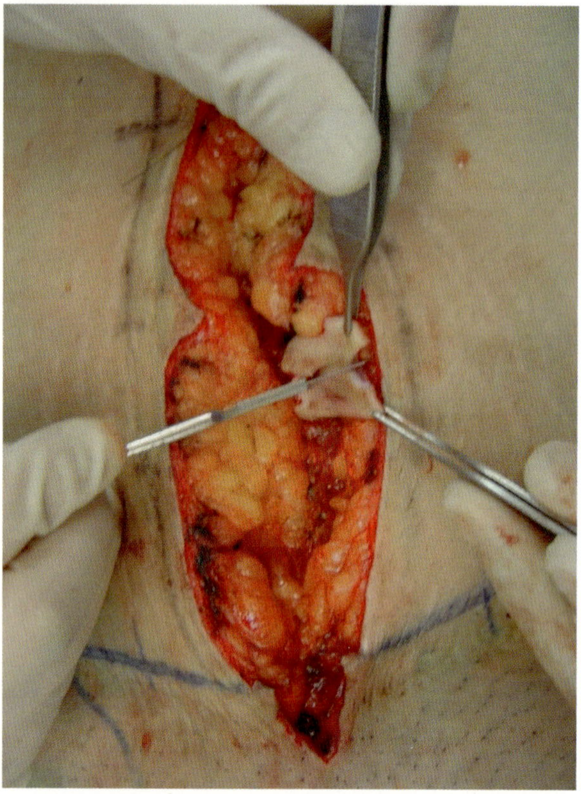

Fig. 44.5 The umbilical stump is biparted on its laterals, preserving a central segment of approximately 0.5 cm

could obtain an umbilical scar too large (Figs. 44.17 and 44.18), or small if the base is inferior to 1.5 cm. The thickness of the adipose layer of these flaps also must be preserved, because it offers deepness to the new umbilical scar, aggregating aesthetic quality. The height of umbilical stump is also an important technical detail, where the depth may be at the level of the aponeurosis or up to 1 cm above. For thicker abdominal flaps, this relation must be increased, in a way to avoid a resulting belly button that is too deep.

We found some technical limitation on those cases where the umbilical scar is flat or there is low skin flabbiness on the abdominal wall. The possibility of performing a plicature of rectus abdominis muscles may correct these situations, facilitating the performance of this omphaloplasty technique.

On secondary cases where we assess too much abdominal tension at the umbilical level, with the enlargement of it, it seems to us that this technique is a contraindication, as well as keloid scars with difficult control.

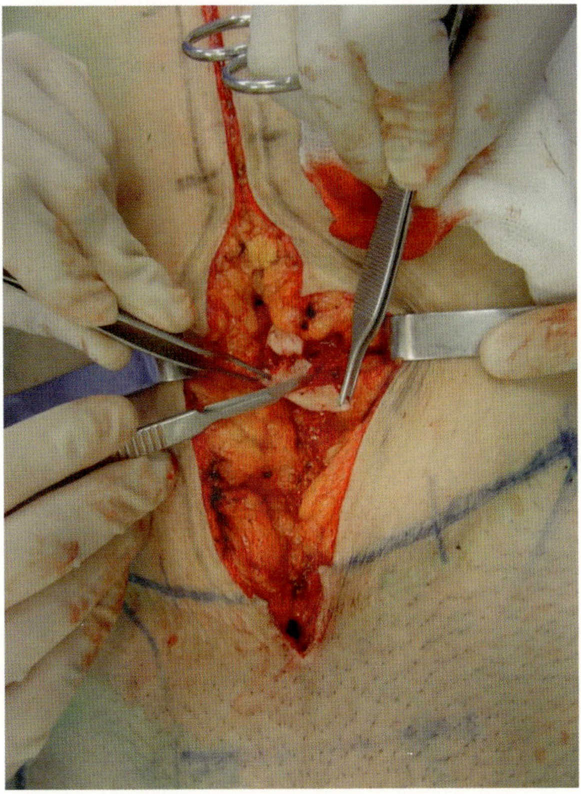

Fig. 44.6 Resecting the skin excesses of umbilical stump

Postoperatively, we could maintain a small silicone or plastic mold on the umbilical scar to compress and keep its form, but nowadays we do not use anything besides a gauze turunda for up to 15 (fifteen) days.

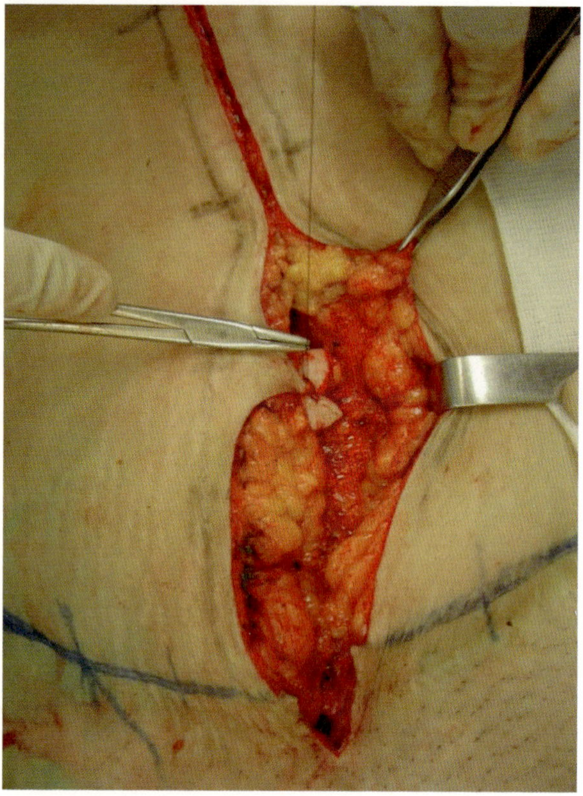

Fig. 44.7 Suturing of the extremities of the lateral flaps to the umbilicus

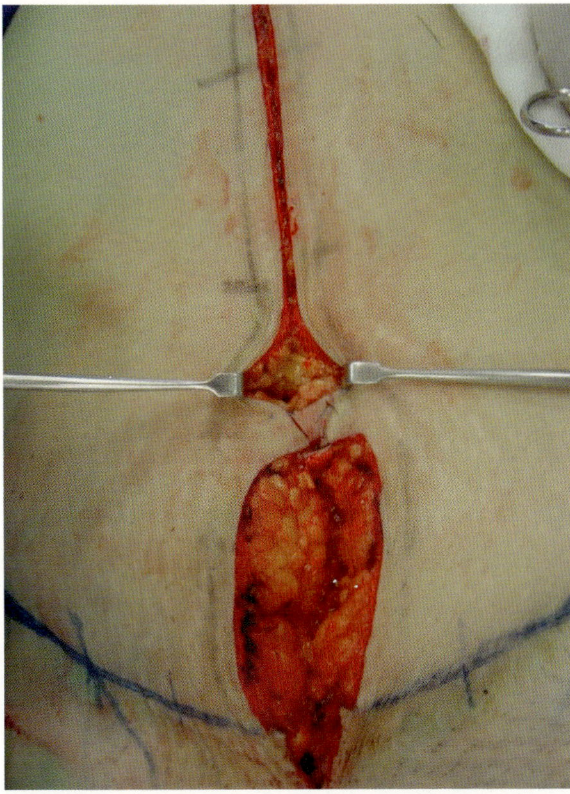

Fig. 44.8 Suturing the extremities of the umbilical flaps to the middle portion of the lateral flaps. Then, finalizing the vertical suture with compensation stitches between the base of umbilical flaps and the lateral portions of the lateral flaps

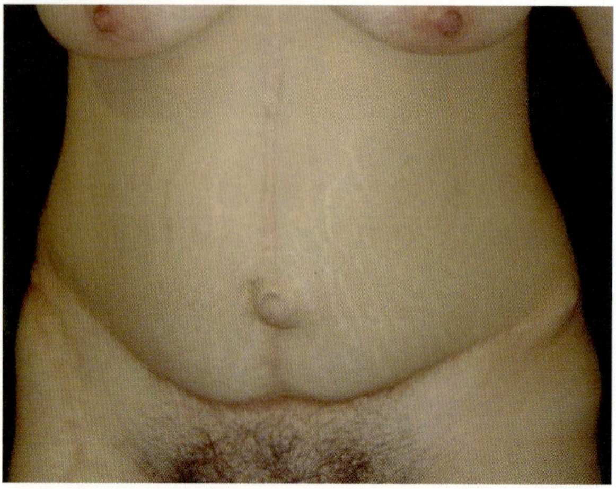

Fig. 44.9 Patient preoperative

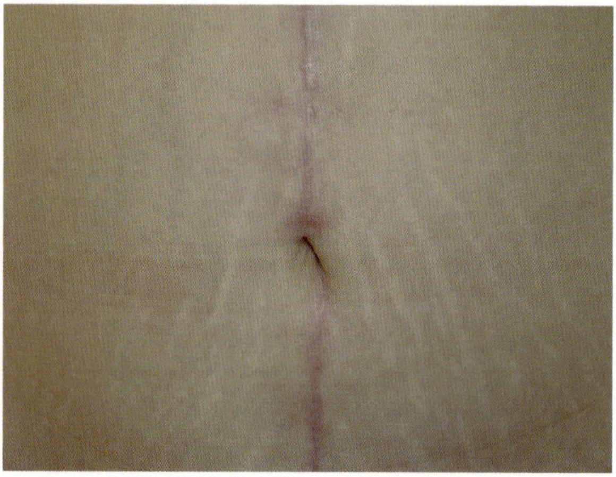

Fig. 44.10 Patient postoperative

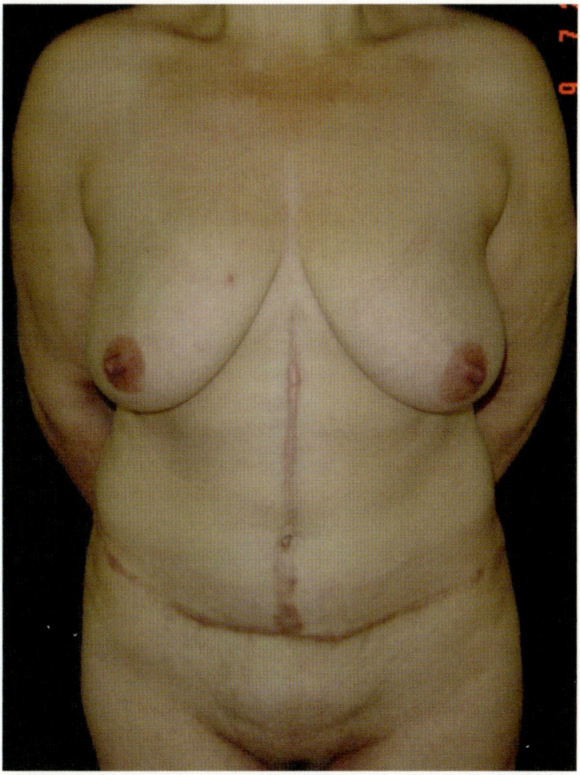

Fig. 44.11 Preoperative

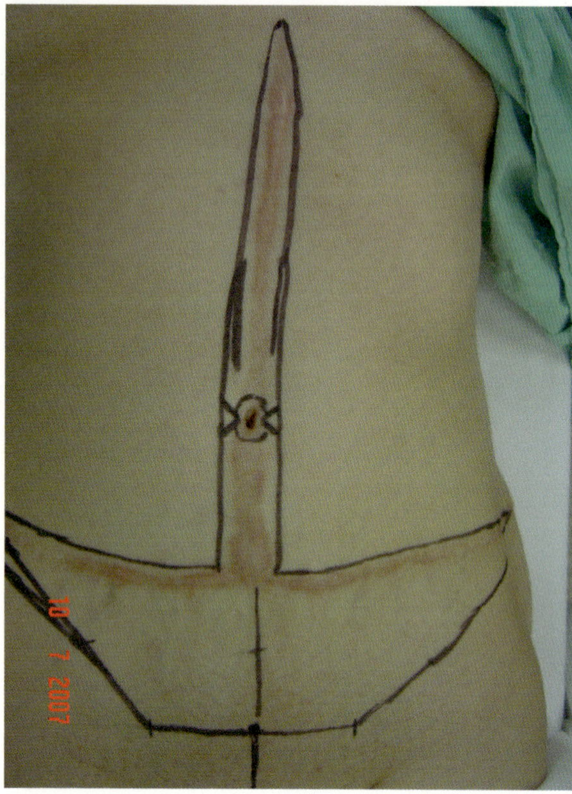

Fig. 44.12 Surgery marking

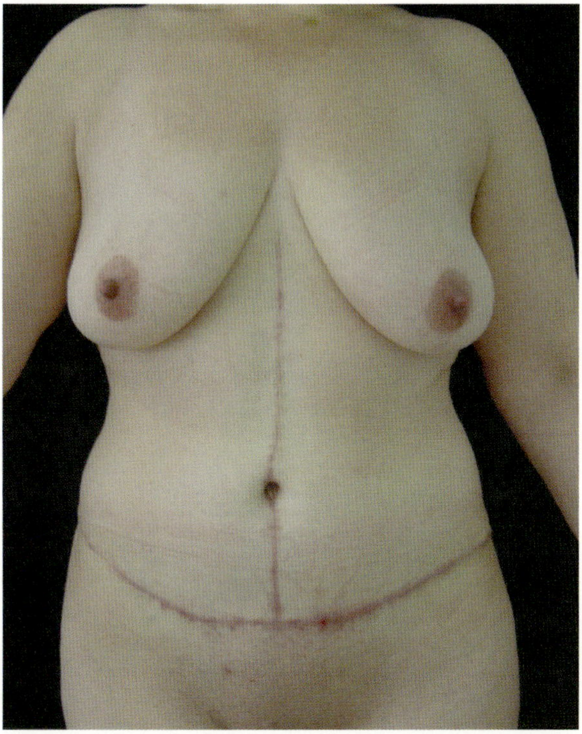

Fig. 44.13 Postoperative

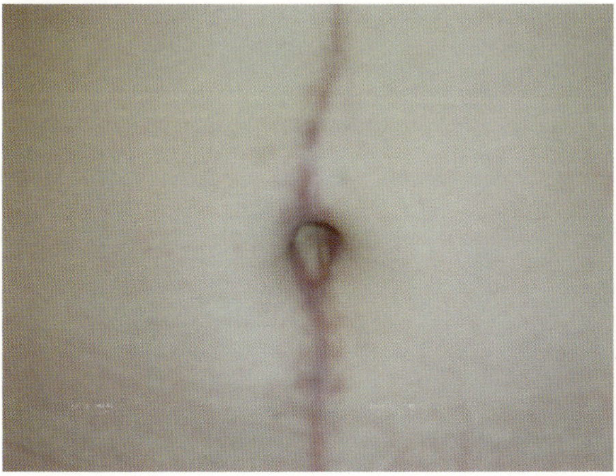

Fig. 44.14 Umbilical closure

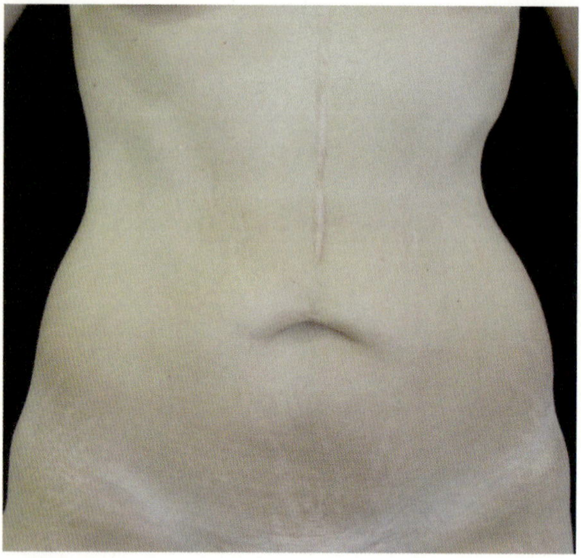

Fig. 44.15 Preoperative

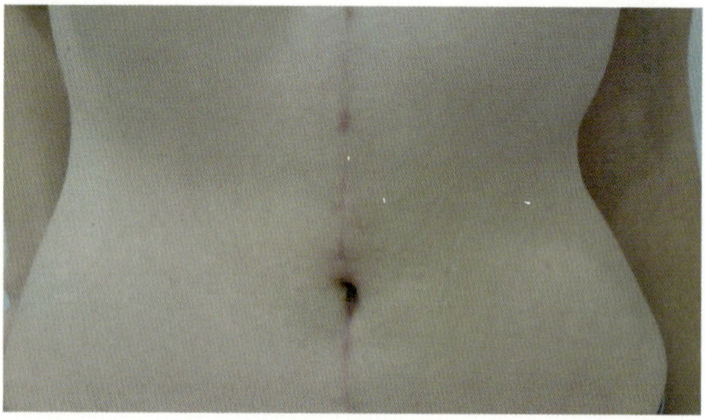

Fig. 44.16 Postoperative

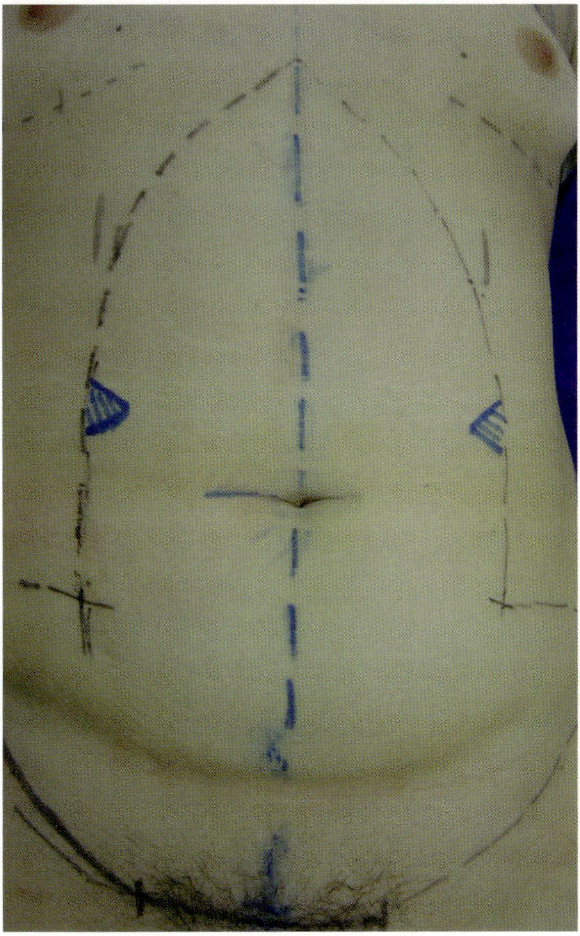

Fig. 44.17 Preoperative markings excessive high position of the lateral flaps

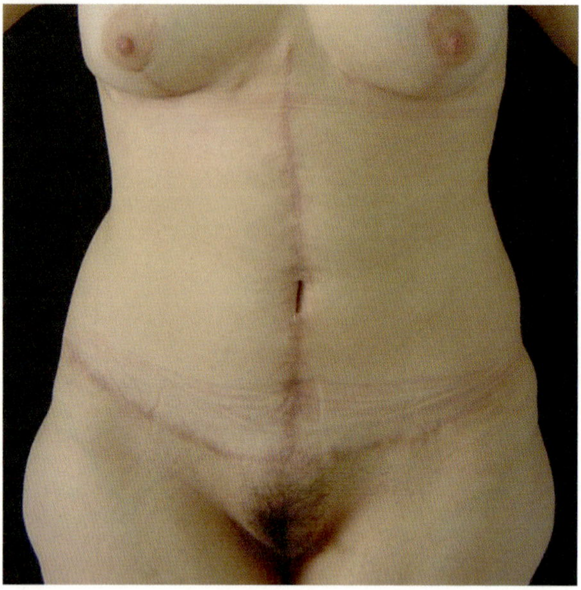

Fig. 44.18 Postoperative. Observe the unaesthetic result obtained due probably to superior tension and lateral flaps too length

44.4 Conclusions

The opposite triangular flaps technique has been our primary indication of omphaloplasty in vertical dermolipectomy, with satisfactory aesthetic results, avoiding stenosis and umbilical scar enlargements, frequent in other techniques. It represents an excellent alternative in secondary cases, or even for neo-omphaloplasty techniques.

Attention to details of this technique as size of flaps, location, and height are important factors on reproducibility of results.

References

1. Yotsuyanagi T, Nihei Y, Sawada Y. A simple technique for reconstruction of the umbilicus, using two twisted flaps. Plast Reconstr Surg. 1998;102(7):2444–6.
2. Malic C, Spyrou G, Hough M, Fourie LR. Patients satisfaction with two different methods of umbilicoplasty. Plast Reconstr Surg. 2007;119(1):357–61.
3. Shinohara H, Matsuo K, Kikuchi N. Umbilical reconstruction with an inverted c-v flap. Plast Reconstr Surg. 2000;105(2):703–5.
4. Sevin A, Sevin K, Senen D, Erdogan B. A new method for umbilicus reconstruction: preliminary report. Aesthetic Plast Surg. 2006;30(5):589–91.

5. Franco D, Medeiros J, Farias C, Franco T. Umbilical reconstruction for patients with a midline scar. Aesthetic Plast Surg. 2006;30(5):595–8.
6. Masuda R, Takeda A, Sugimoto T, Ishiguro M, Uchinuma E. Reconstruction of the umbilicus using a reverse fan-shaped flap. Aesthetic Plast Surg. 2003;27(5):349–53.
7. Amud RJM. Omphaloplasty without scars. Rev Soc Bras Cir Plást. 2008;23(1):37–40.
8. Monte ALR. Treatment of the umbilical stenosis in a vertical dermolipectomy patient. Rev Bras Cir Plást. 2011;26(1):167–70.
9. Pontes R. Abdominoplastia. Ressecção em Bloco e sua Aplicação em Lifting de Coxa e Torsoplastia. Revinter, Rio de Janeiro, Brasil. 2004. p. 25–77.

Part IX
Outcomes

Chapter 45
Umbilical Pilonidal Disease

Mohammad S. Fazeli and Amir Lebaschi

45.1 Introduction

The exact pathogenesis of pilonidal disease remains unknown [1]. Clinical and pathologic observations lend support to the hypothesis of a congenital origin [2], although some experts maintain that the disease is an acquired one [3]. Umbilical pilonidal disease (UPD) is most commonly encountered in adults who have a hair tuft around their umbilicus and is more common in males [3–5]. It is important to differentiate UPD from other umbilical affections by careful clinical observation, and because there is a risk of peritoneal extension of the associated inflammation, UPD should be taken seriously and treated more aggressively than its sacral counterpart [6]. Also, whenever the surgeon comes across a case of resistant or recurrent "omphalitis," UPD should be considered as an alternative diagnosis [7].

45.2 Nonsurgical Management

Nonsurgical measures are usually effective for treatment of mild, minimally symptomatic UPD. Patients with UPD amenable to nonsurgical treatment usually complain of scant, malodorous discharge. These patients frequently have dense hair tufts around the umbilicus. Often there is no sign of infection (redness, swelling,

M.S. Fazeli, M.D. (✉)
Department of Surgery, Imam Hospital Complex, Tehran University of Medical Sciences,
P.O. Box 13145–158, Keshavarz Boulevard, Tehran, Iran
e-mail: mhfazeli@yahoo.com; mhfazeli@sina.tums.ac.ir

A. Lebaschi
Department of Tissue Engineering, Repair, and Regeneration, Hospital for Special Surgery,
New York, NY, USA

M.A. Shiffman (ed.), *Adult Umbilical Reconstruction*,
DOI 10.1007/978-3-319-43887-0_45

and tenderness), and usually no orifice is visible upon inspection of the umbilicus. It is advisable to check other common areas for pilonidal disease to rule out synchronous involvement.

Various techniques have been suggested as treatment option for UPD [5, 8]. The common theme in almost all these measures is decontamination by hair removal, physical cleaning of the umbilicus, and application of antimicrobial agents, including silver nitrate. Our preferred treatment is meticulous hair removal at least three times a week, cleansing of the entire umbilicus with antibacterial soap at least daily, and application of and appropriate antistaphylococcal ointment for 7–10 days. It is important to note that although UPD can occur on the periphery, the most common location is the bottom of the umbilicus. Therefore cleansing and topical antibiotics are not effective if they are not delivered to this area.

Most patients will become asymptomatic after 2 weeks. The patients are recommended to continue maintaining umbilical hygiene for as long as they can.

45.3 Surgical Management

Table 45.1 summarizes the common indications for surgical intervention in UPD. Persistent discharge is the most common underlying complaint in patients undergoing surgical management. In case of cellulitis or abscess formation, infection should be addressed and treated first. For cellulitis, a course of systemic antibiotic is recommended. Authors recommend surgical intervention following the first bout of cellulitis as most of these patients have moderate to severe UPD. In case of abscess formation, urgent incision and drainage in warranted. Systemic antibiotic is usually not necessary unless there are signs of significant cellulitis (more than what is expected to be caused by the abscess formation process), patient is febrile, diabetic, has endovascular implant or is at risk to suffer from bacteremia, or when subfascial extension (SFE) is suspected. Surgical technique described in this chapter should be attempted in the absence of sings of active infection.

Several surgical methods have been advocated ranging from excising the umbilicus without reconstruction [3], sinus excision [9] with cosmetic umbilical reconstruction [7], to total omphalectomy as a primary treatment [2, 10] or for treating recurrent disease. Unlike sacrococcygeal pilonidal disease, where there is ample

Table 45.1 Indications of surgical management in UPD

Failure of medical therapy
Persistent discharge
Recurrence after medical treatment
Cellulitis
Abscess formation
Suspected subfascial extension

space for resection and little concern for cosmetic outcome even in cases with secondary healing, umbilicus is an esthetic structure for not only the abdomen but for the entire body. As such, excisional procedures should be designed in a way that allow reconstruction of an esthetically acceptable (if not pleasing) umbilicus.

45.4 Authors' Preferred Technique

The procedure is performed on an outpatient basis. The patient is prepared and draped in supine position. A curved incision is made along the inferior border of the umbilicus starting at 5 o'clock and extending to 8 o'clock. It is important to adjust the distance of the incision from the center of the umbilicus based on the location of the sinus; if the sinus has a central position, an incision near or at the inferior border of the umbilicus is appropriate. If the sinus is located in the lower half of the umbilicus, the distance of the incision from the inferior border of the umbilicus should be as much as the distance of the sinus from the umbilical center. The incision is deepened to cut the dermis, and the subcutaneous tissue is dissected to arrive at the fascia along the full length of the incision. Then, using scissors to cut through the subcutaneous fat and just superficial to the fascia, a plane is developed around the umbilical attachment to the fascia to encircle this attachment. After full detachment of the umbilical stalk from surrounding subcutaneous tissue, the stalk is cut from its point of attachment to the underlying fascia (Fig. 45.1). The umbilicus is then completely everted by inserting an index finger from underneath and pushing the cut stalk outward while holding the cut edge of the umbilicus with the thumb of the same hand (Fig. 45.2). It is important that one should not lift the umbilical fold too much as in some cases it may affect the blood supply in its most distal part, thereby causing problems associated with necrosis. With this maneuver the sinus becomes everted too, although it may be necessary to use a small-tipped instrument to drive the base of the sinus out. All stalks

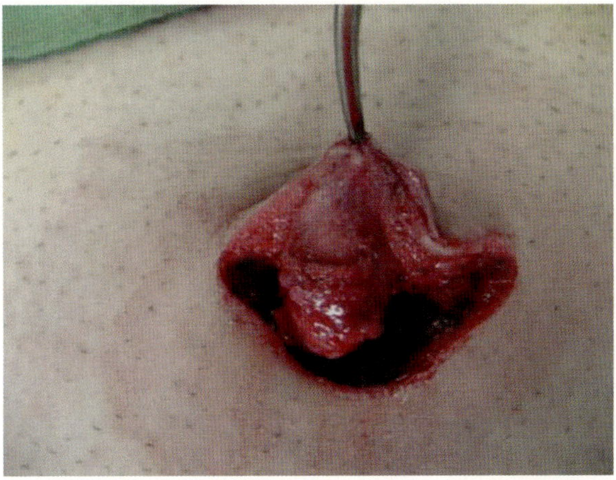

Fig. 45.1 Umbilicus is dissected and detached from fascia (reprinted from Fazeli MS, Lebaschi AH, et al. Evaluation of the outcome of complete sinus excision with reconstruction of the umbilicus in patients with umbilical pilonidal sinus. World journal of surgery 2008;32(10):2305–8, with permission from Springer)

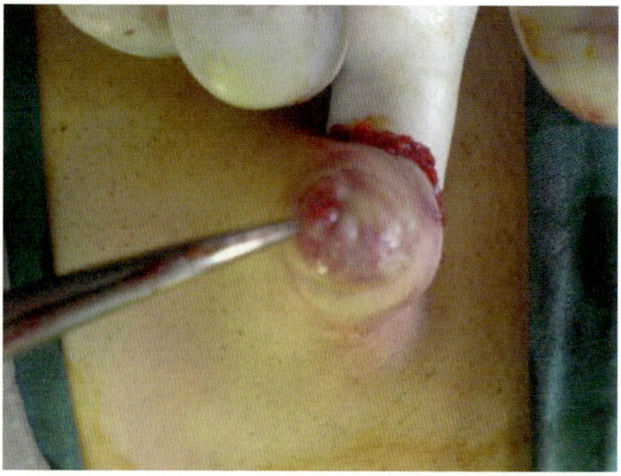

Fig. 45.2 Sinus is completely everted. The whole sinus is now seen (reprinted from Fazeli MS, Lebaschi AH, et al. Evaluation of the outcome of complete sinus excision with reconstruction of the umbilicus in patients with umbilical pilonidal sinus. World journal of surgery 2008;32(10):2305–8, with permission from Springer)

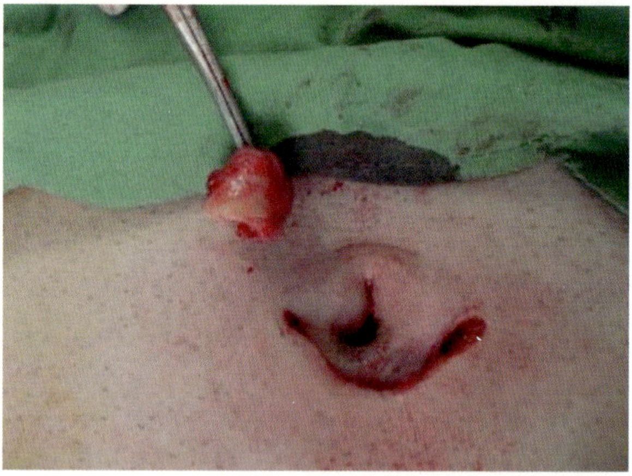

Fig. 45.3 Sinus is completely excised. The defect in the umbilicus is ready to be repaired (reprinted from Fazeli MS, Lebaschi AH, et al. Evaluation of the outcome of complete sinus excision with reconstruction of the umbilicus in patients with umbilical pilonidal sinus. World journal of surgery 2008;32(10):2305–8, with permission from Springer)

should be meticulously checked for potential subfascial extension. In the presence of such an extension, the everted umbilicus will show an orifice, indicating that the tract has penetrated the bottom of the umbilicus and extended into the fascia. A transverse elliptical incision is made on the everted side of the umbilicus, and the sinus is excised completely. The incision should be kept as small as possible to keep umbilical skin loss to a minimum. Also, it is important to observe the traditional rules for designing random flaps and to leave enough width of skin in the resulting circular flap (Fig. 45.3). This elliptical incision is then repaired by separate absorbable sutures from underneath. In most cases, the fascia should be repaired at the site of stalk detachment. This should not be mistaken for subfascial extension. The center of the repaired umbilicus is now secured to the old attachment point on the fascia by a single nonabsorbable or delayed absorbable suture. Then the skin is closed using simple interrupted sutures. Selecting the location of the initial infraumbilical incision is critical to provide an adequate skin margin for closure and maintenance of umbilical symmetry. The new umbilicus will invariably have less depth than the original one [11].

45.5 Postoperative Care

Standard wound care as dictated by good surgical practice is all that is required. It is authors' practice to discharge the patients who do not have SFE with a short course of oral cephalexin the same day. The most dreaded complication from a cosmetic standpoint is the necrosis of the inferior parts of the flap. Therefore it is recommended to check the umbilicus 24–48 hours postoperatively, especially in cases with extensive excision. Subsequently, the patients can be seen 1 week after surgery.

45.6 Subfascial Extension

Subfascial extension (SFE) is violation of the fascia (linea alba) and extension of the sinus into the preperitoneal space with the risk of transperitoneal and intra-abdominal penetration. SFE provides the surgeon with a challenge, especially in cases where the sinus is initially deemed to be limited to supra-fascial region (essentially inside and limited to umbilical stalk) and an outpatient procedure is planned only to discover that the surgery will need to be upgraded to an outright celiotomy. Many of the UPDs with SFE are extensive, but authors have encountered cases in which SFE could not be suspected on clinical grounds at all. Risk factors for development of SFE include long-standing UPD, short umbilical stalk, and low body mass index. Ultrasound scanning and magnetic resonance imaging can delineate the boundaries of SFE and assist the surgeon to have a better surgical planning. Management of umbilical part of a UPD with SFE is essentially the same. Injection of methylene blue dye in the orifice of the sinus at the level of fascia may be useful, but it is usually possible to detect and remove the sinus completely as the preperitoneal space contains little tissue and the sinus will be sharply demarcated. Subsequent to umbilical stalk detachment, a longitudinal incision is made in the fascia superior and inferior to the fascial penetration site. Although inflammatory response in fascia around the sinus tract usually calls for resection of a variable portion of the fascia together with the tract, it is possible to close the fascia primarily without tension. Every effort must be made to leave peritoneum intact. The sinus can be identified easily as it has an appearance similar to an inclusion retention cyst with irregular shape.

45.7 Complications

45.7.1 Wound Infection

Infections following UPD excision and reconstruction should be treated through venting the infection by opening the wound, except for the cases with minor signs of cellulitis and no collection. Even in the absence of SFE, there will be a small defect in the fascia subsequent to stalk detachment in most cases of UPD excision which poses a risk for intra-abdominal extension in the presence of infective processes; hence the importance of drainage cannot be overemphasized. Wound infection can also cause umbilical detachment, leading to a floating umbilicus which may require fixation at a later time. Preventive measures include avoiding surgery in the presence of active infection, prophylactic preoperative antibiotic, and meticulous preparing of the surgical site.

45.7.2 Partial Necrosis

Partial necrosis could be inconsequential or devastating based on the extent of the necrosis. In cases of extensive necrosis, umbilical stenosis, flattening, and other deformities may occur, and later reconstruction may be warranted based on patient's request. In the acute setting, topical antibiotics are recommended till the necrotic potions are sloughed and secondary healing is complete.

45.7.3 Recurrence

Recurrence in any patients with UPD is a possible scenario. Patients should understand that UPD is, at least in part, caused by genetic factors that are not modified or eliminated by any surgical technique, and this fact should be discussed with every patient with UPD well in advance of any surgical intervention.

The authors have not observed any recurrence so far subsequent to application of this technique, perhaps because the technique described in this chapter leads to a shallow umbilicus that is easy to keep clean. We recommend to treat recurrent cases as a new one, although a trial of nonsurgical treatment for mild recurrent cases is probably warranted prior to attempted re-excision.

References

1. Gupta S, Gupta S. Pilonidal sinus of the umbilicus with urachal adenoma. Trop Geogr Med. 1981;33(4):393–6.
2. Tocchi A, Liotta G, Agostini N, Maggiolini F. The umbilical pilonidal cyst: a case report. Comments on its etiopathogenesis and treatment. G Chir. 1994;15(1–2):33–6.
3. Dixit SP. Pilonidal sinus of the umbilicus. Can J Surg. 1976;19(5):422–6.
4. Eryilmaz R, Sahin M, Okan I, Alimoglu O, Somay A. Umbilical pilonidal sinus disease: predisposing factors and treatment. World J Surg. 2005;29(9):1158–60.
5. Abdelnour A, Aftimos G, Elmasri H. Conservative surgical treatment of 27 cases of umbilical pilonidal sinus. J Med Liban. 1994;42(3):123–5.
6. Schoelch SB, Barrett TL. Umbilical pilonidal sinus. Cutis. 1998;62(2):83–4.

7. Colapinto ND. Umbilical pilonidal sinus. Br J Surg. 1977;64(7):494–5.
8. El-Bakry AA. Discharging umbilicus. Saudi Med J. 2002;23(9):1099–100.
9. Al-Naami MY. Outpatient pilonidal sinotomy complemented with good wound and surrounding skin care. Saudi Med J. 2005;26(2):285–8.
10. Sroujieh AS, Dawoud A. Umbilical sepsis. Br J Surg. 1989;76(7):687–8.
11. Fazeli MS, Lebaschi AH, Adel MG, Kazemeini AR. Evaluation of the outcome of complete sinus excision with reconstruction of the umbilicus in patients with umbilical pilonidal sinus. World J Surg. 2008;32(10):2305–8.

Appendix A

Cullen TS. Embryology, Anatomy, and Diseases of the Umbilicus: Together with Diseases of the Urachus. Philadelphia, WB Saunders Co. 1916 pp 350-458

http://www.ebooksread.com/authors-eng/thomas-stephen-cullen/embryology-anatomy-and-diseases-of-the-umbilicus-together-with-diseases-of-t-llu/page-35-embryology-anatomy-and-diseases-of-the-umbilicus-together-with-diseases-of-tllu.shtml

http://www.ebooksread.com/authors-eng/thomas-stephen-cullen/embryology-anatomy-and-diseases-of-the-umbilicus-together-with-diseases-of-the-urachus

UMBILICAL TUMORS.

Hypertrophy of the umbilicus.

Angiomata of the umbilicus; report of cases.

Umbilical lymphocele.

Myxomata.

Fibromata; report of cases.

Papillomata; report of cases.

Lipomata.

Dermoids or atheromatous cysts; report of cases.

Umbilical tumors consisting chiefly of sweat-glands.

An abdominal tumor attached to the inner surface of the umbilicus by a pedicle two inches in diameter.

Papilloma of the umbilicus secondary to papilloma of the ovary.

Benign umbilical tumors:

Hypertrophy.

Angiomata.

Lymphocele.

Benign connective-tissue growths.

Myxomata.

Fibromata.

M.A. Shiffman (ed.), *Adult Umbilical Reconstruction*,
DOI 10.1007/978-3-319-43887-0

Papillomata. *
Lipomata.
Dermoid cysts.
Sweat-gland tumors.
Abdominal myoma springing from the umbilicus.
Papilloma secondary to growth in ovary
Adenomyomata.
Malignant:
Carcinoma of the umbilicus.
A. Primary Squamous-cell carcinoma.
B. Primary Adenocarcinoma.
C. Metastatic
1. From the stomach.
2. From the gall-bladder.
3. From the intestine.
4. From the ovary
5. From the uterus.
6. From other abdominal organs.
D. Sarcoma.
1. Telangiectatic myxosarcoma.
2. Spindle-cell sarcoma.
3. Round-cell sarcoma.
4. Melanotic sarcoma.

* In the ordinary umbilical papilloma the growth is caused by a proliferation of the stroma —the squamous epithelium covering the papillae occupies merely a passive role. It is for this reason that we have grouped these small tumors with the benign connective-tissue growths. Some of these may or may not be malignant.

GENERAL REMARKS.

Many authors who have published cases showing abnormalities of the umbilicus have endeavored to classify satisfactorily umbilical diseases. Probably one of the best articles on the subject is the exhaustive treatise by Nicaise, published in Paris in 1881. In 1883 Codet de Boisse gave a satisfactory resume of the subject, and the following year Reginald H. Fitz, of Boston, published a most instructive article in which he included lesions of the umbilicus owing their origin to persistence of the omphalomesenteric duct.

Villar, in 1886, wrote a thesis on umbilical tumors, going into the subject very carefully, and making a satisfactory classification of the various umbilical tumors. In 1890Ledderhose discussed umbilical diseases very fully and satisfactorily, and in 1892 Pernice published his well-known monograph on Umbilical Tumors. Finally, in 1906, Guiselin, in his Bordeaux thesis entitled Cancer of the Umbilicus, outlined a very practical classification of umbilical tumors. After reviewing the literature on the subject, I have found the above classification the most satisfactory:

LITERATURE CONSULTED ON UMBILICAL TUMORS IN GENERAL.

Codet de Boisse: Tumeurs de l'ombilic chez l'adulte. These de Paris, 1883, No. 311.

Fitz, Reginald: Persistent Omphalomesenteric Remains, Their Importance in the Causation of Intestinal Duplication, Cyst Formation, and Obstruction. Amer. Jour. Med. Sci., 1884, lxxxviii, 30.

Guiselin, E. J. M. J. : Du Cancer de l'ombilic. These de Bordeaux, 1906, No. 47.

Ledderhose, G. : Deutsche Chirurgie, 1890, Lief. 45 b.

Nicaise: Ombilic. Dictionnaire encyclopedique des sc. med., Paris, 1881, xv, 140, deuxieme ser.

Pernice, Ludwig: Die Nabelgeschwiilste, Svo. Halle a. S. 1892.

*Villar, Francis: Tumeurs de 1'ombilic. These de Paris, 1886. No. 19.

HYPERTROPHY OF THE UMBILICUS.

Villar* speaks of hypertrophy of the umbilicus in a patient sixty years of age.

Inasmuch as from the description it is clear that there was a definite umbilical suppuration and the histologic examination showed an inflammatory condition, we should certainly hesitate to class the case as one of true hypertrophy of the umbilicus. I have encountered no other literature on the subject.

ANGIOMATA OF THE UMBILICUS.

Definite literature on the subject is very rare.

Virchow, in 1862, mentions two varieties of umbilical fungi. The one is usually rich in blood-vessels, bleeds readily, and is found after the cord comes away. It consists of granulation tissue, and after the use of astringents soon disappears. He is evidently referring to the simple granulation tissue not infrequently noted after the cord comes away.

The second variety represents a congenital tumor, and in the majority of cases is a remnant of the omphalomesenteric duct. Virchow then refers to cases reported by Maunoir and Lawton.

* Villar: Op. cit., p. 76.

UMBILICAL TUMORS.

Xicaise refers to the subject and mentions three cases from the literature. Ledderhose briefly refers to angiomata of the umbilicus, and says that cases have been recorded by Maunoir, Chassaignac, Lawton, Boyer, and Colombe. Kidd and Patteson, in 1889, in an article on Capillary Angioma of the Umbilicus, reported a case in a child six weeks old. From the description, however, it would seem probable that the tumor consisted of granulation tissue and was not an angioma in the accepted sense of the word, although it must be admitted that granulation tissue in itself at times has such a rich capillary blood-supply that it might with propriety be called an angioma.

Pernice, in his exhaustive monograph on Tumors of the Umbilicus, brieflyconsiders the cases recorded in the literature. He also refers to a case recorded by Boyer. A nine year-old girl from her birth had had an umbilical tumor largely made up of varicose veins. This tumor was pedunculated, like a polyp, grew slowly, was bluish in color, and felt soft. After being repeatedly tied off, it completely disappeared.

Robson, in 1872, reported a somewhat complicated tumor of the umbilicus occurring at birth. The soft and elastic portion of the tumor was of a dirty, livid color and probably represented an area of hemorrhage and not a genuine angioma. The essential points in the case are as follows :

The mother of the child was delivered before Robson arrived, but he noticed an abnormal condition at the umbilicus, three distinct tumors resting on the abdomen, and connected with the umbilicus close to the integument of the navel. The one containing the cord was about the length and circumference of a one-ounce quinin jar, with a continuation of a small, shriveled cord projecting from its extremity. The under part of this tumor consisted of firm, compact tissue; the upper was soft and elastic, without any pulsation, and of a dirty, livid color. Immediately beneath and growing from the first, at its junction with the abdomen, was a second tumor consisting of a transparent, globular mass the size of a arge orange, and a third, the size of a pullet's egg, containing a thick, albuminous substance like jelly. The growths were extirpated.

The tumor consisted mainly of the cord in a spiral form, each coil adhering to the other and thoroughly agglutinated by the albuminous substance. There was extravasation of blood, with here and there organized matter.

In the cases reported by Chassaignac, Lawton, and Colombe, a definite angioma of the umbilicus existed. The first two were noted in infants, but Colombe's case occurred in an adult. As seen from the detailed report, when Chassaignac's patient was twelve days old, a minute nodule was noted at the umbilicus. At six months the tumor was as large as a hen's egg and was non-pedunculated; the overlying skin had a bluish

tinge, and beneath the surface a varicose network of veins could be seen. Where the veins were very near the surface, the bluish tinge of the skin was naturally more accentuated. A large vein appearing to the left of the xiphoid passed downward to the umbilicus and was continuous with the tumor.

Lawton's observation was made on a new-born child, and in addition to the tumor there was an umbilical hernia. The tumor was the size of a jargonelle pear, and darkish in color. It was of the consistence of placental tissue. On microscopic examination, it was found to be composed chiefly of the ramifications of large blood-vessels held together by areolar tissue.

Colombe's patient, when twenty-six years old, noticed a small tumor the size of a grain of wheat at the umbilicus. It gradually increased in size, was purple and soft. When seen ten years later, it was the size of the end phalanx of the little finger. Two years before coming under observation she had had a hemorrhage from the tumor lasting two days. The bleeding was controlled by styptics. Three days before admission the hemorrhage recurred and the bleeding was so excessive that the patient showed marked constitutional symptoms.

The cases of Chassaignac, Lawton, and Colombe are so interesting that I report them in detail:

An Erectile Venous Tumor Developing in the Region of the Umbilicus in a Child Six Months Old.*

The child was six months old. To the left of the umbilicus was attached a tumor the size of a small hen's-egg. This was regular, non-pedunculated, raising the left half of the umbilical margin and the skin, and giving the overlying skin a bluish tinge.

The surface of the tumor was evidently made up of a network of varicose veins (subcutaneous), and had three or four small spots where the bluish tint was more marked. Another bluish spot, with the diameter of a 50-centime piece, had occupied the summit of the tumor. This was crescentic, with the hollow of the crescent directed upward and toward the median line. A large vein appearing to the left of the xiphoid passed downward to the umbilicus and evidently was continuous with the tumor.

Pressure on the tumor produced pallor, but, when the finger was raised again, the color returned with increasing intensity.

The mother noticed, twelve or thirteen days after birth, a small spot the size of a pin-head at the umbilicus. A bandage was applied, but the spot increased in size and became thickened. It was removed satisfactorily. The tumor consisted of two parts — adipose tissue and blood-vessels surrounded by cellular tissue. The vessels were very abundant, and in several places showed varicose dilatations. This tumor was an angioma.

* Chassaignac, M. E.: Traite de l'ecrasement lineaire, Paris, 1856, 535.

A Case of Vascular (Erectile) Tumor in the Sheath of the Cord in a New-born.

Mr. Lawton* * was called to the delivery of a fine male child, and when he proceeded to tie the cord, he found a tumor the size and shape of a medium jargonelle pear with its neck communicating with the cavity of the abdomen through the umbilical opening and strongly adherent to the cord, the covering being common to both. Mr. Lawton divided the cord above the tumor in the usual way. On examination the growth felt tough, rather fleshy, and somewhat like a placenta might feel before degeneration commences — it did not feel at all like intestine, although when the child cried, both it and the investing membrane, together with the tegumentary portion of the umbilicus, enlarged very much — the tumor from being engorged with blood and the membrane from protrusion of intestine. Pressure reduced the one and somewhat decreased the size of the other.

After reduction of the hernia, pressure was applied by means of a pad and banda^-, and it was resolved to wait and see what might be the termination of the case if left to nature, as it was thought that the tumor might dry up and slough with the cord. After a day or two affairs presented nearly the same appearance as at first, and Mr. Lawton determined to explore a little. He did so by carefully dissecting(over the fundus of the tumor) the outer covering, when a clear, yellow serum escaped. He then made a small opening into the second covering, and blood of a dark color flowed pretty freely. A pad and bandage were immediately applied, and the case was allowed to take its course for two days more. On entering the room on the third day the smell of the decomposing membranes was strong, and the integument around the umbilicus much inflamed. The umbilical opening was large enough to receive four fingers, and was more or less oval. At the lower end protruded a knuckle of gut; at the upper end, a non-pulsating, pyriform tumor, and at the right-hand side, the cord, between the knuckle of gut and tumor. The membranes were gangrenous and the fundus of the tumor was bare. It presented a dark color; to the touch it felt firm, unless strongly compressed, when it somewhat diminished in size and was a little flaccid. The crying of the child gave now no impetus to the tumor.

Lawton resolved to return the protruded intestine, and, after applying a ligature around the neck of the tumor, to excise it. After chloroform had been given, a finger and thumb were applied to the neck of the growth and fully compressed it. The operator made a slight incision in the fundus of the tumor, and on careful relaxation of the pressure, the blood was inclined to flow very freely. A ligature was then applied around the neck of the growth, but the membranes, being gangrenous, it cut through them, and, the abdominal muscles becoming rigid at the same time, from eight to ten inches of gut protruded. The tumor was excised above the ligature, the cord tied as low down as possible, and after careful and patient manipulation the protruded intestine was returned. The opening was closed as far as possible by passing through four common needles in place of harelip pins; a pad and bandage were applied in the usual way. The child's bowels were not moved for three days after the operation, when they acted freely. The little patient had no bad symptoms, and at the time of the report was quite well.

Microscopic examination by Dr. J. Braxton Hicks showed that the whole mass was penetrated by large blood-vessels, of the ramifications of which it was principally composed, coupled with areolar tissue, in the network of which were nucleated cells of round or oval form, generally in groups of four or five. There was in some parts, however, an excess of the connective-tissue elements so as to form solid portions. The tumor was an angioma.

* * Lawton: London Obstet. Trans., 1866, vii, 210.

A Vascular Tumor of the Umbilicus.***

The patient was a woman, thirty-six years of age, in good health. She had had a child at nineteen. Ten years before she had noticed a small tumor the size of a grain of wheat at the umbilicus. It had gradually increased in size. It was purple, rather soft, painless, but made her uncomfortable. About the week before she was seen, it was the size of the end of the phalanx of the little finger. Two years before there had been a hemorrhage from the tumor, the bleeding coming in jets of the diameter of a pin. The hemorrhage lasted two days, was not continuous, and was controlled by perchorid of iron. Three days before admission she had a second hemorrhage and perchloric! of iron was used, the flow ceasing just as the astringent was employed. The volume of bleeding could be compared to that from the femoral artery; the bleeding, however, was intermittent. The patient was in a sea of blood. She was pale and apparently in a serious condition. Forceps were applied, and the arealigated en masse, but with difficulty, as the bleeding came from the bottom of the umbilicus. Seven days later the bleeding again recurred. A ligature was applied, and the bleeding stopped and never returned. The tumor disappeared.

*** Colombe: Tumeur vasculaire de l'ombilic, hemorrhagic, guerison. Gaz. med. de Paris, 1887, lviii, 245.

LITERATURE CONSULTED ON ANGIOMATA OF THE UMBILICUS.

Chassaignac, M. E.: Traite de l'ecrasement lineaire, Paris, 1856, 535.

Colombe: Tumeur vasculaire de l'ombilic, hemorrhagie, guerison. Gaz. med. de Paris, 1887, lviii, 245.

Kidd and Patteson: Capillary Angioma of the Umbilicus. Illustrated Med. News, 1889, iv, 148.

Lawton: Case of Vascular (Erectile) Tumor in the Sheath of the Cord in a New-born. London Obstet. Trans., 1866, vii, 210.

Ledderhose, G.: Chirurgische Erkrankungen des Nabels. Deutsche Chirurgie, 1890, Lief. 45 b.

Nicaise: Ombilic. Dictionnaire encyclopedique des sc. medicales, Paris, 1881, 2. ser., xv, 140.

Pernice, L.: Die Nabelgeschwulste, Halle, 1892.

Robson, R.: Disease of the Funis Umbilicalis. Medical Examiner, Chicago, 1872, xiii, 33.

Virchow: Die krankhaften Geschwulste, 1862-63, hi, erste Halfte, 467.

UMBILICAL LYMPHOCELE.

Koeberle,* in 1878, speaking of ovarian cysts, said that sometimes the lymphatic vessels beneath the umbilicus take on an excessive development and the umbilicus becomes the site of a tumor consisting exclusively of the sac-like dilatations of the lymphatic vessels.

* Koeberle: Nouveau dictionnaire de med. et de chir. prat., 1878, xxv, 522.

Codet de Boisset quotes a letter from Koeberle to Blum in which Koeberle* stated that in his Cases 49 and 50 he had removed growths of this character when operating for ovarian tumors. One of these umbilical tumors was 8 cm. in diameter.

He further drew attention to the fact that similar tumors had never been described.

They are evidently very rare, as I have not found mention of any in the literature.

In a very large series of patients from whom ovarian tumors have been removed at the Johns Hopkins Hospital we have never seen umbilical growths of this character.

BENIGN CONNECTIVE-TISSUE GROWTHS OF THE UMBILICUS.

Under this head are included myxomata, fibromata, papillomata, and lipomata.

As a rule, papillomata are classified with epithelial growths. In umbilical papillomata, however, the connective-tissue growth is the essential feature, the epithelium playing a passive role §. I have accordingly included them under connective-tissue growths.

Myxomata of the Umbilicus.

These tumors are exceptionally rare. According to Ledderhose %, J Weber collected three cases — those of Fischer-Coin, Busch, and his own. In Busch's case the tumor was the size of a goose's egg. Its surface was ulcerated.

§Quoted by Pernice: Die Nabelgeschwiilste, Halle, 1892, 21.

% Ledderhose, G.: Deutsche Chirurgie, 1890, Lief. 45 b.

UMBILICAL TUMORS

Mori* described a sessile umbilical tumor the size of a cherry, which had ulcerated at its most prominent part. Histologically, it consisted of fibrous and myxomatous tissue. He gives a very good picture of the microscopic appearance. In Pernice's** monograph will be found the best description of this class of umbilical tumors. He says that myxoma of the umbilicus was first described by Weber, and was supposed to originate from portions of Wharton's jelly. The rendition is very rare, only nine cases being found in the literature. On section the tumors look like white pork, are pale, edematous, and gelatinous. Some are soft. others hard, according to the amount of connective tissue. They vary in size from that of a hazelnut to that of a goose's egg. In four cases the tumors were pedunculated and the pedicle came directly from the umbilical scar. In two cases the tumors lay on the top of an umbilical hernia. Pernice points out that only the cases since Weber's time have been examined microscopically. The blood-vessels are abundant. The vessel- walls are thick and lie in a connective-tissue framework consisting chiefly of spindle-cells and sometimes of round-cells. There is an intercellular substance. In other words, the ground-substance is like that encountered in embryonic tissue. Most of these tumors are covered over with normal skin, and only rarely is the surface ulcerated. The prognosis is good.

Pernice then goes on to record cases reported by Weber, Maunoir, Chassaignac, Lawton, Villar, Virchow, and Leydhecker. In only a few of the cases are the microscopic reports of any value.

Fibromata of the Umbilicus.

Growths of this character are likewise rare. Although the majority occur in middle life and in males, they are sometimes found in infants. The size of the tumors reported varied greatly. One was as large as a bird's egg, another the size of a walnut, another as large as an apple. The largest was said to be the size of an infant's head at term. They are usually oval or round and more or less pedunculated, the pedicle springing from the umbilical depression. Sometimes, however, the umbilicus may be recognized as an irregular slit in the center of the tumor.

The growth is usually covered with normal or slightly atrophic skin. On account of the exposed site of the tumor, its more prominent surface may be excoriated, presenting blackened points; or the injured areas may be covered with crusts. On section, the growth usually presents a grayish-white or whitish-yellow surface, with a definite fibrous arrangement. In a few instances one or more small cysts containing serous fluid were found, or a small quantity of fat was detected in the tumor.

Histologic examination shows that the skin covering the growth is normal or atrophic, or that there is some thickening of the squamous layers. In the last type the papilla are much elongated. The stroma of the tumor consists, as a rule, of typical fibrous tissue containing a varying number of spindle-shaped nuclei. Some of the growths, particularly where there has been an irritation of the surface, show marked small-round-cell infiltration in the vicinity of the point or points of such irritation. Here, as in other parts of the body, the diagnosis between a very cellular fibroma and a spindle-cell sarcoma is fraught with much difficulty or is impossible.

* Mori, A. : Contribute) alio studio dei tumori ombelicali. Gazzetta degli ospedali, Milano, 1902, xxiii, 632.

**Pernice: Die Nabelgeschwulste, Halle, 1892.

On account of the rarity of this condition, I append those cases in which the diagnosis of fibroma of the umbilicus was certain, or at least highly probable.

Cases of Fibroma of the Umbilicus.

Fibroma of the Umbilicus.

Legrand* reported from Sappey's service the case of a man fifty-one years of age. When the patient was thirty-nine years old a tumor the size of a hazelnut had been observed at the umbilicus. This was soft and covered with skin of a natural color. For five months before the patient came under observation it had been increasing rapidly, becoming more than two- thirds larger. Later, small excoriations were noticed on the surface. These were covered with crusts.

On admission to the hospital an ovoid tumor, about seven or eight inches in its vertical diameter, was found in the umbilical region. It was somewhat pedunculated, and with the patient- lying down reached to within 1 cm. of the xiphoid. The pedicle was inserted in the umbilical scar. The tumor itself was hard, smooth, round, and in its right third bossed and ulceiated. In other portions it was covered with brownish-yellow crusts alternating with a purple discoloration of the skin. At some points fluctuation was noted, but there was no hemorrhage from the surface. The patient's general condition was good. The tumor was removed and recovery followed. The tumor on section was whitish in color, homogeneous, and very hard. It contained a small, cyst-like cavity with serous fluid contents. Robin, who made the histologic examination, said that it was a fibroplastic tumor and not a cancer.

A Fibro nucleated Tumor at the Umbilicus.**

The patient was thirty years of age, and the tumor had been noticed for three months. On admission to the hospital in April, 1857, the tumor was the size of an orange and situated beside the umbilicus. It had evidently developed in the umbilical wall, and was firm and fibrous in character. The general health was good. On histologic examination the tumor was found to be composed of fibrous tissue. Bryant t draws attention to the fact that such tumors are evidently rare.

Fibrolipoma of the Umbilicus. J

Hugh G., aged thirty, seven years before had noticed a small lump about the size of a walnut at the site of the navel. It increased gradually for two years, when a surgeon, probably a quack, "put it back," but it soon returned. Until six months before Barton% saw him the tumor had increased only gradually, but since then had doubled in size. It was so large that it prevented the patient from walking. It was oval, and extended across the abdomen from the umbilicus to the left anterior superior spine. It was slightly constricted at its base, measured 23 inches in circumference, and was fixed to the skin only at the umbilicus. On removal it was found attached to the underlying tissue at only one point. The abdomen was not opened. No histologic examination is mentioned.

Fibromata of the Umbilicus.

Damalix§ treats the subject in general, and says that Sappey and Limange report cases in which the pedicle came from the umbilicus.

* Legrand: Tumeur volumineuse de la region ombilicale de nature fibroplastique, prise pour une tumeur encephalolide. Gaz. des hop., 1850, 29.

**Pernice: Die Nabelgeschwulste, Halle, 1892.

t Bryant, T.: Guy's Hospital Reports, 1863, ix, 245.

% Barton: Reported by Bennett: Dublin Jour. Med. Sci., 1882, lxxiv, 239.

§ Damalix: Etude sur les fibromes de la paroi abdominale anterieure. These de Paris, 1886, No. 148.

A Fibroma of the Umbilicus. *

A woman, twenty- two years of age, entered the Hotel-Dieu on May 20, 1888. In February, 1887, one month after her child had been weaned, an umbilical tumor was first noticed. This was the size of a hazelnut, and could be rolled between the fingers. For a time it grew slowly, but after six months rapidly. At the umbilical site was a tumor the size of the head of a child at term. Its summit was divided by the distended umbilical cicatrix. The tumor was hard, with several points of softening. It was irregular and bossed. The skin covering was normal, without any marked dilatation of the veins. It slid readily over the tumor.

The growth was easily dissected out, but was found intimately adherent to the peritoneum. Recovery followed. The tumor was hemispheric, irregular, about 10 cm. in diameter; it had a whitish surface, and presented an irregular, bossed appearance in the depth, where there were several depressions dividing it into lobules. On section it was whitish and smooth; in the deeper portion, yellowish in color. Here it had a definite fibrous arrangement.

Histologically, the tumor was composed exclusively of fibrous tissue, wavy threads for the most part running parallel to one another, but with no characteristic arrangement. The cells were abundant and in general well developed. They were fusiform in shape. The tumor seemed to have originated from the aponeurosis. It was a fibroma.

Fibrous Tumors in the Umbilicus.

Pernice** says this form of tumor cannot be sharply differentiated histologically from those of inflammatory origin. It may originate from three different parts of the umbilicus: (1) From the dense connective tissue of the umbilical scar; (2) from that of the skin which, as we have seen, is really scar tissue covered with epithelium; (3) in young individuals from myxomatous connective-tissue remains of the cord.

Fibroma of the Umbilicus [?].

This case occurred in Volkmann's private practice. E. H., aged forty-two, had at the umbilicus a hard, slightly lobulated, broad-based tumor the size of an apple. This was thought to be a fibroma. On histologic examination, however, it proved to be a spindle-cell sarcoma. The spindle-cells were relatively small and had large nuclei. The abdomen was not opened. The woman was well at the end of ten years. [A sarcoma occurring in the abdominal wall is so intimately associated with the surrounding tissue that one would hardly expect a permanent recovery, such as occurred in this case. This fact would rather indicate a cellular fibroma. — T. S. C]

A Fibroma of the Umbilicus [?].§

A man, forty-nine years of age, entered Polaillon's service at the Hotel-Dieu March 25, 1895. Eighteen months before he had noticed at the umbilicus small tubercles, which had caused pain and inconvenience.

Attached to the lower border of the umbilicus was a pedunculated tumor, cylindric in form, 5 cm. long and 12 or 13 mm. in diameter. Its free end showed a small crust covering a healed area of ulceration. The skin covering it was delicate and reddish in color.

On taking the tumor between the fingers it gave the sensation of the finger of a glove filled with nuts. The skin surrounding the tumor contained seven or eight pinkish tubercles about the size of green peas. The skin alone was involved, as the tumor was movable on the underlying aponeurosis. No enlarged glands were detected, and the general health was good. The diseased area was removed. Histologic examination of the main tumor and of the small nodules showed sarcoma fusocellulare covered with skin. The superficial half of the skin seemed to have been the starting-point of the tumor, which tended to pass out and become pedunculated.

[The growth may equally well have been a fibroma associated with secondary small nodules. The microscopic examination is not conclusive. — T. S. C]

* Pic, Adrien: Lyon med., 1888, lix, 546.

** Pernice, L.: Die Nabelgeschwülste, Halle, M. Niemeyer1892.

§ Sourdille, Gilbert : Sarcome pedicule de la peau de l'ombilie. Bull, de la Soc. anat. de Paris, 1895, lxx, 302.

Probably a Fibroma of the Umbilicus.*

J. W., ten months old, was brought to the clinic February 27, 1896. He had remains of the omphalomesenteric duct at the umbilicus, as recognized by a reddish tumor covered with ntestinal mucosa. In addition there was a smooth, cap-like area partly coveringthis reddish tumor, which was composed chiefly of fibrous tissue. [Evidently a true fibroma. — T. S. C]

A Small Fibroma Associated with an Umbilical Concretion.

Coenen** reports cholesteatomata of the umbilicus, and in his Fig. 2 shows a definite but small fibroma occupying the umbilical cicatrix. It is covered over with many layers of squamous epithelium. The central portion consists of fibrous tissue, and scattered throughout it are many small round-cells, indicating- recent inflammation. The inflammatory reaction was evidently started up by the umbilical concretion.

Papillomata of the Umbilicus.

Probably the first case of this character recorded was that of Fabricius von Hilden, published in 1526. From that time on isolated cases of papilloma of the umbilicus have been recorded, but, as in the majority of these no microscopic examination was made and as the gross picture was not sufficiently convincing, we have omitted most of these, confining our attention chiefly to those cases in which a careful histologic description has been given. Most of the tumors have been noted between the twenty-fifth and fiftieth years. In Broussolle's case, however, in a child only two months old, a typical papilloma, 5 mm. in diameter, occupied the umbilical depression. Ordinarily one would consider this small nodule in such a young individual as a mass of granulation tissue left after the cord had come away, or as a remnant of the omphalomesenteric duct. Broussolle, however, distinctly says that its surface was covered with squamous epithelium analogous to that of the skin. From the limited number of cases it is difficult to draw any definite conclusion, but papillomata seem to be equally frequent in both sexes. As a rule, they are of slow growth and vary from 5 mm. in diameter to the size of a walnut. They are usually pedunculated, but in the case reported by Peraire the papillary growth had spread out for a considerable distance into the surrounding- abdominal wall.

* Sauer, F.: Ein Fall von Prolaps eines offenen Meckelschen Divertikels am Nabel.

Deutsche Zeitschr. f. Chir., 1896-97, xliv, 316.

** Coenen, H.: Uber Das CholesteatomDes Nabels. Münch. Med. Wochenschr., 1909, 56. Jahrg., 1583.

Where the growth is small, it frequently looks red and reminds one of a raspberry, and on examination with a magnifying-glass it is found to be composed of blunt papillary masses. As the growth increases in size the portion near the pedicle may have a violet tint, while the superficial portion is pinkish in color.

In Segond's case, reported by Villar, the growth consisted of rounded projections varying greatly in size. The largest nodule was bean-shaped and contained a small cyst; another was the size of a pea, and lying between them were smaller ones. As a rule, when the tumor reaches its full size it resembles a large wart. Its surface is covered with myriads of papillae, and these are flattened laterally, owing to the close juxtaposition. On section the papillary or tree-like arrangement is clearly evident, and the stroma of the nodule and of its pedicle is seen to consist of fibrous tissue. Histologic examination shows that the surface of the papillae is covered with squamous epithelium, in which epithelial pearls can occasionally be demonstrated. Where there has been much irritation, the epithelium may be thickened and the skin papillae greatly lengthened. The stroma of the papillary growth consists of fibrous tissue. Just beneath the epithelium this may show marked infiltration and greatly dilated blood capillaries. The general appearance, both macroscopically and microscopically, is similar to that of skin papillomata in any part of the body.

Cases of Papilloma of the Umbilicus.

Papillomata of the Umbilicus[?].

Küster* cites a case seen by Fabricius von Hilden and recorded in 1526. A man, twenty-five years of age, well nourished, had a fungating excrescence at the umbilicus which had developed in about six months. The tumor was the size of a walnut, bright red in color, and emitted an odor like that of foul cheese. At first it was painless; later there were severe pain and two hemorrhages. Fabricius considered the growth a carcinoma. On exposing the tumor he found that it consisted of three portions, each with a delicate pedicle. He ligated the pedicles and the patient was well five months later. [This does not seem to have been carcinoma, but suggests rather a papilloma with inflammation of the umbilicus due to accumulation of foul material. Of course, at that time no histologic examination was made. — T. S. C]

In Küster's Case 8 a man, thirty-six years of age, had had a specific ulcer on the glans penis eight months before. Six weeks prior to observation he noticed that the umbilicus was moist. In the left umbilical fold was a small tumor which grew rapidly. Astringents proved of no value. On examination, in the left side of the umbilical cavity was a pedunculated tumor the size of a phalanx of the little finger; it was movable, and discharged a foul-smelling fluid. It was covered with small red bodies (papillae) and looked like a raspberry. When the umbilicus was split open small papillary outgrowths were found springing from it. [On histologic examination the mass was found to be a simple papilloma covered over with several layers of epithelium. In some places there were epithelial pearls.]

Papilloma of the Umbilicus. — Tillmanns,** after saying that Kiister had described a papilloma of the umbilicus, mentions a case seen by Wilms.

Papilloma of the Umbilicus. ±

In a woman, fifty-four years of age, a tumordeveloped from a congenital umbilical nevus. This tumor became excoriated, and there was a discharge of bloody fluid.

It reached the volume of an egg, and two enlarged glands were noted in the inguinal region. The tumor and the glands were removed. Demarquay%says the inguinal glands were not malignant, but that the enlargement was due to irritation from the growth. On histologic examination the growth proved to be a papilloma

* Küster: Die Neubildungen am Nabel Erwachsener und ihre operative Behandlung.

Langenbeck's Arch. f. klin. Chir., 1874, xvi, 234.

** Tillmanns: Deutsche Zeitschr. f. Chir., 1882-83, xviii, 161.

% Demarquay: Bull, de la Soc. de chir., 1870-71, 2. ser., xi, 209.

Papilloma of the Umbilicus.*

The patient, a concierge, forty-three years of age, a year before he entered the hospital had noticed an irritation of the umbilicus. In the umbilical depression there were small elevations the size of pinheads. They had gradually increased in size, until six months later the tumor had emerged above the level of the umbilical depression and there were excoriations. At operation the growth was the size of a franc piece, round, with a narrow base. Microscopic examination showed that it was a fibropapilloma of the umbilical cicatrix.

Papilloma of the Umbilicus.

Broussolle** reported a case of a child, two months old, who suffered from suppuration at the umbilicus. There was a minute umbilical tumor, reddish in color, 5 mm. in diameter. Microscopic examination showed that it was a true papilloma composed of connective tissue only slightly organized. Its surface was covered with squamous epithelium analogous to that of the skin.

Papilloma of the Umbilicus.

This case was communicated to Villar% by E. Launois. M. H., aged forty-six, was operated upon by Dr. Segond for a very large fibroma of the uterus. At the umbilicus also she had a lobulated tumor, which occupied all the cavity of the umbilical depression. This tumor had first been noticed six years previously. It had increased slowly in volume, its development occurring chiefly in the appearance of small lobules. The mass was very tender on pressure and on palpation. On examination it was found to consist of a series of small elevations juxtaposed to one another. Above and below were two rounded masses. The upper one was the size of a pea, the lower one presented the form and volume of a bean. Between the two were other lobules. The surface of the two voluminous portions was covered with skin which had retained its characteristic appearance, but was wrinkled. The small granulations had a blackish-violet appearance. At first sight the growth suggested a melanotic tumor. The umbilical nodules were included in the abdominal incision when the uterine tumor was removed.

At the base of the tumor were a number of vascular orifices distended with blood.

The mass, which was the size of a pea, consisted of a small cyst containing yellowish liquid.

Histologic Examination. — The tumor was divided into three fragments. The first contained the cyst which has been described. The walls were composed of dense connective tissue. At several points in the cyst were remnants of epithelium. The second fragment comprised all the small elevations between the two larger ones. They were composed of a series of papillae. Each papilla was formed of dense connective tissue containing a few nuclei. The skin covering the surface presented the usualcharacteristics. The Malpighian layer was thicker than usual, and many cells contained yellowish-brown pigment. In each of the papillae were numerous capillary vessels anastomosing with one another. The third fragment consisted of the inferior elevation, and was much larger than the first; it was formed of dense connective tissue, and the skin covering was somewhat thinner. The entire growth was evidently a papilloma.

* Nicaise, M. : Fibro-papillome de la cicatrice ombilicale. Revue de chir., Paris, 1883, iii, 29.

**Broussolle, E.: Des vegetations de I'ombilic. Revue mens, des mal. de l'enfance, 1886, iv. 314. '

% Villar: Tumeura de I'ombilic. These de Paris, 1886, obs. 38, p. 71.

Papilloma of the Umbilicus.

Ledderhose* says that Rizzoli had a patient, fifty-one years old, with an ulcerating papilloma at the umbilicus which was removed with zinc paste.

Fibropapilloma of the Umbilicus. **

M. K., a fireman, aged thirty-five, three months before admission and shortly after a blow in the umbilical region, had noticed a small tumor at the umbilicus. This had steadily increased in size, and latterly caused much inconvenience and at times a dull, throbbing pain. The umbilical cavity was completely obliterated by a prominent, firm growth the margin of which was continuous with the skin of the abdominal wall. This growth was circular, with a diameter of 1% inches. Its surface presented a warty appearance, and was covered with elongated papillary growths varying in size and flattened laterally by mutual compression. The surface of the tumor was pinkish in color, intact, and free from discharge of any kind.

This prominent and warty growth was seated on and continuous with a very hard, thick growth extending all around and into the umbilicus, and forming a subjacent swelling about three inches in diameter. The whole mass was freely movable in all directions. When the growth was removed, the abdomen was examined and found perfectly normal.

On section the tumor was of a dull white color, and its substance, which was of almost cartilaginous hardness, was directly continuous without well-defined margins. It had extended into the surrounding fat and other tissue..The peritoneum was adherent to the tumor and drawn up into it. The entire tumor presented to the naked eye an appearance very similar to that of a recent specimen of cancer of the mamma.

On histologic examination it was found to consist of fibrous tissue fully developed. The growth was a so-called fibropapilloma. [Smith's description is a particularly good one. — T. S. C]

Papillary Fibromata of the Umbilicus.

In the literature Pernice% found only seven definite cases of papilloma of the umbilicus, and he added one from the Halle clinic. [These cases did not impress us very definitely as being instances of simple papilloma.] Pernice says that the outer surface of the papilloma, as well as the stroma, is similar to that found in other parts of the body. Where an ulcerated papilloma of the umbilicus exists, a lymphatic swelling of the inguinal glands may follow, but this does not necessarily indicate that carcinoma exists. Where a papilloma is not pedunculated, the diagnosis may be difficult prior to operation. The clinical course of papilloma is benign throughout. He then goes on to report the cases of Kuster, Weber, Billroth, Blum, Villar, and mentions some reported by Duges. In very few of these is it absolutely clear that a careful histologic examination was made. In a second case of Kuster 's the microscopic examination showed that the growth was a simple papilloma. Pernice also reports some rather indefinite cases from the clinic at Halle.

* Ledderhose: Deutsche Chirurgie, 1890, Lief. 45 b.

** Smith, J. : The Lancet, 1890, i, 1013.

% Pernice, L. : Die Nabelgeschwtilste, Halle, 1892.

Pernice says that when his article was already in the printer's hands he had an opportunity of seeing a rare case of papilloma of the umbilicus observed in a patient coming under the care of Dr. Harttung, of Frankfort. This patient was a woman, fifty-two years old, very corpulent, and previously healthy. Four years before, the umbilicus, which was markedly funnel-shaped, had commenced to be moist. The patient was not cleanly. After some time there was a reddening in the depth with much irritation and itching, which caused the patient to rub the umbilicus. Later on a wart-like appearance was noted. The secretion was much more abundant, and the patient complained of pain.

On examination the umbilicus was found to be much drawn in, very much reddened, and there were excoriated places on the skin about the size of a mark. In the center of this eczematous area was the umbilicus. It was covered with a large number of papillary-like growths, each being about the size of half a grain of wheat. These papillomata resembled in their color and arrangement pointed condylomata. When the abdominal walls were drawn apart, a large number of smaller papillomata were seen and there was a purulent secretion.

No induration could be made out at the base of the tumor, the axillary and inguinal glands were not swollen, and there were no symptoms referable to other organs.

The diagnosis of papilloma of the umbilicus was made, and the growth removed. The tumor was about 2 cm. in height and the skin of the part was raised. From the center of the tumor sprang about 20 or 30 wart-like growths of soft consistence. These were covered with smooth epidermis, and all their ends were somewhat pointed. These papillary masses filled the entire umbilical pocket, which was 2 to 3 cm. deep. Their epidermis was not ulcerated at any point.

The microscopic picture was very simple, and corresponded identically with the picture of the soft warts — in other words, the growth was a true papilloma. Along the edge was perfectly normal skin; toward the center the epidermis became thicker, and between the papillae of the skin the epithelial projections were irregular, sometimes longer and narrower, and at other times thick and plump. The papillary masses consisted of a connective-tissue groundwork with an epithelial covering. The epithelium was here more irregular, and sometimes sent prolongations downward. The masses were, however, simple throughout. On the surface the hornification was somewhat advanced. The connective tissue of the tumor and also of the surrounding skin showed abundant small-round-cell infiltration.

Papilloma of the Umbilicus.*

R. A., aged twenty-seven, had had a swelling at the umbilicus for four months, which discharged a serosanguineous fluid. On admission a tumor, the size of a walnut, was found situated in the center of the umbilicus. At its base it had a violet tint, and at its summit was grayishwhite. It was sessile, soft, and round, resembling a wart. It was very painful on palpation. It was thought to be a papillofibroma of the umbilicus, and was removed under local anesthesia.

The microscopic examination was made by Professor Cornil. The skin was very irregular and in the form of papillae. The papillae on the surface of the tumor were very long, very abundant, tree-like, and formed the depression penetrating the connective tissue. They were composed of dense connective tissue supporting the blood-vessels and were covered with epithelium. Between the epithelial cells were leukocytes. The tumor was a fibropapilloma showing inflammatory reaction, Peraire remarks that this variety of tumor is rare. Villar reported only four cases — those of Kiister, Blum, Nicaise, and Segond.

* Peraire, Maurice: Fibro-papillome de l'ombilic. Bull, de la Soc. anat. de Paris, 1902, lxxvii, 346.

Papilloma of the Umbilicus.*

Mrs. B. C. C, aged forty-two, a patient of Dr. W. T. Watson, was admitted to the Church Home and Infirmary October 26, 1910. During the abdominal preparation prior to removing the appendix and shortening the round ligaments, we noticed a small papillary mass at the umbilicus. It was excised.

The specimen is 5 mm. broad, 4 mm. long, slightly pedunculated. Its surface is divided into three lobules, which are perfectly smooth and remind one very much of a small fibroma.

Histologic Examination. — The greater part of the specimen imbibes hematoxylin with avidity. The surface is covered with very atrophic squamous epithelium, the superficial portion of which is hornified. The deepest layer contains yellowish and brownish pigment in places, and reminds one of the skin of a colored person, although the patient is white. Beneath the epithelium is a narrow zone of connective tissue, poor in cell elements, and beneath this again fibrous tissue, literally packed with cells containing oval or round, uniformly staining nuclei. Dividing the fibrous tissue into alveoli are minute arterioles. Small papilloma in the umbilical depression central portion of the specimen is made up of fibrous tissue poor in cell elements. The picture at first suggests sarcoma. The surface epithelium is, however, everywhere intact. The nuclei of the stroma cells, although exceedingly abundant, there is no evidence of nuclear figures. The surface of each lobule are uniform in size. In addition, the clinical history shows that the patient had had this small nodule for years. It is a simple papilloma of the umbilicus.

LIPOMATA OF THE UMBILICAL REGION.

In the umbilical depression there is little or no fat, consequently we should not expect to find any fatty tumors in this situation. Tillmanns,** however, points out that Wrany has drawn attention to the fact that, where there is a dilatation of the umbilical ring, some of the subperitoneal fat may escape through the hernial ring, producing an " adipose hernia " or a lipoma, which may be confused with an omental hernia.

A reference to Levadoux's*** masterly article on the Anatomy of the Umbilicus clearly shows just how such a hernial protrusion may occur at or near the umbilicus.

* Cullen, Thomas S.: Personal observation.

** Tillmanns: Ueber angeborenen Prolaps von Magenschleimhaut durch den Nabelring (Ectopia ventriculi), und iiber sonstige Geschwiilste und Fisteln des Nabels. Deutsche Zeitschr. f. Chir., 1882-83, xvhi, 161.

*** Levadoux: Varietes de l'ombilic et de ses annexes. These de la Fac. de med. et de pharm. de Toulouse, 1907, No. 711.

LITERATURE CONSULTED ON BENIGN CONNECTIVE-TISSUE GROWTHS OF THE UMBILICUS.

Barton: Fibrolipoma of the Umbilicus. Dublin Jour. Med. Sc, 1882, lxxiv, 239.

Bennett: See Barton.

Bryant, T. : A Fibronucleated Tumor. Guy's Hospital Reports, 1863, ix, 245.

Broussolle, E. : Des vegetations de l'ombilic. Rev. mens, des mal. de l'enfance, 1886, iv, 314.

Coenen: Das Nabelcholesteatom. Munch, med. Wochenschr., 56. Jahrg., 1909, 1583.

Cullen Thomas S. : Papilloma of the Umbilicus.

Damalix: Etude sur les fibromes de la paroi abdominale anterieure. These de Paris, 1886, No. 48.

Demarquay : Cancer de l'ombilic. Bull, de la Soc. de chir., 1870-71, 2. ser., xi, 209.

Green, CD.: Trans. Path. Soc. of London, 1899, 1, 243.

Küster, E. : Die Neubildungen am Nabel Erwachsener und ihre operative Behandlung. Langenbeck's Arch. f. klin. Chir., 1874, xvi, 234.

Ledderhose, G.: Deutsche Chirurgie, 1890, Lief. 45 b.

Legrand: Tumeur volumineuse de la region ombilicale de nature fibroplastique, prise pour une tumeur encephaloi'de (fibrome de l'ombilic). Gaz. des hop., 1850, 29.

Mori, A.: Contributo alio studio dei tumori ombelicali. Gazz. degli ospedali, Milano, 1902, xxiii, 632.

Nicaise: Fibro-papilloma de la cicatrice ombilicale. Rev. de chir., Paris, 1883, hi, 29.

Peraire, Maurice: Fibro-papillome de l'ombihc. Bull, de la Soc. anat. de Paris, 1902, lxxvii, 346.

Pernice, L. : Die Nabelgeschwulste, Halle, 1892.

Pic, Adrien: Lyon med., 1888, lix, 546.

Sauer, F.: Em Fall von Prolaps eines offenen Meckel'schen Divertikels am Nabel. Deutsche Zeitschr. f. Chir., 1896-97, xliv, 316.

Smith, J.: Fibroma of the Umbilicus. The Lancet, 1890, i, 1013.

Sourdille, G. : Sarcome pedicule de la peau de l'ombilic. Bull, de la Soc. anat. de Paris, 1895, lxx,

Tillmanns: Deutsche Zeitschr. f. Chir., 1882-83, xviii, 161.

Villar, F. : Tumeurs de l'ombilic. These de Paris, 1886, No. 19.

DERMOIDS OR ATHEROMATOUS CYSTS OF THE UMBILICUS.*

Judging from the number of cases reported one would infer that dermoids at the umbilicus are by no means rare. Nevertheless, on carefully following the clinical histories and checking up the pathologic findings, one finds that in nearly all the cases the supposed dermoid cyst was nothing more than an umbilical concretion, in the majority of the cases associated with suppuration, and that the diagnosis of dermoid cyst has erroneously been made owing to the presence of the sebaceous material and hairs in the discharge from the infected umbilicus. Villar, in 1886, pointed out this erroneous conception, and several others have also mentioned it.

* In this connection we used the words dermoid and atheromatous as synonymous terms.

After carefully analyzing the cases of supposed dermoids or atheromata of the umbilicus that are available in the literature, I have found among them only six that were true umbilical dermoid cysts. These were reported by Kiister, Lotzbeck, Morestin, Lannelongue and Fremont, Hue and Guelliot. These atheromatous tumors were all noted in young patients. In three they were found at birth, in one after the cord came away, and in the remaining two they had been present since childhood.

A dermoid cyst may spring from the umbilical cicatrix or from the side of^the umbilicus. It may reach the size of a walnut and tend to become pedunculated. It may be tense or occur as a flaccid sac. It contains sebaceous material, which, on histologic examination, yields epithelium, fat-droplets, and frequently cholesterin crystals. The cyst-walls examined histologically have shown an inner lining of squamous epithelium devoid of hairs or glands of any sort, and in none of the cases have hairs been detected in the cyst contents.

The skin covering these cysts is, as a rule, unaltered. In Morestin's case, however, as a result of the rubbing of the clothing, it had become reddened at one pointand slight suppuration had occurred, followed by discharge of the characteristic cyst contents.

Detailed Report of Cases of Dermoid or Atheromatous Cysts of the Umbilicus.

Dermoid Cyst at the Umbilicus.*

In July, 1872, Küster saw a woman, twenty-one years old, who had a tumor at the umbilicus. This had been noted since birth. It was round, soft, and attached to the umbilicus by a pedicle. It sprang from the left of the umbilical depression, and was easily shelled out. It had thin walls, and the sac was filled with atheromatous material, fat, epithelial cells, and cholesterin crystals. No microscopic examination was made of the nodule. It was probably, as Küster thought, a dermoid.

A Pedunculated Sebaceous Cyst of the Umbilicus.**

A man, twenty-seven years of age, entered the service of Pean. At birth he had had at the umbilicus a tumor the size of a hazelnut. Within five or six weeks before he entered, as the result of pressure produced by a belt, it had increased to four times its original size; it had become red at its prominent part, slightly ulcerated, and a whitish, thick, granular, or clotted material had escaped from it. On examination the tumor was found to be the size and shape of a small fig, and was attached to the umbilical cicatrix. It was lax, a little wrinkled, and gave the sensation of a half-empty pouch. It was not painful on pressure.

The skin covering it was thin. The patient refused operation. A congenital sebaceous cyst was diagnosed.

Cyst of the Umbilicus, Possibly a Dermoid.

Ledderhose,*** after saying that the literature on the subject, is scanty, refers to a case reported by Lotzbeck, in which Bruns removed a multilocular tumor the size of a ist from a child two and one-half years old. This had been noticed immediately after birth, and was then the size of a walnut. It contained fluid which was partly clear amber yellow, somewhat alkaline, and partly thick, honey-brown, and gelatinous. The tumor lay between the skin and the rectus. The connective-tissue wall of the cyst contained small, thread-like, cartilaginous deposits, and was lined with a simple squamous epithelium. The contents were fat, cholesterin, and numerous cells.

A Congenital Dermoid Cyst.§

A child, nine years old, presented in the middle of the umbilicus a hemispheric protuberance the size of half a walnut. The skin had not changed color. The central portion of the tumor was soft and fluctuating. It was circumscribed, but in the deeper portion adherent. It was not enlarged by crying, was irreducible, and was found to be a cyst. It had been noted immediately after the cord came away, and had enlarged rapidly during the first five or six months of life. At operation it was found to contain sebaceous material.

* Kiister: Die Neubildungen am Nabel Erwachsener und ihre operative Behandlung. Langenbeck's Arch. f. klin. Cbir., 1874, xvi, 234.

**Guelliot: Observation de kyste sebace pedicule de l'ombilic. Revue de chir., 1883, iii, 193.

*** Ledderhose: Deutsche Chirurgie, 1890, Lief. 45 b.

§ Lannelongue et Fremont: De quelques varietes de tumeurs congenitales de 1'ombiUc et plus specialement des tumeurs adenoides diverticulaires. Arch. gen. de med., 1884, 7. ser., xiii, 36.

A Dermoid Cyst at the Umbilicus.

Hue* noted a dermoid cyst of the umbilicus as large as a pigeon's egg. It had been taken for an umbilical hernia. The patient, a girl of nineteen, had carried it from childhood, and had only suffered from some slight inconvenience. The umbilical depression had been replaced by this round tumor. The skin covering it was normal, but the tumor was attached to the umbilical cicatrix by a flattened pedicle. It was soft, painless, and irreducible, but was easily removed. At the meeting of the Medical Society Hue showed photographs of the case. I wrote asking Dr. Hue if he could send me a photograph of the tumor. He replied saying that the photographs had been mislaid, but as soon as he found them he would gladly send me one, but thus far I have not received a second communication from him.

Deve found it to be a cyst covered over with normal skin, and containing a whitish, creamy material without any development of hair. The cyst-wall was scarcely 1 mm. thick, composed of fibrous tissue, and lined with squamous epithelium without hair or glands of any sort. Hue thought it had originated from a nipping-off of a fragment of skin in the umbilical cicatrix following the dropping-off of the cord.

A Dermoid Cyst of the Umbilicus **

The patient was a male, nineteen years old. Since childhood he had had a small round tumor attached to the umbilicus. A few days before Morestin saw him it had become tender, more prominent, and pink or reddish in color. It had occasioned some suffering. On the night after admission a whitish material was seen escaping from a small opening at the point where the redness had developed. On examination the nodule was found to be the size of a walnut, whitish red, and occupying the center of the umbilical region. It was attached by a pedicleto the center of the umbilicus. The surrounding skin was normal. The growth was removed under local anesthesia, but the peritoneal cavity was not opened. The cyst contained some greasy whitish material. There were no hairs. Mallet made slides and found an epithelial lining, but no hairs and no glands. He felt sure that the tumor was a dermoid cyst.

A Possible Dermoid of the Umbilicus.%

In this case of Villar's it is impossible to determine accurately whether or not the cyst was in reality atheromatous in character. It did not seem to be in any way associated with an inflammation of the umbilicus.

Yillart reports a case of dermoid cyst occurring in the service of Professor Verneuil. M. 0., a Russian officer twenty-seven years old, was seen in consultation June, 1886, for a small tumor of the umbilicus situated exactly in the left of the umbilicus and passing off from the umbilical depression. The tumor was the size of a walnut and semifluctuant.

On pressure it did not change in volume. It had been present for a little more than two years and had not increased in size until a short while before. On pressure it was painful. The diagnosis lay between a small umbilical hernia, a cyst, and a lipoma. The tumor was opened with a bistoury and there escaped a clear liquid; a cystic sac remained. The

histologic examination was made by Clado. The tumor was as big as a large walnut, was whitish blue, and fibrous in character. The inner surface presented a granular appearance and had a caseous-like covering; the contents were liquid and seropurulent. Microscopic examination showed white blood-corpuscles in large numbers and also some red blood-corpuscles, numerous very attenuated hairs, and small cholesterin crystals. Cultures from the liquid yielded a diplococcus. Examination of the cyst-wall was difficult. In the wall there were neither glandular elements nor hair-follicles. [The origin of this cyst does not seem to be perfectly clear.]

* Hue, F.: Kyste dermoide de l'ombilic. La Xormandie medicale, 1909, xxiv, 28.

** Morestin, H.: Kyste dermo'ide de l'ombilic. Bull, de la Soc. anat. de Paris, 1909, annee 84, 742.

% Villar: Tumeurs de l'ombilic. These de Paris, 1886, 66.

LITERATURE CONSULTED ON DERMOID CYSTS OF THE UMBILICUS.

(See also the literature on Umbilical Concretions)

Bondi, J.: Zur Kasuistik der Nabelcysten. Monatsschr. f. Geb. u. Gyn., 1905, xxi, 729. (From Schauta's clinic.)

Guelliot: Observation de kyste sebace pedicule de l'ombilic. Revue de chir., 1883, iii, 193.

Hue, F. : Kyste dermoiide de l'ombilic. La Normandie medicale, 1909, xxiv, 28.

Ktister, E. : Die Neubildungen am Nabel Erwachsener und ihre operative Behandlung. Langenbeck's Arch, f.klin. Chir., 1874, xvi, 234.

Lannelongue et Fremont: De quelques varietes de tumeurs congenitales de l'ombilic et plus specialement des tumeurs adenoiides diverticulaires. Arch. gen. de med., 1884, 7. ser., xiii, 36.

Ledderhose, G.: Deutsche Chirurgie, 1890, Lief. 45 b.

Morestin, H.: Kyste dermoi'de de l'ombilic. Bull, de la Soc. anat. de Paris, 1909, annee 84, 742.

Pernice, L. : Die Nabelgeschwulste, Halle, 1892.

Villar, F. : Tumeurs de l'ombilic. These de Paris, 1886.

UMBILICAL TUMORS CONSISTING CHIEFLY OF SWEAT-GLANDS.

Three cases have been recorded in which the tumor was supposed to have originated in whole or in part from sweat-glands. These were reported by Wullstein, von Noorden, and Ehrlich. In Wullstein's and also in von Noorden's case there is some doubt, and from the histories it seems to me that the growths probably originated from Miiller's duct or from uterine mucosa. This point the reader can decide for himself, as they are reported in full on p. 384 and p. 387.

In Ehrlich's case part of the growth consisted of sweat-glands, the remaining portion of uterine glands. The sweat-glands were gathered into definite colonies. Each colony was embedded in a stroma, which was sharply differentiated from the surrounding stroma, although essentially similar in character to it. The epithelium lining the glands was of the characteristic low cuboid variety. Some of the glands were dilated. I have referred to a small aggregation of sweat-glands occurring in an adenomyoma of the umbilicus that came under my personal observation. This case reminds one somewhat of the gland grouping found in fibromata of the breast. Although, as a rule, there are no sweat-glands in the umbilicus, nevertheless, the normal skin is so close to it that a tumor consisting of sweat-glands might soencroach upon the umbilicus that it could not be distinguished from one growing in the umbilical depression.

In the specimen recently sent me by Dr. Edward G. Jones of Atlanta I found sweat-glands and glands resembling those of the body of the uterus. Part of the small umbilical tumor, which was three-quarters of an inch in diameter, undoubtedly consisted of sweat-glands.

LITERATURE CONSULTED ON UMBILICAL TUMORS CONTAINING SWEAT-GLANDS.

Wullstein, L.: Arbeit-en aus dem Path. Inst, in Gottingen, R. Virchow, zum 50. Doctor-Jubilaum, 1893, 245.

Von Xoorden: Deutsche Zeitschr. f. Chir., 1901, lix, 215.

Ehrlich: Arch. f. klin. Chir., 1909, lxxxix, 742.

AN ABDOMINAL TUMOR ATTACHED TO THE INNER SURFACE OF THE UMBILICUS BY A PEDICLE TWO INCHES IN DIAMETER.

From the description of this case one gathers the impression that the tumor was a myoma. It may have been a myoma that had engrafted itself upon the umbilicus.

A few details in the description point to the possibility that the growth was an adenomyoma ("ferous matter"). We know that a small adenomyoma with glands identical with those of the uterine mucosa may be found at the umbilicus. In the cases recorded the growths have been on the outer or skin surface of the umbilicus, but there seems to be no adequate reason why they might not just as well project from the inner or peritoneal side of the umbilicus, producing, as in this case, an abdominal tumor with its pedicle attached to the umbilicus. In the umbilical adenomyomata reported, however, the tumors have always been of small size.

A Hydrops Ascites From a Tumor Depending from the Navel Internally.*

A multipara, about forty-three years of age, was thought to be pregnant. After going a year she had labor-like pains for eighteen hours. Her periods returned and continued to be regular for eight or nine months. There was then one flooding, after which no further periods were noted. She complained of fulness in the abdomen. Six years later she was tapped, large quantities of fluid being removed from time to time.

The patient finally died. A large carnous excrescence was found depending from the umbilicus by a pedicle two inches in diameter. The tumor was adherent to several parts of the peritoneum, but these adhesions were easily separated with the hand. Xo vessels were seen except those in the pedicle of the tumor. The tumor appeared to be composed of cells communicating with each other. Some contained "ferous matter," others were full of a substance of the consistence of "marrow." From these cells tubes as large as goose-quills and full of the same material passed out into the umbilicus, being contained in a thick, muscular substance of which the neck of the tumor was principally composed. The entire tumor weighed eight pounds. Nothing widely deviating from the ordinary structures was noted in the abdominal viscera.

[At this time no careful histologic examinations were made. The muscular character of the tumor, coupled with the appearance of "ferous matter" and of spaces as broad asgoose-quills filled with the same material, strongly suggests to us the possibility of an adenomyoma. Of course, this is merely surmise. The presence of ascites with a parasitic myoma is not of rare occurrence. — T. S. C]

* Johnston, William: Medical Essays and Observations, Edinburgh, 1744, v, part ii, 640.

PAPILLOMA OF THE UMBILICUS SECONDARY TO PAPILLOMA OF THE OVARY.

This is the only case of this character of which we have any record. As will be noted from the history, papilloma of the ovary and secondary abdominal nodules were found at operation in 1898. The patient was seen from time to time, and about six and a half years later a small, partially ulcerated, umbilical nodule was removed. On histologic examination the superficial portions of the nodule showed some inflammatory reaction. The remaining portions were composed of papillary masses covered over with cylindric epithelium and conforming exactly in appearance to the histologic picture of papilloma of the ovary, but differing totally from a primary papilloma of the umbilicus. The relatively benign character of the growth is evident, as the patient was in fair condition over six years after partial removal of the papillary masses from the abdomen.

Papilloma of the Umbilicus Secondary to Papilloma of the Right Ovary. F. M., a woman, was admitted to the Johns Hopkins Hospital on May 18, 1898. An exploratory laparotomy was made, and a large sac was removed, together with papillary masses from the peritoneum. The growth proved to be papillary in origin and came from the right ovary.

November 18, 1898: Two liters of ascitic fluid were removed. November 13, 1899: The abdomen was opened for papillomata of the ovary involving the peritoneum, and also for post-operative ventral hernia. November 7, 1900: An exploratory operation was performed, and 14 liters of ascitic fluid were evacuated. There was a papilloma of the right ovary the size of a child's head and also papillary growths in the parietal peritoneum. In the pelvis was a subperitoneal cystic growth surrounding the rectum on both sides. It did not seem to be made up of papillary masses, but appeared to be due to an effusion of serous fluid beneath the peritoneum. The parietal peritoneum was roughened and reddened.

March 13, 1901: Ascitic fluid was removed. March 20, 1901 : The fistulous opening in the abdominal wall was excised. March 19, 1905 : A small umbilical nodule was removed by Dr. Hunner.

The superficial portion consists of granulation tissue. Thesurface is covered with hyaline material embedded in which are a large number of polymorphonuclear leukocytes; beneath this is canalized fibrin, also containing polymorphonuclear leukocytes, and in the depth are dilated capillaries surrounded by young connective-tissue cells. The central portions are well organized. The more protected parts consist of typical papillary masses, large and small. They are covered over with one layer of cylindric ciliated epithelium. The epithelium varies considerably; in some places it is exceedingly high, and in others cuboid. The nuclei may be oval and uniformly staining, or oval and vesicular. The tumor presents the typical picture of papilloma of the ovary, although found at the umbilicus. Some of the papillary masses are well organized. In places the stroma has been replaced by hyaline tissue. In short, we have at the umbilicus a papilloma identical with an ovarian papilloma. On account of irritation from the clothing, the superficial portion has become inflamed and is partly replaced by granulation tissue. It is remarkable that the woman has lived so long, particularly with such wide-spread papillary masses. Some of these patients, however, live for a great many years.

In 1894 I* reported a case of double papillocystomata of both ovaries. Fifteen years later I heard from the same patient. She was well and had gained 49 pounds.

* Cullen, Thomas S.: Johns Hopkins Hosp. Bull, November, 1894, No. 43, 103.

ADENOMYOMA OF THE UMBILICUS.

Historic sketch.

Report of cases.

Personal observations.

UMBILICAL TUMORS CONTAINING UTERINE MUCOSA OR REMNANTS OF MULLER'S DUCTS.*

While gathering together from the literature the numerous cases of primary tumor of the umbilicus I found several that did not seem to belong to any of the classes hitherto recognized, and yet all of these cases in one or more points bear a certain amount of resemblance to one another. Finally, the picture of this new group became so firmly fixed in my mind that when reading the description of a case recorded in 1899 by Dr. Green, of Romford, England, I felt so sure that his case came under this category that I wrote him, asking if perchance he still had a section of the tumor. An examination of the slide which he kindly furnished me showed that we were right in our surmise. In brief, the clinical histories in this class of cases, coupled with the gross appearances of the tumors, leave no doubt that we are dealing with a variety of umbilical tumor never before clearly understood.

The composite picture of such tumors — which were found only in women — is as follows: At some time between the thirtieth and fifty-fifth year a small tumor develops at the umbilicus, reaching its full size in the course of a few months. It is usually described as being the size of a small nut. Sometimes it is painful, especially at the menstrual period, and in at least one instance there was a brownish, bloody discharge from the umbilicus at such times. The overlying skin is usually pigmented, and there may be one or two bluish or brownish cysts just beneath the skin. These may rupture and discharge a little brownish fluid— old blood. On section the nodule is found to be intimately attached to the skin, is very dense, and is traversed by glistening bands of fibrous tissue. Scattered throughout the nodule one sometimes finds small spaces presenting a sieve-like appearance. These spaces are filled with brownish fluid. Occasionally there may be a small cyst, several millimeters in diameter, filled with brownish contents. Exceptionally, grayish, somewhat homogeneous areas are distinguishable in the tumor. On histologic examination the superficial squamous epithelium is usually found intact. It may be normal or thickened. The stroma of the growth is composed of dense fibrous tissue. Sometimes a few bundles of non-striped muscle are noted here and there in the fibrous stroma. In other specimens the non-striped muscle is much more abundant than the fibrous tissue. Scattered throughout the field are glands, round, oval, or irregular. They occur singly or in groups, and are lined with cylindric epithelium. When occurring singly, they frequently lie in direct contact with the fibrous tissue, but when found in groups, are usually surrounded by a characteristic stroma that stains more deeply and is much more cellular than the surrounding fibrous tissue. The cells of this stroma between the glands usually have oval or round vesicular nuclei. Frequently some of the glands are dilated and their epithelium is somewhat flattened. The cyst spaces, noted macroscopically and filled with brownish fluid, are likewise dilated glands, and the fluid is old blood. The stroma around the glands frequently shows fresh hemorrhage or remnants of old blood, to be recognized by the deposit of blood pigment.

From the above description it is clearly seen that the gland picture is that of the uterine mucosa with its typical glands and its characteristic stroma, and further that the typical menstrual reaction is often present, as evidenced by the pain in the nodule at the periods, the accumulation of old menstrual blood with the formation of small cysts, and in at least one instance by the occasional discharge of blood from the umbilicus. In this case one or two of the glands opened directly on the surface, thus allowing free escape of the menstrual blood.

* Shortly after the appearance, in Surgery, Gynecology and Obstetrics (May, 1912, 479), of my article on Umbilical Tumors Containing Uterine Mucosa or Remnants of Miiller's Duct, I received the following, in a letter from Dr. S. W. Goddard, of Brockton, Mass., dated September 10, 1912: "After reading your recent article in Surgery, Gynecology and Obstetrics on Umbilical Tumors and noting a similarity to two I have published, I am sending you a reprint of the same in hopes that they may be of interest to you, and, if of any value, would be glad to have you make use of them in connection with your work, as I infer that you are specially interested in the subject. I have not seen any similar cases since."

These two cases reported by Dr. Goddard belong to the same group as those I have collected. That he clearly recognized the source of origin of these glands is also evident from the title of his article: Two Umbilical Tumors of Probable Uterine Origin. I had overlooked Dr. Goddard's article completely. To him undoubtedly belongs the credit for having drawn attention to the probable origin of the glands in these cases. Dr. Goddard's cases, one recently recorded by Barker,and one examined by me for Dr. Jones, of Atlanta, are recorded at the end of the chapter.

In all, nine cases have been recorded. Green's case, Mintz's first and third cases, and Ehrlich's case owe their glandular origin without doubt to the uterus or to a portion of Miiller's duct from which the uterine mucosa originally comes. Although the cases reported by Wullstein, Giannettasio, von Noorden, and Mintz (Case 2) also probably belong to the same group, the evidence is not quite so clear, and without the opportunity of carefully studying the original sections I should not feel justified in including them as certain instances.

The most common glandular elements at the umbilicus are remnants of the omphalomesenteric duct. These are usually identical in structure with the glands of the small intestine, and never give rise to the cystic dilatations noted in the group of cases under discussion; moreover, hemorrhage into the stroma is exceptional. They differ totally both in their gross and histologic appearances.

We have in this group of cases glandular elements that from their histologic appearance and arrangement correspond exactly with those found in adenomyoma of the uterus, and in one case at least (Green's) the surrounding stroma was composed chiefly of non-striped muscle, making the growth essentially an adenomyoma. In the majority of the cases, however, the stroma consisted of fibrous tissue, but little muscle being present. These growths are benign, and if removed in toto, provided no other embryonic foci exist, give rise to no further trouble. In Mintz's first case, four years after thefirst nodule had been removed, two others developed. These were also extirpated.

In Ehrlich's case, in addition to typical uterine mucosa, there was a definite tumor formation that had originated from sweat-glands.

In order that the reader may gain a clear insight into each of the cases, they are reported in detail, together with the comments on each case. The descriptions of the illustrations naturally differ from those given by the various authors. I have redescribed each picture in the light of our new knowledge of the subject.

A Small Umbilical Tumor Containing Uterine Glands.*

[The author very kindly placed a section of the growth at my disposal. There is no doubt that the gland elements in this case are identical with those of the uterine mucosa. — T. S. C]

The patient, a woman fifty years of age, had complained of irritation about the umbilicus for about two and a half years, and there had been an occasional discharge, brownish in color. When Dr. Green saw her, fourteen months before the growth was removed, there was some eczematous irritation of the skin in the neighborhood, but no projecting growth could be observed at that time. The bottom of the umbilical depression had an irregular, wart-like appearance. The surrounding eczema soon yielded to treatment, but there was from time to time an irritating discharge from the umbilicus, which the patient declared was always worse during her menstrual periods.

The umbilicus with the growth and a portion of the surrounding skin was removed. The omentum was not adherent to the umbilicus, and no intestine was seen at operation. The wound healed by first intention and there was no subsequent trouble, so far as could be learned.

On microscopic examination the skin was found to be normal. The stroma of the growth was made up of fibrous tissue and non-striped muscle, scattered among which, without any definite arrangement, were numerous gland elements. Some of these were very near the free surface, others more deeply placed. They were for the most part tubular and lined with columnar epithelium showing large, deeply staining nuclei. They were thought to be reproductions of Lieberkiihn's crypts, but differed from them in their exaggerated dimensions. Some of them were so large that they might almost have been described as cysts. [Dr. Green thought that the growth was a remnant of the vitello-intestinal tract.]

On reading this history I noted that there had been some discharge of blood from the umbilicus, as indicated by the brownish color, and, furthermore, that the patient had always been worse at the menstrual periods. This made me suspect the possible presence of uterine glands at the umbilicus. I wrote Dr. Green and early in July received the following reply:

The Ferns, Romford, England, June 22, 1911.

Dear Sir: In reply to your query about my case of umbilical growth, I am pleased to be able to send you a section from the same, so that you may form your own judgment as to its histology. I did not think it was malignant. I last heard of the patient two and a half years after the operation. She was then alive and well. This, I think, shows that the growth was not secondary to an undiagnosed growth within the abdomen. Owing to removal, I have not subsequently heard of her, so I cannot say what ultimately happened to her. I inclose a copy of my paper which I happened to have kept.

Yours faithfully,

Charles D. Green.

* Green, Charles D.: A Case of Umbilical Papilloma Which Showed Some Activity of Growth in a Patient Fifty Years of Age and Which was Due Apparently to Inclusion of a Portion of Meckel's Diverticulum. Trans. Path. Soc. London, 1899, 1, 243.

We were particularly fortunate in obtaining this specimen from Dr. Green, in the first place, because it was twelve years since the case had been reported.

A Small Umbilical Tumor Containing Glands and Stroma Identical with Those of the Uterine Mucosa.

The slide was kindly furnished me by Dr. Charles D. Green, of Romford, England, and is from the umbilical growth reported by him in the Transactions of the Pathological Society of London, 1899. The squamous epithelium is intact, and apart from some thickening appears normal. Scattered throughout the underlying stroma are oval, round, or irregular glands occurring singly or in groups; there are also a few cystic spaces. Some of the glands lie directly beneath the skin. Two of the glands open directly upon the surface of the umbilicus. The photomicrographs of this series were made by Mr. H. H. Hart.

Dr. Green's specimen, The skin surface is intact and practically normal, although at a few points the epithelium is considerably thickened. In one or two places directly beneath the skin there is small-round-cell infiltration, chiefly in foci. At one point the surface epithelium extends a short distance into a cavity. In the lower portion of the cavity the lining consists of cylindric epithelium, one layer in thickness. Around this area the stroma shows a considerable amount of hemorrhage. It is from this point that there was undoubtedly bleeding at the menstrual periods. The underlying stroma consists to a large extent of non-striped muscle. Scattered here and there throughout the muscle

Glands from a Small Umbilical Tumor.

The normal character of the surface epithelium is clearly seen. The gland spaces vary considerably in size and shape and are lined with cylindric epithelium. Those in the picture lie in direct contact with the dense surrounding stroma. are glands. They are small, round, oblong, irregular, or large. A few of them occur singly and lie in direct contact with the surrounding stroma. The majority, however, occur in groups or in chains, and are separated from the surrounding stroma by a definite stroma of their own, which is recognized by its deeper stain and its abundance of vesicular nuclei, which are oval or round. Some of the glands are very much dilated. Where such dilatations have taken place the surrounding stroma frequently shows a good deal of hemorrhage.

Were it not for the presence of the skin surface one would immediately diagnose the specimen as an adenomyoma of the uterus. The growth is an adenomyoma of the umbilicus. Dr. Green at the time felt sure that the condition was a rare one, as indicated from a second communication dated August 4, 1911:

Dear Dr. Cullen:.... I am glad you found my specimen so interesting. I had some photographs prepared, but the Committee of the Pathological Society did not think them of sufficient interest to insert them in the Transactions. I was a little disappointed at the time, for I thought that the condition was uncommon.

Yours faithfully,

Charles D. Green.

Typical Uterine Mucosa in a Small Umbilical Tumor

The three large glands in the right-hand part of the picture, in shape and arrangement, resemble those found in an adenomyoma of the uterus: separating them from the dense tumor growth is a definite and characteristic stroma. The group of glands in the middle of the picture is even more characteristic, one of the glands being dilated. All are lined with cylindric epithelium, and the contrast between the surrounding stroma and the dense growth is very clearly marked. Afl noted in the description, non-striped muscle was found scattered throughout the nodule.

[On looking up the Transactions, I found that two of the committee diagnosed the growth as a columnar-cell carcinoma, but whether primary or secondary they were unable to decide. The chairman of the committee said some of the members present who examined the specimen were not inclined to regard it as malignant. There is little wonder that at that time confusion existed, and had it not been for the specially favorable opportunity I had had of examining so many cases of adenomyoma, I should have undoubtedly overlooked the true origin. — T. S. C]

Adenomyoma of the Umbilicus.*

In 1883 a woman acquired an umbilical hernia after labor. Ten years later, within the space of about two months, a dark-blue tumor the size of a hazelnut developed on the umbilical elevation. This had two cystic areas on its surface. During menstruation the tumor swelled and the cysts ruptured. They contained blood-tinged fluid.

The tumor was extirpated and the hernia repaired. This tumor on section presented a cavernous appearance, but no microscopic examination was made. In 1897, four years later, there was a return of the hernia, and at the umbilicus were two hard nodules about the size of hazelnuts. On microscopic examination they were found to contain glands lined with cylindric epithelium and surrounded by a definite stroma. Here and there bundles of non-striped muscle were in evidence. The dilated glands contained blood-pigment. Mintz thought he was dealing with remains of the omphalomesenteric duct.

[When discussing this case some three years ago, just after making theabstract, I made the following note:

"The clinical history, the macroscopic appearance, the picture of the glands, the stroma, and the contents of the dilated glands all point to aclenomyoma, although adenomyoma of the I, umbilicus has never been reported." — T. S. C]

*Chil. f. klin. 1909 lxxxix 385.

We are fortunate in again hearing from Mintz* on this subject. Ten years later he published an article. The outlying connective-tissue stroma is very iriegular. Occupying the lower half of the field are glands showing some branching. They are lined with one layer which separates them from the fibrous tissue. There is cylindric epithelium that lie in a characteristic stroma. He describes, more in detail, the tumor. The entire picture reminds one to a large extent histologic findings of the Same Case. That of adenomyoma of the uterus. He says :

" The ground substance of the growth consists of connective tissue not very rich in cells. They cross one another or run parallel with one another in cords. Here and there in the scar tissue one sees gland tubules in either transverse or longitudinal section. They are surrounded by young, very cellular connective tissue, which passes very gradually into the old scar tissue. The glands are lined with one layer of cylindric epithelium. Their lumina are collapsed and contain blood pigment or reddish-colored contents. In some places the tubules lie close, at other points they are separated. The newly formed connective tissue surrounding them has changed into old connective tissue poor in cell nuclei. Some of the glands are dilated and their epithelium is flattened. The lumina appear to be filled with detritus. Here and there the cylindric epithelium is unrecognizable and the cavity contains blood-pigment. W'here the dilatation has occurred, the epithelium has disappeared; in this way are to be explained the cysts with blood contents which were noted when the patient first entered the hospital. Between the glandular portion of the tumor there are at some points groups of non-striped muscle-fibers that have no definite topographic arrangement in relation with the glands. The microscopic examination shows an adenomatous growth in the scar tissue. This has stimulated the growth of the scar tissue, and thus originated the young connective tissue surrounding the new glands. In the mean time the periphery of the nodule in the scar has been converted into sarcoma."

* Mintz, W.: Das wahre Adenom des Xabels. Deutsche Zeitschr. f. Chir., 1899, li, 545.

[After giving this description he says in a foot-note that at the time of writing (that is, ten years later) the tumor had not returned. The explanation of the origin of this tumor he gives as persistent remains of the omphalomesenteric duct which had remained latent for forty-two years in the umbilical scar, and under the influence of chronic injury (a ten-year persistnt. It could not be regarded as an exudate. The physician was interested to find out whether there was any connection between the two tumors; in other words, whether the umbilical growth was a metastasis. Wullstein examined a Muller's fluid specimen. It was everywhere covered with skin. It had a semicircular form and was about the size of a thaler. The umbilicus was raised 1 cm. above the surrounding abdominal skin, and its surface showed numerous shallow furrows. The umbilical furrow was recognized as an irregular, transverse cleft, which divided the umbilicus into two unequal portions, it becoming deeper and deeper in the middle until there was a depression 11 mm. in depth. About the middle of the under surface of the tumor was a cord about 1 cm. long, hardly as thick as a straw. This was solid and composed of connective tissue. The tumor itself was about 3 cm. long and averaged 1.5 cm. in thickness. On section it was seen that the umbilicus was everywhere covered with skin, which in all portions was thickened and markedly pigmented.

From the bottom of the umbilical depression and running parallel were thick bundles of dense connective tissue. The tumor consisted of numerous dense, hard, glistening connective-tissue bundles, which enclosed more or less long or round areas of loose tissue, grayish in appearance, and in the interior in places were small lumina.

Subcutaneous fat was absent. In the vicinity of the umbilical scar the tissue was sieve-like. The spaces of the meshwork were filled with dark-brown masses about the size of poppy-seeds. The meshwork consisted of firm connective tissue. Microscopic examination of a section from the middle of the tumor showed that the epidermis was thickened. The deepest cells of the stratum mucosum were granular, and contained everywhere brown pigment. Only at the base of the umbilicus, where the papillae were not markedly formed, was the pigment absent. Everywhere in the corium and in the subcutis were numerous mast cells. Hair and sebaceous glands were nowhere to be found. The deeper layers of the skin contained normally formed sweat-glands. The tumor consisted chiefly of a connective-tissue stroma and of cavities varying in size and form. The stroma, which in amount predominated over the alveolar tissue, was composed of broad, thick, dense connective tissue, which contained a few cell-elements with spindle-shaped nuclei. Only around the spaces there was present a connective tissue which was very delicate and whose fibers formed a network partly as fine bundles. The numerous nuclei were oval and frequently almost round. Immediately around the alveoli the connective-tissue threads formed a thick layer, really a membrana propria. The cavities were lined with cylindric cells placed at right angles to the basement-membrane. Their height was not always in proportion to the size of the cavity, but seemed to depend on the pressure of the gland contents. In a few places the tubules were filled with epithelium. The gland tubules were usually cut either obliquely or longitudinally. The gland lumina near the periphery of the tumor in width resembled normal sweat-glands. On the other hand, those in the middle of the tumor were markedly dilated and round; in the latter the tissue was frequently infiltrated with cells. The majority of the glands were filled with a secretion composed of a most delicate, rather granularnetwork of thread mixed with epithelial cells. The entire tumor was permeated by a thick network of capillaries which surrounded the individual gland tubules. In many places in the connective-tissue stroma in the neighborhood of the blood-vessels were remnants of old and fresh blood.

In the preparations taken from the lateral portion of the tumor accumulations of round cells and blood-vessels were seen. The cystic dilatation of the canals had evidently been produced by pressure from within. The cavities were lined with endothelium, and the walls of these new cavities had projections into them. These cavities were due to the confluence of the neighboring small cavities. The origin of these in some places could be followed. At several points between the blood- spaces were dilated tubules lined with cylindric epithelium, usually filled with secretion, and surrounded by the characteristic connective tissue which sometimes reached as far as the endothelium of the blood-spaces. A few of the gland-like cavities also contained blood. At no point, however, was this adherent.

After these findings we must ask: Are we dealing here with an individual tumor or is there a combination of two tumors? Further, under what category does this tumor formation belong? Wullstein held it to be a combination of cystadenoma of the sweat-glands with cavernous angioma.

He says that what makes him think there is a combination of two tumors is the fact that there is a different lining to the large spaces, the one being lined with endothelium and the other with cylindric epithelium. No less typical is the relation of the surrounding connective tissue to the spaces. The differences even with the low power are easily recognized, through the various microchemical reactions in color with methylene-blue. The above already described delicate bluish connective tissue is independent of the sweat-glands and their tributaries in the specimen, and is present only in the vicinity of the tubules lined with cylindric epithelium, whereas the spaces lined with endothelium are always surrounded by a thick, fibrillated tissue which stains intensely red. He thinks that the largecavernous spaces in the first place are due to circulatory disturbances.

He says we must look upon the sweat-glands as the point of origin for the epithelium of the new-growth, on account of the position of the tumor beneath the skin, the presence of cylindric epithelium, and the absence of squamous epithelial nests. Its origin from the epidermis or from the hair-follicles or the sebaceous glands is excluded. On the other hand, we must ask whether it may not be due to some embryologic deposit. Three things have to be thought of: the umbilical canal, the urachus, and the omphalomesenteric duct. Have we in this mixed tumor a purely accidental combination of an adenomatous cyst of the sweat-glands and a cavernous angioma? or do the two varieties bear a causal relation one to the other? In conclusion, he says, the old and fresh hemorrhages in various portions of the tumor have followed as a result of hyperemia — perhaps the menstrual hyperemia. [Wullstein's tumor also occurred in a woman. He speaks of its characteristic connective tissue separating the glands lined with cylindric epithelium from the surrounding stroma. Further, in his last paragraph he speaks of the hemorrhage through the tumor being due to hyperemia, possibly menstrual in origin. We believe that here he has the clue and that, in all probability, the glands in this case were also uterine glands. Although the description of the histologic appearances in this case is in places somewhat involved, we have in our translation held closely to the text in orderthat the points favoring the uterine origin of the glands might not be unduly accentuated. I wrote Professor Orth, of Berlin, and he in turn referred me to Dr. Wullstein, who at the time this case was published (1893) was an assistant of Professor Orth and occupied the room next to mine in the Gcittingen Laboratory. Dr. Wullstein kindly sent me the reprint of his article, but I was unable to get the specimen, and consequently cannot speak with absolute certainty.— T. S. C]

N. Giannettasio,* in an article, gives a resume of the literature on tumors of the umbilicus, and reports a case in a multipara aged forty-four. A year and a half before she came under his observation the patient noticed a small tumor the size of a walnut at the umbilicus. This was solid, immobile beneath the skin, and occasionedno discomfort. It occupied the lower andleft side of the umbilical depression.

It was removed, and the patient was perfectly well twenty-five months later. He gives a very good plate, but the text is not satisfactory. The nodule, however, he says, contained "cytogenous" connective tissue. The plate shows normal skin, dilated blood-vessels, and gland-spaces lined with apparently cuboid epithelium, and surrounded by a stroma, the picture somewhat suggesting uterine glands.

Probably Uterine Glands in a Small Umbilical Tumor **

In the beginning of his article von Noorden states that he is going to demonstrate a tumor which, from its characteristics and anatomic picture, leaves no doubt that it originated from the sweat-glands, and that, so far as he knew, no similar case was on record. On October 1, 1898, a thirty-eight-year-old multipara told him that for two months she had had a slight unevenness in the middle of the umbilicus. Eight days previously a physician had observed a pea-sized enlargement in the floor of the umbilicus. Clinically it suggested a nevus, and on account of the dark pigmentation von Noorden thought of melanosarcoma. On October 14, 1898, the tumor was larger than a pea, semicircular, and not sharply defined from the surrounding umbilical tissue. In its center it had a small, wart-like elevation. There were no inflammatory changes in the vicinity. The skin over the tumor was somewhat uneven, grayish in color, and here and there more deeply pigmented than the floor of the umbilicus. No pulsation was noted, no variation on pressure. The umbilicus was removed. Two and a half years later the patient was perfectly well.

The umbilicus on section showed a drawing in of the skin, and in the depth there was a wart-like projection. The tissue of the umbilicus itself was very hard. On section a pea-sized, light brownish, pigmented area was observed, which was not sharply defined from the surrounding tissue.

Microscopic Examination. — The nodule was made up of a loose connective tissue with numerous large cells. It contained a large number of capillaries. Within this connective tissue were slit-shaped cavities lined with cylindric epithelium which had become loosened irregularly from the wall. Some of these cavities had become dilated into irregular cystic spaces, which here and there showed clearly a lining of cylindric epithelium, while in other places they had completely lost it. The contents of these cavities had dropped out in some places; in others it consisted of cylindric epithelium, and in numerous cases of an irregular, structureless network. Further sections were made, and the squamous epithelial layer over the entire nodule was found to be intact. Over the most prominent part it was three times as thick as at the periphery. Where the cells were most abundant, the deepest layers showed pigmentation. At one point "the sweat-glands ' ' could be traced almost to the surface, being covered only with a few layers of cells.

* Giannettasio, N. : Sur les tumeurs de l'ombilic. Arch. gen. de nied., 1900, n. ser., iii, 52.

** von Noorden, W. : Ein Schweissdrusenadenom mit Sitz im Nabel und ein Beitrag zu den Nabelgeschwtilsten. Deutsche Zeitschr. f. Chir., 1901, lix, 215.

The stroma consisted of three definite kinds of tissue : normal, dense fibrous, and mucoid-like tissue. The chief interest lay in the sweat-glands; roots of hairs were nowhere to be found, and sebaceous glands were reduced to a minimum. The search for muscle-fibers in the reticulate.d tissue was fruitless. No elastic fibers were found. In general it may be said the sweat-glands were normal in the subcutaneous layer and were arranged in groups. Then in one section one would find two large openings and three or four glands, and in another section groups of from two to four glands. Some were cut in such a manner that 9 to 15 round lumina were in a A Small Umbilical Tumor Containing Numerous Glands. (After von Noorden.). The growth is covered with squamous epithelium. Scattered throughout the stroma are quantities of glands. In form they bear a closer resemblance to uterine glands than to sweat-glands. At one point the glands almost reach the surfaceline or in the form of a hook. The groups lay, as a rule, very close to one another. The normal sweat-glands lay partly in the fibrous connective tissue, others — and this is to be noted — were separated by a rather broad layer of cells from the normal corium. The nuclei of this zone were pale and less abundant than in the remaining corium. This zone suggested the above-mentioned mucoid tissue, in which in part the altered glands lay. This tissue appeared always to penetrate between the normal gland grouping, and had separated the glands from one another. The gland epithelium was not changed. In addition to this slightly normal and slightly changed skein-like gland there were in the corium a number of cavities and tubules. These extended from near the surface of the papillary masses to the vicinity of the subcutaneous fat. The cavities and the tubules are to be seen in Figs. 178 and 179. [We do not clearly understand what von Noorden means by corium. It seems, however, that he uses the term instead of stroma. His general description is somewhat hazy throughout. — T. S. C]

He gives a resume of his description: The tumor is made up of many roundish and often dilated, cyst-like portions which lie deeply seated in the corium. In intimate relation to these, or independent of them, are tubular channels with numerous corkscrew-like windings. These extend toward the epidermis. The cystic and also the tubular pictures are surrounded by dense and loose connective tissue which separates them from the surrounding connective tissue and are without any definite capsule. In the above-described coil we can with certainty recognize the sweat-glands.

On p. 229 he reports one of Mintz's cases and says that possibly the new-growth had developed from the glandular portion of the skin; for example, from the sweat glands. He says: "I will also not assume this, but will say that portions of my tumor in respect to form, grouping, contents, and relation of the cells, both in the description and in the picture, produce a very similar appearance to the case reported by Mintz, and had it not been possible to establish a relation to the sweat-glands I should in all probability have followed the views of Mintz. Mintz found smooth muscle-fibers in the connective tissue at several points. The explanation as to the origin is difficult. "

In conclusion, von Noorden says: "From the above findings a true benign adenoma springing from the sweat-glands can be diagnosed."

[As will be noted from the history, the patient was a woman thirty-eight years of age. There was no evidence of inflammation. Histologic examination in some places showed groups of glands lying in a stroma differing from the ordinary surrounding stroma. These groups of glands were lined with one layer of cylindric epithelium, and the cavities of some of the dilated spaces contained cells that had taken up blood-pigment.

Yon Noorden draws attention to the fact that his case bore a marked resemblance in many ways to Mintz's case. There remains little doubt in my mind that the glands resemble those found in the body of the uterus, and the thickened, dense stroma around them bears a marked resemblance, even with the very low power, to the stroma of the uterine mucosa. The picture, at any rate, is much more suggestive of a glandular growth of uterine origin than of one coming from the sweat-glands. I endeavored, through

Professor Doderlein, of Munich, to locate Dr. von Noorden, and, if possible, secure a section of this growth, but have not been successful. — T. S. C]

After Glands in a Small Umbilical Tumor. von Noorden.

The glands in the lower half of the picture bear quite a resemblance to uterine glands. Those in the center of the field remind one of the pictures seen in the depths of uterine glands, where there is some reduplication of the folds. The gland in the left part of the field is markedly dilated and contains much detritus. It is rather difficult to classify this tumor reported by Villar, but as it presentsa few clinical and histologic points suggestive of the group under consideration, I mention it here, although it is not considered in the digest.*

L. L.. aged forty-six. entered the service of Professor Guyon September 17, 1886.

In the month of December, 1885, nothing abnormal was noticed in the umbilical region, but shortly afterward her corsets produced pain in this region and she discovered a small tumor the size of a pin-head, reddish in color, in the umbilical depression. This tumor increased very slowly, and in May, 1886, she went to the hospital for examination. She continued under treatment, and in the month of August entered the hospital. At that time at the umbilical depression was a tumor the size of a bird's egg. It was conic. Its base was continuous with the cicatrix,and was somewhat constricted by the depression. It had a very narrow, but relatively large pedicle. It was in reality sessile, firm in consistence, but elastic and reddish in color. At the top was a blackish point, 2 mm. in diameter. The any liquid. Two or three days after she entered the hospital the blackish point ruptured and there was an escape of tarry blood. The patient experienced no pain and there was no glandular enlargement.

Histologic Examination by Clado. — The tumor is situated in the center of the umbilicus and has developed in the depth of the cicatrix. It is covered with skin. In consistence it is a little less firm than a fibroma. On section one finds a capsule which surrounds the central mass. The tumor is whitish-gray, with numerous dark spots not any larger than the head of a pin scattered throughout it. Microscopic examination shows that the tumor is formed of sarcomatous tissue, the cells being fusiform in shape.

Some of the spaces are round, others oval, and have anastomosed with one another. Some of the canals are lined with pavement epithelium. Between the cystic spaces one finds stroma containing a small number of vessels. The skin which composes the outer covering of the tumor is exceedingly thin, but presents the characteristic appearance. There has been extravasation of blood at the center of the tumor.

[This woman, as above noted, was forty-six years of age. The history does not convince one absolutely that this was a sarcoma. It might very well have been a fibroma. It resembles in a few particulars those tumors of the umbilicus that contain uterine glands or glands somewhat resembling them. — T. S. C]

Further Cases of Adenomyoma of the Umbilicus.

These four cases have come to my knowledge since this chapter was prepared. They bear a striking resemblance to those already discussed in the preceding pages :

Two Umbilical Tumors of Probable Uterine Origin. **

" In the surgical service of Drs. Munro and Bottomley, at the Carney Hospital, there recently occurred within a few weeks of each other two examples of umbilical tumor, the striking similarity and unusual histologic structure of which warrant their publication.

* Villar: Tumours de l'ombilie. These de Paris, 1886, obs. 68.

** Goddard, Samuel W. Surg., Gyn. and Obst,, August, 1909, 249-252.

"Because of the comparative rarity of these cases the clinical histories are set forth in considerable detail :

"Case 1. — Miss S., a housekeeper, forty-four years of age, and born in New Brunswick, entered the Carney Hospital May 22, 1907. Her family and past history have no bearing on her condition at that time. A year previously, during a catamenial period, she noted some redness and tenderness about the umbilicus; two months later, at a similar time, a small tumor appeared in the abdominal wall close to the umbilicus. This tumor increased in size but slightly, and most of the increase came in the two weeks just preceding her admission to the hospital. The tenderness and pain, which at first were evident only during the menstrual periods, had been constant for some months, though most marked just before, during, and for a week after menstruation. Her menstrual history was not otherwise remarkable. An abdominal bandage, her only treatment, had given her some relief. There had been some little loss of weight and strength. For two months the tenderness had kept her from her usual work. No symptoms referable either to the gastro-intestinal or to the urinary tract had been noted.

"About and including the umbilicus was a rather deep-seated, spheric, slightly tender, fixed mass, of rather firm consistence, and about 2 cm. in diameter. In the navel itself was a thin, yellowish crust; a sinus could not be demonstrated; the skin over the tumor was not red. Examination of the abdomen was otherwise negative. Examination per vaginam showed only vaginismus and a moderately retroverted uterus.

"On May 23d Dr. Munro excised the growth (including the navel) with a portion of the adjacent peritoneum and sheath of the rectus muscle. The former was not involved in the growth; to the latter the growth was adherent. The convalescence was without note, and the patient was still free from recurrence one year after operation.

"Case 2. — Mrs. D., a housewife, entered the Carney Hospital June 23, 1907.

She was born in Ireland forty-two years before that time, and came of healthy stock. Her menstrual history previous to her marriage was entirely normal in every way. Married seventeen years, she had borne four children. Following her first confinement she had had a ' milk leg. '

"For six years previous to entering the hospital a slight bloody discharge from the navel without pain or tenderness had come with each menstruation. The discharge came only at that time. Independent of the umbilical disorder she had had in the past three years attacks of sharp pain beneath the right costal border, accompanied by vomiting, chills, and jaundice.

"The patient was rather obese, and showed distinct tenderness beneath the right costal border. At the umbilicus was a small, irregularly shaped papillomatous tumor, 2 cm. in diameter, with three distinct projections covered with normal appearing skin. At the top of the largest projection was a pin-hole opening capped with dried blood. The tumor was soft, freely movable, not tender, and apparently superficial.

"On June 24th the umbilicus with the tumor was excised by Dr. Bottomley. The tumor was confined to the skin and fat outside the aponeurosis. The peritoneal cavity was opened, and the gall-bladder and stomach regions were explored; these were found normal. Convalescence was uneventful except for the development of malaria on the ninth day, which promptly yielded to treatment. The patient was discharged, relieved, on July 11th, and when heard from, one and a half 3 r ears later, there had been no recurrence.

"For the microscopic study of these tumors, in the laboratory of Dr. Henry A. Christian at the Harvard Medical School, a large number of sections were taken from different planes and four different methods of staining were used for each section.

"So closely do the tumors resemble each other microscopically that no evident difference between them can be determined. The arrangement and construction, both in general and particular, are nearly identical. For descriptive purposes a median longitudinal section of Case 2 will be used. To the naked eye it presents an irregularly convex surface covered with true skin. Underlying this at each extremity are what appear to be sweat-glands, and in another part, chiefly in the center, are numerous vacuolated structures varying in size from a pin-point to a pin-head. The intervening structure cannot be definitely determined. Microscopically, the tumor is seen to be covered with normal epidermis, but varying in thickness. Below this, at either end, are numerous sweat-glands, thickly grouped, and around these is an abundance of fibrous connective tissue. The vacuolated or glandular structures found throughout the tumor vary in size, and for the most part are of rounded contour, while some are elongated. Some, especially the larger ones, are discrete, while others are aggregated into small groups. Some are immediately surrounded by fibrous tissue, while others are embedded in cellular tissue. There are none which appear to have any connection with the epidermis. All the gland-spaces are lined with epithelium. They are either devoid of contents, or contain a granular, structureless material in which are often found groups of red blood cells. The epithelium varies in the different glands and even in the same gland, from the low, flattened variety to the tall, columnar cells with all the intermediate forms. The tall, columnar variety is for the most part closely compacted, with long, narrow nuclei and with no visible cell membrane. Most of them have a distinct top plate, and many show cilia of considerable length and uniformity, while others have only a suggestion of striae. The cilia in some places are from one-fourth to one-third the length of their cells, and in others their extremities end in a globular, deeply staining tip. At irregular intervals among the nuclei of the columnar cells are larger rounded and more faintly stained nuclei. In some places the epithelium is distinctly cuboid, the nuclei clear and rounded, and the whole cell clearly defined. There is a larger group of glands which presents the flattened epithelium. The epithelium lining the glands, whether flattened, cuboid, or columnar, is for the most part in single layers. In some places the glandular epithelium is immediately supported by fibrous connective tissue, but in others the underlying structures are decidedly cellular. The cellular tissue is more compact the nearer the glandular tissue is approached, i. e., the most cellular tissue is found in close connection with the gland-spaces. The nuclei are rounded or elongated and deeply stained, the protoplasm and cell membrane not being distinct. In the immediate neighborhood of some of the gland-spaces are large hemorrhagic areas in which large quantities of red blood-cells are scattered freely and intermingled with the cellular structures. These areas seem to have no direct relation to blood-vessels, which are not superabundant or enlarged. The fibrous connective tissue shows nothing of interest throughout the section. There is an abundance of smooth muscle whichis closely interwoven with the connective tissue."

The microphotographs accompanying Goddard's article bring out clearly the structure and arrangement of the tumors, and emphasize the points mentioned above.

Adenomyoma of the Umbilicus; also a Small Adenomyoma near the Anterior Iliac Spine.*

Case 3. — "A woman, aged thirty-seven, came to me on September 2, 1908, for advice about a small tumor of the umbilicus which she had noticed during the last few months. The lump was about the size of a filbert, and lay in the lower part of the navel. It was irregular in outline, but smooth, and was of a bluish-purple color, suggesting a melanotic sarcoma. There were no abdominal symptoms or signs and no secondary deposits in the inguinal glands or elsewhere. A few days later I removed the whole navel and adjacent skin widely between two elliptic incisions, opening the abdomen on either side and taking away the intervening peritoneum. There were no traces of growth within the peritoneal cavity. The wound was stitched up in layers and healed absolutely by first intention. The specimen was given to Air. Lawrence, the curator of our museum, for examination. Sections showed to the naked eye a hard, fibrous structure, the superficial parts of which, under the epithelial covering of the navel, were pigmented. In the deeper parts of this fibrous tissue were many islands of tubular glands lined with columnar epithelium and filled with epithelial debris. Some were cut obliquely and showed a looser areolar investing layer outside the membrana propria. The latter was not penetrated by the cells, so that one sign of the benign character of the tumor was present. Nor were there any other signs of the spread of the growth beyond the limits of the tubules. I therefore, put it down as an adenoma derived from remnants of the vitelline duct, of which I had read but never seen.

"I saw no more of this lady until January, 1913, when she consulted me about a little nodule seated in the subcutaneous fat, about two inches internal to the left anterior iliac spine. It felt about the size of a pea, and was hard. On gently pinching the skin the latter puckered over the nodule. There were no enlarged inguinal glands or other signs of infiltration. This knot was removed shortly after by Mr. F. Hinds, of Worthing, and was sent to me. Mr. Lawrence kindly prepared several microscopic sections of it. They showed precisely the same structure as the first nodule, except that the fibrous tissue, which made up the bulk of the mass, was more dense and fewer connective-tissue corpuscles were scattered through it.

"The reappearance of this small knot, repeating the structure of the first nodule at the umbilicus, suggests, of course, strongly that the first was malignant and has recurred in the lymphatics of the subcutaneous tissue of the abdominal wall. Then the question arises, Was the original lump in the umbilicus a primary growth in some of the glandular remnants of the umbilicus enumerated above, or could it be a nodule secondary to some visceral carcinoma within the abdomen? This latter view is one adopted by Mr. Shattock, to whom I sent sections of both the first nodule removed and that obtained four and a half years later, and who was kind enough to write to me fully on the subject. It may be correct, but so far the lady has shown no evidence of visceral trouble — nearly five years after the appearance of the first nodule in the umbilicus. Time alone will show. In the meanwhile I am inclined to negative the visceral theory."

* Barker, A. E. : Three Cases of Solid Tumours of the Umbilicus in Adults. The Lancet, London, July 19, 1913, 128.

In answer to a request from me, Dr. Barker very kindly sent the only section of the umbilical tumor which the curator of the museum still possessed.

Description of the slide sent me by Dr. Barker. — The section of the umbilical nodule has a normal covering of squamous epithelium. The underlying tissue shows no evidence of glandular tissue. Dr. Barker, however, in his description of the case, says that this tumor contained glands, and, furthermore, that the glands near the anterior-superior spine were similar in character to those found at the umbilicus. Dr. Barker was good enough to also send me several slides from

Adenomyoma in the Abdominal Wall near the Anterior Iliac Spine.

This is a photomicrograph of a portion of the small nodule furnished me by Mr. Arthur E. Barker, London, England. Near the center of the field are two glands. Their epithelium has been slightly strengthened to bring them out more distinctly. The glands are lined with one layer of cylindric epithelium. Surrounding them is a zone of stroma cells. This zone is continuous with a large, irregular area of stroma just below and to the left of the glands. In the upper part of the field is another gland, which lies in direct contact with the tissue of the tumor. The greater part of the nodule consLsts of non-striped muscle and fibrous tissue. In the outlying portions of the field is adipose tissue. The growth is a typical adenomyoma, with glands similar to those of the uterine mucosa. Mr. Barker, in his description of the case, says that the umbilical nodule and the one here depicted were identical in character; consequently the umbilical growth was also an adenomyoma with glands and stroma identical with those of the endometrium of the uterus.

The growth near the anterior-superior spine. In one section I found not only myomatous tissue, but a triangular area of stroma with tubular glands at one end Tig. 180;. This area was sharply defined from the surrounding tissue. In another section was what appeared to be fibrous tissue, and possibly a little muscle. Here we had irregular, triangular areas of stroma, sometimes without any glands, sometimes with tubular glands identical with those of the uterine mucosa. At other points the glands lay in direct contact with the muscle. Surrounding the entire growth was adipose tissue. The picture in the main is analogous to that which we have described as representing adenomyomaof the umbilicus. Mr. Barker's case is particularly interesting in that he had not only a tumor of this character at the umbilicus, but also a nodule near the anterior iliac spine.

A Small Umbilical Tumor Consisting i n Part of Sweat-glands and in Part Apparently of Uterine Glands.

While in Atlanta, at the meeting of the Southern Surgical Association in December, 1913, Dr. Edward G. Jones, of Atlanta, told me that he had recently seen an umbilical tumor in which I might be interested. On December 22, 1913, he wrote: "I am sending under separate cover a section of the umbilical tumor. Unfortunately, I cannot give you any clinical data. The nodule was three-quarters of an inch in diameter, and gave the patient some discomfort at times." Later Dr. Jones discovered that, according to the patient's account, the tumor seemed to her to enlarge at the time of menstruation.

The specimen sent me by Dr. Jones is covered over with squamous epithelium-which contains pigment in the deeper layers. The underlying tissue consists in a large measure of fibrous tissue. The capillaries scattered throughout it are in many places surrounded by round cells. Here and there throughout the fibrous tissue are groups of sweat-glands. These are separated from the fibrous tissue by a definite stroma.

At other points are large glands lined with cylindric epithelium. Some of these glands lie in direct contact with the fibrous tissue; others have a definite stroma, separating them from the connective tissue. This stroma stains more deeply than the connective tissue, and its nuclei are oval and stain deeply.

The tumor is evidently made up of two distinct varieties of glands: some corresponding to sweat-glands and others bearing a marked resemblance to those of the uterine mucosa. There is little doubt that part of this growth consists of uterine glands. The section was, unfortunately, too thick to supply a satisfactory photomicrograph.

PERSONAL OBSERVATION.

In 1900 Mrs. E. J. D., aged thirty-eight, was admitted to Dr. Howard A. Kelly's Sanitarium on account of a retroflexed uterus and a relaxed vaginal outlet. A small round nodule was at the same time detected at the umbilicus. The nodule was removed, the uterus brought up into position, and the perineum repaired. Her convalescence was prolonged on account of phlebitis in both legs.

This patient was the mother of four children. Her menses began at thirteen, were fairly regular, and lasted from three to five days. About two years before admission the patient first felt a little pain in the umbilical region. During the last year this had become very severe and the small umbilical growth had developed. There was no reddening at the umbilicus, and the general health had not been affected.

This small umbilical tumor was brought over to the gynecologic laboratory of the Johns Hopkins Hospital and carefully examined. For some unforeseen reason it was not indexed, and, consequently, when we were getting together all our umbilical material, was overlooked. It was accidentally discovered when class sections were being gone over a few days ago (March 3, 1915). Dr. Elizabeth Hurdon, who examined the specimen at the time, drew special attention to the fact that the glands in the growth weresimilar to those of the endometrium, and that some of them were surrounded by the characteristic stroma of the uterine mucosa. The tumor averages 1.5 cm. in diameter.

A Small Umbilical Tumor Containing Glands Similar to those of the Body of the Uterus.

The low-power photomicrograph of a section of the entire umbilical nodule showsthe skin covering is normal. Occupying the lower half of the field is a somewhat circular growth, denser in structure than the surrounding stroma. It consisted of fibrous tissue and non-striped muscle. Scattered throughout the tumor are glands. Some occur singly, others in groups. Some of the smaller glands are surrounded by a dark zone — a zone of characteristic stroma. Many of the glands are dilated and partially filled with blood. In the upper part of the field are aggregations of sweat-glands.

Adenomyoma of the Umbilicus.

This picture gives an enlargement of the adenomyoma. The stroma of the growth consists of non-striped muscle and fibrous tissue. Occupying the center of the field are several glands. They were lined with one layer of cylindric epithelium, on which cilia were here and there demonstrable. The glands are separated from the muscle by a definite stroma. This, with a higher power, was found to be identical with that of the endometrium of the uterus. In the left upper corner of the picture is a markedly dilated gland. This and other dilated glands contained old blood and exfoliated epithelial cells, which had taken up blood-pigment and had become spheric. The entire picture of the umbilical tumor is analogous to that of an adenomyoma of the uterus. Its outer surface is covered with normal-appearing skin. On section it presents a dense fibrous structure.

On histologic examination the skin surface is found intact and normal. The stroma of the growth consists of fibrous tissue with a moderate amount of non-striped muscle distributed throughout it. Scattered here and there throughout the nodule are round or tortuous glands. Some of these occur in groups, others are single (Figs. 181 and 182). The glands are lined with one layer of low cylindric epithelium, which in a few places shows definite cilia. Some of the gland cavities are empty, others are dilated and filled with old blood, and in a few are exfoliated epithelial cells which have become spheric and have taken up the blood-pigment. Some of the glands lie in direct contact with the muscle or fibrous tissue; others are separated from the dense tissue by a definite stroma, which is very cellular. The picture is that of a typical adenomyoma with glands identical with those of the uterine mucosa.

A Group of Sweat-glands in an Umbilical Tumor.

At one point is an aggregation of glands of a totally different type. These glands are small, round, and have a lining of two layers of low cuboid cells. They closely resemble sweat-glands. This is another definite example of an adenomyoma of the umbilicus. It will be remembered that in several of the recorded cases the sweat-glands were markedly increased in number.

LITERATURE CONSULTED IN THE PREPARATION OF UMBILICAL TUMORS CONTAINING UTERINE MUCOSA OR REMNANTS OF MULLER'S DUCT.

Barker, Arthur E.: Three Cases of Solid Tumours of the Umbilicus in Adults. Lancet, London, July 19, 1913, 128.

Cullen, Thomas S.: Umbilical Tumors Containing LTterine Mucosa or Remnants of Midler's Ducts. Surg., Gyn. and Obstet., May, 1912, 479.

Ehrlich: Primares doppelseitiges Mammacarcinom und wahres Nabeladenom (Mintz). Aus von Eiselsberg's Klinik. Arch, f.klin. Chir., 1909, lxxxix, 742.

Giannettasio : Sur les tumeurs de l'ombilic. Arch. gen. de med., 1900, n. serie, iii, 52.

Goddard, Samuel W.: Two Umbilical Tumors of Probable Uterine Origin. Surg., Gyn. and Obstet., August, 1909, 249.

Green: Trans. Path. Soc. London, 1899, 1, 243.

Herzenberg: Ein Beitrag zum wahren Adenom des Nabels. Deutsche med. Wochenschr., 1909, i, 889.

Mintz, W.: Das wahre Adenom des Nabels. Deutsche Zeitschr. f. Chir., 1899, li, 545.

von Noorden, W. : Ein Schweissdrtisenadenom mit Sitz im Nabel und ein Beitrag zu den Nabel-geschwulsten. Deutsche Zeitschr. f. Chir., 1901, lix, 215.

Villar, Francis: Tumeurs de l'ombilic. These de Paris, 1886.

Wullstein, L.- Eine Geschwulst des Nabels. (Kombination von Cystadenom der Schweiss- driisen mit cavernosem Angiom.) Arb. a. d. Path. Inst, in Gottingen, R. Virchow, zum 50. Doctor-Jubilaum, 1893, 245.

CARCINOMA OF THE UMBILICUS.

General consideration.

Classification.

Primary squamous-cell carcinoma of the umbilicus.

Primary adenocarcinoma of the umbilicus; report of cases.

Carcinoma of the umbilicus secondary to carcinoma of the stomach; symptoms; treatment; detailed report of cases.

Carcinoma of the umbilicus secondary to cancer of the gall-bladder; report of cases; personal observation.

Carcinoma of the umbilicus secondary to cancer of the intestine; report of cases.

Carcinoma of the umbilicus secondary to ovarian carcinoma; report of cases; personal observation.

Carcinoma of the umbilicus secondary to carcinoma of the uterus.

Cases of secondary carcinoma of the umbilicus in which the source of the primary growth was not determined.

A retroperitoneal carcinoma accompanied by cancer of the umbilicus.

In an article on Surgical Eiseases of the Umbilicus which I read before the Surgical Section of the American Medical Association in June, 1910, and which waspublished in the Journal of February 11, 1911, the subject of umbilical cancer was briefly referred to, and several cases that had come under my observation were reported. In the present article cancer of the umbilicus will be much more fully considered, and the cases hitherto recorded in the literature brought together. Associated intimately with the early development of the subject. of carcinoma of the umbilicus are the names of Parker,* Chuquet,f Villarj Feulard,§ Burkhart,|| Ledderhose,** Neveujt Morris,|J Pernice,§§ Quenu and Longuet,|||| Le Coniac,*** and Besson.tft Many other authors have enriched the literature by publishing individual cases.

Before discussing the malignant epithelial growths occurring at the umbilicus,it may be well to refresh our minds as to the histologic appearance of the normal umbilicus and as to the umbilical lymphatics. The umbilical scar is covered over with a very thin squamous epithelium and is devoid of hair-follicles, sweat-glands, and sebaceous glands.

* Parker, W. : Excision of Umbilicus for Malignant Disease. Arch. Clin. Surg., New York. 1876-77, i, 71.

t Chuquet : Du carcinome generalise du peritoine. These de Paris, 1879, No. 548.

i Yillar, Francis: Tumeurs de 1'ombilic. These de Paris, 1886.

§Feulard: Fistule ombilicale et cancer de l'estomac. Arch. gen. de med., 1887, 7. ser., xx, 158.

|| Burkhart, 0.: Ueber den Nabelkrebs. Inaug. Diss., Berlin, 1889.

** Ledderhose, G.: Deutsche Chirurgie, 1890, Lief. 45 b.

ffNeveu: Contribution a l'etude des tumeurs malignes secondaires de l'ombilic. Paris, L890.

%X Morris:. Malignant Disease of the Navel as a Secondary Complication. Verhandl. d. 10. Internat. Med. Cong., 1890, Berlin, 1891, iii, 7. Abth., 122.

§§ Pernice, L.: Die Nabelgeschwiilste, Halle, 1892.

Qu£nu and Longuet : Du cancer secondaire de l'ombilic. Rev. de chir., 1896, xvi, 97.

"* Le Coniac, H. C. J. : Cancer secondaire de l'ombilic, consecutif aux tumeurs malignes de l'appareil utero-ovarien. ThSse <\<- Bordeaux, 1898, No. 19.

tft Besson, E.: Cancer de l'ombilic. These de Paris, 1901, No. 263.

In a few cases remnants of the omphalomesenteric duct have been detected at the umbilicus. These may be recognized as small fistulous tracts or as cysts lying between the peritoneum and the rectus muscle, or just beneath and communicating with the skin. In a few instances remnants of the omphalomesenteric duct have been present as small tubular glands opening directly upon the surface of the umbilical depression. Such a case has been particularly well described by Fox and MacLeod*.

From the above description it is evident that, while, as a rule, we have only a very attenuated squamous epithelium at the umbilicus, in some cases cylindric epithelium is present. Consequently we can have two varieties of primary carcinoma in this region.

The careful study of many umbilical lesions in the past has demonstrated that,when the liver is involved in a malignant growth which has extended to or encroached upon the suspensory ligament, the growth tends to pass by way of the lymphatics out along the suspensory ligament to the umbilicus. Where a malignant pelvic growth extends to the umbilicus, it usually follows the lymphaties found in the course of the remnants of the obliterated umbilical arteries and urachus upward to the umbilical depression. If the umbilicus is the seat of a malignant growth, either the inguinal or axillary glands may be secondarily involved, according as the growth occupies the upper or lower part of the umbilicus. The lymphatics of the umbilical region are considered at length in Chapter II.

* Fox and MacLeod: A Case of Paget's Disease of the Umbilicus. Brit. Jour. Dermatol., 1904, xvi, 41.

From a study of the literature it is found advisable to divide carcinomata of the umbilicus into two main groups — those that are primary, and those that are secondary to some intra-abdominal tumor. Each of these groups may be subdivided as follows :

A. Primary umbilical carcinoma.

1. Squamous-cell carcinoma.

2. Adenocarcinoma.

B. Secondary umbilical carcinoma, i

1. From the stomach.

2. From the gall-bladder.

3. From the intestine.

4. From the ovaries.

5. From the uterus.

6. From other abdominal organs.

i Walshe: Nature and Treatment of Cancer, London, 1S46, 92. 27

Cancer of the umbilicus, whether primary or secondary, is exceptionally rare.f Thus, according to Parker (1876), Walshel states that Tanchou found that the mortuary register of Paris and two adjacent arrondissements yielded 9118 deaths from cancer between the years 1830-40 inclusive, and that in only two instances was the umbilicus the seat of the carcinoma. With the early recognition of abdominal lesions and their timely surgical treatment, carcinoma of the umbilicus will in all probability diminish instead of increase.

1 1 have carefully read Sir William Osier's splendid series of lectures on the Diagnosis of Abdominal Tumors, published in vols, lix and lx of the New York Medical Journal, 1894. but failed to find any case in which the umbilicus was the seat of a secondary carcinoma.

PRIMARY SQUAMOUS-CELL CARCINOMA OF THE UMBILICUS.

Malignant squamous-cell growths occurring at the umbilicus are exceedingly rare. Hannay,* in 1843, reported a case of scirrhous cancer of the umbilicus. A microscopic examination was. however, not given, and it is impossible to determine whether or not the growth was primary.

Pernice'sf Case 77 from Yolkmann's clinic is more suggestive. The patient for a long while had had an umbilical stone. A carcinoma developed, and there was a purulent secretion. When Volkmann saw him, there was an ulcerated area the size of a thaler. On account of the cauliflower-like walls the growth was diagnosed as a cancroid (squamous-cell) carcinoma. The diagnosis was probably correct, although we have no data as to any histologic examination. It would seem that in this case the constant irritation of the foreign body had stimulated the development of a malignant growth.

Pernice, in his Case 79, reports another carcinoma, also from Yolkmann's clinic. The patient was a man, fifty-nine years of age, and of uncleanly habits. Not long before admission he had noticed a large number of brownish-looking spots all over the body. These varied in size from a finger-nail to a lentil. When the crusts were removed, there was free bleeding. For six or eight years he had noticed moisture around, and an odor from, the umbilicus. He consulted a physician, who removed several small particles of secretion. The walls of the umbilicus formed a cuff of cancroid or epithelial cancer. When Volkmann saw the patient, it was the size of a thaler and secreted a great deal. There was marked infiltration of the abdominal wall. The abdomen was opened during the operation. The patient died of sepsis in thirty-six hours. No further details of this case are given. The growth was evidently a primary carcinoma of the umbilicus, and in all probability had developed from the squamous epithelium, as indicated by the mode of origin and the slow growth. These are the only cases I could find suggesting a primary squamous-cell carcinoma of the umbilicus.

In the cases reported in the literature it is very difficult to determine accurately-whether the umbilical tumors were primary or secondary. Where the patient gave no history of any abdominal lesion, and where careful abdominal inspection before and at operation brought to light no evidence pointing to the existence of any other primary abdominal growth, one may, with a relative degree of certainty, conclude that the tumor was primary at the umbilicus. Still it must be remembered— as was clearly demonstrated in Valette's case — that, although a careful visual and manual examination may fail to reveal any priman* cancer in the stomach, such a growth may nevertheless exist. In Valette's case, when the umbilical growth was removed, the stomach was brought up into the wound for examination, and was apparently free from disease. The patient died of peritonitis, and at

autopsy a latent carcinoma of the stomach was found. The absence of any * abdominal symptoms for a period of two or three years after a removal of an umbilical carcinoma is the most certain proof that the growth has originated in the umbilicus.

* Hannay: Edin. Med. and Surg. Jour., 1843, lx, 313.

t Pernice, L. : Die Nabelgeschwiilste, Halle, 1892.

Pernice found in the literature 21 cases of what he considered primary carcinoma of the umbilicus. In this number he included both the squamous-cell and the glandular variety. I have discarded several of the cases included in his group, and have added several recorded since his valuable monograph was written in 1892; and still the actual number of cases remains uncertain. In the cases reported by Dejerine and Sollier, Bonvoisin, Forgue and Riche, Hue and Jacquin, Maylard, Parker, and Tillaux and Barraud, the growths seem, without a doubt, to have been primary. The growths reported by Ajello, Burkhart, Despres, Dannenberg, Demarquay, Giordano, Guiselin, Heurtaux, Ippolito, Jores, Lewis, Stori, and Wagner were also probably primary adenocarcinomata of the umbilicus, although the evidence in these cases is not quite so convincing. In Besson's case the picture suggested to some extent the presence of an umbilical tumor containing uterine glands. Hertz's case need be only mentioned here. From the description the growth does not seem to have been a carcinoma, but resembled in some degree the type of umbilical tumors containing uterine glands.

Pernice's Case 78 bears a striking resemblance to that reported by Fox and MacLeod. The man was seventy-two years of age, and the commencement of the umbilical growth dated back five or six years. It was the size of a two-mark piece, and was here and there covered with hard crusts. It looked very much like a rodent ulcer. On microscopic examination it was found to be a slowly growing, relatively benign carcinoma of the epithelium. Here and there a definite tendency toward gland formation was noted. It is quite possible that these glands were remnants of the omphalomesenteric duct, and that the proliferation of the squamous epithelium was similar to that noted in the case reported by Fox and MacLeod, and designated as Paget's disease of the umbilicus.

In Doderlein's case and in Pernice's Case 76, although the umbilical growths were considered as primary, they would seem to have been secondary to an abdominal lesion.

Primary adenocarcinoma of the umbilicus usually develops as a very small nodule in the umbilical depression, which may grow slowly or rapidly. In some cases it has not been larger than a small nut; in others it has reached the size of a walnut or a hen's egg. Such a tumor has been known to grow to the size of a five-franc piece in the course of six months. It may be smooth or have a slightly papillary surface. With the increase in size there is a tendency for the surrounding tissue to become infiltrated. The central portions of the nodule tend to ulcerate, and these areas of ulceration may be covered over with crusts. The ulceration is naturally accompanied by serous secretion, and occasionally by some bleeding.

Histologically nearly all these growths have been put down as adenocarcinomata of the type usually developing from the small intestine. This is but natural, as they originate from remnants of the omphalomesenteric duct.

Age. — In the cases which I have collected and in which the age was given, the youngest patient was thirty-seven, the oldest, seventy-six.

Under 40 years 2 cases

Between 40 and 50 2 cases

" 50 and 60 7 cases

" 60 and 70 6 cases

" 70 and 80 5 cases

Sex. — Of 20 patients of whom I have records on this point, 9 were men and 11 women. This tends to show that the disease is equally prevalent in both sexes.

Treatment. — This naturally consists in the wide removal of the umbilicus, care being taken not to spread the carcinoma cells into the surrounding healthy abdominal wall. The inner surface of the umbilicus should be carefully examined to see if adhesions exist, and then, after fresh abdominal dressings have been applied, a systematic inspection of the abdominal viscera should be made to exclude the possibility of carcinoma of the stomach, intestine, or pelvic organs. If no abdominal focus be found, and provided a wide removal of the growth has been possible, the prognosis is relatively good.

Detailed Report of Cases of Primary Adenocarcinoma of the Umbilicus.

In the majority of the cases the umbilical tumors were undoubtedly primary, but in several it is not certain that they were not secondary to some intra-abdominal growth.

A Primary Adenocarcinoma of the Umbilicus.

Ajello's* patient was a woman, sixty-four years old, from whom an umbilical growth was removed. He gives a picture of the outer surface and also of the smooth peritoneal surface of the tumor.

Histologic examination showed a definite regular glandular growth. Ajello then discusses the literature.

Primary Cancer of the Umbilicus.

Bessonf reports the case of a woman thirty-seven years of age. The patient's father had died of some pulmonary trouble, the mother of cancer. This woman, ten years before, on making an extra effort, had complained of intense pain at the umbilicus, and later noticed a small tumor developing in the umbilical cicatrix. It was the size of the last phalanx of the index-finger, and was hard in consistence. Elevation of the arms increased the sensitiveness at the umbilicus. The region was also somewhat painful at the menstrual period. The patient had been assured that the tumor was not reducible. It had increased in size quite slowly. According to the patient, during the last four months it had become painful and larger, and the skin had become violet in color. There had been some emaciation, associated with paleness. When the patient entered the hospital, the umbilical cicatrix formed a crescent with the concavity directed downward. Palpation showed that this elevation was produced by a solid tumor which was hard and about the size of a mandarin orange. The skin was not movable over the tumor, as it was adherent at the umbilical cicatrix. The tumor was removed, and the patient made a good recovery.

Histologic examination showed that it was composed of fibrous tissue and of a glandular growth similar to that developing from intestinal glands. When seen four years later, the patient was perfectly well. The growth was diagnosed as a cylindric-cell carcinoma. It had developed at the umbilical cicatrix, and was covered with skin. It consisted of fibrous tissue and glands lined with cylindric epithelium resembling that of the adult or embryonic Lieberkuhn's glands. The epithelial cells had infiltrated into the stroma, and there was a tendency to invade the surrounding tissue.

* Ajello: Contribute alia genesi embrionale di un adeno-epitelioma cistico primitivo dell' ombelico. From Tansini's Clinic. j La Riforma medica, 1899, anno 15, iii. 663.

f Besson : Cancer de l'ombilic. These de Paris, 1901, No. 263, 66.

Primary Adenocarcinoma of the Umbilicus.

Bonvoisin,* after citing a case already described by Tillaux, reports a second also from Tillaux's service. The patient, a man sixty-four years of age, had the general appearance of a sick person. He had been ill for about two months. At the umbilicus was a brawny excrescence. There was no history of injury. When the nodule was first noticed it was the size of a small pea. In about fifteen days it commenced to ulcerate and the physician thought it was eczema. At the time of Tillaux's examination the umbilicus had disappeared and had been replaced by a shallow area of ulceration covered with a blackish crust surrounded by an area of inflammation several millimeters in diameter. The total zone of inflammation was the size of a five-franc piece and about 1 cm. broad. The mass was immobile vertically, but could be pushed from side to side. There was no enlargement of the axillary or inguinal glands.

The umbilicus was removed, but the patient died. Autopsy failed to reveal any peritonitis, and the peritoneal portion of the growth was free from adhesions. The stomach and intestines were normal. The growth was a primary adenocarcinoma of the umbilicus and had evidently originated from remains of a fetal structure. Ducellier made the microscopic examination in Prof. CorniFs laboratory.

Primary Carcinoma of the Umbilicus.

Dannenberg f reports the case of a day laborer, seventy-one years old, operated upon by Maas. For three months before admission he had complained of pain in the umbilicus, and now showed an umbilical tumor 3 cm. broad, 2.5 cm. long, and raised 5 mm. above the surface of the abdomen. There was a dark-red, funnel-shaped ulceration in the middle. The tumor was firm in consistence and the surrounding tissue was infiltrated. There was pain on contraction of the abdominal muscles, and swelling in the inguinal glands, more marked on the left than on the right side. The appetite was good. When the tumor was removed, the peritoneum was found perfectly free at the umbilicus. The patient made a good recovery.

Microscopically, solid nests were here and there visible, and at other points cavities lined with one layer of cylindric epithelium. The tumor was diagnosed as a scirrhous carcinoma, but from the description it would seem to have been an adenocarcinoma. [Although there are many points suggesting a primary growth in this case, in the absence of a most thorough abdominal examination it is impossible to say that it might not have been secondary. — T. S. C]

Primary Adenocarcinoma of the Umbilicus. t

At an autopsy on a man, fifty-four years of age, who had had tabes for eleven years, a tumor of the umbilicus was found, circular in form, about 7 or 8 cm. in diameter and 5 to 6 cm. thick. It lay in front of the aponeurosis, and had not encroached on the peritoneum. It was an adenocarcinoma. There was no evidence of metastases. This tumor was looked upon as a primary carcinoma of the umbilicus.

Carcinoma of the Umbilicus.

Demarquay's § patient, fifty-four years of age, had a tumor the size of an egg at the umbilicus. She had had a congenital nevus at the umbilicus, and this had started to increase in size two years before her admission.

The tumor had become excoriated, was painful, and there was a small amount of hemorrhage. Demarquay hesitated to operate on account of two small tumors in the inguinal region. These, however, were looked upon as papillomata of the inguinal glands, not malignant, but caused by irritation from the umbilical growth. The general health of the patient became poor, and a fatal issue seemed probable.

* Bonvoisin, G. : Etude pathogenique et histologique sur une variete de l'epitheliome de l'ombilic. These de Paris, 1891, No. 305.

f Dannenberg, O. : Zur Casuistik der Nabeltumoren insbesondere des Carcinoma umbilicale. Inaug. Diss., Wurzburg, 1886.

t Dejerine et Sollier: Bull. Soc. anat, de Par., 1888, 649.

§ Demarquay: Cancer de l'ombilic. Bull. Soc. de chir. de Par. (1870), 1871, 2. ser., xi, 209.

Carcinoma of the Umbilicus (Primary or Secondary?).*

The patient, a man of seventy-four years, complained of pain when the clothes came in contact with the umbilicus. Situated in the umbilicus was a reddish nodule the size of a pea, which was slightly blood-tinged. The tumorincreased rapidly and reached the size of a two-franc piece. It was removed, and examination proved it to be an adenocarcinoma. There were no signs of any other growth.

Primary Adenocarcinoma of the Umbilicus.

Doederlein's t patient was a woman fifty-five years of age. Three months before admission she had first noticed a small, hard, painful tumor at the umbilicus. Four weeks before coming under observation the tumor had shown a small ulcer on its surface. The physician that saw her had diagnosed inflammation of the umbilicus, and ordered moist applications. The condition had become worse, and several other ulcers had developed around the umbilicus. When Doederlein saw her, the umbilicus was funnel-shaped and drawn in. The entire skin of the umbilicus was very thick, and the underlying parts were fixed. The surface was ulcerated, and there was a serous secretion. In the vicinity of the umbilicus were numerous dilated blood-vessels. Diffusely scattered, particularly toward the symphysis, were small hard nodules in the skin, the size of millet-seeds or linseeds. These on pressure were not painful. In both inguinal regions were hard packets of tumors the size of a goose's eggs. They were somewhat movable, and on pressure were not painful. Under anesthesia the umbilicus was widely removed. When the abdomen was opened, the peritoneum in the vicinity of the umbilicus was found to contain numerous small nodules. The umbilical tumor was removed, and the inguinal growths were dissected out. The patient died ten days later in collapse.

The portion of the abdominal wall removed was 20 by 12 by 4 cm., and the umbilical funnel was 2.5 cm. deep. The skin over the prominence of the umbilicus was somewhat stretched. On both sides of the umbilical depression were small superficial ulcers. These had irregular margins and somewhat reddened and dirty surfaces. In general the condition suggested that the depth of the umbilicus had consisted of small tumors which had pressed the skin forward and tended to break through. On palpation one could feel the nodules beneath the surface of the skin, and in the umbilical depression they merged with one another, forming a hard mass. A sharp outline between the skin and the tumor was macroscopically impossible.

On histologic examination the umbilical growth was found to be an adenocarcinoma; the enlargement in the inguinal glands was also due to carcinomatous involvement. The liver contained about 20 irregular, small metastases on its surface. These varied from a millet-seed to a bean in size. There was also one on the anterior surface of the gall-bladder. The gall-bladder contained stones. In the visceral peritoneum were about 60 or 80 nodules.

Doederlein came to the conclusion that the growth in the gall-bladder was a secondary one. [From the evidence at hand it is impossible for us to determine whether the umbilical carcinoma was primary or secondary. — T. S. C]

* Despres: Bull, et Mem. Soe. de chir. de Par., 1883, ix, 245.

t Doederlein, F.: Ein primares Adenokarzinom des Nabels. Inaug. Diss., Erlangen, 1907.

Primary Adenocarcinoma of the U mbilicus.

Forgue and Riche* report the case of a woman, aged fifty-six, who six months before coming under observation had noticed a reddish point at the umbilicus. At the time she was operated on it was the size of a five-franc piece and indurated, and for four months there had been a slight ulceration which emitted at times a bloody discharge. No abdominal tumor could be demonstrated at operation. The pelvis was empty; no enlarged glands could be detected. The tumor was removed 1, and on microscopic examination proved to be a typical adenocarcinoma. The glands in some places resembled those of Lieberkiihn.

The patient was well twenty-two months after operation. This tumor would seem to have been a primary adenocarcinoma which had probably developed from remains of the omphalomesenteric duct.

Probable Primary Carcinoma of the Umbilicus.

The patient, a porter aged thirty-eight, had a papillary-like growth at the umbilicus from which there was bloody discharge. The growth varied from 10 to 15 mm. in diameter. The pictures given by Giordano t are excellent. He thought he was dealing with a primary carcinoma of the umbilicus. He gives a short review of the literature.

Primary Carcinoma of the Umbilicus.

Guiselin + reports a case observed by Villar that had not yet been published. The woman was sixty-four years of age, a music teacher. Her father had died at seventy of cancer of the tongue. For five months she had noticed a small, painless enlargement at the umbilicus. The tumor had increased gradually in size and had become reddish in color during the two months before she was seen by Guiselin. On examination theumbilicus was found to be violet in color, and a tumor, the size of a hazelnut, occupied the umbilical depression. It presented bosses, was hard, adherent, and reducible. When the abdomen was opened, no tumor could be made out in the intestinal tract, stomach, liver, or genital organs.

Histologic examination showed the growth to be epithelial in character and of a cylindric type. It appeared to be a primary adenocarcinoma of the umbilicus.

Adenocarcinoma of the Umbilicus. §

The woman, fifty-eight years of age, had a tumor the size of a small hazelnut at the umbilicus. This was very soft and reddish gray in color. Microscopic examination showed gland-spaces surrounded with loose connective tissue. The epithelium in some places was one and in others several layers in thickness. There were also " Schichtungsperlen, " but a real hornification did not exist. In other places there was a definite malignant growth of the glands. Hertz says that, although the growth was malignant, it must have developed from the epithelium of the intestine or of the omphalomesenteric duct. [The growth strongly suggests an umbilical tumor containing uterine glands. — T. S. C]

* Forgue et Riche: Alontpellier med., 1907, 2. s., xxiv, 145-169.

t Giordano, D. : Sopra un caso di cancro dell' ombelico. La Medicina Italiana, 1911, ix, 6.

+ Guiselin: Du cancer de l'ombilic. These de Bordeaux, 1906, No. 47.

§ Hertz: L'eber einen Fall von Adenocarcinom des Nabels bei einer 5S-Jahrigen Frau. Inaug. Diss., Wurzburg, 1905.

Carcinoma of the Umbilicus.*

The patient was fifty-one years old. A small tumor had developed at the umbilicus a few months after she had received a blow. Microscopic examination showed that it was a cylindric-cell carcinoma.

Probable Primary Cancer of the Umbilicus.t

The patient, a soldier forty-five years of age, had a nodule at the umbilicus. This was opened and was thought to contain pus, although there was only a slight discharge. It became fungating, and grew as large as a fist. There was bladder involvement. Whether the growth was primary or not was uncertain.

Microscopic examination showed that it was a carcinoma, apparently of the adenocarcinomatous type. Autopsy revealed no growth in the intestine or stomach.

The fungating process was probably hastened as a result of the cutting; consequently I omit any description of the umbilicus.

Adenocarcinoma of the Umbilicus.

Ippolito i gives a brief review of the literature and then reports the case of a woman fifty-one years of age. An umbilical growth was removed, which microscopically proved to be an adenocarcinoma of the intestinal type. Ippolito thought it was primary, but there is no note made of any careful abdominal examination. [Possibly it was a secondary growth.— T. S. C]

Probable Adenocarcinoma of the Umbilicus. § — The tumor was removed by Professor Witzel; it was the size of a walnut. The peritoneum was intact. The tumor on section was hard, firm, and appeared to be encapsulated in fibrous tissue. On microscopic examination it. proved to be an adenocarcinoma of the type resembling that usually found developing in the stomach. Examination of the patient did not give any evidence of cancer in the abdomen. This was probably a primary growth.

A Malignant Tumor in an Umbilical Hernial Sac. ||

The patient was sixty-seven years of age and had had an umbilical hernia for fifteen years. No truss had been used, but the hernia had been reduced without difficulty until a year before. Pain in the umbilicus increased rapidly and radiated to the stomach and the pelvic region. The patient lost flesh and strength and had frequent vomiting, with constipation and diarrhea.

On examination a hard, nodulated, bluish-red tumor was found at the umbilicus.

Its surface was slightly ulcerated. The sac contained omentum, which was not diseased, and also subperitoneal tissue infiltrated as far as a finger could reach.

The growth was removed, but the patient died of shock six hours later. Microscopic examination showed a malignant growth, which the author thought was a sarcoma connected with Lieberkiihn's glands, although he questioned whether or not it might represent remains of the omphalomesenteric duct. The case is not very clear, but the tumor was evidently malignant.

* Heurtaux: Epitheliome de l'ombilic. Gaz. med. de Nantes, 18S6, iv, 46.

t Hue et Jacquin: Cancer colloid e de la l'ombilic et de paroi abdominale anterieure ayant envahi la vessie. L'Union med., 1868, 3. ser., vi, 418.

i Ippolito: t it caso d'epitelioma dell'ombelico. Gazz. Internaz. di med., 1901, iv, 302.

§ Jores: Cylinder-Epithelkrebs des Nabels. Vereins-Beilagc der Deutsch. med. Wochenschr., 1899, xxv, 22.

|| Lewi.-,: Med. Record, 1889, xxxvi, 394.

Cylindric-cell Carcinoma of the Umbilicus.*

The specimen was from a man sixty-five years of age. For two months before admission he had complained of pain in the lumbar region. He had not noticed the umbilical nodule until it was pointed out to him by the doctor. A small projection the size of a pea was readily seen and felt in the pit of the umbilicus. On deep palpation it appeared to be larger. It was removed through an elliptic incision. The peritoneal surface was puckered. On section, the tumor presented a solid appearance.

Microscopic examination showed a cylindric-cell carcinoma. Maylard suggested that it had developed from the omphalomesenteric duct. Macewen, in the discussion at the Glasgow Path, and Clin. Society, before which this case was reported, said he had seen two similar cases, but when brought to him both patients already had advanced peritoneal disease. Each of the umbilical growths was considered primary. In one case pain in the back was thought to be due to the involvement of the liver, as found at autopsy.

Primary Carcinoma of the Umbilicus. t

A woman seventy-six years of age, had a malignant growth at the umbilicus. The disease gradually progressed and she died. At autopsy the feasibility of an operation for the removal of the mass forcibly impressed itself on Parker. The growth was evidently primary.

Primary Carcinoma of the Umbilicus. J Case 76.

Volkmann removed from a man, seventy-four years of age, a squamous-cell carcinoma the size of a hen's egg from the umbilicus. The omentum was already degenerated with carcinomatous nodules, and death followed five months later with abdominal carcinoma and ascites. The growth was not glandular.

Primary Carcinoma of the Umbilicus. §

Case 78. — A forester, seventy-two years of age, came to Volkmann suffering from an ulceration at the umbilicus the size of a two-mark piece, which had first begun some five or six years previously. Here and there it was covered with hard crusts. The condition strongly suggested a rodent ulcer. On microscopic examination it proved to be a slowly growing, relatively benign, carcinoma. The slightly thickened walls of the ulcer were excised, the abscess was cureted out and freely cauterized, and a plaster laid over it. The wound healed speedily, and the man had no return of the growth, but died of pneumonia four or five years later. Examination of the tumor showed no evidence of a horny layer or of nests of cells resembling those of the rete Malpighii. Here and there was a definite tendency toward gland formation.

[It is quite possible that in this case there were remains of the omphalomesenteric duct at the umbilicus, as seen in Fox and MacLeod's case, which they diagnosed as Paget's disease of the umbilicus. — T. S. C]

Adenocarcinoma of the Umbilicus. ||

The patient, sixty-eight years of age, for nearly a year had complained of discomfort just above the umbilicus, which was continuous and independent of digestion. At the umbilicus was an indurated area, the size of a pigeon's egg. When seen at operation, it was ovoid in form, 6 cm. in itslongest diameter,and 4 cm. broad. It seemed to be a primary tumor of the abdominal wall. It was removed, and the patient died of peritonitis. Microscopic examination showed that the growth was an adenocarcinoma. [Whether this was primary or secondan- is uncertain. — T. S. C]

* Maylard: Trans. Glasgow Path, and Clin. Soc, 1886-91; 1892, iii, 294.

t Parker: Excision of Umbilicus for Malignant Diseases. Arch. Clin. Surg., Xew York, 1876-77, i, 71.

J Pernice, L. : Die Nabelgeschwulste, Halle, 1892.

§ Pernice, L.: Op. cit.

|| Stori: Contribute alio studio dei tumori dell'ombelico. Lo Sperimentale, Arch, di biologia normale e patologia, 1900, liv, 25.

Carcinoma of the Umbilicus Developing in the Depth of an Umbilical Diverticulum.* The patient, a woman forty years of age, entered the hospital for an umbilical tumor. In childhood she had had no serious diseases. Seven months previously, while bathing, she had noticed a small crust at the umbilicus. This she had removed, and had seen a small, dark-red tumor the size of a lentil. There was no ulceration and no discharge. It had increased steadily in size and had been cauterized, but had reappeared as a small but rapidly growing tmnor. At the end of three weeks it had ulcerated, and there had been slight hemorrhages. On admission the entire umbilicus was found transformed into a tumor about the size of a ten-centime piece. It was.circular and bulging. It was dark red, ulcerated, and cup-shaped over an area the size of a five-centime piece. The surrounding tissue was indurated. No axillary or inguinal gland enlargement was noted. The patient was in good condition and had no indigestion. An extensive removal was made. The omentum was not adherent, and no abdominal lesion was noted. Recovery followed.

Cornil made the following report: "The tumor consists of a cylindric-cell epithelioma. The epithelioma is analogous to that which develops primarily in the intestinal glands." [Of course, the length of time — about four months — was too short to warrant a final prognosis. — T. S. C]

Carcinoma of the Umbilicus f

A woman, aged forty, who had had 12 children, two years previously had noticed two pea-sized bodies in the skin on the left side of the umbilicus, winch had grown gradually for eighteen months. Blisters had formed and broken, discharging a foul-smelling pus. On admission the tumor was 43^ inches in its longest diameter and 11 inches in circumference; it was lobulated and had a dirty, ulcerated surface, covered with a foul-smelling discharge. Xo other local manifestations were detected. The growth was removed in 1816 and the patient recovered. Naturally, at that time there was no microscopic examination. [The duration is strongly indicative that this growth was primary, in view of the fact that, when the umbilical growth is secondary, the primary tumor usually causes death in the course of five or six months. — T. S. C]

A Supposed Sub malignant Adenocarcinoma of the Umbilicus.

From the history this growth seems to have been primary. Its situation and relation would suggest its origin from the urachus, but Koslowski i says that the glands in it were of the intestinal type. It is probable that it had developed from extraperitoneal remnants of the omphalomesenteric duct. As it does not nsemble any case heretofore described, I have allotted it a separate place.

Koslowski'si patient was operated upon in October, 1902. Five weeks before, he had noticed, in the mid-line, between the symphysis and umbilicus, a small painful tumorwhich grew to the size of a walnut. The abdominal pain radiated. On examination the man, although only fifty-five years old, was markedly emaciated and looked as if he were about seventy. He had had frequent diarrhea. He was bent over as if guarding the abdominal muscles. Between the umbilicus and the symphysis, near the mid-line, was a tumor reminding one of a patella. The overlying skin was free. The tumor was very painful and slightly movable. It felt dense and gradually merged into the surrounding tissue. Toward the umbilicus was a cord the size of a goose-quill. The growth was thought to be a malignant epithelial tumor of the urachus.

A median incision showed that the tumor had grown through the linea alba and the sheath of the rectus. A portion of the rectus muscle, of the transversalis fascia, and of the peritoneum were removed. After the abdomen had been opened and the tumor had been drawn up, fibrous cords were seen passing from the umbilicus. The upper one was the size of a goose-quill, firm and infiltrated; the lower contained a venous cord, was less firm, and passed into the vesico-umbilical ligament. The peritoneum covering the posterior surface of the tumor showed evidence of scarring and of ulceration. The patient made a good recovery.

The tumor in form, as mentioned above, resembled a patella. The peritoneum was firmly attached to it, and the surrounding muscle had been penetrated by it. On microscopic examination the growth was found to be made up of glands varying in size between that of a urinary tubule and that of a gland large enough to be seen with the naked eye. The diagnosis was fibro-adenocarcinoma submalignum. The glands resembled those of the intestinal type

* Tillaux and Barraud: Epithelioma de l'ombilie, developpe aux depens d'un diverticule intestinal; omphalectomie, guerison. Annales de Gyn., Paris, 1887, xxvii, 401.

f Wagner: Abtragung eines carcinomatosentarteten Nabels. Med. Jahrb. d. k. k. oster.

31 lates, Wien, 1839, n. F., xviii, .585-589.

i Koslowski: Ein Fall von wahrem Xabeladenom. Deutsche Zeitschr. f. Chir., 1903, lxix, 469.

LITERATURE CONSULTED ON PRIMARY CARCINOMA OF THE UMBILICUS.

Ajello: Contributo alia genesi embrionale di un adeno-epiteliorna cistico primitivo deU'ombelico (from Tansini's clinic). La Riforma medica, 1899, Anno 15, iii, 663.

Besson, E. : Cancer de l'ombilic. These de Paris, 1901, No. 263.

Bonvoisin, G. : Etude pathogenique et histologique sur une variete de l'epitheliome de 1'ombilic. These de Paris, 1891, No. 305.

Burkhart, O.: Ueber den Nabelkrebs. Inaug. Diss., Berlin, 1889.

Chuquet: Du carcinome generalise du peritoine. These de Paris, 1879, No. 548.

Dannenberg, O. : Zur Casuistik der Nabeltumoren insbesondere des Carcinoma umbilicale. Inaug. Diss., Wiirzburg, 1886.

Dejerine et Sollier: Bull. Soc. anat. de Paris, 1888, 649.

Demarquay: Cancer de l'ombihc. Bull. Soc. de Chir. de Par. (1870), 1871, 2. s. xi, 209.

Despres: Bull, et Mem. Soc. de chir. de Paris, 1883, ix, 245.

Doederlein, F. : Ein primares Adenokarzinom des Nabels. Inaug. Diss., Erlangen, 1907.

Fox and MacLeod: A Case of Paget's Disease of the Umbilicus. Brit. Jour. Dermatol.1904, xvi, 41.

Forgue et Eiche: Montpellier med., 1907, 2. s., xxiv, 145-169.

Feulard: Fistule ombilicale et cancer de l'estomac. Arch. gen. de med, 18S7, 7. ser., xx, 158.

Giordano, D.: Sopra un caso di cancro dell'ombilico. La Medicina Italiana, 1911, ix, 6.

Guiselin, E. J. M. J. : Du cancer de l'ombihc. These de Bordeaux, 1906, No. 47.

Hertz, W. H.: Uber einen Fall von Adenocarcinom des Nabels bei einer 58-Jahrigen Frau. Inaug. Diss., Wiirzburg, 1905.

Heurtaux: Epitheliome de l'ombilic. Gaz. med. de Nantes, 1886, iv, 46.

Hue et Jacquin: Cancer colloide de l'ombihc et de la paroi abdominale anterieure ayant envahi la vessie. L'Union medicale, 1868, 3. ser., vi, 418.

Ippolito, G. : Un caso epitelioma dell'ombelico. Gaz. internaz. di med., 1901, iv, 302.

Jores: Cylinder-Epithelkrebs des Nabels. Vereins-Beilage der Deutsch. med. Wochenschr., 1899, xxv, iv, 22.

Koslowski: Ein Fall von wahrem Nabeladenom. Deutsche Zeitschr. f. Chir., 1903, lxix, 469.

Ledderhose, G. : Deutsche Chirurgie, 1890, Lief. 45 b.

Lewis, D.: A Malignant Tumor in an Umbilical Hernial Sac. Medical Record, 1889, xxxvi, 394.

Le Coniac, H. C. J.: Cancer secondaire de l'ombilic, consecutif aux tumeurs malignes de l'appareil utero-ovarien. These de Bordeaux, 1898, No. 19.

Maylard: Cylinder-celled Epithelioma of the Umbilicus. Trans. Glasg. Path, and Clin. Soc, 1886-91; 1892, iii, 294.

Morris, R.: Malignant Disease of the Navel as a Secondary Complication. Verhandl. d. 10. Internat. Med. Cong., 1890, Berlin, 1891, iii. Abth., vii, 122-126.

Neveu, v. : Contribution a l'etude des tumeurs malignes secondaires de l'ombilic. Paris, 1890.

Osier, Sir William: Lectures on the Diagnosis of Abdominal Tumors. New York Med. Jour., 1894, lix; lx.

Parker, W. : Excision of Umbilicus for Malignant Disease. Arch. Clin. Surg., New York, 1876- 77, i, 71.

Pernice, L. : Die Nabelgeschwiilste, Halle, 1892.

Quenu et Longuet: Du Cancer secondaire de l'ombilic. Revue de Chir., 1896, xvi, 97.

Sollier, Paul Henri: See Dejerine.

Stori, T.: Contributo alio studio dei tumori dell'ombelico. Lo Sperimentale, Archivio di biologia normale e patologia, 1900, liv, 25.

Tillaux and Barraud: Epithelioma de l'ombilic, developpe aux depens d'un diverticule intestinal; omphalectomie; guerison. Ann. de Gyn., Paris, 1887, xxvii, 401.

Villar, F. : Tumeurs de l'ombilic. These de Paris, 1886.

Wagner: Abtragung eines carcinomatosentarteten Nabels. Med. Jahrb. d. k. k. oster. Staates, Wien, 1839, N. F., xviii, 585-589.

CARCINOMA OF THE UMBILICUS SECONDARY TO CARCINOMA OF THE STOMACH.

In 27 cases we have found fairly conclusive evidence that the umbilical growth was secondary to carcinoma of the stomach.

Age. — In 23 of these we have definite data as to the age of the patient. The youngest patient was twenty-six, the oldest seventy-two, years of age.

26 years old 1 case

Between 30 and 40 1 "

" 40 and 50 4 cases

" 50 and 60, 10 "

" 60 and 70 5 "

" 70 and 80 2 "

From the above it will be seen that the age distribution corresponds to that in which carcinoma of the stomach is usually found.

Sex. — Of the 27 cases, data as to the sex are given in 23. Ten of the patients were men and 13 were women, indicating that men are nearly equally liable to this affection.

Trauma. — Occasionally, as in the cases reported by Attimont, Burkhart, and Wulckow, and in my own Case G., the patient attributed the umbilical lesion to an injury. Attimont's patient dated her symptoms from the time she had hurt her abdomen on the edge of a tub. Burkhart's patient noticed an umbilical nodule four months after her abdomen had been accidentally and forcibly compressed; Wulckow's patient, as he was going home on a dark night, struck his abdomen against a stony projection and complained from that time on. My patient, shortly before the umbilical growth was noticed, had been struck in his umbilical region by a boot, which was probably not unusual for him, as he kept a shoe-store.

Gastric Symptoms. — In about two-thirds of the cases symptoms suggestive of deranged digestion were noted. In some there was loss of appetite, in others indigestion accompanied by more or less epigastric pain; some vomited food, and in one case at least the vomitus contained blood.

A deep-seated tumor in the pyloric region was detected in several cases, and the condition was so clear that the physician diagnosed cancer of the stomach. In a few cases a definite enlargement of the liver was found, and in several instances the abdomen contained ascitic fluid. Quite a number of the patients, however, gave no gastric symptoms whatsoever, but felt weak and looked cachectic. In at least one case (Valette's) there was not the slightest evidence at operation of any other abdominal lesion. It will be noted that the umbilical growth was the size of a 50-centime piece, and that its central portion was ulcerated, and, moreover, that it was firmly fixed. During removal of the tumor the abdomen was inspected and small peritoneal metastases were found. The stomach, however, appeared to be normal. The patient died on the eighth day, and at autopsy a primary carcinoma was found in the stomach.

The umbilical nodule, when first noted, may not be larger than a grain of wheat. In the course of a few months it has increased in some cases to the size of a small nut, in others to that of a chestnut. Sometimes it is first noted in the umbilical depression; in other instances in the umbilical wall or in the tissues immediately adjacent to the umbilicus. At first these tumors may be sharply circumscribed, the overlying skin being free. But with the growth of the nodule the skin soon becomes adherent and the tumor may show a bluish-violet or brownish-red discoloration. The more prominent portions of the tumor tend to become ulcerated, and may discharge a serous or purulent fluid or be covered with crusts. In a few instances there have been several small hemorrhages from them. With the continued growth of the nodule the central portion may be deeply ulcerated, and surrounding the ulcer papillary or cauliflower-like masses may form and the nearby skin show considerable infiltration, frequently of an inflammatory character.

In Cannuet's case there was a small umbilical hernia. This contained incarcerated omentum, in which was found a carcinomatous nodule. In a case which I have recently seen the patient had had an umbilical hernia for thirty-two years. A few months before coming under my care the hernial mass had become hard, and on palpation definite firm nodules could be felt scattered throughout it. At operation I found an ovarian tumor, general peritoneal carcinosis, and a markedly thickened omentum. The portion of the omentum incarcerated in the umbilical hernia also contained carcinomatous nodules. The primary growth in this case was apparently in the ovary.

There is another group of cases presenting a totally different picture. The umbilicus may or may not be the seat of a nodule, but a slight tumefaction of the region is noted. The swelling increases in amount and abscess is suspected. In some cases the picture is that of an acute phlegmon. On the supposition that the condition was inflammatory, several of the tumors were opened. The incision in some yielded nothing but blood and serous fluid; in others small foci of pus were found. In a short time the supposed inflammatory area would undergo gradual dissolution or necrosis en masse, and a fungating base be left at the site of the umbilicus. A little later gas-bubbles would be noted, and ere long stomach-contents would commence to pass through the fistulous opening. The margins of the fistulous opening in some cases were surrounded by large papillary or fungoid growths. In these cases the carcinoma had not extended to the umbilicus by way of the suspensory ligament, but by direct continuity. The carcinoma of the stomach had become adherent to the abdominal wall at or near the umbilicus, and by direct extension had caused a gradual disintegration until the surface of the abdomen had been reached.

If the carcinoma is situated at or near the pylorus and becomes adherent to the abdominal wall, it is only natural that the attachment should be in the umbilical region. If the disease, however, be in another part of the stomach, the abdominal wall may be attacked at another point, as was well shown in the following case :

Mrs. B., seen in consultation with Dr. Edwin B. Fenby July 8, 1910. Thispatient had been seized that evening with sudden abdominal pain about an inch and a half above and to the left of the umbilicus. She had a temperature of 100° F.; pulse, 116. "When I saw her, she was rather pale. Appendicitis was ruled out, but some malignant growth was suspected. She had a leukocytosis of 15,000. She was at once removed to the hospital' for observation. Ten days later we made an incision through the left rectus, and on cutting down to the fascia found some edema. On going into the peritoneal cavity we found that the stomach had become adherent to the anterior abdominal wall. After adhesions had been liberated, the parts were walled off as thoroughly as possible, and a tract 3 mm. in diameter was found passing from the stomach directly to the abdominal wall. In other words, there was a perforation of the stomach at this point. We gradually loosened the organs from the surrounding indurated tissue, which in some places was fully 2 cm. thick and as hard as gristle. The stomach was brought out and was found to be indurated in every direction. The growth was a carcinoma. The area of induration in the anterior wall was 7 by 5 cm., and just beneath the point of perforation there was a punched-out area in the carcinoma 2 cm. long. It was at the thinnest point of this that the perforation had taken place. We removed about half of the stomach. The patient made a very satisfactory recovery, and for a year there were no definite signs of a return of the growth. These, however, developed later and she died on November 12, 1911.

In those cases in which the disease reaches the umbilicus by way of the suspensory ligament the peritoneal surface of the umbilicus is usually smooth, because the lymphatics are extraperitoneal. On section an intact carcinomatous nodule of theumbilicus does not resemble cancer, but we find what looks like a diffuse fibrous thickening, and one can hardly realize that it is fairly riddled with glands. Where ulceration exists, however, the true character of the growth is more manifest. On histologic examination the tumor is found to consist of fibrous tissue with myriads of carcinomatous glands scattered throughout it. The gland type is identical with that found in the original gastric tumor, and where ulceration has occurred, the usual picture of gland disintegration, together with polymorphonuclear leukocytes and small-round-cell infiltration, is noted on the surface.

Treatment. — If a patient has given definite signs of carcinoma of the stomach, by the time an umbilical nodule has developed the malignant process has become so wide-spread that operative interference is of no avail. In those cases in which the cancer has extended to the abdominal wall by continuity and has broken down, causing a gastroumbilical fistula, operation is out of the question. There are a certain number of cases, however, in which, even when a secondary abdominal nodule exists, gastric symptoms are lacking. Here the surgeon will naturally remove the umbilical growth in the hope that it may be a primary lesion. In all such cases, when the abdomen is opened, a careful survey of the stomach and abdominal contents should be made to determine if any visceral carcinoma exists.

Prognosis. — Where an umbilical carcinoma is secondary to carcinoma of the stomach, practically all the patients speedily succumb.

Cases of Carcinoma of the Umbilicus Secondary to Cancer of the Stomach.

In the majority of the cases here detailed the diagnosis is certain, as proved at operation or at autopsy. In a few of the cases such absolute proof was wanting, but the clinical picture strongly suggested the stomach as the source of the primary tumor.

Carcinoma of the Umbilicus Secondary to Carcinoma of the Stomach.

Attimont's* patient was a woman fifty-three years of age. She had enjoyed good health until three months before he saw her, and dated her gastric symptoms from the time she hit her abdomen on the edge of a tub. On palpation no internal tumor could be found, but at the umbilicus were two small nodules the size of grains of wheat. At the end of two months the patient returned emaciated. The nodules at the umbilicus had increased in size, one being as large as a small walnut. It was hard, and the overlying skin was adherent. The umbilical mass was removed and proved to be an adenocarcinoma.

Autopsy at a later date showed carcinoma of the lesser curvature of the stomach, with secondary nodules on the surface of the liver and uterus and cancerous masses between the folds of the suspensory ligament.

Cancer of the Stomach; Gastro-abdominal Fistula. f

A woman, forty-nine years of age, complained of epigastric pain, difficult digestion, and frequent vomiting. Blood had never been noted in the vomited material or in the stools. On palpation an ill-defined tumor was found in the epigastric region which was painful on pressure. Cancer of the stomach was diagnosed. Some time after the patient entered the hospital she had fever at night. The tumor rapidly increased in size. The abdominal wall became a little red, was painful on pressure, and fluctuation was detected. On making an opening with the bistoury odorless pus escaped. A sound could be passed inward for 5 or 6 cm. The fever disappeared and the patient ate without vomiting or pain. A month later the skin around the incision was thinner, reddened, and an area of ulceration the size of a five-franc piece existed. In the depression were fungoid masses which gave off a fecal odor. Two weeks later all trace of the umbilicus had disappeared and there was an area of ulceration as large as the palm of the hand, and three fungoid masses, forming a tumor the size of a fist, presented. The discharge was so fetid that the patient was isolated. Gas and particles of stomach-contents escaped. The mushroom growths increased rapidly and broke down easily. Hemorrhages resulted, whichwere controlled with difficulty. The patient became very cachectic, and died two weeks later.

At autopsy the abdomen contained clear yellow fluid. The intestines were small in caliber, but not adherent. The anterior part of the stomach was adherent to the ulcerated abdominal wall. The opening was near the pylorus; the area round it was hard and infiltrated. The subcutaneous abdominal tissue was necrotic. The right lobe of the liver contained cancerous masses. In this case the carcinoma of the stomach had become adherent to the umbilicus and the opening between the stomach and the umbilicus had resulted.

* Attimont, A.: Remarques sur le cancer de l'ombilic. Gaz. med. de Nantes, 1887-88, vi, 137; 149.

f Auger, M. G.: Cancer de l'estomac fistule gastro-abdominale. Bull. Soc. anat. de Paris, 1875, i, 708.

Carcinoma of the Stomach with Perforation of the Abdominal Wall.*

The patient was a weakly woman, fifty-two years of age, and the mother of 17 children. In the spring she had complained of pain in the abdomen, and in July had had to give up work. She was very anemic and wasted. In August she had had severe colicky pains in the region of the spleen; in September these had migrated to the umbilical region. At this time there could be felt a tumor the size of a fist deep in that region. The tumor descended until it lay behind the umbilicus, forming a mass about 5 inches in diameter, with the umbilicus in the center. It became softer, and a few days later a small area sloughed, and the stomach-contents escaped. The opening rapidly increased in size and the patient soon died. The growth was a carcinoma of the stomach which had opened near the umbilicus.

Carcinoma of the Umbilicus Probably Secondary to Carcinoma of the Stomach. f

A delicate, poorly nourished woman, fifty-nine years of age, entered Bergmann's clinic. Some time before, her abdomen had been accidentally compressed, and four months later she had noticed a painless but hard nodule at the umbilicus. The skin covering it was smooth. Three months later the tumor was the size of a hazel-nut. On examination the umbilicus was elevated. The tumor was the size of a two-mark piece and could be sharply outlined. The surface was very red and nodular, and suggested dense granulation tissue. It secreted pus. Operation was not advised, but was insisted upon by the patient. She left the hospital before any local return had occurred.

The growth was a glandular carcinoma and probably secondary to carcinoma of the stomach.

Carcinoma of the Umbilicus Secondary to Carcinoma of the Stomach. t

A farmer, aged seventy-two, for six months had been complaining of gastric disturbances. Ten weeks before coming under observation he had noticed a moistness at the umbilicus and a discharge of a tarry-looking, brownish secretion. Later there had been ulceration, which had gradually increased. The patient was well nourished and strong. At the umbilicus was an irregular ulceration the size of a two-mark piece. It was hard and seemed unattached. At operation it was necessary to remove the ligament um teres to the liver. The patient died one month after. A carcinoma the size of a three-mark piece was found near the pylorus; it was adherent to the liver, and in the liver diffuse carcinomatous infiltration was present.

* Balluff: Magenkrebs, Erweichung unci Aufbruch desselben durch die allgemeinen Bauchdecken, Magenfistel. Correspondenzbl. des Wiirtemberg. arztl. Vereins, Stuttgart, 1854, xxiv, 37.

f Burkhart: Ueber den Nabelkrebs. Inaug. Diss., Berlin, 1889.

t Burkhart: Op. cit.

Carcinoma of the Liver with Carcinoma of the Omentum; Incarcerated Umbilical Hernia. Cannuet* reported the case of a patient with carcinoma of the liver probably secondary to carcinoma of the stomach. There was an umbilical hernia containing incarcerated omentum, and in this incarcerated omentum was a cancerous nodule.

Carcinoma of the Umbilicus Secondary to Carcinoma of the Stomach f

A man, sixty-three years of age, had had pain in the abdomen, complained of indigestion, and later had noticed a tumefaction at the umbilicus. He had diarrhea and vomiting and a supposed abscess of the abdominal wall. This was opened and bloody fluid escaped. Later there was the characteristic fetid cancerous discharge from the umbilicus. At autopsy a carcinoma of the pylorus was found adherent to the umbilical tumor.

Carcinoma of the Umbilicus Secondary to Cancer of the Stomach. J

In a woman, twenty-six years of age, a fistula developed at the umbilicus. There was no vomiting, but emaciation. Just above the umbilical cicatrix was a reddening. The skin was distended, hot, and painful and serous or purulent fluid escaped from the opening. At autopsy cancer of the pyloric region was found. On the outer surface of the pylorus were cancerous vegetations. These had become adherent to the abdominal wall; suppuration had followed, and an opening had developed at the umbilicus.

Carcinoma of the Umbilicus Secondary to Cancer of the Stomach. — Fischer § operated on a woman fifty-two years of age who had a carcinomatous tumor of the umbilicus which had extended as far as the interior of the abdomen. On opening the abdomen he discovered that the anterior part of the stomach was perforated and transformed into a large carcinomatous ulcer, which penetrated directly into the transverse colon. The patient had never manifested any gastric symptoms. Fischer removed the entire anterior portion of the stomach and the diseased colon. The patient made a good recovery, but developed other stomach symptoms and died five months later.

Carcinoma of the Umbilicus, Secondary. ||

A woman, fifty years of age, had had a warty, nodular growth at the umbilicus for two or three months and was not in good health. No abdominal lesions being noted, Hutchinson made an elliptic incision and removed the growth. It extended to but had not invaded the peritoneum. Two months later there was a nodular thickening of the liver, great irritability of the stomach, and the patient died four months after operation. Hutchinson thought that the umbilical growth was secondary to that in the liver. In two other of his cases, he says, a carcinoma of the umbilicus had developed secondarily to a growth in the liver. [Of course, the majority of the cases of cancer of the liver are secondary to those of the stomach.— T. S. C]

Carcinoma of the Umbilicus Secondary to Cancer of the Stomach.**

A man, forty-four years of age, gave a history of vomiting and loss in weight. At theumbilicus was a tumor 5 cm. in diameter. Its central portion was ulcerated and surrounded by a zone of induration. At death the growth was found extending to the peritoneal surface, but there was no adhesions. The patient had cancer of the stomach, which had extended to the liver. There were numerous other Secondary nodules.

* Cannuet: Bull. Soc. anat. de Paris, 1852, xxvii, 274.

f Codet de Boisse: Tumeurs de l'ombilic chez l'adulte. These de Paris, 1883, No. 311.

J Feulard: Fistule ombilicale et cancer de l'estomac. Arch. gen. de med., 1887, 7. s., xx, 158.

§ Fischer (Breslau) : Resection de l'estomac. La Semaine med., Paris, 1888, viii, 134.

|| Hutchinson, Jonathan: Arch, of Surgery, 1893, iv, 153 (1 pi.).

** Largeau, R.: Cancer de l'ombilic. Bull. Soc. anat. de Par., 1884, lix, 210-212.

Carcinoma of the Umbilicus Probably Secondary to Cancer of the Stomach or Liver. Ledderhose,* after giving a survey of the literature, reports a case communicated to him by A. Cahn. L., fifty-eight years of age, complained of gradually increasing lack of appetite and of the development, a few months later, of edema of the lower extremities and varicose veins in the leg. Still later the scrotum and the abdominal wall became edematous and there was also ascites with complete loss of appetite and intestinal obstruction. At the umbilicus was a hard, semicircular nodule. By deep ballottement, enlargement of the hardened liver could be made out. A provisional diagnosis of carcinoma of the liver with peritonitis was made. No microscopic examination is given.

In all probability the umbilical growth was secondary to a carcinoma of the stomach with implication of the liver. Ledderhose follows this by two other observations; in none of the cases, however, was any autopsy made.

Carcinoma of the Umbilicus Secondary to Carcinoma of the Stomach. f

A man, forty-five years of age, gave a history of vomiting for a year. He was well nourished and of good color, but had lost 24 pounds. At the upper and left side of the umbilicus was a small tumor the size of a bean; the overlying skin was free. In two weeks the tumor had become adherent to the skin and had increased in size. Two months later the abdomen was distended with ascitic fluid, and the patient died soon after the fluid had been removed.

Autopsy showed carcinoma of the lesser curvature of the stomach and compression of the portal vein; no involvement of the liver was found. No microscopic examination of the abdominal tumor is recorded.

Umbilical Fistula Due to Latent Cancer of the Stomach.

Monod's t patient was a woman sixty-six years of age. She was cachetic, but had had no vomiting. At the umbilicus was a fistulous opening of recent date. A diagnosis of latent cancer of the stomach was made. At autopsy in the region of the umbilicus Monod found a compact mass consisting of the stomach, liver, transverse colon, and duodenum. The lesser curvature of the stomach was adherent to the liver. The anterior surface of the stomach was involved in the cancer, which extended to the posterior surface; the fistulous opening reached the umbilicus. The transverse colon communicated by an oblique opening, measuring 5 x 6 cm., with a pocket formed by the stomach and the left lobe of the liver.

Cancer of the Umbilicus Secondary to Cancer of the Pylorus. §

A woman, seventy years of age, came with a diagnosis of cancer of the pylorus. Six months from the beginning of her symptoms she had begun to have pain at the umbilicus and noticed a small lump there. This became very hard, was about as largeas a chestnut, bluishred in color, and had a smooth surface, which was somewhat ulcerated and discharged a little straw-colored serum. Morris removed the diseased umbilicus and found that it was not in contact with anything but normal structures. The patient died two months later with the ordinary symptoms of cancer of the pylorus. No autopsy, however, was permitted. The umbilical growth was an adenocarcinoma.

* Ledderhose : Chirurgische Erkrankungen des Nabels. Deutsche Chirurgie, 1890, Lief. 45 b.

f Mirallie: Reported by Attimont.

t Monod: Fistule Ombilicale; cancer latent de l'estomac. Bull. Soc. anat. de Paris, 1877, lii, 38.

§ Morris, Robert : Lectures on Appendicitis and Notes on Other Subjects, 1895, 95.

Cancer of the Pylorus; Secondary Growth at the Umbilicus.

Morris * cites an extract from a letter from Dr. Grinnell, of Burlington, Vermont. The patient was a man sixty-eight years of age who had symptoms of cancer of the pylorus. Eight months before death the umbilicus became hard and painful and there was a malodorous discharge from it. Five months before death enlargement of the liver was noted; the death was caused by cancer of the liver, as determined at autopsy.

Carcinoma of the Umbilicus Probably Secondary to Cancer of the Stomach f

Case 109 was a personal communication received by Pernice from R. Volkmann. The man was tapped on account of the presence of ascitic fluid, which proved to be hemorrhagic in character. After the removal of the fluid a tumor could be palpated. The umbilicus, stomach, and liver region were involved, and at the umbilicus were adhesions to the skin. The patient died without operation and no autopsy was allowed.

Secondary Carcinoma of the Umbilicus. J

A woman, aged fifty-nine, entered the Frauenklinik in Breslau. About six or nine months before, she had noticed below the umbilicus a small, hard nodule, that gave rise to little trouble and did not interfere with her work. She suffered from lack of appetite, vomiting, and constipation. The nodule grew rapidly and commenced to give trouble. The umbilicus became reddened and inflamed. On admission she looked frail and cachectic. The swelling at the umbilicus had extended to the surrounding parts, and the tissue was very hot and painful. On examination there could be felt in the depth a tumor the size of an ostrich's egg. On both sides the tumor extended 5 cm. from the umbilicus and could be sharply outlined. About 3 cm. above the umbilicus were several other fluctuating nodules. An exploratory operation was made, and three small abscesses, containing purulent, smeary masses were removed. The abdomen was opened, and the tumor was found to involve the stomach.

Resection of the stomach was done, and the patient died of shock. In this case there was a primary carcinoma of the stomach and a secondary growth at the umbilicus. It will be noted that the primary tumor in the beginning had given hardly any symptoms.

Secondary Carcinoma of the Umbilicus. §

This case was reported from the Universitatsklinik in Halle. A man, fifty-eight years of age, had been strong and healthy until he began to complain of pain in the abdomen and of a brownish vomitus. Later he had pain in the region of the umbilicus and then a nodule was detected. The patient on admission was very feeble, and the skin had a jaundiced tint. The umbilicus was somewhat distended by a nodule the size of a 10-pfennig piece. It was very hard and painful, brownish red, and on the surface slightly ulcerated. In this case there was probably a carcinoma of the stomach with secondary carcinoma at the umbilicus. Operation was refused.

* Morris: Op. cit., 114.

f Pernice: Die Nabelgeschwulste, Halle, 1892.

J Pernice: Op. cit., obs. 110.

§ Pernice: Op. cit., obs. 123.

Carcinoma of the Umbilicus Secondary to Cancer of the Stomach.*

For about a year a woman, sixty-two years of age, had had symptoms of cancer of the stomach. For four months she had noticed a hardening at the umbilicus. This was prominent; the skin was reddened, the surface of the tumor uneven and very dense. It was sharply defined and showed no ulceration.

Carcinoma of the Umbilicus Secondary to Abdominal Carcinoma. f

A woman, forty years of age, suffered from a malignant disease in the abdomen and had been frequently tapped. At autopsy carcinoma of the liver, omentum, and peritoneal surfaces of the intestine was found, and the uterus and ovaries formed one mass. At the umbilicus was a circumscribed tumor the size of the last phalanx of the thumb, looking like an umbilical hernia. This was also a carcinoma, evidently secondary to the abdominal tumor, which had probably originated in the stomach.

Carcinoma of the Umbilicus Secondary to Cancer of the Stomach.

Tillmannsi X said he saw a case of carcinoma of the stomach with a secondary growth at the umbilicus.

Secondary Carcinoma of the Umbilicus. §

A farmer, aged fifty-two, for two months had noticed an enlargement at the umbilicus which had increased rapidly in size and become ulcerated. The patient was slightly emaciated. The inguinal glands were enlarged. Peritoneal carcinosis, which had probably originated from the stomach, was found at operation. No microscopic examination was made.

Cancer of the Umbilicus Secondary to Cancer of the Cardiac End of the Stomach. ||

The patient, fifty years of age, was admitted to the service of Damaschino. Cancer of the stomach could be definitely made out. Later on, just beneath the umbilicus, one could feel with the ends of the fingers a hard tumor occupying the lower portion of the epigastric region. This tumor had a regular surface and presented the characteristics of a secondary neoplasm. Still later, at the umbilical cicatrix, there appeared a small,violet-colored tumor. This was covered over with a delicate crust. Microscopic examination showed that the tumor of the stomach and omentum, the abdominal glands, and the growth in the umbilical cicatrix were of precisely the same type of cancer.

Carcinoma of the Umbilicus Secondary to Carcinoma of the Stomach.

The report of the case was communicated to Villar** by Broussolle. X. entered the service of Professor Le Fort in 1885. There had been no digestive disturbances. The patient had come to Paris to consult a surgeon on account of a vegetative, ulcerating tumor situated in the umbilical region.

On admission to the hospital he was very feeble, and this feebleness was attributed to the fatigue of the journey. In the epigastric region and encroaching on the umbilicus was a vegetating tumor which was ulcerating and bled. At first sight it appeared to be a phlegmon, but on careful examination was found to present special characteristics. Some time afterward cancerous nodules appeared in the liver. At autopsy cancer of the pylorus was found and cancerous masses of the liver and plaques of carcinoma, which occupied the umbilicus and a certain portion of the anterior abdominal wall.

* Schlesinger : Die Bedeutung cler Nabelmetastasen ftir die Diagnose abdomineller Neoplasmen. Wien. med. Wochenschr., 1911, No. 8, 519.

f Storer: Circumscribed Tumor of the Umbilicus Closely Simulating Umbilical Hernia, etc. Boston Med. and Surg. Join -., 1864, lxx, 73.

X Tillmanns, H.: Ueber angeborenen Prolaps von Magenschleimhaut durch den Nabelring (Ectopia ventriculij, und iiber sonstige Geschwulste und Fisteln des Nabels. Deutsche Zeitschr. f. Chir., 1882-83, xviii, 161.

§ Tisserand: A propos de deux cas de cancer secondaire de l'ombilic. La Loire med., St. Etienne, 1906, xxv, 131.

|| Villar: Tumeurs de l'ombilic. These de Paris, 1886, obs. 79.

** Villar: Op. cit., obs. 85.

Carcinoma of the Umbilicus Secondary to Latent Carcinoma of the Stomach.

Valette* gives a list of the cases of primary and secondary carcinoma of the umbilicus, and then cites the history of a woman, sixty-one years old, who entered the hospital on August 16, 1896. In March of the same year she had noticed a small lump at the umbilicus. Later this had become painful, in some weeks had reached the size of a large nut, and ulcerated.

On admission the umbilical depression was found replaced by an elevation of the skin with an ulceration in the center and fungus-like margins. The growth was the size of a 50-centime piece (about 2 cm. in diameter). The ulceration had extended to the aponeurosis and the tumor was fixed. The inguinal glands were not enlarged. The question arose as to whether the growth was primary or secondary. The patient gave no history of stomach trouble and had had no vomiting, but the appetite was slightly diminished and she had lost weight in the last six months. At operation the peritoneal surface of the umbilicus was found smooth. There were small metastases in the peritoneum. The stomach was apparently normal. The patient died on the eighth day. At autopsy an adenocarcinoma of the stomach was found. The growths in the abdomen and at the umbilicus were similar to that in the stomach and were evidently secondary. This case demonstrates very clearly the fact that a malignant growth in the stomach may be unrecognizable during life, and be detected only at autopsy.

Carcinoma of the Umbilicus Secondary to Carcinoma of the Stomach. f

The patient was a man, thirty-three years of age, of strong build. When going home one dark night he struck his abdomen in the region of the stomach against a stony projection and was never well afterward. Early next year he consulted his physician for indigestion. In the fall of the same year he noticed that the umbilicus was inflamed, but there was no pain. When seen by Wulckow the umbilicus was slightly raised above the surrounding skin and was reddened. Along the margins were rough excrescences, and where the skin was gone the surface was moist. The entire mass was the size of a large plum. The skin around the umbilicus was reddened over an area the size of a two-thaler piece (about 6 cm. in diameter). The growth could be lifted up from the underlying abdominal contents. The patient died of hemorrhage of the stomach. At autopsy carcinoma was found in the stomach and at the umbilicus. The umbilical growth was in all probability secondary to that in the stomach.

* Valette: Contribution a. 1' etude du cancer secondaire de l'ombilic. These de Paris, 1898, No. 550.

f Wulckow: Beitrag zur Casuistik der Xabelneubildungen. Berlin, klin. Wochenschr., 1875, xii, 533.

LITERATURE CONSULTED ON CARCINOMA OF THE UMBILICUS SECONDARY TO CARCINOMA OF THE STOMACH.

Attimont, A. : Remarques sur le cancer de I'ombilic. Gaz. med. de Nantes, 1887-88, vi, 137; 149.

Auger, M. G.: Cancer de l'estomac, fistule gastro-abdominale. Bull. Soc. anat. de Paris, 1875, 1, 70S.

Balluff: Magenkrebs. Erweichung und Aufbruch desselben durch die allgemeinen Bauchdecken, Magenfistel. Med. Correspondenzbl. des Wurtemberg. arztl. Vereins, Stuttgart, 1854, xxiv, 37.

Burkhart, O.: Ueber den Nabelkrebs. Inaug. Diss., Berlin, 1889. Cannuet: Bull. Soc. anat. de Paris, 1852, xxvii, 274.

Codet de Boisse: Tumeurs de I'ombilic chez l'adulte. These de Paris, 1883, No. 311.

Feulard, H.: Fistule ombilicale et cancer de l'estomac. Arch. gen. de med., 1887, 7. ser., xx, 158.

Fischer: Resection de l'estomac. La Semaine med., Paris, 1888, viii, 134.

Hutchinson, J. : Carcinoma of the Umbilicus, Secondary. Arch, of Surgery, 1893, iv, 153 (1 pi.).

Largeau, R. : Cancer de I'ombilic. Bull. Soc. anat. de Paris, 1884, lix, 210-212.

Ledderhose, G. : Chirurgische Erkrankungen des Nabels. Deutsche Chirurgie, 1890, Lief. 45 b.

Mirallie: Reported by Attimont.

Monod, E.: Fistule ombilicale; cancer latent de l'estomac. Bull. Soc. anat. de Paris, 1877, lii, 38.'

Morris, Robert T. : Lectures on Appendicitis and Notes on Other Subjects, 1895, 95.

Pernice, L. : Die Nabelgeschwulste, Halle, 1892.

Schlesinger: Die Bedeutung der Nabelmetastasen fur die Diagnose abdomineller Neoplasmen. Wien. med. Wochenschr., 1911, No. 8, 519.

Storer, H. R. : Circumscribed Tumor of the Umbilicus Closely Simulating Umbilical Hernia, etc. Boston Med. and Surg. Jour., 1864, lxx, 73.

Tilhnanns, H: Ueber angeborenen Prolaps von Magenschleimhaut durch den Nabelring (Ectopia ventriculi), und iiber sonstige Geschwulste und Fisteln des Nabels. Deutsche Zeitschr. f. Chir., 1882-83, xviii, 161.

Tisserand, G. : A propos de deux cas de cancer secondaire de I'ombilic. La Loire med., St. Etienne, 1906, xxv, 131-136.

Valette, A.: Contribution a 1' etude du cancer secondaire de I'ombilic. These de Paris, 1898, No. 550.

Villar, F. : Tumeurs de I'ombilic. These de Paris, 1886.

Wulckow: Beitrag zur Casuistik der Nabelneubildungen. Berlin, klin. Wochenschr., 1875, xii, 533.

CARCINOMA OF THE UMBILICUS SECONDARY TO CANCER OF THE GALL-BLADDER.

Inasmuch as primary carcinoma of the gall-bladder is relatively rare, we should not expect to find many growths of the umbilicus secondary to it. Ledderhose, in 1890, reported a case that he had observed in Kussmaul's clinic. A woman, fifty-six years old, was brought to the hospital on account of jaundice. It was impossible to detect any growth in the liver either by palpation or percussion. At the umbilicus, however, was a bean-sized, hard tumor which suggested the diagnosis of carcinoma of the liver or of the gall-bladder. Subsequently it became possible to detect large and irregular masses with nodular margins in the liver. At autopsy a primary carcinoma of the gall-bladder was found which had given rise to the umbilical growth.

In 1901 Besson gave a splendid resume of the literature on secondary carcinoma of the umbilicus, and cited a case of carcinoma of the gall-bladder with a secondary growth at the umbilicus. The umbilical growth was the size of a small hazelnut. The histologic pictures from this case are given in Figs. 225, 226, and 227 of Cornil and Ranvier's Manuel d'histologie pathologique, published in the same year.

Tisserand, in 1906, reported a case of this character. A woman, fifty-four yearsold, the mother of four children, had had pain for five months in the umbilical region, but her general health had been good. On abdominal examination the cicatrix of the umbilicus seemed to be simply inflamed. It was very red, slightly painful, and indurated. An exploratory operation was performed. The patient died suddenly on the tenth day. There was a carcinoma of the gall-bladder with biliary stones. The glands along the suspensory ligament of the umbilicus showed a bead-like involvement. No trace of cancer could be found in any other organ. In this case there was a definite carcinomatous extension along the lymphatics.

Schlesinger, in 1911, reported a case of primary carcinoma of the gall-bladder with a secondary nodule at the umbilicus. In this connection the following case of biliary fistula reported by Gross may be of interest:

Biliary Fistula at the Umbilicus.*

A man, aged forty- four, two months before had noticed a small lump at the umbilicus; it was not painful, but caused a continuous pricking sensation. The lesion had progressively enlarged, and on admission the umbilical growth was the size of a large red buttonand the man had a continuous dull pain. For a month it had been severe enough to prevent him from sleeping. The patient had become emaciated, but had had no intestinal disturbances.

On admission he was thin, and grayish in color. On January 29th a tumor covered by intact red skin was removed. It was adherent to the peritoneum. Microscopic examination showed it to be a cancer. The patient developed pneumonia, but recovered from it. On February 18th, an irritating biliary discharge was noted, but no inflammatory reaction. He left the hospital on March 11th well of his pneumonia, but with a biliary fistula.

Gross thinks that the gall-bladder had become adherent to the umbilicus, and after operation a small abscess had developed and perforation of the gall-bladder had taken place. [It is just possible that a primary carcinoma of the gall-bladder existed in this case.— T. S. C]

While reviewing the literature on diseases of the umbilicus I was asked to see the following case, and profiting by the knowledge gleaned from the literature, at once ventured a provisional diagnosis of either carcinoma of the stomach or of the gall-bladder with gall-stones and a secondary malignant growth at the umbilicus.

Adenocarcinoma 'of the Umbilicus Secondary to Carcinoma of the Gall bladder. f

Mrs. B., aged fifty-eight, was seen in consultation with Dr. George L. Wilkins and admitted to the Church Home and Infirmary April 24, 1910. The patient showed a slight bulging at the umbilicus on standing. This was painful when the clothes rubbed against it. It had been noticed first in December, 1909, that is, about four months before examination. For some months the patient had suffered at intervals with pain in the region of the gall-bladder and had been jaundiced. The pain had radiated to the back and to the right shoulder. At the time of examination there was some tenderness in the gall-bladder region. She had suffered from the presence of gas and from constipation. No clay-colored stools had been noted. The heart, lungs, and kidneys were normal.

From the history and general condition a provisional diagnosis was made of either cancer of the stomach or of the gall-bladder, associated with a secondary nodule at the umbilicus. On examination of the umbilicus there was just a slight rolling-out, but nothing to suggest a nodule until one picked the umbilicus up between the fingers, when marked sensitiveness became apparent.

Operation. — April 25, 1910. On making a right rectus incision I at once encountered little nodules in the lesser omentum. The gallbladder contained numerous stones and also a new-growth. The latter was firm and had extended to the lymph-glands around the portal vein. One of these was over 3 cm. in diameter. We were dealing with a carcinoma of the gallbladder, together with metastases in the lesser omentum and the umbilicus. On account of the marked involvement of the lymph-glands complete removal of the primary growth was impossible. As the patient had had a great deal of pain in the umbilicus, this was removed. The inner or peritoneal surface of the umbilicus was free from adhesions. The patient made a good temporary recovery and was discharged May 9, 1910.

She subsequently developed large secondary nodules in the abdominal cavity, and died on September 16, 1910.

Pathologic Examination: The specimen consists of the umbilicus and surrounding skin. It is 7 cm. in length, 5 cm. in breadth. The umbilicus is slightly prominent. It is commencing to unfold a little. The parts are slightly distorted from the action of the hardening fluid and the umbilicus comes out more prominently than it really did in the patient. There is, however, a slight unfolding of the umbilicus, and one part seems somewhat raised. The umbilicus itself, however, was perfectly intact. A transverse section through the umbilicus. The half to the left is more prominent and represents the elevation noted in the umbilical depression. The surface, however, is intact. There is an increase in the amount of connective tissue, but no evidence of any definite nodule. Histologic examination showed that this area was everywhere infiltrated with carcinomatous glands.

It was not quite so prominent, however, in the fresh state. The nodule could be readily felt on lifting the umbilicus up with the fingers. It appeared to be about 1 cm. or more in diameter. In the hardened specimen the tissue was contracted, bringing the tumor out more prominently. The skin was everywhere intact. The peritoneal surface was slightly puckered, but was free from adhesions. On section of the umbilicus the tissue looked fibrous and in its middle portion was what appeared to be a little area of hemorrhage about 2 mm. in diameter. At first sight one would not for a moment suspect the presence of carcinoma.

Histologic Examination. The squamous epithelium is intact, and immediately beneath it in a few places are some sweat-glands. Approaching the peritoneum colonies of glands are found closely packed together with very little connective tissue between them. The gland epithelium is for the most part one layer in thickness. In some places it is cuboid, at other points cylindric, and there are very minute glands. The nuclei of the epithelial cells stain uniformly, but vary considerably in size. In some places the epithelial cells seem to have a tendency to be arranged in single rows. The growth is without doubt a carcinoma. The small metastatic nodules found in the lesser omentum in the neighborhood of the gallbladder present a precisely similar appearance. We are undoubtedly dealing with a primary carcinoma of the gall-bladder, involving the lymphatics around the portal vein. There have been metastases in the lesser omentum and also involvement of the umbilicus.

Treatment. When the diagnosis is perfectly clear, operation is not indicated, as it is impossible completely to eradicate the disease. In my case the operation was undertaken solely on account of the severe pain caused by the umbilical nodule.

* Gross, G.: Neoplasme de l'ombilic. Revue med. de Test., Nancy, 1898, xxx, 559.

f I reported this case in Jour. Amer. Med. Assoc, 1911, lvi, 391.

LITERATURE CONSULTED ON CARCINOMA OF THE UMBILICUS SECONDARY TO CANCER OF THE GALL-BLADDER.

Besson, E.: Cancer de l'ombilic. These de Paris, 1901, Xo. 263.

Cornil et Ranvier: Manuel d'histologie pathologique, 3. ed., Paris, 1910, i, 493.

Gross, G. : Xeoplasme de 1'ombilic. Revue med. de Test., Nancy, 1898, xxx, 559.

Ledderhose, G. : Deutsche Chirurgie, 1890, Lief. 45 b.

Schlesinger: Die Bedeutung der Nabelmetastasen fur die Diagnose abdomineller Xeoplasmen. Wien. med. Wochenschr., 1911, Xr. 8, 519.

Tisserand, G. : A propos de deux cas de cancer secondaire de 1'ombihc. La Lone med., St. Etienne, 1906, xxv, 131-136.

CARCINOMA OF THE UMBILICUS SECONDARY TO CANCER OF THE INTESTINE.

I have found five cases of this character in the literature, those of Lage, Chuquet, Villar, Pernice, and Barker. It is quite probably that Plagge's case also belongs to this group, although the tumor was described as a myxosarcoma. In Chuquet's case the carcinoma was situated in the rectum.

On reading the histories of these cases it will be seen that in the majority of the cases, in addition to the primary growth, there were wide-spread abdominal metastases facilitating extension of the carcinomatous process to the umbilicus.

Histologically, the umbilical growths conform exactly to the type of the original intestinal tumor.

Cases of Carcinoma of the Umbilicus Secondary to Cancer of the Intestine.

Carcinoma of the Large Bowel "With Metastases at the Umbilicus.*

The patient died of carcinoma involving nearly all of the large bowel. There were metastases in the mesenteric glands. At the umbilicus was a brownish red. mottled growth. The umbilicus felt like a broad, hard, flat surface. The growth was probably a carcinoma secondary to that of the large bowel.

Carcinoma of the Rectum With Secondary Carcinoma at the Umbilicus f

This case had been reported by Lebert (Bull. Soc. anat. de Paris). A woman, fifty-four years of age, six weeks before coming under observation had- commenced to have violent colic and pain at the umbilicus with digestive disturbances. On admission she looked cachectic and the abdomen was much distended. Beneath the umbilicus was felt a hard, cartilaginous plaque which at its prominent part raised the skin nearly 3 cm.

At autopsy small carcinomatous masses were found scattered over the peritoneum and there was a scirrhous carcinoma of the rectum. The umbilical growth had developed in the linea alba. [Although the growth was probably secondary to that in the rectum, one cannot feel absolutely sure. — T. S. C]

Carcinoma of the Umbilicus Secondary to Carcinoma of the Transverse Colon.

Villar % describes a case occurring in the sen-ice of Damaschino. The patient, fifty-three years of age, had a cancer of the transverse colon involving the omentum, cancerous nodules in the peritoneum, ulceration and cancer of the umbilicus, and seconda^ nodules in the liver.

During the progress of the disease a hard mass developed in the umbilical region, and in two months the umbilical depression was effaced by a violet mass which reached the dimensions of a two-franc piece. This was covered with a thick crust. When this was removed, the new-growth was found to be nodular, irregular, and reddish. On palpation one could feel in the umbilical region, over an area 10 cm. in diameter, a hard, slightly movable, mass. At autopsy it was found that the tumors of the omentum and of the peritoneum, as well as the umbilical mass, were of exactly the same structure as the intestinal growth.

Cancer of the Transverse Colon with Secondary Carcinoma of the Umbilicus.§

Case 1. — "A man, aged thirty-seven, admitted to the University College Hospital February 3, 1910. In March, 1909. he noticed occasional pains around the navel irrespective of food. These lasted three or four months. In the July following he entered a country hospital, having noticed for about a fortnight a swelling in the abdominal wall at the umbilicus. This was opened with the knife on July 24th and was said to have given exit to pus and to have healed again in a week. In the September following the swelling increased again and burst, and has been discharging ever since. On admission on February 3d he was well nourished. Below and to the left of the navel was a discolored and irregular prominence about 2 inches in diameter, with a wound discharging through the old scar. On palpation the induration was much larger- than it looked. It extended downward for several inches in the left rectus muscle and was everywhere very hard. Except to the skin over the most prominent part, it showed no attachment anteriorly, but was incorporated with the rectus. The discharging sinus led downward and outward about 2. inches. To be quite sure of its nature, which was believed to be cancerous, I made an incision into the swelling, and, finding it unmistakably so, prepared for removal. This was done on February 20th, between two long elliptic incisions from above downward, opening the abdomen and including most of the left rectus muscle. The tumor was then seen to be obviously a growth of the transverse colon fungating through the umbilicus. I then clamped the colon on each side and removed it with about I-2 inches on both sides of the growth — about seven or eight inches in all. The ends of the divided bowel were brought together in the usual way, and the wound was only partially closed, as there was little or no muscle to fill it. Some suppuration followed, as I expected, from the foul state of the breaking-down growth, and a fecal fistula formed for a little while, but soon closed and the wound granulated up. On May 6th I removed a nodule of growth, cutting the skin and inserting a delicate wire netting. Since then all has gone well, and I have recently seen the man — more than three years after the operation — quite free from any sign of recurrence. He plays golf and performs on a wind instrument; he has no hernia.

"The growth was a typical columnar carcinoma, and corresponded to an ulcer on the mucous surface of the free side of the transverse colon, as large as a crown piece, with everted edges. There were no tangible glands in the mesentery or any other signs of generalization."

* Lage: Krebshafte Entartung eines grossen Theils des Dickdarms. Schmidt's Jahrbuch, 1847, Iv, 295.

fChuquet: Du carcinome generalise du peril oine. These de Paris, 1879, No. 548, obs. 18.

% Villar, F. : Tumeurs de l'ombilic. These de Paris, 1886, obs. 78, 112.

§ Barker, A. E.: TheLancet, London, July 19, 1913.

Secondary Carcinoma of the Umbilicus.*

Case 129, reported from the Frauenklinik of Breslau. A woman, fifty-two years of age, complained of a sticking, burning pain, which was more marked on pressure. The abdomen was much distended. In the vicinity of the stomach and also in the region of the umbilicus nodules could be made out. The patient looked weak and cachectic. In the umbilical region there was marked resistance. This extended three fmgerbreadths to the right and over a handbreadth and a half to the left. On account of the ascites, nothing more could be made out. There was a small umbilical tumor. At an exploratory operation carcinomatous nodules were found on the intestine, and the omentum was everywhere covered with small carcinomatous nodules.

A Case of Myxosarcoma of the Umbilicusf

In childhood the man had difficulty in digestion, and later vomiting and diarrhea. In the summer of 1887 he had pain in the stomach for the first time and noticed a small tumor at the umbilicus. By November of the same year the tumor had reached the size of a hazelnut, and four weeks later a nodule the size of a pea below and to the left, close to the linea alba, could be felt. The patient became emaciated and died on March 14, 1888. At autopsy the umbilicus showed a thickening, the size of a five-franc piece, raised 2 cm. above the abdominal level. Above and below, the thickening could be followed 5 cm. in each direction. The skin was movable over the area of thickening. When the abdomen was opened, a nodule 2 mm. in diameter was found in the umbilical region. In the ligament passing from the umbilicus were small nodules. The omentum, diaphragm, and intestine were implicated.

The stomach was normal. Microscopically, a diagnosis of myxosarcoma was made.

[The clinical picture in no way indicated a primary growth. The condition resembles in some degree a case of a colloid carcinoma of the intestine with secondary growths at the umbilicus. — T. S. C.l

* Pernice, L.: Die Nabelgeschwiilste, Halle, 1892.

f Plagge, H.: Em Fall von Myxosarcoma des Xabel. Inaug. Diss., Freiburg i. B., 1889.

LITERATURE CONSULTED ON CARCINOMA OF THE UMBILICUS SECONDARY TOCANCER OF THE INTESTINE.

Barker, A. E.: Three Cases of Solid Tumors of the Umbilicus in Adults. The Lancet, London, July 19, 1913.

Chuquet, A. : Du carcinome generalise du peritoine. These de Paris, 1879, No. 548.

Lage: Krebshafte Entartung eines grossen Theils des Dickdarms. Schmidt's Jahrbuch, 1847, lv, 295.

Pernice, L. : Die Nabelgeschwulste, Halle, 1892.

Plagge, H. : Ein Fall von Myxosarcom des Nabel. Inaug. Diss., Freiburg i. B., 1889.

Villar, F. : Tumeurs de l'ombilic. These de Paris, 1886, obs. 78.

CARCINOMA OF THE UMBILICUS SECONDARY TO OVARIAN CARCINOMA.

I have found several cases of this character in the literature, and two have been observed in the Gynecological Department of the Johns Hopkins Hospital. A very careful review of the subject was given by Le Coniac in his thesis published in 1898. The youngest of the patients here recorded was thirty-two years of age; the oldest, sixty-eight. Five of the nine patients were between fifty and sixty years of age.

Most of the umbilical growths were small, and some of them were very hard. In Gueneau de Mussy's case the growth was pedunculated. A small umbilical hernia had existed, and a month before the patient came under observation it had become irreducible. It then became very hard, and was evidently infiltrated with cancer. In Burkhart's case, in addition to the umbilical nodule, there was also one attached to a rib. The umbilical nodule in one of Demons and Verdelet's cases was ulcerated. In one of our cases (Gyn. No. 6150) there was a round, ulcerated area with sharply cut edges and a granular base. As seen from Fig. 185 (p. 432) the floor of this ulcer consisted of carcinomatous tissue. In Aslanian's case the carcinoma had extended to the inguinal glands.

It is hardly necessary to analyze the histories of these cases, as the findings are common to those ordinarily noted where carcinoma of the ovaries, together with wide-spread peritoneal carcinosis, is present. It will be noted that in all but one of the cases there was a wide-spread peritoneal carcinosis, and consequently secondary involvement of the umbilicus was relatively easy.

The histologic picture of these umbilical nodules naturally corresponds to that present in primary ovarian tumors. We see the edge of the carcinomatous nodule. The growth can be traced through the abdominal wall as far as the epithelial covering of the umbilicus. Over the area of ulceration the skin covering had disappeared entirely and the carcinomatous tissue formed the floor of the ulcer. Any operative treatment in these cases is of little or no value.

Cases of Carcinoma of the Umbilicus Secondary to Ovarian Carcinoma.

Carcinoma of the Umbilicus Secondary to Carcinoma of the Ovaries.

Aslanian* covers the literature on peritoneal carcinosis very thoroughly. He cites the following case: A woman, aged thirty-five, had cancer of the ovaries with metastases to the abdominal peritoneum. Eleven months before she had given birth to a child. Fifteen days later she had commenced to suffer with abdominal pain and developed an induration at the umbilicus. The umbilical growth had finally ulcerated, and it was for this that the patient entered the hospital. During surgical intervention metastatic nodules were noted in the parietal peritoneum. The patient recovered from the operation, but did not improve. The appetite diminished more and more, and she became thin. She returned to the hospital on account of the abdominal pain and another growth in the umbilical region. At the site of the umbilicus the scar contained a soft tumor the size of a walnut. In both inguinal regions the glands were enlarged and formed two elongate tumors parallel with the inguinal folds. One could detect beneath the integument of the abdominal wall some small nodules the size of lentils or peas, and over these the skin was adherent. To the left of the tumor was. a hard cord, 3 to 4 cm. long, which terminated in the enlarged glands. Deeper down, nodules could be made out in the hypogastrium. At the level of the umbilicus on the right was a deep-seated induration. Palpation was not painful, and there was an accumulation of ascitic fluid.

All the time the patient was in the hospital she continued to complain of pain. The emaciation increased, and toward the end of her illness there was edema of the feet.

At autopsy the peritoneal cavity was found to contain 300 c.c. of reddish fluid. In the pelvis the normal relations were markedly altered. Both ovaries had been converted into hard tumors the size of apples. They were nodular and had uniform surfaces. The left ovary presented a small cyst. On section, the tumors were found to have a uniform, hard, grayish surface, with yellowish areas scattered here and there through them. The Fallopian tubes showed hypertrophy. Their extremities -were free, but the mucosa of the fimbriae contained cancerous nodules which were yellowish in color, very hard, and simulated eruptions of tubercles. The entire peritoneum was involved in the cancer. The neck of the cervix was hard and infiltrated in its entire thickness with numerous cancerous nodules, some as large as a pea. In addition to the wide-spread peritoneal involvement, the omentum was contracted into numerous folds and contained cancerous nodules. It was adherent to the abdominal wall at the umbilicus. At this point the cancerous nodules were very abundant. The small intestines did not show any secondary nodules, but there were some in the mesentery. The liver was voluminous and nodular, and occupied all the epigastrium. Glisson's capsule did not contain any nodules, but in the hepatic tissue there were 15 secondary growths varying from the volume of a pomegranate to that of a peach in size. On the inferior surface of the diaphragm on the right side were cancerous plaques. On the anterior abdominal wall were whitish cords. These were cancerous lymphatics, following the direction of the umbilical arteries, and terminating at the umbilical tumor where the omentum was adherent to the abdominal wall. The nodules at this point varied from the size of a pin-head to that of a pea. Cancerous nodules were present in the thorax.

On histologic examination, the ovary, uterus, intestine, muscle, and peritoneum of the umbilical tumor all showed an alveolar carcinoma. Aslanian says that pregnancy played a large role in the provocation of the generalization of the cancer, not only on the serous surfaces, but also in the generative organs and in the anterior abdominal wall. His article is a very thorough one.

* Aslanian, G.: Contribution a l'etude de la peritonite cancereuse. These de Paris, 1895, No. 150, obs. 70.

Carcinoma of the Umbilicus Secondary to Ovarian Carcinoma.

Burkhart* reports Kiister'sf case of a woman, fifty-seven years of age, who had had several labors. Two years before she had complained of a dull feeling in the lower abdomen, and six months before a small nodule had been detected at the umbilicus; two months before coming under observation nodules had been noted on the ribs near the sternum. At the time of the patient's death the tumor at the umbilicus was the size of a nut. The overlying skin was movable. The malignant growth had involved the uterus and ovaries. It had originally been an ovarian cyst and had become carcinomatous.

Carcinoma of the Umbilicus Secondary to Carcinoma of the Ovary %

Case 1. — A woman, forty-five years of age, for a month had had an abdominal enlargement. She was thin, and the abdomen contained an accumulation of fluid. At the umbilicus was a small tumor. Deep palpation revealed a large tumor attached to the uterus. At operation the abdomen was found to contain pelvic tumors. There were papillomata involving the intestine and the omentum, and converting the ovaries and uterus into one mass. The fluid was removed, and the umbilical tumor taken away. The histologic picture noted in the umbilical tumor was identical with that frequently found in the ovary.

Cancer of the Ovaries with a Secondary Growth at the Umbilicus.§

Case 2. — A woman, fifty-three years of age, for nine months had had abdominal pain. Shortly after falling on her abdomen she had noticed a small, non-painful enlargement. The abdomen increased in size and the patient became emaciated. On examination abundant free fluid was found. At the umbilicus was a small tumor which was not ulcerated and lay beneath the skin. Hard, fixed masses could be felt in the lower abdomen. Vaginal examination revealed a nodular, irregular tumor. The condition was diagnosed as carcinoma of the ovaries with secondary carcinoma of the umbilicus. At operation 12 liters of ascitic fluid were removed. Tumors were found filling Douglas' cul-de-sac. Attached to the parietal peritoneum were several secondary nodules, and the omentum formed a tumor mass. The umbilical growth was removed and the abdomen closed.

Probable Carcinoma of the Ovary with a Secondary Growth at the Umbilicus. ||

A woman, sixty-eight years of age, a year before admission had had abundant uterine hemorrhages and since then had been ill. The abdomen was slightly distended. Her appetite had gone, she was constipatecl, and had been gradually wasting away. She had pain in the abdomen. Two months previously she had first noticed at the umbilicus a hard, irregular tumor, which soon ulcerated. Eight days before admission jaundice had become pronounced. On examination the abdomen was found distended, tympanitic, and at the umbilicus was a small, indurated tumor with diffuse margins. It was ulcerated. A diagnosis of cancer was made. In Douglas' pouch was a tumor. The outlines were not clear. The patient was too weak for operation. The condition was diagnosed as cancer of the ovaries with secondary growths at the umbilicus. [Of course, there is a chance for error in this case, as no operation was performed. — T. S. C]

* Burkhart, ().: Uebcr don Xabelkrebs. Inaug. Diss., Berlin, 1889.

f Krister: Beitrage z. Geb. u. Gyn., 1875, iv, 6.

% Demons et Verdelet: Cancer secondaire de l'ombilic. Congres pcriodique de gyn.,

d'obstet. et de paed., 1898, ii, 344.

§ Demons et Verdelet: Op. cit.

|| Demons et Verdelet: Op. cit.

Probable Carcinoma of the Umbilicus Secondary to Carcinoma of the Ovaries.*

A woman, fifty-nine years of age, for three months had been supposed to have influenza. Two months before coming under observation she had become yellow and had had pain in the abdomen. On admission she was jaundiced, had lost weight, vomited bile, and gave a history of vomiting blood on one occasion. At the umbilicus was a knob-like hardness drawn inward, as if pulled by something from within. At autopsy carcinoma of both ovaries was found. There were small nodules in the peritoneum and pleurse. The gall-bladder was small and filled with stones. The common duct was compressed by cancerous nodules. The growth at the umbilicus was apparently secondary to that in the ovaries.

Carcinoma of the Umbilicus Secondary to Cancer in the Pelvis.

Gueneau de Mussy's t patient, a woman fifty-nine years old, was suffering from an obscure abdominal lesion. At the umbilicus was a small, hard disc, the size of a large almond, attached by a pedicle in the umbilical ring. The patient said she had had a small hernia, easily reducible, but for the past month it had been hard and remained outside.

At autopsy, several months later, an abdominal carcinoma was found. The pelvis contained a mass the size of a new-born child's head, and other foci existed.

Probable Adenocarcinoma of the Umbilicus Secondary to Carcinoma of the Ovary.

Mrs. C. W., aged thirty-two. Admitted to the Johns Hopkins Hospital May 25, 1893. Operation by Dr. Kelly. The abdomen contained about 8 ounces of ascitic fluid; the peritoneum was dark in color. The right ovary was the size of an orange, and was surrounded by a capsule 34 m ch in thickness. This was easilytorn. Several small nodules were felt in different portions of the peritoneum; in the median line and around the umbilicus was a loosely encapsulated white lump the size of a shell-bark nut. This was not removed, on account of the presence of secondary nodules. The liver was covered with whitish nodules, similar in character; these extended from the liver down to the umbilicus.

The specimen consists of the ovary, tube, and a portion of the broad ligament. The ovary is very much enlarged and contains three or four cysts. The surface is irregular in outline. There is a dense, hard capsule with several small cysts showing through the outer surface. At the inner end of the ovary is a cyst, 2 cm. in diameter, filled with clear, watery fluid. The cysts are confined to the superficial portion of the ovary. On section, the greater portion of the mass appears to be made up of translucent, grayish tissue having an edematous appearance, and running through this in every direction is dense fibrous tissue. There are ecchymotic patches here and there throughout the specimen. The broad ligament is thickened and contains numerous hard masses varying from a pin-head to a lima bean in size. On histologic examination the matrix of the tumor is found to consist of very edematous fibrous tissue. Scattered sparsely or abundantly throughout the stroma are colonies of carcinomatous glands. The gland type in some areas is very well preserved. At other points the carcinoma seems to form solid masses.

* Liveing: The Lancet, 1875, ii, 8.

t Gueneau de Mussy : Cancer du peritoine. Clin, med., Paris, 1875, ii, 28.

Carcinoma of the Umbilicus Secondary to Carcinoma of the Ovaries.

The umbilicus has been converted into a round, ulcerated area, with sharp edges and a granular base. The picture is taken from the indurated tissue near the edge of the ulcer. To the left is squamous epithelium, which in places is much thickened, but in the upper part of the picture is normal in thickness. On the surface is some exfoliated and partly hornified epithelium. Immediately beneath the skin the stroma shows considerable small-round-cell infiltration. The right half of the field consists of nests of cancer-cells. The floor of the ulcer to a large extent is made up of cancerous tissue. In many portions of the growth the typical glandular character of the tumor was evident. It was an adenocarcinoma.

There is no trace of ovarian stroma remaining. The growth is a virulent adenocarcinoma of the ovarjr. It is exceptional with such an early tumor to find such widespread metastases. The nodule at the umbilicus, although not examined histologically, was undoubtedly similar in origin. Whether the umbilical growth was due to extension upward from below or from above is problematic, but with metastases in the liver and extending down along the suspensory ligament to the umbilicus it looks very much as if the growth were secondary to the liver nodules.

Adenocarcinoma of the Ovary; Metastases to the Peritoneum and to the Umbilicus.

Admitted to the Johns Hopkins Hospital June 6, 1898. The patient, fifty-five years of age, was married twenty-six years ago. She has had no children and no miscarriages. The present illness began over a year ago. She has gradually grown weaker, and has not been able to work for a long time. She complains of abdominal enlargement, of marked constipation, and of a growth at the umbilicus. At operation the parietal peritoneum was studded with small, whitish elevations, and the abdominal cavity contained several cystic masses reaching to the umbilicus. They could not be removed. The umbilicus itself had been converted into a round, ulcerated area with sharp edges and a granular base. This was excised when the abdomen was opened. The patient was much relieved by the operation and the tenderness over the abdomen disappeared.

The specimen consists of fluid from the peritoneal cavity, of a small section of a cyst wall, and of the umbilicus.

Section from the Umbilicus. — The skin surrounding the umbilicus is perfectly normal. As one approaches the area of ulceration it is raised somewhat and becomes thickened, and the papillae extend a certain distance downward. The tissue beneath the squamous epithelium is normal, but as one approaches the area of ulceration it shows small-round-cell infiltration around the capillaries. Near the edge of the ulcerated area one finds nests of epithelial cells which have retracted somewhat from the surrounding stroma. In certain areas one can make out a definite gland arrangement. The growth is an adenocarcinoma with a tendency to form solid nests. As one passes to the ulcer, the squamous epithelium disappears. The surface is covered with fibrin, polymorphonuclear leukocytes, and small round-cells. The nuclei of the cancer-cells vary considerably in size. Some cancer-cells are large, stain deeply, and contain irregular masses of chromatin. The entire floor of the ulcer is made up of granulation tissue and nests of cancer-cells. The line of junction between the surface epithelium and the cancer is very sharply defined. In the depth of the ulcer the tissue consists almost entirely of nests of cancer-cells. The process has undoubtedly extended up from the abdomen as a wedge and raised the squamous epithelium. Over the area of carcinoma the skin has given way and an ulcer has resulted. The umbilical growth is identical in character with the ovarian tumor from which it originated.

After the book was in type and shortly before going to press the following interesting case came under my care:

Adenocarcinoma in the Omentum Incarcerated inan Old Umbilical Hernia

The primary growth was apparently in the ovary, possibly in the uterus. Mrs. Annie E., aged seventy- two, referred to me by Dr. Albert Singewald, was admitted to the Church Home and Infirmary September 28, 1915. The patient had had two children and one miscarriage. The menopause had occurred at forty.

Present Illness. — About four years before she had noticed vaginal bleeding, which had persisted up to the time of admission. For the last two or three months she had had profuse bleeding, lasting from three to four days. Between these attacks there had been a continuous thin, pinkish discharge. For the last two months she had suffered a great deal with pain over the sacrum and in the lower abdomen, and during the same time there had been pain on voiding. She had lost 25 pounds within the last two months.

The patient was a very large woman, weighing 235 pounds. She looked relatively well. On physical examination the abdomen was found much distended, but there was some laxness in both flanks. An umbilical hernia (Plate V) was noted, which presented a somewhat unusual appearance. It seemed somewhat lobulated, and the umbilicus itself was crescentic. The entire raised area measured about 5 cm. from above downward and about 4 cm. from side to side. It did not present the uniformity of outline so frequently noted in umbilical hernise. On palpation it felt hard, and one could detect definite nodular thickenings in the hernial mass. These were apparently four or five in number, and immediately suggested metastatic nodules.

On carefully questioning the patient we learned that she had had an umbilical hernia since she was forty; in other words, for thirty-two years. During the last three months she had noticed that the hernia, which hitherto had been quite soft, had become gradually hard and nodular.

On abdominal palpation a definite tumor mass could be felt to the left of the umbilicus. Its exact dimensions could not be determined on account of the abdominal distention. In either flank fluctuation could be elicited.

I kept the patient in the ward several days, while debating whether any operative-procedure should be undertaken. She was so anxious for relief that I finally consented to make an exploratory incision.

Operation October 1, 1915. — An elliptic incision was made around the enlarged and nodular umbilicus, and in the abdominal muscles just above the umbilicus was found a definite nodule, about 1 x 1.5 cm. After the umbilical growth had been freed from the abdominal wall, a tongue of omentum was discovered that passed into the hernial sac. This portion of omentum was intimately blended with the umbilicus and was removed with the sac. The parietal peritoneum everywhere was studded with carcinomatous nodules varying from 1 to 6 mm. in diameter. To the left of the umbilicus was an ovarian tumor which appeared to be about 16 cm. in diameter. The omentum was markedly thickened, and the greater part of it lay rolled up above the umbilicus. Loops of small bowel were adherent to the anterior abdominal wall near the symphysis, and also at other points, and here and there, plate v.

Cancer op the Umbilicus Apparently Secondary to a Tcmor of the Ovary.

At the umbilicus was the hard umbilical hernial mass containing cancerous nodules, and at operation a cancerous nodule was found in the mid-line just above the umbilicus. To the left of the umbilicus was an ovarian tumor apparently cystic. The greater part of the omentum was rolled up and formed a tumor mass about midway between the xiphoid and the umbilicus. As there was a general peritoneal carcinosis and many adhesions, a more extended examination was not made.

The umbilical area is sharply raised from the surrounding abdominal walls, and the umbilical depression is represented by a crescentic slit. In this tumor four or five very hard nodules could be distinctly made out, at once suggesting malignancy.

Occupying the left side of the lower abdomen is an ovarian cyst. This below and posteriorly is adherent. The omentum above the umbilicus is greatly thickened as a result of involvement in the carcinomatous process. The lower end of the omentum fills the umbilical hernial sac. This portion of the mentum is also much thickened and has become intimately blended with the hernial walls. The incarcerated omentum is riddled with cancer. In the lower part of the omentum, that lies in the hernia, is a small cyst.

We see small carcinomatous nodules in the- parietal peritoneum of the anterior abdominal wall. The omentum (6) projects into, completely fills, and is intimately blended with the hernial sac. In the upper part of the picture, where a catgut ligature is seen, the omental fat can still be fairly well recognized, but most of the omentum in the hernia looks very much like fibrous tissue. It was everywhere invaded by adenocarcinoma. The cyst was lined with one or more layers of cancer cells,

Cancer of the Umbilicus Apparently Secondary to a Tumor of the Ovary.

Carcinomatous nodule with peritoneum intact. Ornentum where such adhesions existed, the bowel was covered over with flakes of fibrin. Further examination being impossible, the abdomen was closed as soon as the umbilical growth had been removed.

The patient rallied remarkably well and left the hospital on October 23, feeling very much relieved.

Sections involving the entire hernial mass show that the omentum which had extended into the hernia has become blended with the walls of the hernial sac, and that very little adipose tissue remains, the stroma consisting almost entirely of fibrous tissue, rich in spindle cells. Scattered through this are many glands occurring singly or in groups. In some places they are lined with one layer of epithelium, the cells being somwhat cuboidal or roundish and manifesting a tendency to drop off. In other places there are colonies of glands, some of the gland-spaces being partially or completely filled with epithelial cells. The nuclei of the epithelial cells vary markedly in size. Some of them contain large masses of deeply staining chromatin. The picture is that of an adenocarcinoma of a type usually noted in the ovary. The cyst-like space noted at one end of the umbilicus is lined with epithelium. In some places this is almost flat; in other places it is drawn up in papillary-like folds. In this case we have a definite adenocarcinoma of the umbilicus.

From the foregoing it is perfectly clear that the primary cancer was either in the ovary or in the uterus. The type of gland found in the carcinoma might well have been from either the body of the uterus or from the ovary. Uterine hemorrhage extending over a period of four years is somewhat unusual in so old a patient unless some serious uterine trouble exists. On the other hand, we all know that uterine hemorrhage is not infrequently associated with an ovarian tumor.

The presence of the ovarian tumor, with apparently thick walls, would strongly suggest the ovary as the primary seat of the trouble. Further, metastases from an ovarian carcinoma are not uncommon. Peritoneal metastases of such a character following a carcinoma of the body of the uterus I have never seen. In all probability, then, this patient had a primary carcinoma of the left ovary; general peritoneal metastases had developed, and finally the omentum in the umbilical hernia had been invaded by carcinomatous nodules. Here they could be palpated with the utmost ease.

LITERATURE CONSULTED ON CARCINOMA OF THE UMBILICUS SECONDARY TO OVARIAN CARCINOMA.

Aslanian, G.: Contribution a P etude de la peritonite cancereuse. These de Paris, 1895, No. 150.

Burkhart, 0.: Ueber den Nabelkrebs. Inaug. Diss., Berlin, 1889.

Cullen, Thomas 8.: Gyn. Xo. 2004, from the records of the Johns Hopkins Hospital; Gyn. No. 0150, from the records of the Johns Hopkins Hospital.

Cullen, Thomas S. : Cancer of the Uterus, 1900.

Demons el Verdelet: Cancer secondaire de Pombilic. Congr. periodique de gyn., d'obstet. et de paod., 1898, ii, 344.

Gueneau de Mussy: Cancer du peritoine. Clin, med., 1875, ii, 28.

Liveing: Cancer of Ovaries and Peritoneum and Umbilicus. The Lancet, 1875, ii, 8.

CARCINOMA OF THE UMBILICUS SECONDARY TO CARCINOMA OF THE UTERUS.

Extension of carcinoma of the uterus to the umbilicus is exceptionally rare. In the examination of an unusually large number of cases of uterine cancer I have never detected an umbilical involvement. Le Coniac,* in his thesis on cancer of the umbilicus secondary to primary uterine or ovarian growths, says that in one case there existed between the cancer of the uterus and the umbilical tumor a chain of nodules along the anterior abdominal wall.

Catteau f in his thesis in 1876, described the case of a young woman who had carcinoma of the body of the uterus. There were two nodules in the abdomen and a tumor the size of a filbert at the umbilicus. The inguinal glands were enlarged. In this case the umbilical growth was in all probability secondary to that in the terus. These are the only two cases that I can find in any way suggesting cancer of the umbilicus secondary to a primary growth in the uterus.

Quenu and Longuet, X however, in their paper mention two cases of cancer of the uterus with secondary nodules at the umbilicus.

CASES OF SECONDARY CARCINOMA OF THE UMBILICUS IN WHICH THE SOURCE OF THE PRIMARY GROWTH WAS NOT DETERMINED.

These cases closely resemble those of secondary carcinoma of the umbilicus already considered. A few, however, present particularly well some of the salient points and other features not illustrated by the preceding cases.

In Bantigny's case a small, ovoid, sessile nodule was present at the umbilicus. The inguinal, axillary, and subclavicular glands on both sides were implicated.

In Chuquet's Case 3, at the umbilicus was a cancerous plaque, 10 by 5 cm., which was continuous with the induration in the suspensory ligament.

My case (G) was unusual, in that the umbilical changes had become apparent exceptionally early, there being merely a delicate papillary growth in the umbilical depression. This growth on section clearly shows the fibrous appearance of these tumors. The specimens from three others of these cases came under my personal attention. In Dr. W. T. Willey's case the growth was bluish red and very prominent. It showed areas of ulceration. Operation was contraindicated, and we were unable to get an autopsy. In Irving Miller's case the umbilical growth reached the surface of the umbilicus. Haggard's case is particularly striking on account of the large dimensions of the umbilicus, its general contour being still preserved. This tumor on section also clearly showed the apparent fibrous character of these growths. The carcinomatous structure would not for a moment be suspected from such a picture.

Secondary Carcinoma of the Umbilicus.

Bantigny's patient, § a man fifty-three years of age, six months before coming under observation, had noticed a tumor the size of a pea in the center of the umbilical depression. His digestion had been poor for some time, and he had had radiating pains in the umbilical region. There had been loss of appetite and progressive emaciation for two months. At the time of operation the umbilical nodule was the size of a small walnut, ovoid in form, and with a broad pedicle. It was purple in color, ulcerated, but apparently movable. The inguinal glands on both sides were enlarged. The subclavicular and axillary glands were also involved.

At operation the omentum was found adherent, and at its extremity was a small tumor the size of a pea, hard, and manifestly cancerous. Bantigny held that the umbilical cancer was secondary to some visceral growth.

* Le Coniac, H. C. J. : Cancer secondaire de l'ombilic, consecutif aux tumeurs malignes de l'appareil utero-ovarien. These de Bordeaux, 1898, No. 19.

f Catteau, J. F. : De l'ombilic et de ses modifications dans les cas de distension de l'abdomen. These de Paris, 1876.

X Quenu et Longuet: Du cancer secondaire de l'ombilic. Rev. de chir., 1896, xvi, 97.

§ Bantigny, A. : Un cas de cancer de l'ombilic. Jour, des sci. med. de Lille, 1898, 2. s., xxi, 91.

Carcinoma of the Umbilicus Secondary to Peritoneal Carcinosis.

Chuquet* bases his paper on general carcinosis of the peritoneum on 46 cases.

Case 3. — A woman, sixty years of age, two and one-half months before, had begun to complain of severe pain in the legs and in the inguinal region. At that time a painful, hard, and ulcerated enlargement at the umbilicus had been noticed. The ulceration was superficial and covered with a crust which dropped off at intervals. At the same time she had had a diarrhea lasting three weeks.

The abdomen was enlarged, and on examination an area of induration, 5 by 6 cm., could be felt at the umbilicus, and in the abdomen hard masses could be detected. Several glands were palpable in the inguinal region.

At autopsy several liters of ascitic fluid were found. The intestines were studded with small cancerous nodules. A large tumor was present in the omentum, which was adherent to the anterior surface of the stomach. At the umbilicus was an indurated plaque, 10 cm. long by 5 cm. broad, continuous with an induration in the suspensory ligament of the liver. The ulceration of the umbilicus was only superficial. Nodules were present in the pelvis and the liver. The mucosa of the stomach had not been invaded. [Of course, in this case the primary site is still in doubt. — T. S. C]

A Malignant Growth of the Umbilicus, Apparently a Carcinoma Secondary to Some Abdominal Growth.

Mrs. J. J., aged eighty, seen in consultation with Dr. W. T. Willey, October 5, 1910. This patient has had indigestion for years, more marked during the last few months. She rises early for her breakfast and then goes to bed for several hours on account of the uncomfortable sensation in the abdomen. For about ten years she has had uterine hemorrhages at irregular intervals. Her chief complaint is of pain and enlargement at the umbilicus.

Examination. — The umbilicus is rolled out and its right side is occupied by a bluish-red nodule, 3.5 cm. in diameter. This presents a glazed appearance. In some places it is covered over with skin, but at a few points are little areas of ulceration, which, however, do not bleed much. If one attempts to roll the tumor out of the umbilicus, some pus escapes from the crevices. Surrounding the umbilicus is a zone of induration about 1 cm. in diameter. The umbilical tumor seems to be fairly well fixed. On pelvic examination the uterus is found to be about four times the natural size. The cervix is normal.

It looks very much as if the growth at the umbilicus is a carcinoma, and that it is secondary to some abdominal growth. It is just possible that it may come from a carcinoma of the body of the uterus, but it is more probable that it is secondary to some growth in the stomach.

After considering the matter fully I decided against operation on account of the patient's age, and because there existed some inoperable growth in the abdomen. The patient died a few months after my visit. No autopsy was permitted.

* Chuquet, A. : Du carcinome generalise du peritoine. These de Paris, 1879, No. 548.

Carcinoma of the Umbilicus Secondary to an Abdominal Growth.

(Personal communication from Dr. Irving Miller.) E. M.was operated on at the Church Home and Infirmary on August 31, 1909. She was a woman fifty-eight years of age, married, and had had one child. At the lower end of the umbilical depression was a painless growth the size of a lentil, grayish red in color. There was a considerable amount of moisture. No nodule could be detected in the abdomen, and the patient had no indigestion. During the removal of the growth nodules were found in the omentum and mesentery. These varied from the size of a pea to that of a hazelnut. The peritoneum was free and there was no hernia.

A Malignant Growth of the Umbilicus, Apparently a Carcinoma Secondary to Some Abdominal Growth.

This photograph of Dr. Willey's patient was made by Dr. Cecil Vest. A growth occupies the site of the umbilicus; this is several centimeters broad, as indicated by comparing it with the fingers. The skin is still intact, but very thin, and over the dark areas is almost wanting.

Dr. Miller thought that the umbilical growth was secondary, but could not locate the original tumor. It did not emanate from the pelvis.

The specimen measures 3 by 1 cm., and consists of tissue covered over with skin. Occupying the umbilical region is a firm nodule which, on section, has a whitish, fibrous appearance. The entire specimen resembles a large umbilicus.

On histologic examination the squamous epithelium in the vicinity of the umbilicus is perfectly normal and the underlying stroma unaltered. It ends abruptly, and coming up from below and reaching the surface is a cancerous growth. This is glandular in character, and consists of long, finger-like folds or of papillary masses or groups of glands. The cells are very regular, but mitotic figures are very abundant. Only at one point over a verylimited area is the skin lacking. Here the cancerous tissue reaches the surface. It is covered with a moderate amount of fibrin in which are a few leukocytes. Certain portions of the tumor show small areas of calcification. It is without doubt a secondary carcinoma of the umbilicus. The picture present resembles very closely that found in cancer of.the body of the uterus. It is impossible for us, however, to determine absolutely the original source of the growth.

Adenocarcinoma of the Umbilicus Secondary to an Intra-abdominal Growth.

(Specimen sent by Dr. Irving Miller, Baltimore.) The surface on the left is covered over with squamous epithelium, which shows little deviation from the normal. As we pass to the right the squamous epithelium gradually disappears, and on the extreme right the surface is composed of cancerous tissue. The right half of the picture shows a definite papillary or finger-like character of the growth. It is an adenocarcinoma. Along the advancing margins of the cancer the stroma shows much small-round-cell infiltration.

Secondary Carcinoma of the Umbilicus; Metastases in the Right Inguinal Glands.

Mr. G.,* forty-two years of age, was seen in consultation August 30, 1904. The patient was well nourished, and complained of a discharge from the umbilicus. Six weeks before he had been struck in the abdomen with a shoe and the umbilicus had commenced to discharge three weeks later. The umbilicus itself presented a granular appearance and the tissue surrounding it was indurated. The patient had had dyspepsia for years; also pain in the lower abdomen over the appendix. He was admitted to the Church Home. Under anesthesia the inguinal glands were carefully palpated. A definite enlargement was found in the right side. An incision 10 cm. in length was made and the inguinal glands were removed, together with the surrounding fat. I then made a long elliptic incision around the umbilicus and removed the umbilical tumor, giving the hardened area a wide berth. The growth at the umbilicus closely resembled a retracted nipple. The patient took the anesthetic badly, and consequently I could not make as thorough an abdominal exploration as I desired. With the finger carried in all directions I was unable to detect any thickening.

* This case was reported by me in the Jour. Amer. Med. Assoc., 1911, lvi, 391.

Adenocarcinoma of the Umbilicus.

The umbilicus looks very much like an inverted carcinomatous nipple. The margins present a fine nodular appearance. The dotted line indicates the limits of the incision. On the right is shown a longitudinal section through the umbilicus. There is much thickening due to carcinomatous infiltration. The peritoneum beneath the umbilicus was free from adhesions.

Histologic Examination. — The umbilical growth proved to be a typical adenocarcinoma. The squamous epithelium in many places was normal, but along the edge of the growth it was impossible to distinguish between the cells of the adenocarcinoma and those of the squamous epithelium. There was as yet little breaking down. The growth in the inguinal glands macroscopicalfy looked like cancer. On histologic examination it presented exactly the same pattern as that noted at the umbilicus.

On January 25, 1905, the patient was in fairly good health; but was still constipated and had great difficulty in defecation. On February 24th a firm globular mass fully 10 cm. in diameter was found occupying the middle of the abdomen and the left inguinal glands were considerably enlarged. The umbilical growth was undoubtedly secondary to the intra-abdominal cancer. In May, 1905, 1 again saw the patient. His bowels had not moved for ten days, and he was so emaciated that one could hardly recognize him. Nodules were palpable everywhere in the abdomen. He died a few days later.

Cancer of the Umbilicus.

Haggard * reports the case of a man fifty-nine years of age. Three months before admission the patient had noticed a hard nodule the size of a hickory-nut just above the umbilicus. The hardness gradually increased, and the umbilicus commenced to bulge. The tumor was slightly tender, and there was a sense of uneasiness; it was the size of a goose's egg, was stony hard, and the skin could not be moved over it. The mass was fixed. The patient commenced to lose flesh.

Haggard removed the umbilicus February 17, 1904, making an elliptic incision. The resultant opening gaped nearly as large as a saucer. The stomach, gall-bladder, and liver were examined for cancer, but none was found. The gall-bladder was very hard and thickened and contracted down on a stone; this was removed and the gall-bladder drained. The peritoneum could not be approximated. The omentum was turned up and sewed to the serous margins of the incision. With considerable difficulty the fascia and muscle were partly brought together with interrupted sutures of catgut. The edges of the wound were still about 13 inches apart. The silver wire filigree of Willard-Bartlett was used. This was laid on corduroy sutures of catgut, the edges resting between the fat and the fascia, and the skin was closed. The wound healed without incident.

Secondary Adenocarcinoma of the Umbilicus. t

The specimen sent me by Dr. Haggard, of Nashville, Tenn., in April, 1910, consists of the umbilicus with a good deal of surrounding tissue. The entire specimen measures 10 cm. in length, 7 cm. in breadth. The umbilicus is 2.5 cm. across and is covered with skin. It presents a rather uneven, nodular surface, and is much more prominent than usual, having welled up in the center. There is no evidence of ulceration at any point. On section the distance between the umbilicus and the peritoneal surface is 2 cm. The tissues look fibrous, and in the vicinity of the umbilicus show infiltration, apparently with fibrous tissue. At one point is an area of what looks like localized fibrous thickening, 2.5 cm. in diameter. The adipose tissue has been almost entirely replaced at this point.

* Haggard, W. D. : Cancer of the Umbilicus. Amer. Jour. Surg, and Gyn., St. Louis, 1903-04, xvii, 196.

t This case was reported by me in Jour. Amer. Med. Assoc, 1911, lvi, 391.

The Section Shows Carcinoma of the Right Inguinal Glands. Scattered throughout the adipose tissue are several solid areas. Those indicated by a are small lymph-glands. The lymph-gland at b is greatly enlarged, and everywhere infiltrated by carcinoma which is invading the surrounding tissue; c is alsoan area of carcinoma.

Secondary Carcinoma of the Umbilicus.

(Specimen sent by Dr. W. D. Haggard of Nashville, Tenn., April, 1910.) The umbilical fold is much widened, and the umbilicus is shallower than usual. It resents a somewhat uneven and nodular appearance, but is everywhere intact. On the right is shown a longitudinal section through the umbilicus. There is a deep cleft along the skin surface, and the umbilical fold is deeper than usual. The fat in the depth has been replaced to a large extent by fibrous tissue, which is everywhere infiltrated with carcinoma. The peritoneal surface, which is to the left, is perfectly smooth; there is no evidence of any adhesions.

Histologic Examination. — The squamous epithelium is intact, and there is pigmentation in the deeper layers, suggesting that the specimen has come from a colored patient. The tissue immediately beneath the skin in some places is normal; at other points it shows some small-round-cell infiltration. Scattered everywhere throughout the thickened fibrous tissue are glands. Some of them are small and round, others elongated or tubular; others are dilated. The glands are lined with cylindric or cuboid epithelium, which in most places is one layer in thickness. The nuclei of the epithelial cells are for the most part oval and stain uniformly. A few of the epithelial cells have very large and deeply staining nuclei. Where the glands are dilated, the epithelium tends to become cuboid. At other points the glands are very abundant, are undergoing disintegration, and are filled with mucus. In some places the epithelium is several layers in thickness. Here and there gland epithelium has proliferated to such an extent that new glands are being formed. The growth is undoubtedly a carcinoma of a glandular type and similar to one originating either in the stomach or intestine.

Encephaloid Cancer of the Umbilicus.*

The umbilicus of an old man was occupied by a tumor the size of a fist, and presenting a bluish aspect. It was apparently adherent to the peritoneum and to the skin at the umbilicus. It was soft, but could not be moved at all without displacing the abdominal wall. The patient had lancinating abdominal pains. Demarquay diagnosed cancer of the umbilicus, but did not operate. The patient died.

Cancer of the Umbilicus.

Demarquayf with Dr. Roger saw a patient, sixty years of age, who had a soft and somewhat fluctuating tumor at the umbilicus. It was the size of two hands. It had originated at the umbilicus. It was opened at several points and fungating masses grew from it. A diagnosis of encephaloid cancer was made. The patient died. No histologic examination is reported.

Cancer of the Omentum and Umbilicus Simulating Hernia. %

Mary T., aged sixty-six, the mother of four children, had been in good health until four years previously, when she had noticed a projection at the umbilicus. This was the size of a finger-tip, and was pressed on by her stays. The bowels had been regular until one month before, when diarrhea had commenced. This had ceased without any treatment, but had returned two weeks later, accompanied by pain in the abdomen, especially at the umbilicus. Vomiting had then started, and the patient had rapidly grown worse.

After admission she vomited frequently. The vomitus had an offensive but non-fecal odor. The patient had an anxious expression. She was stout and well nourished; the abdomen was distended, tympanitic, and tender. There was a nodular projection in the left half of the umbilicus, half an inch in diameter. The overlying skin was normal, but immediately beneath the umbilicus and in the abdominal cavity was an ill-defined, very hard, slightly movable tumor, apparently continuous with that of the umbilicus. The patient on the twelfth day developed a temperature of 104° F. and died.

Autopsy showed invasion of the peritoneum by cancer. The mass involving the omentum had extended into the umbilicus. [This case at first simulated a small, strangulated umbilical hernia. There is no note as to the original site of the cancer. — T. S. C]

Carcinoma of the Umbilicus §

A stout woman, forty-nine years of age, had had an umbilical hernia for a long time. Six months before she had received a slight injury of the umbilicus, and from that time the hernia had increased in size. On admission it was as large as an egg, hard, painful on pressure, and irreducible.

* Demarquay: Bull. Soc. de chir., 1870, 2. ser., xi, 209. Seance du 8 Juin.

f Demarquay: Op. cit.

% Forster, J. Cooper: Guy's Hospital Reports, 1874, 3. s., xix, 4.

§ Gallet, M. A. : Epithelioma de l'ombilic. Jour, de chir. et ann. Soc. beige de chir., Bruxelles,

The umbilical growth was removed. The omentum was found adherent, and in it were enormous cancerous masses. Two large ovarian cysts were removed at the same time. At autopsy gall-stones were found. The intestinal tract was normal. Gallet thought the cancer was primary in the umbilicus. No microscopic examination, however, was given, as the case was reported at the society on the day of the operation. [The umbilical growth was probably secondary. — T. S. C]

Carcinoma of the Umbilicus.

Kuster* reports a case personally communicated to him by Wilms. An old Israelite had a carcinoma of the umbilicus and died in consequence of digestive disturbances. The general history suggests that the umbilical growth was secondary.

Cancer of the Umbilicus. f

A young married woman, twenty-seven years of age, had a tuberculous peritonitis with effusion. In the region of the umbilicus was an ulcerated and hemorrhagic area. McMurtry opened the abdomen, evacuated the contents and took the umbilicus out through an elliptic incision. He diagnosed the case as one of fibroid carcinoma. [In the absence of mention of a microscopic examination a possible tuberculous character of the umbilical lesion cannot be absolutely excluded. — T. S. C]

Carcinoma of the Umbilicus. J

A man, fifty-four years of age, had carcinoma of the glands of the left groin for two years and intra-abdominal symptoms of malignant disease. For four weeks a small, very painful, fungating mass had been developing at the umbilicus. The umbilicus as a whole was not enlarged or hardened. From its center sprang a tuft of purplish-red granulation about as large as a small pea. Morris removed the umbilicus, and at the same time made an exploratory opening for examination of the abdomen. The omentum was the seat of a colloid carcinoma, but there were no adhesions of the omentum to furnish a route for infection to the umbilicus. The umbilical growth was an adenocarcinoma.

Cancer of the Umbilicus.

Nelaton§ speaks of a scirrhus of the umbilicus in a patient sixty years of age. It was spheric, regular, about 2.5 cm. in diameter. No microscopic examination was made.

Carcinoma of the Umbilicus Secondary to Abdominal Carcinoma. ||

A woman, fifty-one years of age, had had an abdominal enlargement for fifteen months. In the right iliac fossa was a round enlargement increasing in size. Her digestion was poor, and she suffered from nausea and vomiting and lost weight. Blood and pus were present in the stools. One of the left inguinal glands was enlarged to the size of a hazelnut. The point of origin of the tumor was not certain. At the umbilicus was also a carcinomatous nodule the size of a walnut, hard and purple in color. In the vicinity there was another nodule.

The growth was an adenocarcinoma. Neveu then goes on to give a general resume of the subject.

* Kuster, E. : Die Xeubildungen am Xabel Erwachsener unci ihre operative Behancllung.

Langenbeck's Arch, f.klin. Chir., 1874, xvi, 234.

f McMurtry, L. S.: Louisville Monthly Jour, of Med. and Surg., 1902-03, ix, 492.

J Morris, R.: Lectures on Appendicitis and Xotes on Other Subjects, 1S95, 96.

§ Nelaton: Squirrhe ombilical. Gaz. des hop., Paris, 1860, xxxiii, 294.

|| Xeveu, V.: Contribution a l'etude des tumeurs malignes secondares de l'ombilic, Paris, 1890, No. 50.

Secondary Carcinoma of the Umbilicus.

Pernice* cites a case reported by Bergeat (Inaug. Dissert., Munich, 1883). A woman, sixty-one years old, for three years had had a tumor at the umbilicus which had ulcerated. The inguinal glands were swollen. At autopsy a tumor the size of a child's head was found, which projected into the abdomen. The gall-bladder was adherent and had opened into the tumor.

Excision of Umbilicus for Malignant Diseases. f

The patient, thirty-seven years of age, was thin and cachectic. At the umbilicus was a nodule the size of a hen's egg. It had been growing rapidly, was painful and ulcerated. Operation was advised, but the patient disappeared.

Secondary Carcinoma of the Umbilicus. X

A woman, fifty years of age, had been in perfect health until six months before, when she commenced to lose her appetite and have vomiting spells. In less than two months she had lost 15 kilos. A month before admission she had noticed a moderate-sized induration at the umbilicus. A few days later it had become dark red. She never had had any pain. The umbilicus was removed. No tumor was detected in the abdominal cavity. The specimen consisted of a violet-colored mass which had ulcerated, and there was induration of the surrounding tissue. On cutting through there was a gritty-like feel suggestive of carcinoma. The peritoneum covering the under surface was indurated, but smooth. There was no evidence of neoplasmin the abdomen. On histologic examination the growth proved to be a cylindric-cell carcinoma. From the findings thus far the tumor might have been considered as primary. Three months later, however, the patient was suffering from hemorrhage from the bowels. The inguinal glands on both sides were enlarged, forming a definite mass. The patient became cachectic and soon died. The umbilical growth had evidently been secondary.

Quenu and Longuet gave the following data concerning cases with secondary carcinoma of the umbilicus In 32 cases in which the sex is recorded, 23 of the patients were females — a proportion of 70 per cent. (To explain this Damaschino expressed the opinion that carcinoma of the umbilicus occurs secondarily to carcinoma of the uterus or the ovaries.) In 19 out of 36 cases in which accurate data were given, the primary growth was in the gastro-intestinal tract. Of these 19 cases, in 14 the growth was primary in the stomach, in 4 in the intestine, and in 1 in the stomach and intestine. In two cases the primary cancer was in the uterus, and in three cases the original tumor was found in the ovaries.

Secondary Carcinoma of the Umbilicus.

Verchere§ gives a short review of the literature and reports the case of a woman, fifty-five years of age, who for several days had had signs of intestinal obstruction. Her general health up to that time had been good. The abdomen was distended, and at the umbilicus was a tumor slightly smaller than half an apple. It was hard, red, and ulcerated, but on the surface was smooth and regular. It was surrounded by a deep funnel, the walls of which were composed of healthy skin. Verchere thought it was a secondary growth, and made a rectovaginal examination, inquired for gastric and intestinal symptoms, and examined the anterior surface of the liver. All these examinations gave negative results. At operation he found, on the peritoneum of the anterior abdominal wall, many small, whitish-yellow, cancerous nodules. The primary source of the abdominal growth which had given rise to these metastases and to the secondary carcinoma at the umbilicus could not be located.

* Pernice, L. : Die Nabelgeschwtilste, Halle, 1892.

f Parker, Willard: Arch. Clin. Surg., New York, 1876-77, i, 71.

X Quenu et Longuet: Du cancer seconclaire de l'ombilic. Rev. de chir., 1896, xvi, 97.

§ Verchere: De hi valeur si'meiologique du cancer de l'ombilic. Rev. des mah cancereuses, 1895-96, i, 81.

Adenocarcinoma of the Umbilicus.*

The patient was sixty-eight years old, and for nearly a year had had discomfort just above the umbilicus. This was almost continuous and was independent of digestion. At the umbilicus was an indurated area the size of a pigeon's egg. When the patient came under observation the induration was ovoid in form, 6 cm. in its longest diameter, and 4 cm. broad. It seemed to be a primary tumor of the abdominal wall. It was removed but the patient died of peritonitis.

On microscopic examination, according to Stori, the growth proved to be an adenocarcinoma.

A Retroperitoneal Carcinoma Associated with Cancer of the Umbilicus.

From the accompanying history it appears that the primary growth was retroperitoneal. From what epithelial structure it originated, it is, however, impossible to say.

MacMunn's f patient was a woman sixty-three years of age. She was cachectic and had a "mouse smell. " The lymphatics in the left groin were of stony hardness and considerably enlarged. At the umbilicus was a hemispheric tumor, purplish in color, the size of a plum. It was firm, and had on its surface two small ulcers. When lifted up, the tumor could readily be isolated from the deeper structures.

At autopsy the umbilical growth was found to be bluish or grayish white and hard; it projected through the abdominal wall, raised the peritoneum slightly, but was not adherent to the structures. A few small, whitish nodules were found between the umbilicus and the pubes. The omentum contained nodules, the largest 23^ by 3^2 inch. Secondary growths were also present in the mesentery. The umbilical growth was undoubtedly secondary to the retroperitoneal tumor.

* Stori, Teodoro: Contribute) alio studio dei tumori dell' ombelico. Lo Sperimentale, Arch, di biologia normale e patologia, 1900, liv, 25.

f MacMunn: Case of Retroperitoneal Cancer Accompanied by Cancer of the Navel. Dublin Jour, of Med. Sci., lxii, 1876, 1.

LITERATURE CONSULTED ON CASES OF SECONDARY CARCINOMA OF THE UMBILICUS IN WHICH THE SOURCE OF THE PRIMARY GROWTH WAS NOT DETERMINED.

Bantigny, A. : Un cas de cancer de 1'ombilic. Jour, des sci. med. de Lille, 1898, 2. s., xxi, 91.

Chuquet: Du carcinome generalise du peritone. These de Paris, 1879, No. 548.

Cullen, Thomas S. : Dr. W. T. Willey's case: Secondary Carcinoma of the Umbilicus.

Cullen, Thomas S. : Dr. Irving Miller's case: Secondary Carcinoma of the Umbilicus.

Cullen, Thomas S.: Personal case.

Cullen, Thomas S.: Surgical Diseases of the Umbilicus. Jour. Amer. Med. Assoc, February 11, 1911, lvi, 391.

Haggard, W. D.: Cancer of the Umbilicus. Amer. Jour. Surg, and Gyn., St. Louis, 1903-04, xvii, 196.

Deniarquay : Cancer de l'ombilie. Bull. Soc. de chir., 1S70, 2. ser., xi, 209. (Seance du 8 Juin.)

Forster, J. C: Cancer of the Omentum and Umbilicus Simulating Hernia. Guy's Hospital

Reports, 1S74, 3. s.. xix. 4.

Gallet. M. A.: Epitheliorue de l'ombilie. Jour, de chir. et arm. Soc. beige de chir., Bruxelles, 1901, i, 565.

Exist er, E.: Die Xeubildungen am Nabel Erwachsener und ihre operative Behandlung. Langenbeck's Arch. f. klin. Chir., 1874, xvi, 234.

McMurtry, L. S.: Cancer of the Umbilicus. Louisville Monthly Jour. Med. and Surg., 1902-03, ix, 492.

Morris, R.: Carcinoma of the Umbilicus. Lectures on Appendicitis and Notes on Other Subjects, 1S95, 96.

Nelaton: Squirrhe ombihcal. Gaz. des hop., Paris, 1860, xxxiii, 294.

Neveu, V. : Contribution a l'etude des tumeurs mahgnes secondaires de l'ombilie. Paris, 1890.

Pernice, L.: Die Nabelgeschwulste, HaUe, 1892.

Parker, W. : Excision of Umbihcus for MaUgnant Diseases. Arch. Clin. Surg., New York, 1876-77. i. 71.

Quenu et Longuet : Du cancer secondaire de l'ombilie. Rev. de chir., 1896, xvi, 97.

Stori, T. : Contributo alio studio dei Tumori dell' ombelico. Lo Sperimentale, Arch, di biologia normale e patologia, 1900, liv, 25.

Verchere, F. : De la valeur semeiologique du cancer de l'ombilie. Rev. des maladies cancereuses, 1895-96, U, 81.

SARCOMA OF THE UMBILICUS.

Telangiectatic myxosarcoma.

Spindle-cell sarcoma of the umbilicus: report of cases.

Round-cell sarcoma of the umbilicus.

Melanotic sarcoma of the umbilicus.

The literature on this subject is in a very chaotic condition. From the recorded cases it is possible to make the following classification :

1. So-called telangiectatic myxosarcoma occurring at or near the time of birth. This in reality is not malignant.
2. Spindle-cell sarcoma.
3. Round-cell sarcoma.
4. Melanotic sarcoma.

At best my description of sarcoma of the umbilicus will be fragmentary andincomplete. I shall give abstracts of the more characteristic cases recorded, so that the reader may draw his own conclusions. After careful histologic studies of such cases in the future it is to be hoped that before many years the subject of sarcoma of the umbilicus will be placed on a clear and satisfactory basis.

TELANGIECTATIC MYXOSARCOMA.

Cases of this nature have been reported by Virchow, Kaufmann, and von Winckel. In 1864 Gerdes saw a child, a few hours old, with a horn-like projection from the umbilicus. It was four inches in length and about the thickness of the index-finger, and gradually tapered to the end. At first it was bright red in color, later dark. It was very smooth, had an abundant blood-supply, was rather firm, had no pulsation, and on compression did not diminish in size. The growth was composed of spindle-cells separated from each other by a mucous intercellular substance. Virchow termed it a telangiectatic myxosarcoma.

In Kaufmann's case, reported in 1890, the tumor was likewise present at birth, and in the course of a few days was observed to grow gradually. It projected 6 cm. from the abdominal wall and was 16 cm. in circumference. It was partly covered with skin, partly with amnion. Its outer portion was dense; its central part cavernous. On histologic examination the former was found to consist of spindle-cells, the latter of myxosarcomatous tissue. The angiomatous appearance in the central portion was due to the great dilatation of the arteries.

Von Winckel in 1893 observed a red tumor at the umbilicus in a new-born child. This tumor (Fig. 194) was 4 cm. long, and at the umbilicus 2.8 cm. in diameter. It was bright red in color. Its surface was covered with what appeared to be a hyaline membrane. The growth was composed chiefly of spindle-shaped cells. There was an abundance of large blood-vessels, and, in addition, large lymph-spaces. At certain points the endothelium of the lymph-spaces had proliferated.

These endothelial cells were markedly enlarged and projected into the lumina of the lymphatics. The stroma-cells in the vicinity were very large, but the majority of them contained no nuclei and looked more like cells undergoing degeneration. This case, apart from dilatation of the lymphatics, bore a striking resemblance to those reported by Virchow and Kaufmann. Abstracts of Kaufmann's and von Winckel's cases are appended.

A Congenital Umbilical Tumor.*

On the second day after birth Lissner saw the child. The mother was forty-eight years of age, strong, and well nourished. The patient was the twelfth child. The labor had been easy, and the umbilical tumor had caused no hindrance. At first it was small, but by the end of twenty-four hours had grown markedly. When seen, it was the size of an apple, reddish in color. The skin of the abdomen extended up for some distance on the sides of the tumor. The remaining portion of the tumor was covered over with amnion, which was continued upon the umbilical cord. The tumor was firm in consistence, and on pressure could not be rendered smaller. After six days it had grown a good deal and there had been bleeding from it, which had been checked by the use of styptics. Under chloroform narcosis three needles were passed through the base of the tumor and a bichlorid silk thread was tied around it. The tumor was then cut away, and the wound dressed antiseptically. Six days later the remnant of the tumor was recognized as a thick, brown, hard, dry, mummified crust, which came away readily. Healing took place rapidly.

The tumor was firm in consistence, almost round, 16 cm. in circumference, and reached a height of 6 cm. At its base, where it passed to the umbilical ring, were seen cross-sections of the umbilical arteries and of the umbilical vein. The latter contained a red thrombus. In addition there were cross-sections of other blood-vessels.

Xear the surface the tumor is everywhere dense and fibrous. In the middle portion it is of a myxomatous character, and in this myxomatous tissue are numerous blood-vessels, some of which present a cavernous appearance. Beneath the surface epithelium the cells are partly round, but to a great extent spindle-shaped. These spindle-cells are narrow and often long, resembling muscle-fibers, but the nuclei are more delicate. From the picture Kaufmann concludes that it is a spindle-cell sarcoma. As one nears the center of the tumor the spindle-cells become more sparse and we have a picture of myxomatous tissue. It is in the myxomatous portion of the tumor that the blood-vessels have increased in size and that a cavernous appearance is noted. Some of the blood-vessels show many branchings — some narrow, others wide. A few of the vessels are still filled with blood. The cavernous appearance is due to dilated arteries. Kaufmann designates the tumor as a myxosarcoma telangiectodes, and speaks of its resemblance to the case reported by Virchow.

* Kaufmann: Ueber eine Geschwulstbildung des Xabelstrangs. Virchows Arch., 1890, cxxi, 513.

A Congenital Solid Tumor of the Umbilical Portion of the Cord.

On December 16, 1893, von Winckel* saw a female child, 49 cm. long and weighing 2500 grams. At the margin of the umbilical cord, immediately after labor, a tumor had been noted. This was firm in consistence, bright red in color, and had here and there a bluish, translucent surface. Near the free end were two fine threads with small bodies the size of linseeds on their surfaces. The entire tumor was 4 cm. long, at its base, 2.8 cm. thick, and near the end, 1.6 cm. in diameter. The tumor was removed with the cautery, and the peritoneum opened for a breadth of from 2 to 5 mm., a small quantity of serous fluid escaping. The operation did not last over fifteen seconds. A compression band was applied, and the child made a satisfactory recovery. Fourteen days later, however, she died suddenly of pneumonia.

The outer surface of the tumor was covered with what appeared to be hyaline membrane, which contained connective-tissue nuclei in large or small numbers. Beneath the surface there was a net-like arrangement of threads consisting of connective-tissue nuclei and leukocytes. In the superficial layers of the tumor there was an abundance of large blood-vessels. In addition there were lymph- vessels showing a definite endothelial lining;. These contained fibrin threads and leukocytes. The endothelium of the lymphatics appeared to be proliferating. The endothelial cells were markedly enlarged and projected into the lumen; here and there they contained mitotic figures. In the vicinity of these lymph-spaces, in the connective tissue, spindle-shaped cells were seen, between which there appeared to be some fluid. There were also large epithelioid cells in the stroma.. These stained with hematoxylin-eosin a diffuse violet. The majority contained no nuclei and resembled degenerated tissue-cells. In the pedicle of the tumor a similar structure was noted. The large, deeplytinged cells, however, were lacking. The blood-vessels were abundant. Von Winckel said that, from the description of his case, there was no doubt that he was dealing with a telangiectatic myxosarcoma similar to those reported by Virchow and Kaufmann.

From a careful study of these cases it would appear that they bear a marked resemblance to those considered under angiomata of the umbilicus, and that, in all probability, they should be included in that class. They do not seem to be malignant

* von Winckel: Ueber angeborene solide GeschwiiLste des (perennirenden) Theiles der Nabelschnur. Sammlung klin. Yortrage, n. F. No. 140. (Gyn. Nr. 53.)

SPINDLE-CELL SARCOMA OF THE UMBILICUS.

Only a few instances have been recorded, and, as pointed out by Nicaise, Perniee, and others, even in such cases careful histologic reports are usually lacking. Spindle-cell sarcoma of the umbilicus would appear to be the most common variety, and the growth has been designated as a spindle-cell sarcoma, a fibrosarcoma, a myxosarcoma, or a sarcoma fibrocellulare.

Firm connective-tissue growths of the umbilicus are relatively rare. They may occur in the young, middle-aged, or old. They usually are oval or round, and may-slowly or rapidly reach the size of a fist or an orange. As a rule, they have an intact skin covering. This may be normal, have large veins coursing over its surface, or the skin may show a purple discoloration. Occasionally, as a result of irritation, the surface of the tumor may be slightly ulcerated. The tumor may be sessile or somewhat pedunculated.

Clinically, it is almost impossible to determine whether such a growth is a fibroma or a spindle-cell sarcoma unless metastases occur; and, even if a nodule develops in the abdominal wall, several months or a year or more after the tumor has been removed, there is still the possibility that this second nodule may be a fibroma.

On section, most of these tumors have a fibrous appearance, few of them presenting the homogeneous, pork-like surface so characteristic of sarcoma. If, on histologic examination, the cells contain large, irregular nuclei with deeply staining chromatin, or if nuclear figures are abundantly distributed throughout the tumor, the diagnosis of sarcoma is clear. If, on the other hand, only quiescent spindle-cells are in evidence, it is absolutely impossible to make the diagnosis from the histologic findings, and the surgeon remains in the dark as to the exact character of the tumor, unless its malignancy is clearly shown by the later development of metastases.

Where the sarcoma of the umbilicus is secondary, the growth may tend to spread out into the abdominal wall and wall not be so prominent and well defined.

Cases Reported as Instances of Spindle-cell Sarcoma of the Umbilicus.

Some of these tumors were clearly sarcomatous; others in all probability were fibromata. The reader can draw his own conclusions as to the proper diagnosis in each case. Those cases that were clearly instances of fibroma, although previously classified as sarcoma, are included under fibromata, while quite a number in which not even a probable diagnosis could be made have been entirely omitted.

Spindle-cell Sarcoma of the Umbilicus.*

This tumor was removed by Wehsarg from the umbilical region of a poorly nourished girl aged fourteen. The tumor had grown slowly until three or four years before, when it had suddenly become painful and rapidly grown to the size of a fist. At operation it was round and the size of an orange, smooth, smaller at its base, and slightly pendulous, the umbilicus being pushed down. The skin over the tumor was very thin, bluish red in color, and there were numerous dilated veins. The lower part of the tumor showed several excoriated ulcerated plaques covered with clots and pus. The tumor was removed. It lay on the superficial fascia of the abdominal wall. On section it was yellow, homogeneous, and resembled pork, with here and there darker places surrounded by vessels. Microscopically it proved to be a spindle-cell growth.

Possible Sarcoma of the Umbilicus.

Villarf describes the case of a woman aged forty-six who entered the service of Professor Guyon, September 17, 1886. About December, 1885, she had noticed that her corsets produced pain in the umbilical region, and on examination had found a small, reddish tumor the size of the head of a pin in the umbilical depression. This tumor grew slowly. In May, 1886, the patient presented herself at the hospital for examination. In August, after she had been using iodin without any results, she again came to the hospital. Examination at this time showed that, at the umbilical depression, was a tumor the size of a small bird's egg, but different in form. It was conic, with its base continuous with the umbilical cicatrix. It was slightly pedunculated, firm in consistence, but elastic and reddish in color. At its top was a blackish point 2 mm. in diameter. There was no discharge from the tumor. Two or three days later the blackish point ruptured and there was an escape of dark blood. No glandular enlargement was detected. The tumor was removed. The tumor in question was a little less firm than a fibroma. On section a capsule was found surrounding the central mass. The tumor was whitish gray and had numerous dark spots no larger than the head of a pin scattered throughout it.

Histologic examination showed that the capsule was formed of connective tissue. The central portion of the tumor was composed of sarcomatous tissue, the cells being fusiform. In the center of the tumor there were cavities lined with pavement-cells. These cavities presented various forms. Some were round, others were oval and had anastomosed with one another. In the stroma between the spaces were a small number of blood-vessels. The skin covering the outer surface of the tumor was exceedingly thin, but presented the usual appearance. In the center there had been some extravasation of blood recognizable by deposits of pigment.

(This woman was forty-six years of age. Although the description is not perfectly clear, it bears somewhat the ear-marks of the ease reported by Mintz — a case that proved to be an adenomyoma of the umbilicus. It does not tally with our usual idea of sarcoma. — T. S. C]

* Leydhecker, F. : Zur Diagnose der sarcomatosen Geschwiilste, Giessen, 1856.

f Villar, Francis: Tumeurs de l'ombilic. These de Paris, 1886, obs. 68.

A Case of Myxosarcoma of the Umbilicus.

Plagge* reports the case of a man, twenty-two years of age, who in childhood had had difficulty in digestion and later vomiting and diarrhea. In the summer of 1887 he had pain in the stomach for the first time and noticed a small tumor in the umbilicus. By November, 1887, the tumor was the size of a hazel-nut. Four weeks later there was a nodule the size of a pea below and to the left, close to the linea alba. The patient was much emaciated. He died on March 14, 1888. At autopsy, at the umbilicus a thickening the size of a five-mark piece was noted rising 2 cm. above the abdominal level. Above and below, this thickening could be followed 5 cm. in each direction; the skin was movable over it. On examination of the abdominal cavity in the region of the umbilicus was a nodule, 2 mm. in diameter. In the ligament passing from the umbilicus was a small nodule. The omentum, diaphragm, and intestines were involved. The stomach was normal.

Microscopic examination showed that the growth was a myxosarcoma. [If this had been a primary malignant growth, why had it not broken clown? The clinical picture in no way indicates a primary growth. The histologic appearance suggests very much a colloid carcinoma of the intestine with a secondary growth at the umbilicus. — T. S. C]

Sarcoma at the Umbilicus, f

An East Indian male, aged twenty-four years, was admitted on June 2, 1889. Several weeks before, April 5th, he had exposed himself to the night air after returning from a party. The next morning he felt pain in and around the umbilicus. Two weeks later a small, hard swelling was detected in the navel, and in a few days an unpleasant sensation in this region caused vomiting. The swelling was considered inflammatory in origin, and local applications were made. On examination a subcutaneous growth the size of a hen's egg was found situated exactly at the umbilicus. The skin covering it was deep purple and firmly adherent. The growth was apparently deeply attached by a pedicle fixed to the right side of the umbilicus. A few hard bosses were noted over the surface of the tumor, and a nodule the size of a hazel-nut, detected on the right abdominal wall, was apparently connected with the tumor. This nodule was situated about three and a half inches from the umbilicus. The secondary growth had only recently been noted. Both tumors were tender to the touch.

The main growth and the secondary nodule were removed, but the abdomen was not opened. The patient did not improve, but became profoundly cachectic. About a month after operation a small, freely movable nodule was felt in the subcutaneous connective tissue, about an inch from the abdominal incision below the umbilicus. Soon after, another was noted in the left rectus, close to the cartilage of the ribs. This increased rapidly; there was great nausea and occasional vomiting, suggesting dissemination in the diaphragm. [Microscopic examination showed that the umbilical growth was a fibrosarcoma. The abdomen was not opened. The secondary growth proved the malignancy of the condition, and the vomiting and loss of weight strongly suggested a primary abdominal growth with secondarj^ manifestations at the umbilicus.]

* Plagge, Heinrich: Ein Fall von Myxosarconi des Nabels. Inaug. Diss.. Freiburg, 1889.

f O'Brien, Surgeon- Maj or: Indian Med. Gaz., 1889, xxiv, 215..

A Supposed Sarcoma of the Umbilicus.

Neveu* reported an unpublished case of Monnier's. The patient was a woman fifty years old. She had a uterine growth which extended to the umbilicus. The curet showed sarcoma fusocellulare. Implicating the umbilicus was a mass the size of a hazelnut. No microscopic examination of the umbilical growth was made.

[It is often very difficult, when examining a submucous myoma, to determine whether it is really a spindle-cell sarcoma or a simple myoma. Without an examination of the umbilical nodule we should hesitate to accept this as representing a nodule secondary to the growth in the uterus. — T. S. C]

Sarcoma of the Umbilicus.

Pernicef reports the cases of Blum, Bryant, and Villar. None of the descriptions seem to me to be convincing enough to warrant the growths being included as sarcomata.

Pernice then reports from the Halle Clinic the case of R. Schroeder, aged nineteen. As a child she had a small tumor at the umbilicus. It was not painful and did not grow until the thirteenth year; it was then extirpated. Two years later a new tumor appeared, and, when she was admitted to the hospital, it was the size of a baby's head and was covered with intact umbilical skin. The tumor shone through the skin and was hard. The inguinal glands were not enlarged. The abdomen was widely opened during removal of the tumor, and the patient recovered. About three years later she was in good condition, but shortly afterward a return of the growth was noted. This tumor was the size of a small apple when the patient came back to the hospital. It was situated in the upper angle of the previous incision.

No histologic examination was given. This tumor had not yet been removed when Pernice f reported the case.

[Pernice then goes on to report several other cases, none of which would appear to be an undoubted instance of sarcoma. Although it is quite possible that the growth reported by Pernice was a sarcoma, we must remember that it may equally well have been a fibroma. Where one fibroma develops, others are prone to occur. — T. S. C]

Possibly a Sarcoma of the Umbilicus.

Sourdille + reports the case of a man, forty-nine years of age, who entered Polaillon's service at the Hotel-Dieu March 25, 1895. Eighteen months before he had noticed at the umbilicus small tubercles. These caused him some pain and inconvenience. On admission, attached to the lower border of the umbilicus was found a pedunculated cylinclric tumor, 5 cm. long and 12 to 13 mm. in diameter. Its free end was covered with a small crust over a healed ulceration. The skin covering it was delicate, thin, reddish in color. When grasped between the fingers, the tumor gave the sensation of a finger of a glove filled with hazelnuts. The skin surrounding the tumor contained seven or eight pink tubercles, about the size of green-peas. The skin was movable on the underlying aponeurosis. No enlargement of the glands could be made out. The patient's general health was good. The diseased area was removed.

On histologic examination the main tumor and the small nodules gave a picture of sarcoma fusocellulare covered -with skin. The superficial half of the skin seemed to be the starting-point of the tumors, which tended to pass out and become pedunculated. [This growth may equally well have been a fibroma with very small nodules. The microscopic examination was not very extensive.]

* Neveu: Contribution a l'etude des tumeurs malignes secondares de l'ombilic, Paris, 1890.

f Pernice, L. : Die Xabelgeschwulste, Halle, 1892.

+ Sourdille, Gilbert: Sarcome pedicule de la peau de l'ombilic. Bull, de la Soc. anat. de Paris, 189.5, lxx, 302.

Primary Sarcoma of the Umbilicus.

Gamier * reports for Blanc the case of an otherwise healthy man fifty years old. Six months previously he had noticed a small, hard, painless tumor in the right border of the umbilical depression. It was independent of the skin, and was the size of a hazelnut. The patient had some colic, but no constitutional trouble. He thought that the pain in the pyloric region was due to pressure of the growth on the pylorus. He had lost in weight in the last month.

On admission the tumor was the size of a mandarin orange, round, and was carrying the unfolded umbilicus on its surface. It was hard, painless, and firmly fixed by the contraction of the abdominal muscles. The overlying skin was purple.

At operation it was found that the tumor had developed in the deeper layers. The underlying peritoneum was perfectly smooth, and the tumor was easily removed. Blanc regarded it as a great rarity, this being the first instance observed. He based his assumption that the growth was primary on the absence of functional trouble and on the relative integrity of the patient's general condition.

[He does not mention the examination of the abdominal cavity at the time of operation, and furthermore does not account for the sense of discomfort experienced in the region of the stomach; nor do we know the final outcome. — T. S. C]

On microscopic examination the growth was found to be composed of myriads of small cells separated from one another by a delicate stroma. The cells in general were round or fusiform and had but little protoplasm. Histologically, the growth appeared to be malignant and was a sarcoma. It had developed from the fibrous tissue of the abdominal wall.

ROUND-CELL SARCOMA OF THE UMBILICUS.

The following case represents the only definite instance of round-cell sarcoma of the umbilicus with which I am familiar. The umbilical growth was a secondary one.

Pernicef reports a secondary sarcoma of the umbilicus (Case 71, from the Breslau Gyn. Clinic). The patient was a woman thirty-two years of age. The umbilicus was lifted 3 cm. above the surface of the abdomen. It had the form of an egg-cup, was very hard, but covered with normal skin. There was marked ascites, which made palpation useless. At operation eight liters of hemorrhagic fluid were removed and the omentum protruded. Scattered over it were tumors the size of plums. The umbilical tumor was completely isolated and was removed. It was in no way connected with the omentum. The primary tumor could not be discovered. Microscopic examination showed that the tumors were large round-cell sarcomata.

MELANOTIC SARCOMA OF THE UMBILICUS.

Pernice draws attention to two cases — -one observed by Volkmann, the other by Olshausen. Volkmann's case occurred in a young girl who had an umbilical tumor not larger than a cherry. Notwithstanding the wide removal of the growth, countless secondary tumors were soon noted and the girl died.

* Garnier: Cancer [Sarcoma] primitif de l'ombilic. La Loire medicale, 1910, xxix, 503.

f Pernice, L. : Op. cit., obs. 71.

Olshausen's patient was a woman twenty-one years of age. She had at the umbilicus a melanotic sarcoma the size of an apple. It had been noted first a year and a half before she came for operation. The growth was removed, but twenty-one months later the patient died, with brain symptoms strongly indicative of cerebral metastases.

Catoir* also reports a case of melanotic sarcoma of the umbilicus. The patient was a man sixty-five years old. He noticed a slight, faintly blood-tinged discharge from the umbilicus. At that time there could be seen a simple brownish spot, without any underlying induration. Four months later there was a thickening surrounding the umbilicus. Applications were employed, and an attempt was made to remove the growth with the thermocautery. Two months later the tumor was 3 cm. in diameter. It was raised and formed a semicircle with the umbilicus in the ceEter. The tumor was removed. Xo note is given as to the prognosis.

Microscopic examination corresponded with the clinical diagnosis of melanotic sarcoma. No other primary source of the growth could be found.

[Despite the probability of the correctness of the diagnosis, in the absence of an abdominal exploration it is impossible to feel sure that the growth was primary. — T. S. C]

* Catoir, S.: Sarcome melanique de la region ombilicale chez un homme de 65 ans. Jour. d. sci. med. de Lille, 1899, xxii, 36.

LITERATURE CONSULTED ON SARCOMA OF THE UMBILICUS.

Aveling: Brit. Gyn. Jour., 1886-87, ii, 56; 187.

Berard, P. H.: Fistules urinaires. Diet, de med., Paris, 1840, xxii, 64.

Blum, A.: Tumeurs de l'ombihc ehez l'adulte. Arch. gen. de med., Paris, 1876, 6. ser., xxviii, 151.

Catoir, S.: Sarcome melanique de la region ombilicale chez un homme de 65 ans. Join, des sci. med. de Lille, 1899, xxii, 36.

Dannenberg, O.: Zur Casuistik der Xabeltumoren insbesondere des Carcinoma umbihcale. Inaug. Diss., Wlirzburg, 1886.

Demarquay: Cancer de l'ombihc. Bull, de la Soc. de chir.. 1870-71, 2. ser., xi, 209.

Forgue et Riche: Montpellier med., 1907, xxiv, 145.

Gamier: Cancer [Sarcoma] primitif de l'ombihc. La Loire med., 1910, xxix, 503.

Kaufmann, E.: Leber eine Geschwulstbildung des Xabelstrangs. Virchows Arch., 1890, exxi, 513.

Leydhecker. F.: Zur Diagnose der sarcomatosen Geschwlilste, Giessen, 1S56.

Xeveu, X.: Contribution a l'etude des tumeurs malignes seeondaires de l'ombihc, Paris, 1S90, No. 50.

Nicaise: Fibro-papilloma de la cicatrice ombilicale. Rev. de chir., Paris, 1883, hi, 29.

O'Brien, Surgeon-Major: Sarcoma at the Umbilicus. Indian Med. Gaz., 1889. xxiv, 215.

Pernice, L. : Die XabelgeschwuLste, Halle, 1892.

Plagge, H.: Ein Fall von Myxosarcom des Nabels. Inaug. Diss., Freiburg, 1889.

Quenu et Longuet: Du cancer secondaire de l'ombilic. Rev. de chir., 1896, xvi, 97.

Sourdille, G.: Sarcome pedicule de la peau de l'ombihc. Bull, de la Soc. anat. de Paris, 1895, Lxx, 302.

Tillmanns. H.: Deutsche Zeitschr. f. Chir., 1882-83, xviii, 161.

Yillar, Francis : Tumeurs de l'ombihc. These de Paris, 1886.

Yirchow, R.: Virchows Arch., 1864, xxxi, 128.

von Winckel, F.: Ueber angeborene solide Geschwiilste des (perennirenden) Theiles der Xabelschnur. Sammlung klin. Vortrage, n. F. Xo. 140. (Gyn. Nr. 53.)

Index

M.A. Shiffman (ed.), *Adult Umbilical Reconstruction*,
DOI 10.1007/978-3-319-43887-0

B

E

G

H

M

N

O

P

T

V